SMART MEDICINE FOR A HEALTHIER CHILD

A PRACTICAL A-TO-Z REFERENCE TO NATURAL AND CONVENTIONAL TREATMENTS FOR INFANTS & CHILDREN

JANET ZAND, LAc, OMD
RACHEL WALTON, RN
BOB ROUNTREE, MD

Avery Publishing Group

Garden City Park, New York

The medical information and procedures contained in this book are based upon the research and personal and professional experiences of the authors. They are not intended as a substitute for consulting with your physician or other health care provider. Any attempt to diagnose and treat an illness should be done under the direction of a health care professional.

The publisher does not advocate the use of any particular health care protocol, but believes that the information in this book should be available to the public. The publisher and authors are not responsible for any adverse effects or consequences resulting from the use of any of the suggestions, preparations, or procedures discussed in this book. Should the reader have any questions concerning the appropriateness of any procedure or preparation mentioned, the authors and the publisher strongly suggest consulting a professional health care advisor.

Cover designers: Ann Vestal and Rudy Shur
Front cover photo supply house: Stock Imagery
Front cover photographer: Stephen Whalen
In-house editors: Amy C. Tecklenburg, Marie Caratozzolo, Elaine Will Sparber, and Joanne Abrams
Original illustrations: Edward A. Gallagher
Typesetter: Bonnie Freid

Library of Congress Cataloging-in-Publication Data

Zand, Janet.
    Smart medicine for a healthier child : a practical a to z
reference to natural and conventional treatments for infants and
children / Janet Zand, Rachel Walton, Bob Rountree.
        p. cm.
    Includes index.
    ISBN 0-89529-545-8
    1. Pediatrics—Popular works. 2. Children—Diseases—Alternative
treatment. I. Walton, Rachel. II. Rountree, Bob. III. Title.
RJ61.Z32 1994
618.92—dc20   94-16594
                                                        CIP

Printed in the United States of America.

10 9 8 7 6

Contents

Appendix

Foreword

In medical school, physicians are taught only one "model" for medical care: Wait for someone to get sick, and then give them medicine or operate on them. We doctors are taught to ignore a great deal of wisdom about sickness and health that has developed over thousands of years and that is used by billions of people throughout the world.

We are only now starting to find out that there are many answers to our patients' questions—not just the narrow range of answers we were taught in medical school. For example, consider a recent article in *Pediatrics*. This journal is the official publication of the American Academy of Pediatrics, an organization representing over 32,000 pediatric physicians in America. In a recent issue, *Pediatrics* published a study of homeopathic treatment for diarrhea. The statistics, the experimental methods, and the results were unquestionable: It worked. This is the first time that such an American medical journal has published a clinical trial of this type of alternative care.

Smart Medicine for a Healthier Child is the very first balanced approach to health care I have ever seen. Not only does this book give excellent descriptions of the illnesses and conditions it discusses, it also presents conventional therapy side by side with herbal, homeopathic, acupressure, and nutritional choices.

Choice—that is the key to optimal health for our children and families. Understand health and disease, learn how to prevent illness when possible, and choose the best, least offensive, cure from among all the possibilities available to you.

Conventional Western medicine too often ignores the brilliant wisdom and powers of the human body. A child's immune system will beat almost all common illnesses if given a chance. Very few diseases require immediate treatment with antibiotics or other drugs; there is a vast amount of medical literature that supports the idea that our bodies can usually cure themselves if given a little time.

Of course, there certainly is a place for "modern" medicine, and this book recognizes this as well as any book I've ever seen. Lives *can* be saved in the emergency room or the operating suite. However, lives can also be damaged or lost because of reactions to unneeded medications or unwarranted surgery. Your family will benefit mightily from the balanced approach this book establishes and from the authors' intelligent attitude toward all avenues of prevention and therapy.

Conventional medical care in the 1990s and in the next century will almost certainly continue to emphasize quantity over quality. Doctors are now being asked to see more patients each day than ever before, and they therefore have less time for each patient. Of course, no book—not even a comprehensive reference book with this friendly format—can substitute for a long, far-reaching discussion with a broad-minded health care practitioner. On the other hand, not many people have, or will have, access to that kind of discussion. Perhaps the greatest value of this book will be to show you what has worked for the authors' patients and for many generations of healthy families.

I have been in private practice for fifteen years and have cared for thousands of families. My patients have taught me more than I ever learned in medical school. They have helped me expand my practice by showing me what works for them. I thoroughly enjoyed reading *Smart Medicine for a Healthier Child*, and I learned a tremendous amount about intelligent alternatives to conventional drugs and surgery. Adding this book to your library will make you a better educated medical consumer and more aware of your healthy choices.

Jay N. Gordon, MD
Santa Monica, California

Acknowledgments

To the teachers who inspired me, to the students who challenged me, and to the patients who taught me, I would like to express my endless gratitude.

I would also like to thank Michael McGuffin, who has worked tirelessly to foster the growth of herbal medicine in the United States. I would like to thank Whitfield Reaves, LAc, OMD, whose knowledge, openness, and enthusiasm have made him the ideal colleague.

A special thanks to Dr. Darick A. Nordstrom for his invaluable contribution to all the sections on dental care.

Thank you to Rudy Shur, my publisher, whose vision and support were instrumental in the creation of this book, and to Amy Tecklenburg, my editor, for her hours of diligence and dedication.

And many thanks to my husband, Michael, and my two sons, Christopher and William, for their love, support, and much-needed comic relief.

J.Z.

To Dr. Janet Zand, ND: You have offered your endless eclectic wisdom as a doctor and a friend, and I am forever grateful. Thank you to Dr. Bob Rountree, MD, for your invaluable insights and attention to detail.

Thank you to Dr. Whit Reaves, LAc, OMD, for bringing us together and encouraging me to undertake this project, and then for endless hours of reading and advising. Thank you to Michael McGuffin for his patient support; to David Guenette for his initial and huge input into the breadth and depth of this book; to Nikki Antol for adding energy when we were all very tired; and to our editor, Amy Tecklenburg, for her masterful precision and clarity.

Thank you to the children and families who have touched me and taught me over the years. I am grateful to each one of you. I thank Dr. Jay Wilson, DC, for his brilliant knowledge of and commitment to natural medicine, and for his compassionate doctoring, teaching, and friendship. And thank you to my mother, my father, my brothers Joe and Jimmy, and my beautiful sister Mary, who have each inspired me with love and integrity.

R.W.

My heartfelt appreciation goes out to Janet and Rachel for inviting me along on this wondrous journey. For their invaluable insights and endless handholding I want to thank Linda Pritzker, Wendy Rubin, and Angela Bowman. To Amy Tecklenburg, I say: You are an amazingly patient and skillful editor. And finally, I want to express immense gratitude to my mentors, Jeffrey Bland, Ph D, and Leo Galland, MD. As a young medical resident, fresh out of academia, it was an incredible inspiration to learn from them that there was no inherent contradiction between "science" and holistic medicine. Both then and now, these two individuals serve as living examples of how to successfully integrate different paradigms, which for me is what healing is all about.

B.R.

Preface

*In the history of human thinking, the most fruitful developments
frequently take place at those points where two different lines of thought meet.*

Werner Heisenberg
1932 Winner, Nobel Prize for Physics

Children are full of life. They are resilient, curious, sturdy, and energetic. Nurturing a child's growing awareness of the world is exciting, as we are invited to tap into the creative, playful, vital child inside each of us.

Some of the most important decisions parents have to make in caring for their children concern health care. Yet often, they are not aware of the full range of choices available to them. The goal of this book is to offer you information on a variety of approaches that will help you create vibrant good health for your child. The authors believe in an integrated approach to health care that considers all treatment possibilities and draws on what works. Sometimes this will be an herb, sometimes an antibiotic, sometimes both. We believe it is just as significant that a particular therapy has been used effectively for hundreds or thousands of years as it is that a scientific paper substantiates a particular approach. Taking advantage of one form of knowledge does not necessarily preclude using another.

This book outlines and describes the application of conventional medicine, dietary modifications, nutritional supplements, herbal medicine, homeopathy, and acupressure. We believe that understanding and integrating the full range of health care options offers the most complete and responsible way to a healthy life. We hope to foster an awareness that natural healing therapies and conventional medical treatment, two apparently divergent approaches, can—and should—work together.

Natural healing sciences (including herbal medicine, homeopathy, diet, nutritional supplements, and acupressure) are sometimes called "complementary" medicine. As that name implies, natural medicine and conventional medicine can be used to complement and support each other in helping to create health in a person. Complementary medicine is gaining increasing acceptance in the United States, as evidenced by the many multidisciplinary clinics in which medical doctors, naturopathic physicians, acupuncturists, nutritionists, homeopaths, chiropractors, and counselors work together in an integrated manner, treating the patient as a whole person. Even the United States government has taken notice of these developments. In the fall of 1992, the Office of Alternative Medicine was established at the National Institutes of Health to study the effectiveness of various types of alternative health care. Among the subjects being studied there are homeopathy, acupuncture and acupressure, herbal medicine, reflexology, chiropractic, biofeedback, hypnosis, and relaxation and visualization techniques.

Natural healing systems are much more widely used than many people suppose. The World Health Organization, established in 1948 as a specialized agency of the United Nations, reports that 80 percent of the world's population relies on natural healing as their primary form of health care. And a study conducted at the Beth Israel Hospital in Boston, and published in *The New England Journal of Medicine* in 1993, revealed that one in three Americans tried some form of alternative treatment in 1990 alone. In the same year, Americans made a total of 425 million visits to alternative health care practitioners and spent $13.7 billion on alternative treatments, of which they paid $10.3 billion out of pocket. (Compare this with 399 million visits to conventional medical doctors and $12.8 billion paid out of pocket for conventional medical treatment.)

More and more medical doctors are recognizing the safety and effectiveness of natural medicines. There are physicians who prescribe herbal medicines and homeopathic remedies; many more recommend dietary changes for their patients. By now, a clear link has been established between diet and health. The American Heart Association, the American Cancer Society, and the United States government have all published dietary guidelines to promote health. Conventional and complementary health care practitioners alike emphasize the role of nutrition as fundamental to the healing process.

Homeopathy is an accepted form of medical practice in many parts of the world. Generation after generation of Asian families have turned to acupuncture and acupressure for relief of illness. Even modern pharmacology has deep roots in herbal medicine. The use of the herb ma huang (ephedra), for example, dates back several thousand years; ephedrine, one of its primary ingredients (and pseudoephedrine, a synthetic version of it) is used by pharmaceutical companies today in many over-the-counter cold and allergy medicines.

"The physician treats, but nature heals." This is an often-quoted saying from Hippocrates—known as the "Father of Medicine"—who recognized that the body has a natural tendency toward health and vitality. To nurture this tendency, we need to treat illness in ways that support and strengthen the body's natural processes. Using a complementary approach to health care, we can draw on modern conventional medicine, natural medicine, and ancient healing traditions to find what is most effective and supportive in curing and preventing illness.

Conventional medicine generally works with drugs or surgery to suppress or correct a specific condition. And sometimes, that is exactly what is needed. At other times, however, a natural medical approach makes more sense. Natural medicine works by supporting the body in healing itself. While antibiotics can be used to kill harmful bacteria, for example, the herbs echinacea and goldenseal boost the immune system so that the body is better able to resist infection. These herbs strengthen and support the body in its ability to defend itself against bacterial invasion.

When your child is suffering from a cold, you can choose to give over-the-counter or prescription medications, such as a decongestant or cough medicine, to suppress the symptoms. However, cold medicines can cause side effects, and they do little to strengthen the immune system or address the underlying reason for the cold. Some commonly used ingredients in cold medications can cause restlessness, insomnia, or headaches. And there is nothing in these drugs that can actually *cure* the cold. In contrast, when a cold is treated with herbs to soothe the respiratory tract and boost the immune system, homeopathy to ease the discomforts and prevent recurrences, acupressure to open blocked energy channels, and soups and teas to maintain adequate hydration, the body is supported and strengthened as it works to restore health. For many of the illnesses that afflict us, natural medicine is gentle, effective, and safe. It is an important way to work with the body's ability to heal itself.

When children don't feel well, they somehow seem to know what their young bodies need. They instinctively sleep much and eat little, which permits their bodies to concentrate energy on the healing process. They want comfort, support, and care. The time spent caring for a sick child can be a tender and gentle time, especially as you learn to listen closely, carefully observe signs and signals, and choose ways to comfort and soothe your little one.

We encourage you to allow your child to participate in the healing process. With guidance, simple explanations, and discussion, children learn what does and what does not nourish and support their bodies. Encourage your child's curiosity and exploration of health, illness, and treatment. Observe behaviors and responses. Ask what helps your child to feel better. Teach, listen, and learn together.

Exposing a child to an integrated, complementary approach to health care can make medicine in general less of an unknown and therefore less scary. Instead of worrying when illness strikes, your child will know there is a solution close at hand. Given support and guidance, your child will accept and learn to respect the value of an integrated approach using natural and conventional medicine, and will grow into a healthy, knowledgeable, and responsible young person.

Perhaps the most difficult thing to deal with in treating a childhood illness is not the illness itself, but the expectations parents have of themselves. We want to wave a magic wand, to "kiss it and make it better," and we agonize when we can't do so.

It's natural to feel concern. But a child who sees you fretting and nervous will pick up on your feelings, and will begin to fret and worry also. Developing an attitude of caring, gentleness, and confidence in treating illness may be the healthiest thing you can do as a parent. Once you give a medicine or remedy, remain watchful, but try to relax and feel confident in your ability to observe, respond, and make choices. A positive, optimistic atmosphere promotes a speedy and happy recovery. Further, a relaxed, loving environment promotes a close relationship between parent and child, and teaches your child to love and respect himself and the world around him.

In his book *Health and Healing* (Houghton Mifflin,

1988), Dr. Andrew Weil wrote, "The only prerequisite for learning to take responsibility for one's own health is to discard concepts that stand in the way and adopt more useful ones. . . . Anyone who comes to see healing as an innate capacity of the body, rather than something to be sought outside, will gain greater power over the fluctuations of health and illness."

Being willing to accept responsibility is central to taking an integrated approach to health care. Help your physician, your child, and yourself to develop greater faith in the body's ability to heal itself, when supported and nourished by natural medicines. When faced with illness, use this book to learn and understand the many options for the care and healing of your child. Observe how the natural and conventional medical treatments you choose affect your child's health and well-being. Be both responsible and willing to explore health care options.

With the information in this book, you can learn to be an active participant in your child's health care. As you gain confidence and understanding in the use of natural healing systems for the benefit of your entire family, in concert with conventional medicine when necessary, you will gain greater confidence in optimizing health and managing illness. We invite you to discard the concept that health care is an either-or proposition. It's not. Integrated health care is a remarkably effective and exciting hands-on endeavor.

Using an integrated approach to health care will nourish your child's vitality and curiosity. Taking care of yourself and your family in this way will promote a healthy and responsible relationship between your child and his body; between you and your child; and between your family and your health care practitioner. Your child will learn to pay attention to his body, and to appreciate his own uniqueness and vitality.

Children's bodies are wonderfully responsive. When your child's body is supported with thoughtful integrated care, the best of natural and conventional medicine, it works quickly to attain full health. By giving nature a nudge—by supporting, nurturing, and nourishing the body's capacity to heal itself—you can help create vibrant good health for your child.

How to Use This Book

This is an in-home guide that will help you care for and maintain your child's health, from birth through adolescence, through a unique approach that seeks to combine the best of conventional medicine, herbal medicine, homeopathy, acupressure, diet, and nutritional supplementation. Written by a naturopathic physician, a registered nurse, and a medical doctor, it offers advice and explanations of the full spectrum of options available to parents as they seek to give their children the support they need to be their healthiest, and to treat the common medical problems of childhood.

This book is intended to help parents make informed health care decisions for their children. The information and suggestions presented here are meant to be used in conjunction with the services of a physician or other qualified health care provider. This book is not meant to replace appropriate consultation with health care practitioners, medical investigation or treatment, or emergency first-aid training by qualified professionals. We strongly suggest that anyone who is primarily responsible for the care of a child complete an emergency first-aid course that includes instruction in artificial respiration and cardiopulmonary resuscitation (CPR) for infants and children. Then, should you ever be called upon to practice these techniques, the emergency instructions we provide will help you through the procedure.

The subjects in this book have been divided into three parts. Part One, The Elements of Health Care, discusses the basic history, theories, and practices of conventional medicine, herbal medicine, homeopathy, Bach Flower Remedies, and acupressure. It also covers issues in diet and nutrition, including how to offer your child a safe, beneficial diet; nutritional supplementation; pregnancy safeguards for a healthy baby; newborn care; and things you can do to make your child's environment as healthy and hazard-free as possible.

Part Two, Common Childhood Health Problems,

contains an alphabetic list of the illnesses that commonly afflict children, and outlines the different kinds of treatments appropriate for each. Each entry begins with a discussion of the problem, its causes, and how to identify the signs and symptoms. Treatment options follow, including recommendations for conventional medical treatment, dietary guidelines, and information on nutritional supplementation, herbal treatment, homeopathy, Bach Flower Remedies and acupressure. If emergency treatment is appropriate, this is discussed in an inset in the margin adjacent to the entry and is highlighted in red. Each entry also includes a section on general recommendations that gives a brief listing of the most commonly helpful natural treatments, and advice on prevention.

Part Three, Therapies and Procedures, gives specific instructions to help you use the diagnostic and treatment procedures suggested in Part Two. The use of special diets, the preparation of herbal treatments, the location of acupressure points, and other techniques are explained and illustrated so that you will be able to take advantage of the various kinds of treatments available to you.

Also included, in an appendix, are a glossary of some of the terms used in this book; a list of recommended suppliers of herbal, homeopathic, and nutritional products; a list of helpful resource organizations, with addresses and telephone numbers; and a bibliography for further reading.

Finally, a word about gender. Your child is as likely to be a boy as a girl; however, our language does not provide us with a singular pronoun that includes both genders. To avoid using the awkward "he/she" while still giving equal time to both sexes, the feminine pronouns "she" and "her" and the masculine pronouns "he," "him," and "his have been used in alternating chapters and entries throughout this book. This decision has been made in the interest of simplicity and clarity.

Part One

The Elements of Health Care

The Nuts and Bolts of
Conventional and Natural Treatment

Introduction

Because of your unique and intimate relationship with your child, you play an invaluable role in your child's wellness care. The special bond between parent and child makes you the best judge of your child's health. As you build on the broad and deep understanding you have of your child, you will learn to move from general observation toward identifying the signs and symptoms that reveal an illness or other health problem. Even having a vague sense that your child is just "not quite right" is valid and important. You know your child. You know when something is wrong.

When your child is ill, you want to ease his discomfort quickly and effectively. But conventional and natural therapies alike can seem confusing and overwhelming, just when they are needed most. The approaches to medicine covered in this book include conventional medicine, herbal medicine, homeopathy, acupressure, nutritional supplements, and diet. In Part One you will find historical information, tables, diagrams, and guidelines to help you understand each system of medicine from a conceptual and practical perspective.

Each of the healing systems offers advantages and benefits. Each has drawbacks. This section provides a clear, unbiased look at all protocols. It will help you gain the insight you need to choose an effective course of action and become confident in your ability to provide effective, comforting, and gentle health care for your child.

Conventional Medicine

When most Americans think of health care, they think of conventional medicine. It is without question the dominant approach to medicine in the United States today, and it permeates (often without our being aware of it) even our basic understanding of sickness and health. For example, many people think of health as being the absence of disease, and when they don't feel well, they are apt to ask, "Is there something I can take for this?" Both of these ideas reflect the assumptions of modern conventional medicine, which tends to be oriented toward identifying diseases and prescribing cures, usually in the form of drugs.

THE HISTORY OF CONVENTIONAL MEDICINE

The story of the development of the conventional medical science we know today weaves through many centuries and many cultures. If we go back to the dawn of history, we find that the earliest doctors were shamans, and the first medicines were plants.

It is generally accepted that the history of today's conventional medical science starts with Hippocrates, the Greek physician revered as the "Father of Medicine." Up to the time of Hippocrates (c. 460–370 B.C.), illness was believed to be caused by supernatural forces. Hippocrates taught that all disease was of earthly origin, not visited upon the sufferer by some wrathful god.

It was Hippocrates who set the stage for the scientific procedures of today. He began the practice of bedside observation. He listened and recorded each patient's story—today, we would call it a case history—and considered the effects of diet, emotion, occupation, even climate, in his diagnosis and treatment. Through careful observation and logical reasoning, Hippocrates showed that it was possible to determine the cause of illness, and thereby discern the cure.

Hippocrates believed that health was the result of good balance between a patient's internal nature and his external environment. Illness indicated an imbalance. To restore balance in his patients, Hippocrates designed special diets, mandated exercise, and prescribed botanical medicines, including an occasional purgative or emetic. For digestive troubles (possibly stomach ulcers), he ordered bland drinks. Hippocrates also recognized the importance of stress reduction. He was known to have recommended to certain patients that they relocate to calmer surroundings, or that they take a glass of wine with supper.

Galen (c. 130–200 A.D.), who was known as the "Great Physician," added to the knowledge of medicine and anatomy. He performed experiments and dissections, and wrote prolifically about his discoveries. For example, he is credited with discovering that blood is carried through the body by means of the arteries. Although a Greek by birth, Galen lived and practiced in Rome, where he was personal physician to several Roman emperors.

With the collapse of Rome in the fifth century A.D., Europe descended into a period of turmoil. The anatomical studies and the emphasis on observation and logic of the ancient Greeks and Romans were lost to most of the continent for nearly 500 years. During this time, European medical knowledge for the most part amounted to a mixture of folk art and superstition. The heirs to the knowledge of Hippocrates and Galen were not Europeans, but Arabic and Jewish scholars (although some of the classical practice was preserved in southern Italy). It was through these sources that the medical knowledge of Greece and Rome was eventually reintroduced to Europe. By the year 1000, the medical school at the University of Salerno had an established reputation, and for centuries to come, Italy remained the focal point for medical science in Europe. However, the study of medicine remained primarily an academic discipline, rather than an area of active inquiry, experimentation, or practical application. Not until the Renaissance—when invention, intellectual pursuits, and creativity flourished—did this approach begin to change significantly, ushering in the beginning of what we might recognize as medical science.

Leonardo da Vinci (1452–1519), considered by many to be the first modern anatomist, extensively studied and diagrammed anatomy. Following his initial contributions, other scholars continued to perform dissections and study anatomy, adding to the knowledge of the inner workings of the body. Reason, logic, and observation once again became the foundation of medical learning. The practice of surgery also has its beginnings during this time—despite the lack of anesthesia.

In the century that followed, the mechanisms of blood circulation and respiration came to be understood. Inventions such as the clinical thermometer and the microscope made it possible to observe the workings of the body on an entirely new level; anatomical details such as lymph nodes and red blood cells were appreciated. Certain illnesses were also distinguished, including diabetes mellitus, diabetes insipidus, rickets, scarlet fever, measles, and gout. In the eighteenth century, medical schools were founded in Vienna, Edinburgh, and Glasgow. Although the course of study at the time still emphasized the assimilation of knowledge rather more than experimentation or invention, progress was made in the practice of surgery, amputation, and the treatment of bone fractures, and new diagnostic methods were developed, such as percussion and pulse-taking. Modern immunology also traces its origins back to this period. In 1796, Edward Jenner, an English physician, began a series of experiments that proved that inoculating a person with cowpox provided immunity against smallpox, a dreaded disease that had erupted in epidemics throughout history.

Further dramatic advances and discoveries followed, including the invention of the stethoscope, which made possible more precise diagnosis of heart and lung problems. Huge strides were made in the understanding of anatomy and physiology. Robert Koch—whose bacteriological culture techniques are still used today—identified the bacteria that cause many serious infectious diseases, including anthrax, tuberculosis, and cholera. His work led to an understanding of the importance of water filtration in the prevention of cholera and typhoid. Louis Pasteur made tremendous contributions to our understanding of the causes of disease and the means by which infectious illnesses spread. His study of the activity of bacteria disproved the theory of spontaneous generation (the belief that living organisms can develop from nonliving material) and led to the acceptance of his germ theory of infection. He also invented anthrax and rabies vaccines, as well as the process that bears his name, pasteurization, by which potentially illness-causing microorganisms in food are killed. Soon, many different types of bacteria were identified, including those that cause tetanus, leprosy, typhoid, diphtheria, and gonorrhea.

The acceptance of the germ theory made it possible for surgery to make great leaps forward, because it led to an appreciation of the necessity for sterile conditions during surgery. This new emphasis on aseptic (sterile) technique, plus the development of anesthesia, helped to establish surgery as a viable treatment option, rather than a desperate last resort. (Prior to this time, many people died during or after surgery from infections that were a direct result of a lack of attention to cleanliness.) The germ theory also had great implications for public health policy, which now involved vaccination programs, quarantine measures, and attention to the cleanliness of the water supply.

As understanding of the workings of the body and its systems grew, the latter half of the nineteenth century saw the birth of the fields of neurology (the study of the brain and nervous system), psychiatry, and endocrinology (the study of glands and hormones). In 1895, x-rays were discovered. Medical science continued to follow a path that emphasized the importance of the scientific method—logical study that produces reliable results that can be duplicated. In the last few decades, medicine has made progress that would have been unthinkable just three or four generations ago. The use of insulin injections has allowed people with diabetes to live long and relatively healthy lives; the discovery of antibiotics like penicillin and streptomycin has improved the treatment and prognosis for people with bacterial and tubercular infections; the polio vaccine was developed and has largely eliminated this dreaded disease; and organ transplantation has become an accepted, viable treatment for certain conditions. Increasingly sophisticated diagnostic tools and advances in treatment have been developed. In addition, the course of conventional medicine has included the creation of huge drug companies, health insurance programs, and government agencies like the National Institutes of Health. All of these developments have played a role in shaping the health care system we know today.

Because of the many successes in the treatment of infectious diseases, the emphasis in medical research has now shifted toward the chronic and degenerative diseases, which remain less curable. Heart disease, the various forms of cancer, and acquired immune deficiency syndrome (AIDS) are among the health problems that pose the greatest challenges to medical science today. Since chronic and degenerative diseases are usually the cumulative result of many factors, rather than a reaction to a single agent, practicing preventive medicine—eating a healthful diet, exercising regularly, reducing stress, and making healthy lifestyle choices such as not smoking and limiting alcohol intake—is becoming more and more central to taking care of our health.

CONVENTIONAL MEDICINE TODAY

Most of us grew up with conventional medicine, also called "orthodox," "Western," or "modern" medicine. In the United States, conventional childhood health care usually means a visit to your pediatrician or family physician. Depending on the nature of the problem, your child's doctor may run tests, prescribe a drug, recommend dietary changes and exercise, refer you to a specialist or surgeon, or merely tell you to make sure your child gets extra rest and drinks lots of fluids.

Many sophisticated diagnostic tools are available to medical doctors today. Some are familiar, such as the stethoscope, otoscope, and x-ray. Recent advances also include computerized axial tomography (CAT) scanners, magnetic resonance imaging (MRI), and other laboratory tests. Yet like all healing systems, conventional medical science evolved from a long tradition of careful observation. Even with the tremendous advances of the last 100 years, the most important tool your child's physician has is still his or her willingness to listen closely and observe carefully.

WORKING WITH YOUR DOCTOR

Physicians are here to help you make appropriate decisions in the care of your child, to work with you. Even if you favor a natural approach to health care, there may come a time when only conventional medicine has the cure your child needs. A pediatrician or family physician who knows your child and who has cared for your child from birth through an illness or two is a wonderful backup in case of crisis. When choosing a physician, consider the following guidelines.

- Choose a physician who keeps up to date with the latest treatments. A concerned and knowledgeable physician is an absolute must. New drugs come on the market all the time. The side effects of drugs—especially new ones, which do not have long histories of safe usage—should be understood and carefully considered.

- Find a physician who is open-minded about natural and complementary therapies. Your physician does not necessarily have to prescribe natural medicine, but he or she should at least be willing to listen to your ideas and explore options.

- Find a physician who will work with you as a partner, who believes in making decisions with you, rather than for you.

- Choose a physician who is a good communicator. It is important that a doctor be able not only to explain situations and treatments to you, but also to listen well to your concerns. You want a physician who is competent and supportive, one who will give you enough time so you can ask questions and learn.

- Choose a physician who looks at the "big picture." It is essential to work with someone who acknowledges that your child is not just a case of asthma, but a growing child who is involved with school friends, athletics, and developmental concerns, *and* who has asthma.

- Find a physician who is willing to see you and interact with you as the intelligent, caring person that you are.

You can choose either a pediatrician or family physician to care for your child. Family physicians are trained to diagnose and treat health problems from birth through old age, including all common childhood illnesses. They consider the whole family and the life span when treating a child—how the illness affects the family, whether anyone else in the family is sick, how the illness might affect the family over time, and what impact it might have on the child over the course of her life. Many, however, do not have specialized training in dealing with more serious childhood illnesses. Family physicians often focus their expertise on a specific area of family care. If you choose to work with a family physician, find out about his or her background, special expertise, and experience with children.

A pediatrician is a doctor trained specifically to care for children. He or she works only with children and has specialty training in dealing with more serious illnesses. Pediatricians have a strong background in the growth and development of children. A pediatrician commonly treats a child from birth through adolescence, typically age eighteen for girls and twenty for boys.

Although it is important to have a pediatrician or family physician available to you, you can choose to work with a pediatric nurse practitioner for the bulk of your child's health care needs. Pediatric nurse practitioners are registered nurses who have received additional specialized education that enables them to provide comprehensive assessment and management of well children, children with minor acute illnesses, and children with stable chronic illnesses. Generally, pediatric nurse practitioners have a strong background in growth and development, and are well grounded in disease prevention and health promotion. They usually work closely with or are supervised by physicians, but tend to charge lower fees than either family physicians or pediatricians.

Whatever type of health care provider you choose for your child, it is your responsibility to challenge him or her to know you and your family, to care about your child. That means asking questions, expecting answers, and telling the doctor about natural treatments that have benefitted your child. Actively engage your physician in your child's health care. And if a time ever comes when your child's doctor no longer has your complete trust, or if you feel your doctor doesn't know your child well, it's time to change doctors.

Your child's first encounter with a pediatrician or family physician is likely to come moments after birth. The doctor will perform a physical assessment of your new baby to be sure she is healthy. Following the initial assessment, it is wise to keep regular well-baby and then well-child visits (your doctor will likely recommend an appropriate schedule). If an emerging health problem is discovered during a well-child examination, care and treatment can begin at the optimum moment. In addition, your doctor can reassure you about your child's physical growth and development, and offer guidance concerning cognitive and emotional growth and development. Well-child appointments also enable you to initiate a relationship between doctor and parents and child. You will set the stage for good health for your child.

There may be a time when your doctor recommends a comprehensive health care program for your child. A good doctor will work with you in formulating a regimen that is both effective and manageable. Make sure you fully understand all phases of any program your doctor is suggesting. Ask as many questions as necessary. Don't just agree passively to diet, medication, or lifestyle changes that will be immensely difficult or perhaps even impossible to carry out. Airing your fears and concerns is an important part of your parental responsibility. Without your input, your doctor has no way of knowing that you find a program difficult or impossible to implement. If for any reason you can't carry out the program, or can handle only a portion of it, tell your physician. There are probably workable alternatives.

A good doctor recognizes that a physician-parent partnership is of immense benefit to a child. The physician you choose should want to know your child, welcome your questions, take the time to explain and advise, and be willing to explore natural treatment options. A physician who will work with you in taking an integrated approach to caring for your child is invaluable.

TREATING YOUR CHILD WITH CONVENTIONAL MEDICINE

When you choose conventional medical treatment for your child, an important part of your responsibility as a parent is to thoroughly understand the appropriate use of the medications, both prescription and over-the-counter, recommended by your physician.

Never give your child a prescription drug without first questioning your child's doctor about its purpose, the benefits it offers, the effect it should achieve, how long it will take before you can expect an improvement in symptoms, and possible side effects. For example, the development of a skin rash might be an early warning sign of sensitivity to a particular drug. Unless you are aware that a rash may signal "danger," you could overlook it.

Never give your child an over-the-counter drug without first checking its safety and effectiveness with your physician. Even if the product has been manufactured expressly for childhood conditions, it may not be suitable for your particular child.

When talking with your child's doctor about a medication or over-the-counter product, ask about *all* of the ingredients in it. Many medicines contain significant and often unnecessary amounts of preservatives, dyes, and alcohol. Many prescription and nonprescription medicines also contain sugar to make them taste better. In fact, certain antibiotics and antifungals are suspected of causing tooth decay because they are so laden with sugar. Your doctor should be able to tell you what additives are in a prescribed medication. When selecting an over-the-counter product for your child, read the label carefully. The label should tell you exactly what the product contains, including the sugar content and additives (often listed as "inert ingredients"), as well as how to administer it and possible side effects. If you have any doubts about the safety of giving a particular medication to your child, ask your physician or pharmacist for any further information you need to feel comfortable. We also recommend that you buy or have access to a good reference book on drugs, such as *The Parent's Guide to Pediatric Drugs* by R.M. Bindler, Y. Tso, and L.B. Howry (HarperCollins, 1986) or *The People's Pharmacy* by Joe Graedon (St. Martin's Press, 1985).

Although many prepared medications are sweetened and flavored, *never* tell a child that medicine is "candy" to persuade her to take it. A young child who is taught to think of medicine as candy may one day innocently swallow an overdose. Even vitamin tablets can have toxic effects in excessive doses.

Never give your child a drug that was prescribed for someone else, even if your child's symptoms are identical to those the drug is designed to combat. Even if a child comes down with the same condition as another child in the family, you cannot assume that a drug prescribed for one will be safe for another.

If at any time during the course of treatment your child develops signs of an allergic reaction, such as a rash or difficulty breathing, stop giving the medication and call your doctor immediately. If your child experiences any other new symptoms while taking a drug (such as headache or stomach pains), notify your doctor promptly and ask for advice. It may be advisable to discontinue the medication, or there may be other measures you can take to minimize side effects.

Unless there have been complicating side effects, always continue to administer a prescribed medication—whether a natural or conventional medication—for the full course of treatment ordered by your child's physician. If for any reason your child misses a scheduled dose of medicine, give the next dose at the scheduled time. Do not double the next dose.

When prescribing medication, a doctor may be interested primarily in the effectiveness of a drug, rather than its cost. Your doctor may not even know what a given medication costs, but it is fair and important for you to ask. Drugs can be very expensive. You may wish to ask if a lower priced generic preparation can adequately be substituted for a brand name product.

Common Conventional Medications

The conventional medications most often given to children include analgesics (painkillers), antibiotics, asthma drugs, cold and allergy medicines, and drugs to combat stomach problems and diarrhea. When your doctor writes a prescription or recommends an over-the-counter preparation for your child, refer to the table on pages 8–15 for a quick review of some of these medications, their purposes, and possible side effects.

Administering Conventional Medication

Every parent knows that mixing bad-tasting medicine with something familiar and good-tasting is the easiest way to administer medication to a child. In some cases, however, mixing a drug with food may impede or alter its absorption, making it less effective. Other medications are designed with a timed-release factor that makes certain ingredients exit the stomach and enter the bloodstream at different times. Some drugs work better if taken with a meal; others are more effective if taken on an empty stomach. Some drugs are fine in combination with certain foods, but not with others. Before opening a capsule or crushing a pill and mixing

the contents with food or liquid, check with your doctor or pharmacist to make sure that form of administration is both safe and suitable for that particular medication. Similarly, you should always ask what the best conditions are for giving a particular drug. And you should be especially careful if your child is taking more than one preparation at the same time—whether the medications are conventional or natural, prescription or over-the-counter. Always be sure that your doctor knows about *all* the substances your child is taking.

Following are general recommendations for administering different types of medicines to children.

Liquid Medicines

Almost all of the medications a young child's doctor might prescribe are available in sweetened and flavored liquid form. These are easy to administer. If the taste is too strong, simply dilute the appropriate dosage in a little water, juice, or herbal tea. Give it to your child in a tiny cup, and make sure that she drinks all of it. For an infant, put the medicinal liquid in an eyedropper or empty syringe (without the needle), and gently squirt the liquid inside your baby's mouth.

Tablets

By administering the bitter with the sweet, you can make sure your child receives a full dose of medicine. Some tableted medicines can be crushed and mixed with a spoonful of cream-style cereal or applesauce, or dissolved in grape or apple juice. The natural sugars in fruits make them very good at disguising unpleasant medicinal tastes. As the song says, a little (natural) sugar does help the medicine go down. For a baby not yet on solid foods, crush the tablets and dissolve them in water or juice. Put the dissolved medication in an eyedropper or empty syringe (without the needle), and squirt the liquid inside your infant's mouth.

Some tablets are enteric-coated, and should not be crushed. These tablets are meant to pass through the stomach whole and are absorbed in the intestines. Before crushing tablets to give them to your child, check with your doctor or pharmacist.

Capsules

Capsules slide down much more easily than tablets do. Chances are that an older child may be able to take a capsule even if she can't quite manage to swallow a dry tablet. Unless your physician has given prior approval, *do not* open a capsule and mix the contents with food.

Suppositories

If your child is vomiting and unable to hold anything down, your doctor may prescribe a medicated suppository. To administer a suppository, gently insert it into your child's rectum. To give the suppository time to melt, hold your child's buttocks together for about five minutes.

Because they are designed to melt easily, suppositories should be stored in the refrigerator. To make insertion more comfortable and to shorten melting time after insertion, take a suppository out of the refrigerator about thirty minutes before the scheduled time of administration, so that it can come to room temperature. You can also bring a suppository to a suitable temperature more quickly by rolling it between the palms of your hands.

COMMON CONVENTIONAL MEDICINES

Any medication can cause an allergic reaction. An allergic reaction can happen with the first exposure, or after your child has taken the medication several times. Symptoms of an allergic reaction can include rash, swelling, itching, and/or difficulty breathing. If you think your child is having an allergic reaction, call your physician. If your child experiences difficulty breathing,

Medication	Effect	How Given	How Available
ANALGESICS (PAINKILLERS)			
Acetaminophen (Tylenol, Panadol, and others)	Relieves pain; reduces fever.	By mouth in liquid, chewable, or pill form; in suppository form for infants.	Over the counter.
Aspirin	Relieves pain; reduces fever, inflammation.	Tablet; suppository.	Over the counter.
Codeine	Relieves pain; suppresses cough.	Liquid for coughs; tablet or injection for pain.	By prescription.
Ibuprofen (Advil, Nuprin, and others)	Relieves pain; reduces fever, inflammation.	Tablet.	Over the counter.
ASTHMA DRUGS			
Albuterol (Proventil, Ventolin)	Opens the airway.	Tablet; aerosol inhaler.	By prescription.
Cromolyn sodium (Intal, Nasalcrom)	Prevents spasm of the airway.	Capsule; aerosol inhaler.	By prescription.
Oral steroids (Prednisone and others)	Reduces inflammation of the airway.	By mouth.	By prescription.
Inhaled steroids (AeroBid, Azmacort, Beclovent, Vanceril)	Reduces inflammation of the airway.	Aerosol inhaler.	By prescription.

Injections

Injection of a drug is usually done by a nurse or physician. Should your child ever have an ongoing need for an injectable drug, such as insulin for diabetes, your doctor should make sure you have the training you need to care for your child at home.

Conventional medicine is a broad, ever-expanding field of health care. It is the dominant form of health care in North America, and can be particularly useful in helping you through health crises and acute problems. Develop a trusting working partnership with your doctor. Ask questions, state your concerns and needs, listen, learn—be active in your child's health care. Your child's health can best be supported by integrating conventional medicine with natural medicine.

take her to the emergency room of the nearest hospital. Always follow your doctor's prescription and read package directions carefully to be sure you are giving the medication properly and in the correct dose.

Possible Side Effects	Contraindications	Comments
Reportedly none if taken in recommended doses. Can be fatal if overdosed.	Do not give acetaminophen to a child with liver disease, such as hepatitis or mononucleosis.	In excessive amounts, this drug can cause liver damage. Be careful not to exceed the proper dosage for your child's age and size.
Stomach upset, heartburn, nausea, vomiting, increased chance of bleeding. May cause an allergic reaction.	Do not give aspirin to a child or teenager unless your doctor specifically recommends it. Aspirin has been associated with the development of Reye's syndrome, a potentially life-threatening illness.	Give tablet with food or lots of water to decrease stomach upset. Crush the tablet and mix it in applesauce for children.
Drowsiness, lightheadedness, sedation, upset stomach, constipation, skin rash.	Do not give to a child with a known allergy to codeine or another medication in this family, such as morphine or meperidine.	Give with food to relieve or prevent stomach upset. If your child needs to take codeine, begin anti-constipation measures immediately. Read cough medicine labels carefully; many contain alcohol, which you may not want to give to your child.
Upset stomach, heartburn.	Do not give ibuprofen to a child under 12 years of age without first talking to your physician. Do not take in late pregnancy.	Give with a full glass of water. Giving with food can help prevent stomach upset.
Dizziness, headache, increased heart rate.	Do not give to a child who is allergic to this medicine. Do not give to a child with heart disease.	If your child will be using an inhaler, be sure she understands how to use it properly. Let teachers know your child may need to use this medicine at school.
Throat irritation, dry mouth, nose irritation, stomach upset, chest tightness.	Do not give to a child with a previous allergy to this drug.	Capsule form used only as inhalant.
Suppression of immune system, fluid retention, insomnia, increased appetite.	May be risky in case of serious infections, such as pneumonia, but may be given for bronchitis-complicating asthma.	May cause withdrawal symptoms if stopped abruptly. Dosage must be tapered off gradually.
Oral yeast infection.	May be risky in case of serious infections, such as pneumonia, but may be given for bronchitis-complicating asthma.	Conventional treatment of choice for asthma.

9

Medication	Effect	How Given	How Available
ASTHMA DRUGS (continued)			
Metaproterenol (Alupent, Metaprol)	Opens the airway.	Tablet; syrup; aerosol inhaler.	By prescription.
Terbutaline (Brethaire, Brethine, Bricanyl)	Opens the airway.	Tablet; injection; aerosol inhaler.	By prescription.
Theophylline (Aerolate, Bronkodyl, Duraphyl, Elixophyllin, Primatene, Slo-Phyllin, Tedral, Theolair, Theovent, Umphyl)	Opens the airway.	Capsule; tablet; liquid; injection.	By prescription.
ANTIBIOTICS			
Amoxicillin (Amoxil, Augmentin, Polymox, Trimox, Wymox)	Fights bacterial infection.	Capsule; chewable tablet; liquid.	By prescription.
Ampicillin (Omnipen, Polycillin)	Fights bacterial infection.	Capsule; liquid, injection.	By prescription.
Erythromycin (ERYC, Ilotycin, PCE, Pediamicin, Pediazole)	Fights bacterial infection.	Capsule; tablet; chewable tablet; injection.	By prescription.
Griseofulvin (Fulvicin, Grifulvin, Grisactin)	Fights fungal infection of the skin, hair, and nails; used for ringworm and athlete's foot.	Tablet; liquid.	By prescription.
Mebendazole (Vermox)	Fights worm infection.	Chewable tablet.	By prescription.
Metronidazole (Flagyl, Metric, Protostat)	Fights bacterial infection.	Tablet; injection.	By prescription.

Possible Side Effects	Contraindications	Comments
Headache, nervousness, increased heart rate, flushed face.	Use with caution in a child with heart disease. Do not give to a child with an allergy to this drug.	If your child will be using an inhaler, be sure she understands how to use it properly. Let teachers know your child may need to use this medicine at school.
Nervousness, headache, increased heart rate.	Do not give to a child with an allergy to this drug. Do not give to a child with heart disease.	Can be taken when needed. Keep doses 2 to 3 hours apart. If asthma is triggered by exercise, a dose can be taken 30 minutes before activity to prevent an attack. If your child will be using an inhaler, be sure she understands how to use it properly. Let teachers know that your child may need to take this medicine at school.
Nervousness, headache, irritability, increased heart rate, nausea, diarrhea. Long-term use may be linked to learning disabilities, although recent studies dispute this.	Do not give to a child with an allergy to this drug.	Certain drugs may increase or decrease the effect of theophylline; consult your doctor. Give the drug as prescribed; its effectiveness depends upon achieving a certain level in the blood. Give with food to lessen stomach upset. If using liquid form, shake well before using. If using a sustained-release form, do not crush; granules should be swallowed whole rather than chewed. If your child is vomiting or has a lot of stomach pain, restlessness, or irritability, call your doctor.
Diarrhea, skin rash (hives), yeast infection.	Do not give to a child with a previous allergy to this drug or other penicillin drugs.	Best given 30 minutes before or 1 hour after a full meal (a light snack is okay). If your child develops side effects, call your doctor.
Diarrhea, skin rash (hives), yeast infection.	Do not give to a child with a previous allergy to this drug or penicillin drugs.	Liquid form should be kept in the refrigerator. Do not give with a full meal, as food may decrease absorption of this drug. It is best to give it 1 hour before or 2 hours after a meal. If your child develops side effects, call your doctor.
Upset stomach, skin rash.	Do not give to a child with an allergy to this drug. Poorly tolerated if a child already has nausea or is vomiting.	Do not cut or crush the coated tablets. Talk to your pharmacist about whether or not the brand you are buying can be taken with food. If your child experiences intense stomach pain, discoloration of the skin or eyes, dark urine, or fatigue, call your doctor.
Nausea, vomiting, stomachache, skin rash, increased sensitivity to the sun.	A child with an allergy to penicillin may also be allergic to this drug.	Food increases the absorption of this drug; best given with dinner.
Diarrhea, abdominal pain, fever.	Do not give to a child under 2 years of age.	Can be given at any time during the day. May be chewed, crushed and put in applesauce, or swallowed whole.
Nausea, vomiting, upset stomach, metallic taste in the mouth, headache, dizziness, dark urine, numbness in extremities.	Do not give to a child with an allergy to this drug.	Give with food to lessen nausea. Avoid giving your child alcohol in beverages and medicines when giving this drug.

Medication	Effect	How Given	How Available
ANTIBIOTICS (continued)			
Nystatin (Mycolog, Mycostatin, Mytrex, Nilstat, Nystex)	Fights fungal infection; used for thrush and diaper rashes.	Tablet; liquid; cream, powder.	By prescription.
Penicillin (Bicillin, Pentids, Pen-Vee, Pfizerpen, Veetids, Wycillin)	Fights bacterial infection.	Tablet; liquid; injection.	By prescription.
Sulfamethoxazole + Trimethoprim (Bactrim, Co-trimoxazole, Septra)	Fights bacterial infection.	Tablet; liquid; injection.	By prescription.
COLD AND ALLERGY MEDICATIONS			
Dextromethorphan (Comtrex Cough, Triaminic Multi-Symptom, others)	Inhibits coughing.	Liquid; lozenge.	Over the counter.
Diphenhydramine (Allerdryl, Benadryl, Dytuss, Unisom)	Fights allergic reaction; inhibits coughing; aids sleep.	Capsule; tablet; liquid; cream.	Over the counter.
Guaifenesin (Donatussin, Meditussin, Robitussin AC, others)	Aids in clearing mucus from the respiratory tract.	Capsule; tablet; liquid.	Over the counter.
Phenylpropanolamine (Allerhist, Congesprin, Triaminic, others)	Eases nasal and sinus congestion.	Capsule; tablet; liquid.	Over the counter.
Pseudoephedrine (Novahistine, Sudafed, others)	Eases nasal and sinus congestion.	Tablet; liquid.	Over the counter.
DIGESTIVE MEDICATIONS			
Bisacodyl (Ducolax, Evac-Q-Kwik, X-Prep)	Stimulates bowel movement.	Tablet; suppository; enema.	Over the counter.
Bismuth Subsalicylate (Pepto-Bismol)	Binds with toxins or bacteria in the bowel to fight diarrhea.	Chewable tablet; liquid.	Over the counter.

Possible Side Effects	Contraindications	Comments
Upset stomach.	Do not give to a child with an allergy to this drug.	For oral thrush, the medicine should be swished in the mouth for a couple of minutes. In a young child or infant, it can be painted on the affected area with a cotton swab. Use a clean swab for a second application. Shake the bottle before using. When treating a skin infection, clean the area before applying the cream.
Allergic reaction, skin rash, wheezing, difficulty breathing, swelling of the mouth or throat, upset stomach.	Do not give to a child with an allergy to this or other penicillin drugs. A child with an allergy to cephalosporin drugs may also be allergic to penicillin.	Give 1 hour before or 2 hours after a meal.
Upset stomach, skin rash, anemia, depressed immune system, severe allergic reaction.	Do not give to a child with an allergy to sulfa drugs. Do not give to a child with folate-deficiency anemia.	Give with food to relieve stomach upset.
None reported.	Do not give to a child with a known allergy to this drug.	
Dry mouth, drowsiness; cream can cause hives, rash, itching.	Do not give to a child under 2 years of age unless directed by your doctor. Do not use on an allergic skin disorder, such as poison ivy.	Can be taken with food.
Stomach upset.	Do not give to a child with an allergy to this drug. Do not give to a child under 2 years old.	Encourage your child to drink lots of fluids to increase expectoration.
Restlessness, insomnia.	Do not give to a child with an allergy to this drug. Do not give to a child under 2 years old. Use with caution in a child who has heart disease or high blood pressure.	Takes 30 minutes to 1 hour to work.
Headache, insomnia.	Do not give to a child with an allergy to this drug. Do not give to a child under 2 years old. Use with caution in a child who has heart disease or high blood pressure.	Takes 30 minutes to 1 hour to work.
Diarrhea.	Do not give to a child with a stomachache. Do not give to a child with an allergy to this drug. Do not give to a child under 2 years old, unless prescribed by your doctor.	Do not crush. Do not give with milk or antacid. Suppository takes 15 minutes to 1 hour to work. Tablet will work within 6 to 10 hours. Do not give a child laxatives on a consistent basis.
Constipation.	Do not give to a child with an allergy to aspirin. Do not give to a child under 2 years old.	May cause dark stools. Takes 30 minutes to 1 hour to work.

Medication	Effect	How Given	How Available
DIGESTIVE MEDICATIONS (continued)			
Glycerin (Fleet Babylax, Therevac)	Stimulates bowel movement and softens stool.	Liquid in applicators for rectal use; suppository.	Over the counter.
Kaolin-Pectin (Donnagel, Kaopectate, Parepectolin)	Binds with noxious substances and solidifies stool.	Liquid.	Over the counter.
OTHER MEDICATIONS			
Burow's Solution	Acts as a drying agent for skin problems; fights infection.	Powder, mixed with water and used as a soak.	Over the counter.
Calamine	Acts as a drying agent; relieves itching.	Cream; lotion.	Over the counter.
Hydrocortisone (Alphaderm, Cort-Derm, Cortisporin, Cortril, Hytone, Lacti-Care, Nutracort, Renecort, Synacort, Vioform)	Fights inflammation.	Cream.	Over the counter and by prescription, depending on potency.
Methylphenidate (Ritalin)	Used to treat hyperactivity and attention deficit disorder.	Tablet.	By prescription.
Phenobarbital (Antrocol, Arco-Lase, Belladenal, Donnatal, Donnazyme, Kinesed, Mudrane, Phazyme, Quadrinal, Tedral)	Prevents seizures; acts as a sedative.	Tablet; liquid, injection.	By prescription.
Phenytoin (Dilantin)	Prevents seizures.	Capsule; chewable tablet; liquid; injection.	By prescription.

Possible Side Effects	Contraindications	Comments
Discomfort to rectum.	Do not give to a child with a stomach-ache. Do not give to a child with an allergy to this drug.	Takes 15 minutes to 1 hour to work. Do not confuse this medication with the liquid preparation Glycerol. That is a different medicine, and is not used as a laxative. Do not give a child laxatives on a consistent basis.
None reported.	Do not give to a child with a known allergy to kaolin or pectin.	Takes 1 to 4 hours to work.
None reported.	None known.	Good for weeping eczema and other "wet" skin disorders.
Burning skin rash.	Do not put on open or blistered skin.	Put a thin layer of the cream or lotion on clean skin.
Long-term use can make the skin become very thin and fragile, especially with the high-potency prescription forms.	Do not use on a child under 2 years of age unless directed by your doctor. Do not use on large areas or open areas. Do not use for more than a few days unless directed by your doctor.	Put a light layer on the skin. Leave skin open to air after applying. If the area worsens or shows no improvement after several days of use, call your doctor. Avoid long-term use, especially on the face.
Decreased appetite, nervousness, headache, irritability, difficulty sleeping, slowed growth.	Do not give to a child with an allergy to this drug. Use cautiously in a child with heart disease.	Be sure you obtain an accurate, carefully thought out diagnosis before giving this drug. Monitor your child's growth and weight. Tolerance may develop, requiring changes in dosage.
Sedation and drowsiness; excitability and restlessness.	Do not give to a child with lung disease. Do not give to a child with an allergy to this drug or other barbiturate drugs.	Some medicines may enhance the side effects of this drug; consult your doctor or pharmacist. The effectiveness of this drug depends on building up to a certain blood level, so do not stop giving the drug suddenly. If your child becomes unusally sleepy or unsteady on her feet, call your doctor. Give at bedtime.
Drowsiness, stomach upset, acne, increased facial hair, overgrowth of gums.	Do not give to a child with a known allergy to this drug.	May take 1 to 2 weeks to work. Other drugs affect this drug; consult your doctor or pharmacist. Teach careful oral hygiene and keep regular dental appointments to minimize side effects. Call your doctor if your child develops any of the following: dark urine, yellow skin, decreased appetite, stomach pain, sore throat, bruises, nosebleeds, unusual fatigue, or difficulty walking. Give at bedtime.

Herbal Medicine

Herbalists use the leaves, flowers, stems, berries, and roots of plants to prevent, relieve, and treat illness. From a "scientific" perspective, many herbal treatments are considered experimental. The reality is, however, that herbal medicine has a long and respected history. Many familiar medications of the twentieth century were developed from ancient healing traditions that treated health problems with specific plants. Today, science has isolated the medicinal properties of a large number of botanicals, and their healing components have been extracted and analyzed. Many plant components are now synthesized in large laboratories for use in pharmaceutical preparations. For example, vincristine (an antitumor drug), digitalis (a heart regulator), and ephedrine (a bronchodilator used to decrease respiratory congestion) were all originally discovered through research on plants.

THE HISTORY OF HERBAL MEDICINE

The history of herbology is inextricably intertwined with that of modern medicine. Many drugs listed as conventional medications were originally derived from plants. Salicylic acid, a precursor of aspirin, was originally derived from white willow bark and the meadowsweet plant. Cinchona bark is the source of malaria-fighting quinine. Vincristine, used to treat certain types of cancer, comes from periwinkle. The opium poppy yields morphine, codeine, and paregoric, a treatment for diarrhea. Laudanum, a tincture of the opium poppy, was the favored tranquilizer in Victorian times. Even today, morphine—the most important alkaloid of the opium poppy—remains the standard against which new synthetic pain relievers are measured.

Prior to the discovery and subsequent synthesis of antibiotics, the herb echinacea (which comes from the plant commonly known as purple coneflower) was one of the most widely prescribed medicines in the United States. For centuries, herbalists prescribed echinacea to fight infection. Today, research confirms that the herb boosts the immune system by stimulating the production of disease-fighting white blood cells.

The use of plants as medicine is older than recorded history. As mute witness to this fact, marshmallow root, hyacinth, and yarrow have been found carefully tucked around the bones of a Stone Age man in Iraq. These three medicinal herbs continue to be used today. Marshmallow root is a demulcent herb, soothing to inflamed or irritated mucous membranes, such as a sore throat or irritated digestive tract. Hyacinth is a diuretic that encourages tissues to give up excess water. Yarrow is a time-honored cold and fever remedy that may once have been used much as aspirin is today.

In 2735 B.C., the Chinese emperor Shen Nung wrote an authoritative treatise on herbs that is still in use today. Shen Nung recommended the use of ma huang (known as ephedra in the Western world), for example, against respiratory distress. Ephedrine, extracted from ephedra, is widely used as a decongestant. You'll find it in its synthetic form, pseudoephedrine, in many allergy, sinus, and cold-relief medications produced by large pharmaceutical companies.

The records of King Hammurabi of Babylon (c. 1800 B.C.) include instructions for using medicinal plants. Hammurabi prescribed the use of mint for digestive disorders. Modern research has confirmed that peppermint does indeed relieve nausea and vomiting by mildly anesthetizing the lining of the stomach.

The entire Middle East has a rich history of herbal healing. There are texts surviving from the ancient cultures of Mesopotamia, Egypt, and India that describe and illustrate the use of many medicinal plant products, including castor oil, linseed oil, and white poppies. In the scriptural book of Ezekiel, which dates from the sixth century B.C., we find this admonition regarding plant life: ". . . and the fruit thereof shall be for meat, and leaf thereof for medicine." Egyptian hieroglyphs show physicians of the first and second centuries A.D. treating constipation with senna pods, and using caraway and peppermint to relieve digestive upsets.

Throughout the Middle Ages, home-grown botanicals were the only medicines readily available, and for centuries, no self-respecting household would be without a carefully tended and extensively used herb garden. For the most part, herbal healing lore was passed from generation to generation by word of mouth. Mother taught daughter; the village herbalist taught a promising apprentice.

By the seventeenth century, the knowledge of herbal medicine was widely disseminated throughout Europe. In 1649, Nicholas Culpeper wrote *A Physical Directory*, and a few years later produced *The English Physician*. This respected herbal pharmacopeia was one of the first manuals that the layperson could use for health care, and it is still widely referred to and quoted today. Culpeper had studied at Cambridge University and was meant to become a great doctor, in the academic sense of the word. Instead, he chose to apprentice to an apothecary and eventually set up his own shop. He served the poor people of London and became known as their neighborhood doctor. The herbal he created was meant for the layperson.

The first *U.S. Pharmacopeia* was published in 1820. This volume included an authoritative listing of herbal drugs, with descriptions of their properties, uses, dosages, and tests of purity. It was periodically revised and became the legal standard for medical compounds in 1906. But as Western medicine evolved from an art to a science in the nineteenth century, information that had at one time been widely available became the domain of comparatively few. Once scientific methods were developed to extract and synthesize the active ingredients in plants, pharmaceutical laboratories took over from providers of medicinal herbs as the producers of drugs. The use of herbs, which for most of history had been mainstream medical practice, began to be considered unscientific, or at least unconventional, and to fall into relative obscurity.

HERBAL MEDICINE TODAY

Today, the *U.S. Pharmacopeia*, with its reliance on herbal compounds, has been all but forgotten. Most modern physicians rely on the *Physician's Desk Reference*, an extensive listing of chemically manufactured drugs. It is important to note that each entry in this enormous volume, in addition to specifying the chemical compound and actions of a particular drug, also includes an extensive list of contraindications and possible side effects.

Rather than using a whole plant, pharmacologists identify, isolate, extract, and synthesize individual components, thus capturing the active properties. This can create problems, however. In addition to active ingredients, plants contain minerals, vitamins, volatile oils, glycosides, alkaloids, bioflavonoids, and other substances that are important in supporting a particular herb's medicinal properties. These elements also provide an important natural safeguard. Isolated or synthesized active compounds can become toxic in relatively small doses; it usually takes a much greater amount of a whole herb, with all of its components, to reach a toxic level. Herbs *are* medicines, however, and they can have powerful effects. They should not be taken lightly. The suggestions for herbal treatments in this book are not intended to substitute for consultation with a qualified health care practitioner, but rather to support and assist you in understanding and working with your physician's advice.

There are over 750,000 plants on earth. Relatively speaking, only a very few of the healing herbs have been studied scientifically. And because modern pharmacology looks for one active ingredient and seeks to isolate it to the exclusion of all the others, most of the research that is done on plants continues to focus on identifying and isolating active ingredients, rather than studying the medicinal properties of whole plants. Herbalists, however, consider that the power of a plant lies in the interaction of all its ingredients. Plants used as medicines offer synergistic interactions between ingredients both known and unknown.

The efficacy of many medicinal plants has been validated by scientists abroad, from Europe to the Orient. Thanks to modern technology, science can now identify some of the specific properties and interactions of botanical constituents. With this scientific documentation, we now know why certain herbs are effective against certain conditions. However, almost all of the current research validating herbal medicine has been done in Germany, Japan, China, Taiwan, and Russia. And for the most part, the United States Food and Drug Administration (FDA), which is responsible for licensing all new drugs (or any substances for which medicinal properties are claimed) for use in the United States, does not recognize or accept findings from across the sea. Doctors and government agencies want to see American scientific studies before recognizing the effectiveness of a plant as medicine. Yet even though substantial research is being done in other countries, drug companies and laboratories in the United States so far have not chosen to put much money or resources into botanical research. The result is that herbal medicine does not have the same place of importance or level of acceptance in this country as it does in other countries.

WORKING WITH AN HERBALIST

As of this writing, there is no national licensing or certification for herbalists in the United States. If you wish to locate a qualified herbalist, the best place to start is probably in your local herb shop or health food store. They may be able to refer you to a knowledgeable herbalist who can advise you. If you are unable to locate an herbalist this way, you may wish to contact the Herb Research Foundation, located at 1007 Pearl Street, Boulder, Colorado 80302 (telephone 303–449–2265) for suggestions.

An herbalist may assess your child's health needs in a variety of ways. Along with taking your child's history, methods of observation used by herbalists include pulse and tongue diagnosis, abdominal diagnosis, and iridology, which involves the correlation of minute markings on the iris with specific parts of the body.

After making an evaluation of your child, an herbalist can be expected to suggest individual herbs or herbal combinations known to be beneficial for your child's particular condition. An herbalist will often recommend herbs or herbal combinations to both strengthen the underlying system or organ and to relieve symptoms. Ask your herbalist when the preparation can be expected to effect an improvement in your child's condition. When you administer an herbal prescription, observe how the preparation makes your child feel. Promptly report improvement, lack of improvement, or any side effects to your herbalist. If the specified amount of time passes without any change in your child's symptoms, it is important to report this, too. A change in prescription may be indicated.

TREATING YOUR CHILD WITH HERBS

The power and potency of the healing herbs are very real. Every herbal treatment suggested in this book has specific healing properties, carefully balanced to create a particular action within your child's body.

Natural medicines are not like manufactured drugs. Herbal preparations work gently, so they take time to act internally. When you give your child an herbal preparation, begin with a small amount. Watch closely for signs that symptoms are easing. Observe how the preparation makes your child feel. Using herbal treatment requires observation, coupled with good judgment.

Natural herbal preparations are generally well tolerated by children. Most herbs are nontoxic, with few, if any, harmful side effects. However, it is important to know the action and possible side effects of an herb before you give it. Although it is very unusual, some children may show signs of sensitivity to a particular herb. Reactions can include a headache, an upset stomach, or a rash. If your child has a reaction, discontinue use of the herb.

If your child is responding favorably to the herb, but the reaction is too intense, either decrease the dosage or discontinue use of the herb. For example, say your child is constipated and you administer a laxative herb. If your child begins having diarrhea, you have obviously achieved relief of constipation. It's the right idea, but the reaction is too intense. Use your judgment and discontinue the herb. Likewise, if you are giving an herb with expectorant properties and your child begins coughing up large quantities of mucus, you should consider decreasing the dose so expectoration is manageable.

Herbal treatment is useful for both acute and chronic conditions. It is also valuable in maintaining health and preventing illness. Many of the herbal preparations recommended in this book will help boost the immune response and help arm your child against recurrent infections.

Common Herbs and Herbal Preparations

Herbs are available in a variety of forms, including fresh, dried, in tablets or capsules, or bottled in liquid form. You can buy them individually or in mixtures formulated for specific conditions. Whatever type of product you choose, the quality of an herbal preparation—be it in capsule, tablet, tea, tincture, bath, compress, poultice, or ointment form—is only as good as the quality of the raw herb from which it was made.

Generally, herbs fall into two categories: wild-grown and farm-grown. A wild-grown herb is one that grows naturally, without human intervention. As a result of natural selection, plants tend to be found in places with conditions that optimize their growth. For example, horsetail grows best in moist, swampy areas, while arnica thrives at high altitudes in alpine meadows. The process of gathering herbs from their natural habitats is called *wildcrafting*.

The disadvantage of wild-grown herbs is that there is no guarantee the plants haven't been exposed to chemicals and pesticides. Herbs harvested from a meadow, for example, may have been exposed to chemical drift from a crop-dusted farm nearby. Exhaust fumes from passing traffic may have settled invisibly on plants growing near a country road. Water-loving plants, like horsetail, may be rooted in the bank of a polluted stream.

Because of the possibility of contamination, unless you are very sure of the source of wildcrafted herbs, organic herbs grown commercially may be a better choice. Organic farm-grown herbs are becoming increasingly available, as more and more herb farms are being established. With careful management, organic herb farms can provide a steady supply of quality herbs to the consumer.

To produce top-quality products, herb farmers require a great deal of specialized knowledge. For maximum potency, it is important that particular herbs be harvested at the optimum moment. For example, echinacea is gathered in the spring, winter, and fall, but not in summer, when the plant's energies are concentrated on growth and flowering.

Responsible farmers use compost and organic matter to fertilize and replenish the health of the soil. For obvious reasons, we favor the use of certified organically grown herbs, produced without the use of synthetic fertilizers or chemical pesticides. As of this writing, not all states have agencies inspecting and certifying organic growers, so to be sure you are getting pure, pesticide-free herbs grown without chemical contamination, check the label for the words "certified organic" before you make a purchase. The name of the certifying agency should be specified on the label. Two reliable organizations that certify organic products are the Organic Growers and Buyers Association and California Certified Organic Farmers. Organic products grown in the states of Washington and Texas should be certified organic by the Department of Agriculture of the relevant state. As of this writing, federal legislation on requirements for labeling a product "organic" has been passed, but is not yet being fully implemented. Once it is, it should be easier to be sure that you are buying a genuine organic product. Hopefully this will take place in the next few years.

The herbal treatments recommended in Part Two of this book include teas, baths, compresses, poultices, oils, and ointments. In some instances, you will be starting from scratch and preparing herbal treatments for your child (instructions on how to prepare your own herbal treatments are given in Part Three, Therapies and Procedures). Some of the most commonly used herbal treatments and their applications are reviewed in the table beginning on page 21.

Administering Herbal Treatment

Herbs and prepared herbal compounds are available in different forms, each of which has its own particular characteristics. Your health food store will have individual herbs as well as complex herbal formulations, including raw herbs, tinctures, extracts, capsules, tablets, lozenges, and ointments. Here's a look at what's available.

Tinctures

If the label says *tincture*, the preparation contains alcohol. In a tincture, alcohol is employed to extract and concentrate the active properties of the herb. Alcohol is also a very effective natural preservative. Because a tincture is easily assimilated by the body, it is a very effective way to administer herbal compounds. Tinctures are concentrated and cost-effective. However, the full taste of the herb comes through very strongly in a tincture. Children—and adults, too—may find the taste of some herbs unpleasant. Goldenseal, for example, is bitter-tasting.

Another concern when using tinctures is the presence of the alcohol. If you wish to lessen the amount of alcohol in a tincture before giving it to your child, mix the appropriate dose with one-quarter cup of *very* hot water. After about five minutes, most of the taste of the alcohol will have evaporated away, and the mixture should be cool enough to drink.

Extracts

Extracts can be made with alcohol, like tinctures, or the essence of the herb can be leached out with water. When purchasing a liquid extract of an herb, the only way to be certain of the extraction process (alcohol or water) is to read the label. Extracts offer essentially the same advantages and disadvantages that tinctures do. They are the most concentrated form of herbal treatment and therefore the most cost-effective. They are easy to administer, but have a strong herbal taste.

Capsules and Tablets

Capsules and tablets contain a ground or powdered form of raw herb. In general, there seems to be little difference between the two in terms of clinical results. Because finely milled herbs degrade quickly, it is important that herbs be freshly ground and then promptly encapsulated or tableted, within twenty-four hours of being powdered. When making your selection, read the label to make sure fresh herbs have been used in the product. With the exception of certain herbal concentrates in capsule form, both capsules and tablets tend to be much less strong and potent than tinctures and extracts.

Teas

There are many delicious blends of herbal teas on the shelves of your health food store; they need no introduction here. You'll find loose herbs ready for steeping, herbal formulations aimed at specific conditions, and convenient pre-bagged teas. Some are just for sipping; some are medicinal. When your child is ill, a comforting cup of herbal tea (medicinal or not) is a wonderful way to give additional liquids.

Lozenges

Herbal-based, nutrient-rich, naturally sweetened lozenges are readily available in most health food shops. You'll find cold-fighting formulas, natural cough suppressants, some with decongestant properties. Many are boosted with natural vitamin C. Choose lozenges made without refined sugar.

Ointments, Salves, and Rubs

From calendula ointment (for broken skin and wounds) to goldenseal (for infections, rashes, and skin irritations) to aloe vera gel (to cool and speed the healing of minor burns, including sunburn) to heat-producing herbs (for muscle aches and strains), there's a wealth of topical herbal-based products on the market. Your selection will depend on the condition you are treating.

The Treatment and Care entries in Part Two of this book offer recommendations for herbal treatments for childhood conditions.

When administering herbal treatment, you can follow the same basic suggestions that you would for administering conventional medications. If the taste of an herb is too strong, dilute the appropriate dosage in a little juice or water. Tableted herbs or capsules can be mixed with a spoonful of cream-style cereal or applesauce, or dissolved in sweet fruit juice. For older children, herbal teas can be sweetened with honey (a child under eighteen months old should *never* be allowed to take honey because there is a risk of infant botulism, which can be fatal). For an infant, the herbal tea can be mixed with mother's milk or formula and put into a bottle, an eyedropper, or empty syringe (without the needle), and gently squirted inside the child's mouth. A nursing mother can also take an adult dose of an herbal remedy, and the effect will be transmitted by her breast milk. For instructions on how to make and use different types of herbal preparations, *see* PREPARING HERBAL TREATMENTS in Part Three of this book. Age-appropriate dosage guidelines for herbal treatments may be found in the beginning of Part Two.

When treating your child with herbal remedies, use your judgment and common sense. The herbal treatments recommended in this book are gentle and have been especially selected for use on children. It is still possible, however, for any herb to cause adverse reactions in some children. If your child develops a rash, a stomachache, a headache, or any other new symptom after treatment with an herbal remedy, discontinue using the herb and consult with your health care provider.

Adverse reactions are unusual if herbal remedies are used in recommended doses. Problems are more likely to occur if an herb is overused—if the dosage is too high or if the herb is given continuously for too long. Chamomile, for example, may cause a child to develop an allergy to ragweed if given on a daily basis for too long; the prolonged use of licorice can lead to high blood pressure. This is why, even if an herb is beneficial for a chronic condition, it is not usually recommended that an herbal remedy be given on an ongoing basis, but rather that it be used for set periods of time, or alternated with another remedy or remedies. When using herbal treatment—as with most other aspects of a healthy life—moderation is the key. If you have any question about the use of a particular herb, consult with a qualified herbalist or health care professional.

Herbal medicine has a long history, and a time-tested, valuable place in the treatment of many common health problems. Because they act gently, herbs are particularly suitable for treating children. When using herbs to treat an illness, often you not only help to alleviate symptoms, but also to address an underlying problem and strengthen the overall functioning of a particular organ or system. Herbs are readily available—they can even be grown in your own back yard. To be sure you are getting the best and purest product possible, however, we recommend that you use certified organically grown herbs. The more you use herbs, the more comfortable you will become with this gentle, effective form of health care.

COMMON MEDICINAL HERBS

Any medication, including herbs, can cause an allergic reaction. An allergic reaction can happen with the first exposure, or after your child has taken the medication several times. Symptoms of an allergic reaction can include rash, swelling, itching, and/or difficulty breathing. If you think your child is having an allergic reaction, call your physician. If your child experiences difficulty breathing, take him to the emergency room of the nearest hospital.

Always read package directions carefully to be sure you are giving the preparation properly and in the correct dose. Note that with herbal medicines, side effects are more likely to occur in the case of overdose. When given in recommended doses, toxicity is unlikely.

	Medicinal Use	Part of Plant Used	How Given	Possible Side Effects	Comments
Alfalfa	Tonic; contains natural fluoride, helpful in preventing tooth decay.	Leaf.	Tincture; tea; capsule.	None known.	Excellent for increasing the production of breast milk.
Aloe vera	Topically: Pain reliever, excellent for burns, sore nipples, itching of chickenpox. Internally: Relieves stomach inflammation and constipation.	Pulp from inside leaf.	Liquid applied topically to affected area or taken internally.	None known.	Topically: Use pulp from inside plant leaf. Internally: Use prepared food-grade liquid.
American ginseng	Helps strengthen overall constitution; helpful in relieving fatigue or debilitation after an illness.	Root.	Tincture; tea.	Nervousness, insomnia, diarrhea.	Do not use if a fever is present.
Bupleurum	Liver detoxifier; strengthens immune system; helpful in treating chronic conditions such as allergies, recurring earaches, or runny nose.	Root.	Tincture; capsule (taken in combination with other herbs).	None known.	Most commonly used in combination with other herbs, not by itself. Do not use if fever or other signs of acute infection are present.
Burdock	Blood purifier and cleanser; helpful in treatment of acne.	Root.	Tincture; tea; capsule; fresh cooked root.	Dilated pupils, dry mouth.	Do not use for more than 2 consecutive weeks. Alternate 2 weeks on, 2 weeks off.
Calendula	Antiseptic; speeds tissue healing; useful on cuts, blisters, burns, abrasions.	Flower.	Lotion, cream, or tincture, applied topically to the affected area.	None known.	
Carob	Helps to stop/slow diarrhea.	Pod and seed.	Mix powdered carob with water and drink.	None known.	
Chamomile	Soothes upset stomach; relaxes, induces sleep; helpful for teething.	Flower.	Tincture; tea; capsule; bath.	Allergic reactions in sensitive individuals.	Do not give to a child who is allergic to ragweed.
Dill	Helps to relieve colic, stomach gas.	Leaf.	Tea; in soup or vegetables.	None known.	Increases production of breast milk.

Herb	Medicinal Use	Part of Plant Used	How Given	Possible Side Effects	Comments
Echinacea	Antibiotic; boosts immune system. Useful in treating many infections, insect bites, and stings.	Root.	Tincture; tea; capsule; salve.	None known.	Long-term use not advised. Best used for 5 days to 1 week at a time. Alternate 1 week on, 1 week off.
Fennel	Helpful for colic, stomachache.	Seed.	Tea; capsule.	In large doses, can cause skin irritation, nausea, vomiting.	Do not use during pregnancy.
Fenugreek	Expectorant; helpful in treating sore throat and chest congestion.	Seed.	Tea; capsule.	None known.	May produce unusual body odor. This is only temporary, and not a cause for concern.
Flax	Soothing to digestive tract; relieves constipation.	Seed.	Tea; capsule; oil.	Agitation, excitement, rapid breathing.	Seeds are safe when cooked; leaves can be toxic and are not normally used. May be taken by a breastfeeding mother to relieve infant constipation.
Garlic	Antibiotic, antiseptic, antiworm.	Clove.	Fresh whole herb; capsule; liquid.	Stomach upset, contact dermatitis, flatulence.	Fresh cloves may be used, but odorless capsule form is more palatable for most children.
Ginger	Aids digestion; relieves congestion; promotes perspiration and relieves fever; soothes achy muscles.	Root.	Tincture; tea; bath or oil for achy muscles.	Diarrhea, nausea.	
Goldenseal	Antibiotic; used to treat many infections.	Root.	Tincture; tea; capsule.	Irritation of mouth and throat, nausea, vomiting, diarrhea.	Do not use during pregnancy. Do not take for more than 1 week to 10 days at a time.
Licorice	Tonic; soothing to respiratory tract; increases energy.	Root.	Tincture; tea; capsule.	Can lead to high blood pressure with long-term use.	Use cautiously in pregnancy or in the presence of high blood pressure or heart disease.
Ma huang (Ephedra)	Decreases nasal and sinus swelling and congestion.	Stems, twigs.	Tea; capsule.	Increased blood pressure and heart rate, anxiety, insomnia.	Use cautiously in pregnancy or in the presence of high blood pressure, heart disease, thyroid disease, or diabetes. Not advised for children under 12. Best given before 3:00 P.M. to prevent insomnia.
Marshmallow	Demulcent, helpful for sore throat and lung congestion.	Root.	Tea; capsule.	None known.	

Herb	Medicinal Use	Part of Plant Used	How Given	Possible Side Effects	Comments
Papaya	Aids digestion; relieves indigestion and gas.	Fruit, leaf.	Fruit eaten raw. Leaf in tea form.	Heartburn.	Seeds are used in Asia to eradicate parasites.
Parsley	Increases urination; helpful in treating bladder infection.	Leaf.	Tea; capsule.	Dizziness, headache, warmth, nausea, vomiting, itching.	Use with caution during pregnancy. Excessive amounts will stop milk production in nursing mothers.
Peppermint	Aids digestion; relieves nausea; reduces fever; relieves diarrhea, gas, heartburn.	Leaf.	Tincture; tea; capsule.	In large doses, can cause stomach irritation and coldness of the body.	
Red clover	Blood purifier; helpful in treating acne, boils, skin infections; mild sedative.	Flower.	Tincture; tea; capsule.	None known.	
Rosemary	Antispasmodic, stimulating tonic; helpful in treating colds, sore throats, headaches; increases circulation.	Leaf.	Tea; in soup.	Nausea, diarrhea.	A strong tea can also be used topically to enhance scalp health and hair growth.
Sage	Increases urination; aids digestion; antiseptic; helpful for nasal discharge, sore throat.	Leaf.	Tincture; tea; capsule; topically on cuts or abrasions.	Dry mouth, local irritation.	Can also be used as a gargle for sore throats. Do not use during pregnancy. May decrease milk production in nursing mothers.
Skullcap	Sedative, nerve tonic.	Leaf.	Tincture; tea; capsule.	Giddiness, irregular heartbeat.	Best used in combination with other calmatives. Do not give to a child under 6 years of age.
Slippery elm	Helpful in treating constipation, diarrhea, irritated/inflamed stomach.	Bark.	Mix powdered bark with water and drink.	None known.	
Thyme	Antiseptic; relieves lung congestion, diarrhea, lack of appetite, colic, flatulence.	Leaf.	Tea; in soup.	In large doses, can cause diarrhea.	May be used as a mouthwash.
Yarrow	Useful for colds, flu, fever.	Leaf.	Tea; tincture; capsule.	None known.	Contains small amounts of bioavailable iron. Extended use may make the skin more sensitive to sunlight.
Yellow dock	Detoxifier; mild laxative; antiworm; relieves cough and lymphatic congestion.	Root.	Tincture; tea; capsule.	In large doses, can cause nausea, vomiting, diarrhea.	Encourages perspiration.

Homeopathy

Homeopathy is a system of treatment that uses minute amounts of plant, mineral, and animal substances to stimulate the defensive systems of the body in a very subtle way. It is widely used in Europe, but not as well known in the United States. The theoretical and empirical basis of homeopathy is a concept called the Law of Similars, often summarized as "like cures like." Perhaps more than anything else, what distinguishes the practice of homeopathy from other approaches to medicine is that instead of focusing on the specific *causes* of disease (such as viruses and bacteria), it focuses on the specifics of the *symptoms* of disease, *as they are experienced by the individual patient*.

THE HISTORY OF HOMEOPATHY

Samuel Hahnemann (1755–1843) of Leipzig, Germany, created the practice of homeopathy. A medical doctor, Hahnemann did in-depth studies and wrote extensively on chemistry, pharmacology, and medicine. His study of arsenic, written in 1796, remains an authoritative text.

In 1790, Dr. Hahnemann began to question the accepted medical theories of the time. *Cinchona officinalis*, or Peruvian bark, had been the treatment of choice for malaria since 1700. Conventional medical thought attributed its beneficial action to its bitter and astringent properties. Hahnemann rejected this explanation. He observed that other plants and botanicals had even stronger astringency and greater bitterness, yet did nothing to relieve malaria. In an attempt to better understand how cinchona worked, he experimented by taking some himself. After taking the cinchona compound, Hahnemann promptly developed the symptoms of malaria.

This inspired him to further experimentation with many different plants, chemicals, and minerals. Hahnemann experimented first on himself, then on his family and friends. As his work continued, he noted the same remarkable effect again and again:

Derivatives of certain extracts produced symptoms in the body similar to those produced by certain diseases. Pressing on with his experimentation, Hahnemann found that *minute* doses of extract actually produced the opposite effect. Instead of causing the symptoms of a particular disease, the well-diluted extract reversed the course of the disease. This led Hahnemann to his observation that "like cures like"—that is, a substance that causes a certain set of symptoms in a healthy person will, in minute doses, cure a sick person of those same symptoms. He called this phenomenon the Law of Similars.

Many of Hahnemann's colleagues argued against his practice of using himself as a guinea pig, prophesying dire consequences. But the doctor refused to heed their warnings, saying, "He knows with greatest certainty the things he has experienced in his own person." Through his experiments, Hahnemann learned that a minute dose of a substance would cause illness in a healthy person, but paradoxically effect a cure in a sick individual. For example, a remedy that caused fever, chills, and leg cramps in a healthy person would cure a sick person of similar fever, chills, and leg cramps when given in microdoses.

HOMEOPATHY TODAY

Homeopathy is accepted as an effective form of medicine in many parts of the world today, including Great Britain, France, Germany, Greece, India, and South America. The British royal family has been under the care of homeopathic physicians since the time of Queen Victoria.

Homeopathy is a systematic and precise form of natural medicine that addresses both physical and emotional symptoms. This protocol recognizes that each person is unique and will have an individual disease pattern. The experimentation, documentation, in-depth testing, and recording of the effects of homeopathic remedies did not end with Dr. Hahnemann.

Diagnosis of a specific disease is not the primary concern when treating your child with homeopathics. Rather, the correct remedy is chosen according to the specific symptoms and emotions your child is experiencing.

Homeopathic remedies stimulate the body's vital force, enhancing its ability to heal itself. The "vital force" described by Hahnemann cannot be precisely identified. Even today's most technologically advanced medical detectives do not really understand the ways in which body and mind work together. A complex interrelationship between immune factors and regenerative biological systems, the essential life force locked within body and mind remains a mystery.

Homeopathic remedies work by, in effect, "turning on a switch" that affects both body and mind. Homeopathic compounds somehow send a healing and normalizing message throughout the body. They spark unbalanced internal systems so that they are better able to perform their functions.

WORKING WITH
A HOMEOPATHIC PHYSICIAN

Remedies that may be appropriate for a variety of common childhood health problems are recommended in Part Two of this book. However, because the deeper concepts of homeopathy and the intricacies of the remedies can be difficult to master, you may find it helpful to consult a homeopathic physician. Often, a homeopathic physician can determine a constitutional remedy for your child that will help to balance her entire system.

Homeopathy is on the upswing in the United States. Many different types of health care practitioners use homeopathy. You'll find medical doctors, naturopathic physicians, acupuncturists, herbalists, chiropractors, nurse practitioners, physician assistants, and laypeople who are knowledgeable in the field. Homeopathic pharmacies, even major health food stores, are other resources to explore. They may be able to tell you how to find a practicing homeopath in your area.

There are national organizations throughout the United States that can provide you with a list of homeopaths as well. If you can't readily find a homeopathic physician in your area, you may wish to contact the International Foundation for Homeopathy (2366 Eastlake Avenue E, Suite 301, Seattle, WA 98102-3366; telephone 206–324–8230); the National Center of Homeopathy (1500 Massachusetts Avenue NW, #42, Washington, DC 20005; telephone 202–223–6182); or the Homeopathic Educational Service (2124 Kittredge Street, Berkeley, CA 94704; telephone 415–649–0294).

When choosing a homeopath to care for your child, it is important to select a physician with whom you feel very comfortable. This doctor will question you closely, asking you to reveal very intimate information about your child, and quite possibly about yourself as well. Much of homeopathic diagnosis and treatment depends on your ability to observe and relate specific details, some of which may even seem absurd or irrelevant to you at first.

Your homeopath will want to explore both your and your child's emotional response to her condition, as well as symptomatic details. For example, if your child has a drippy nose or is coughing up phlegm, your homeopath will want to know the color, smell, and consistency of the discharge. You will probably be asked if it is heavier in the morning or evening, after eating, or before eating.

Your homeopath will also consider your child's temperament and the way she responds emotionally to illness. Does your child want hugs and cuddles, or prefer to be left alone? Does your child become whiny and demanding when ill, or quiet and passive? Does she sleep a lot, or become restless and wakeful? Does she want the window open to admit cool, fresh air, or does your child feel chilly even snuggled under a cozy comforter?

How you respond to your sick child is something else your homeopath will ask you to reveal. When a child is ill, some parents become irritated and annoyed, some nervous and anxious. The very fortunate have a deep well of calm and certainty on which to draw. Be truthful when your doctor inquires about this. Emotional responses are not something you necessarily control consciously. Faced with a hectic schedule, many parents have difficulty mustering up as much patience as they would like to comfort and nurture a sick child. All of the physical and emotional factors surrounding your child must be taken into account in determining the appropriate remedy. Because the emotional response of those around an ill child will unavoidably have an impact on her, your homeopathic physician may prescribe a helpful remedy for the primary caregiver as well.

TREATING YOUR CHILD WITH
HOMEOPATHIC REMEDIES

Of all the remedies commonly used in the various medical protocols, homeopathic remedies are unique in that they are symptom-specific. That is, the correct remedy is determined not by the disease, but by the specific complex of physical and emotional symptoms your

child is experiencing. The choice of homeopathic remedies takes into consideration the temperament and
emotional response of the patient, as well as the most
minute details of her physical condition.

For example, the cold that infects your child and a
neighbor's child may be caused by the same virus, but
each child will exhibit a unique set of symptoms and
emotions. One child may have a headache and a runny
nose, feel completely exhausted, and want to eat when
not napping. The other may be clogged and congested,
feel restless, be unable to sleep, and refuse food. Consequently, these two children, although infected by the
same virus, will require entirely different remedies.

Homeopathy respects the complexity and uniqueness of each individual. To identify the correct homeopathic remedy, you must carefully observe your child's
unique—even quirky—behaviors and responses.
Choosing the appropriate remedy requires a parent or
homeopathic physician to match the child's symptoms,
both obvious and subtle, with the remedy.

Based on your child's overall physical, emotional,
and mental constitution, your homeopathic physician
may prescribe a constitutional remedy. An appropriate
constitutional remedy can help prevent illness, as well
as maintain and support optimal health. For example,
if your child is subject to recurrent ear and nose infections, colic, allergies, or digestive disorders, a constitutional homeopathic remedy may be extremely helpful.

The correct constitutional remedy will help
strengthen and stimulate the vital life force. Your child's
response to the remedy will be at once subtle and
profound, on the physical, emotional, and mental levels. Prescribing a constitutional remedy is a complicated art, however. To discover the most helpful
constitutional remedy for your child, consult a homeopathic physician.

Common Homeopathic Remedies

Homeopathic remedies are prepared according to the
standards of the *United States Homeopathic Pharmaco-
poeia*. All remedies are derived from naturally occurring
plant, mineral, or chemical substances. Some of the
most useful homeopathic remedies and their common
indications are described in the table on page 27.

Homeopathic remedies come in different potencies.
Of all of the issues in homeopathy, Dr. Hahnemann's
concept of potency is probably the one that has evoked
the most questions, because it seems somewhat paradoxical at first. In his experiments, Hahnemann noted
that symptoms continued to improve with ever-in-
creasing dilution of a substance. In other words, as the

concentration of the medicinal substance is reduced by
dilution, the remedy becomes increasingly potent. As
yet, there is no satisfactory scientific explanation for
this phenomenon. However, the astounding effectiveness of homeopathic treatment has been empirically
documented around the world.

Commonly available homeopathic remedies come
in several forms: the mother tincture, x potencies, and
c potencies. Homeopathic tablets are made by mixing
diluted remedies with lactose (milk sugar) to make solid
pellets. There are also homeopathic creams, ointments,
and salves, made by mixing diluted remedies with a
cream or gel base.

Mother Tincture

The mother tincture is an alcohol-based extract of a
specific substance, as it comes from the original plant,
animal, or mineral. Mother tinctures are generally used
topically or in a fashion similar to herbal tinctures.

X Potencies

In homeopathic remedies, the x (derived from the Roman numeral decimal system) represents 10. It indicates that the mother tincture has been diluted to one
part in ten. The number preceding the x indicates how
many times the remedy has been diluted. Thus, a 6x
potency represents six such dilutions, beginning with
the mother tincture. Remember that the more diluted
a homeopathic remedy is, the more potent it is. So a 6x
potency remedy, which has been diluted six times, is
more potent than a 3x potency compound, which has
been diluted only three times.

C Potencies

The c, also derived from the Roman numeral decimal
system, represents 100. A c potency indicates that a
mother tincture has undergone dilutions to one part in
100; the number preceding the c indicates how many
dilutions it has undergone. Thus, a 3c potency indicates
that the substance has been diluted to one part in 100
three times. As with x potencies, the higher the number,
the stronger the remedy.

In home treatment, it is usually sufficient to use the
lower potencies, such as 12x, 30x, 6c, and 9c. Many
homeopaths agree that once you have identified the
correct remedy, it will work regardless of potency.

If you are lucky, you may live in an area where you
have access to a homeopathic pharmacy that specializes
in homeopathic remedies. If not, check with your local

COMMON HOMEOPATHIC REMEDIES

Remedy	Indications
Aconite	Very often the first remedy for acute problems, especially if shock or fright is part of the picture.
Antimonium tartaricum	Rattling cough with breathlessness.
Apis mellifica	Insect bites that are red and swollen.
Argentum nitricum	Stomachache from eating sweets; nervousness; for a child who craves fatty foods; for a child who craves stimulation.
Arnica	Bruises; sprains; strains. Can be taken internally or administered topically (but do not use topically if the skin is broken).
Arsenicum album	First remedy for food poisoning; diarrhea with anxiety; a cold with restlessness.
Belladonna	Fever; acute problems with sudden onset, red face, dilated pupils; headache.
Bryonia	Dry cough; constipation; achiness; irritability.
Calcarea carbonica	Teething; digestive problems in babies; for a chubby, chilly infant; for a child who is slow to walk, teethe, read, etc.
Cantharis	Burns; burning sensation associated with urinary tract infections.
Chamomilla	First teething remedy to try; relaxant for teething infant.
Coffea cruda	Difficulty falling asleep due to racing thoughts, such as might occur the night before a big test or other major event in a child's life.
Colocynthis	Menstrual cramps that are sharp and stabbing; diarrhea cramps.
Drosera	Spasmodic, dry cough; coughing that is worse at night.
Dulcamara	Symptoms that are made worse by damp weather or seasonal temperature changes.
Ferrum phosphoricum	Mild fever; nosebleed.
Gelsemium	Cold symptoms that include heavy, droopy eyes, weakness, achy muscles, chills; nervousness before a performance.
Hepar sulphuris	Hypersensitivity to pain; yellow mucus; symptoms that feel worse from cold drafts, better with warmth.
Hypericum	Nerve pain; trauma to nerve endings, especially of the fingers and toes.
Kali bichromicum	A cough with thick, ropy mucus.
Kali muriaticum	Tonsillitis; sinusitis; for a child with yellow mucus.
Ledum	Black-and-blue bruises; puncture wounds; black eye.
Lycopodium	Problems affecting the right side of the body; reactions to food; for a child who looks older than his years.
Magnesia phosphorica	Menstrual cramps that feel better with heat on the lower abdomen, especially cramps on the right side of the body; diarrhea.
Mercurius dulcis	Ear infection.
Natrum muriaticum	Dehydration; emotional upset with strong desire for salty foods; acne; canker sores.
Nux vomica	Hypersensitivity and irritability; indigestion; for a child who likes to go to bed late; for a child who craves rich foods.
Phosphorus	Sore throat; tiredness during the day and difficulty sleeping at night; for a sensitive child.
Pulsatilla	Nasal congestion with yellow mucus; cold symptoms; earache; for a child who cries easily.

Remedy	Indications
Rhus toxicodendron	Chickenpox; poison ivy.
Ruta graveolens	Tendinitis; sprains of wrist or ankle.
Sepia	Menstrual cramps; constipation; for a child who feels better with exercise.
Spongia	Laryngitis; hacking cough.
Sulphur	Pinworms; skin infections; head lice; ringworm.
Thuja	After vaccinations; warts; athlete's foot, thrush.
Urtica urens	Burns; can be taken internally or applied topically.

health food store. Major health food stores across the United States usually carry a comprehensive selection of homeopathic remedies. If you don't find what you're looking for, many health food shops will special-order for you. A list of recommended suppliers of homeopathic remedies is also provided in the Appendix.

Proper storage and handling of homeopathic remedies is extremely important. They are sensitive and a certain amount of care must be taken in order not to diminish their potency or interfere with their action. Keep remedies out of sunlight and extreme heat, and away from strong smells. Avoid touching homeopathic remedies with your hands, and do not put any pellets that fall out of the bottle back in. Also, never touch the inner rim or the inside of a remedy bottle or lid.

Administering Homeopathic Remedies

Many childhood health problems can be treated effectively and gently with homeopathy. Home administration of homeopathic remedies is ideally suited for acute situations—conditions that attack your child suddenly—rather than conditions medically termed chronic (illnesses that develop slowly and persist over a long period of time).

When you give the right remedy, it will work quickly. Experienced homeopathic physicians say that the "wrong" remedy will usually cause no harm. Once your child's symptoms improve, discontinue the remedy. It is possible for a child to experience an aggravation or increase in the symptoms being treated, an effect caused by the Law of Similars. Should your child's symptoms be increased by a remedy, stop administration of the remedy.

Homeopathic remedies come in pellet, tablet, and liquid form. Pellets and tablets are generally the best form of homeopathic remedies to use for children. You should avoid touching them with your hands, as this can decrease their effectiveness. Shake the pellets or tablets into a clean spoon or the top of the bottle, and then place them directly into your child's mouth and tell her to let them dissolve rather than chewing them. Homeopathic pellets and tablets are mostly sweet milk sugar (lactose) that melts in the mouth, so it is generally easy to persuade a child to take them. If you are giving a remedy to an infant, you can dissolve the pellets in water and give the mixture to your child in an eyedropper.

The liquid remedies—homeopathic tinctures—are not generally recommended for children because of their high alcohol content. However, as with herbal tinctures, if you put them in very hot water and let the mixture sit for five minutes, much of the taste of the alcohol will evaporate.

Homeopathic remedies work best when taken at least thirty minutes before or after eating. Clinical practice has shown that strong flavors (such as mint products), odors (paints, perfumes, etc.), foods and beverages that contain caffeine, and camphor or camphor-containing products (such as mothballs or deep-heating ointments—which should not be used on children anyway)—all decrease the effectiveness of the remedies, so all of these substances should be avoided when using homeopathic remedies.

Unless the treatment recommendations in Part Two specify otherwise, use the following guidelines when administering homeopathic remedies.

- **For a severely acute situation.** For a problem such as a headache or fever, give your child one dose, every fifteen minutes, for one hour. If you see no change after four doses, you probably have the wrong remedy and should choose another.

- **For a less acute situation.** For a problem such as a runny nose or a sore throat, give one dose, every two hours. Once symptoms start to improve, you can continue the remedy at less frequent intervals. During this stage, give your child one dose, three times daily.

A homeopathic remedy should be given for as long as it is needed. For example, if your child's headache is gone fifteen minutes after she takes a headache remedy, she can stop taking the remedy. If the headache returns four hours later, try the same remedy again. Once your child feels better, she no longer needs to take the remedy.

Homeopathy is a highly individualized form of treatment that requires careful observation of your child's physical symptoms as well as her emotional reaction to illness. It is a gentle and noninvasive form of natural medicine that can work particularly well for common, acute childhood health problems.

Bach Flower Remedies

The world of natural treatment also includes natural emotion-balancing flower preparations. This system of healing was developed by Dr. Edward Bach (1897–1936). Dr. Bach believed that physical problems were secondary to emotional problems, that physical illness was a manifestation of an emotional imbalance. He taught that physical symptoms could be relieved by altering or alleviating destructive emotions. The various remedies he devised are used to treat illness by easing quite specific types of emotional and mental distress.

The Bach Flower Remedies are dilute essences of plants. Unlike chemical mood-altering drugs, the flower remedies—while effective—are gentle and easy to use.

Although beneficial and benign, these natural flower essences have remarkable emotional and mental balancing effects. Because they act quite gently, they can be used whenever you think they may help your child to feel better. When choosing a Bach essence, match your child's overall temperament, personality, and fears, as well as the particular emotional distress he is experiencing. If no single remedy seems to address all of these concerns, you may combine up to three remedies. (Although there is no danger in blending more than three remedies at any one time, their effectiveness can be diminished in a blend that is too complicated.)

CHOOSING A REMEDY

Once you have identified the primary emotional distress your child is experiencing, use the table on pages 31–34 to find an appropriate remedy. Match the child's personality, temperament, fears, and upset with the suitable Bach Flower Remedy. Bach Flower Remedies are available at many health food stores. If you cannot get them at a store near you, you can obtain them through Ellon Bach USA, Inc. (644 Merrick Road, Lynbrook, NY 11563; telephone 516–593–2206) or Homeopathic Educational Services (2124 Kittredge Street, Berkeley, CA 94704; telephone 510–649–0294).

ADMINISTERING BACH FLOWER REMEDIES

Bach Flower Remedies are essences of flowers that come in tincture form. The bottled remedy you buy at your health food store is called the mother tincture, and is the most concentrated form available. There are two different ways you can administer a Bach remedy to your child.

- Place a drop of the mother tincture into a small glass of noncarbonated spring water and have your child sip this over a period of a few hours. For added benefit, teach him to swish the mixture around in his mouth before swallowing it.

- If you prefer, you can make a diluted mother tincture. Fill a two-ounce glass bottle with spring water. Add three drops of mother tincture and shake gently to blend. When using a diluted mother tincture, give your child two droppersful, three times daily.

After giving your child a flower remedy, observe his response. As his emotional response and behavior change, the need for a particular remedy may cease to exist. Give a remedy until the situation has been resolved. Once your child's mood and emotions have been gently altered, you may need to select another remedy to complete and sustain the alteration. If your child's destructive emotions have eased sufficiently and his emotional and mental state has come into balance, discontinue the remedy.

Of all the Bach Flower Remedies, the overwhelming favorite of many parents is Rescue Remedy. This is a premixed combination remedy made from the essences of cherry plum, clematis, impatiens, rock rose, and star of Bethlehem. It is useful in many crisis situations, such as after hearing bad news, before a test, before going to the dentist, after falling down and getting hurt, or after waking up from a nightmare. It helps to restore balance and relieve apprehension. It will help calm a child who is crying, afraid, panicked, or tense. Rescue Remedy is particularly good in acute situations in which the cause of your child's distress is not clear—when a child begins crying and feeling intensely frustrated for no apparent reason and refuses to be consoled. Put two or three drops of this remedy in half a glass of water and give it to your child to sip as needed, or administer as you would any other Bach Flower Remedy.

Bach Flower Remedies are dilute essences of plants that treat emotional, mental, and physical distress. As with homeopathic remedies, choosing a flower remedy involves close observation of your child's emotional state, and then finding a remedy that matches your observations. Many parents report that these gentle preparations are excellent for alleviating stress and easing a sick, uncomfortable, or unhappy child.

BACH FLOWER REMEDIES

Flower Remedy	Primary Expression of Emotion	Underlying Emotional Concerns
Rescue Remedy (a combination of cherry plum, clematis, impatiens, rock rose, star of Bethlehem)	Fear; panic; apprehension; inconsolable crying; anxiety; tension; night terrors; unexplained screaming.	This premier flower remedy is excellent for alleviating any crisis-caused stress, major or minor. It will help calm an overwrought child, restore balance, and ease apprehension. Whether the cause is an accident, bad news, a nightmare, anxiety over an upcoming test, fear of going to the dentist, an imminent "big day," or anything else, Rescue Remedy calms and alleviates stress. It is particularly useful in acute situations where the cause of a child's distress is unclear, when a child is inconsolable, or appears intensely frustrated and begins screaming for no apparent reason. It is also useful given immediately after a child receives a vaccination. Of all the Bach remedies, parents report being most appreciative of Rescue Remedy.
Agrimony	Outwardly smiling and brave; inwardly, anguished and suffering. Look deep into this child's eyes. The suffering will show.	A determination to appear cheerful, despite suffering going on underneath. The anguish may be due to a family trauma, a significant disappointment, or anything your child may view as "failure."
Aspen	Fearfulness.	Fears that the child can't (or won't) explain, often resulting in many nightmares or difficulty falling asleep.
Beech	Impatience, intolerance.	A tendency to be a perfectionist and to keep to oneself. This type of child is drawn to order, precision, and pure reason, has little patience with others, and rails against an upset in schedule.
Centaury	Shyness; feelings of intimidation.	A weak-willed nature. This child is often pushed around at school or on the playground, has great difficulty standing up for himself, and doesn't want to be noticed.
Cerato	Need for constant affirmation.	Lack of self-confidence; low self-esteem. This child will do a project, then ask you to check it, certain it isn't quite right. He doesn't want to try anything new or go anywhere alone. You may find yourself accompanying this child everywhere.
Cherry plum	Fearfulness.	Fear of situations over which the child has no control. This is the type of child who will never venture onto a roller coaster, for example.
Chestnut bud	Incorrigible behavior.	An inability (or unwillingness) to understand cause and effect or learn from past mistakes. As a result, reprimands may go unheeded. For example, this child may continue hitting a sibling even though he has been punished for it several times. Chestnut bud is especially helpful in alleviating this kind of behavior.

Flower Remedy	Primary Expression of Emotion	Underlying Emotional Concerns
Chicory	Need for constant attention; selfishness; possessiveness; easily hurt feelings.	Insecurity and fear of being rejected. This child has difficulty sharing anything, especially his parents. His feelings are easily hurt and he often feels rejected. He says "mine" a lot, while snatching toys from a sibling or playmate.
Clematis	Indifference; apathy; short attention span.	A tendency to daydream. This child doesn't seem to care very much about anything. He becomes distracted and preoccupied easily, and appears indifferent to his surroundings. It is difficult to capture and hold his attention.
Crabapple	Excessive neatness; compulsive behavior.	An inability to tolerate disorder or untidiness, which may be related to a child's feelings of shame about his physical condition or appearance. This child's striving for neatness may border on compulsive behavior.
Elm	Feelings of incompetence.	Fundamental feelings of inadequacy. This child may often whine, "I can't," and complains of being incapable of doing things he wants (or needs) to accomplish.
Gentian	Need for much praise and encouragement.	A tendency to become discouraged by any setback, no matter how minor. This child requires much encouragement to accomplish anything. He typically tries something once, and if success is not immediate, he is unwilling to try again. Gentian is especially helpful for a child who is discouraged with schoolwork.
Gorse	Feelings of deep despair, usually after a serious family trauma.	Following a traumatic situation, such as a death or divorce, this child knows that "nothing will ever be the same again," and fears that he will never be able to be happy and carefree again. Without denigrating him or denying the child this period of grieving, supply much reassurance. Gorse can help to ease his feelings during this period.
Heather	Self-centeredness.	Utter self-absorption. This child believes the world begins and ends with him. He will talk exclusively (and at length) about his cuts and bruises, problems and concerns.
Holly	Anger; fits of temper.	Insecurity and jealousy, such as a feeling of being displaced after the birth of a new sibling, that come out in displays of anger and bad temper.
Honeysuckle	Obsession with happy times from the past; homesickness.	A feeling that past times were perfect, and an obsession with comparing them to the imperfect present. This child typically talks of times when he was particularly happy, such as when the family went to grandmother's house on holidays, when his parents were still together, or when an older sibling doted on him. Honeysuckle is also helpful for a child who is homesick, perhaps because of being away from home for the first time.
Hornbeam	Exhaustion.	Fatigue and tiredness that keeps a child from joining in family activities or play with other children. As a result, this child misses out on a lot of fun times.
Impatiens	Impatience; nervousness; hyperactive behavior.	Feelings of impatience and tension. This child is easily irritated and nervous. Impatiens is also an excellent remedy for a hyperactive child who can't sit still.
Larch	Lack of self-confidence.	Low self-esteem. This child is self-effacing and fears calling attention to himself. Standing in front of the class and giving an assigned presentation is an ordeal for this child. Larch will help bolster a child's self-confidence before taking a test or giving an oral report.

Flower Remedy	Primary Expression of Emotion	Underlying Emotional Concerns
Mimulus	Frequent expression of fears of one thing or another.	Fearfulness, shyness, and timidity. This child typically talks of being afraid of specific people and/or things, whether teachers, other children, animals, accidents, or monsters. He blushes easily. Unlike the Aspen child, who has fears he can't name, the Mimulus child has fears that are identifiable and well articulated.
Mustard	Sadness.	Sorrow and depression. The cause may not be readily apparent, but often these feelings are related to a loss of some kind.
Oak	Constant busyness and bustling.	A "type-A" personality; a relentless drive to achieve. This child seems to feel he must be a role model for others; he is an overachiever who presses on without letup.
Olive	Exhaustion.	Continual fatigue; a sense of being exhausted to the very core. Gently stimulating olive is the remedy of choice for this child.
Pine	Feelings of guilt.	A deep, internalized sense of shame and remorse. This child may feel he has done something so awful it can never be forgiven; he may blame himself for everything that goes wrong. Even when the fault lies elsewhere, this child feels guilty inside.
Red chestnut	Inappropriate worrying.	Excessive concern over the well-being of others. This child worries constantly.
Rock rose	Absolute terror; panic.	Irrational fears. This child often suffers from nightmares.
Rock water	Inflexibility; unwillingness to forgive.	A rigid, unforgiving nature, and a need to strive for perfection. This child is very hard on himself, as well as on others.
Scleranthus	Feelings of uncertainty; vacillation.	An inability to make a decision, to choose between different courses of action. This child feels torn between choices and often asks, "Should I do this?" or, "Should I do that?"
Star of Bethlehem	Emotional shock following a life-changing experience.	A traumatic and possibly life-changing event, such as sudden or shocking sad news, a severe scare, an accident, or a significant disappointment, that causes feelings of shock and loss. Star of Bethlehem is excellent for alleviating the physical and emotional shock associated with traumatic experiences.
Sweet chestnut	Anguish and torment.	Feelings of exhaustion and alienation. For whatever reason, this child is in torment and feels very much alone.
Vervain	Tension; drivenness.	Perfectionism that causes a child to strive to hard that he becomes nervous and tense. This child may have difficulty sleeping normally.
Vine	Selfishness; ruthlessness.	A need to have one's own way, no matter what. This child will do and say anything to swing others his way, and can be utterly ruthless in pursuit of his desires.
Walnut	Tendency to be very easily influenced.	A nature that is sensitive and easily cowed. Even if a proposed course of action is not to his liking, this child will "follow the leader" rather than following the dictates of his own head and/or heart.
Water violet	A tendency to be alone, removed from peers.	An asocial nature that feels no need or desire to associate with other children. This child prefers to be alone, aloof, and removed, "above" the daily hurly-burly.
White chestnut	Obsessive thinking.	A tendency to dwell on ideas or events without letup. Long after you thought the subject had been forgotten, this child may still be fixated on the same idea. This remedy is very helpful for a child who obsesses about being accepted into a particular group or clique.

Flower Remedy	Primary Expression of Emotion	Underlying Emotional Concerns
Wild oat	Indecisiveness.	A tendency to be fearful and anxious, especially about the future. This remedy is especially helpful for the child at a crossroads who is fearful and indecisive over future plans, such as a teenager who is having trouble deciding on what he wants to do after leaving high school.
Wild rose	Apathy; resignation.	Feelings of tiredness, a lack of vitality. This child seems resigned to just soldier on, placing one foot in front of the other, buffeted by the winds of fate.
Willow	Refusal to be pleased or satisfied.	Resentfulness, bitterness, feelings of dissatisfaction and jealousy. Nothing is ever "good enough" for this child. When ill, he can be very difficult to treat. This child may even refuse to admit to being helped or eased.

Acupressure

Acupressure is a gentle, noninvasive form of the ancient Chinese practice of acupuncture. In acu*puncture*, thin needles are inserted into the body at specific points along lines called meridians. In acu*pressure*, thumb or finger pressure is applied at these same points, but the body is not punctured. In both practices, the aim is to effect beneficial changes and achieve harmony within the body's systems and structure.

THE HISTORY OF ACUPRESSURE

Because acupressure evolved from acupuncture, an ancient Chinese healing practice, the history of this form of treatment begins with traditional Chinese philosophy as it applies to the healing arts. The fundamental principle of Chinese philosophy is the concept of *yin* and *yang*. The yin and yang are two opposite, yet complementary, forever-entwined forces that underlie all aspects of life. Yin-yang is depicted as the subtly curved light and dark halves of a circle. Both proceed from the *t'ai chi* (the Supreme Ultimate).

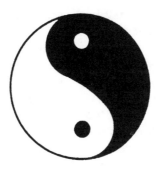

The Yin-Yang Circle

According to this philosophical system, the human body, like all matter, is made up of five elements: wood, fire, earth, metal, and water. Each element corresponds to an aspect of the body, such as the organs, senses, tissues, and emotions, as well as to aspects of nature, such as direction, season, color, and climate (see inset, page 36). The five-element theory, combined with the principle of yin and yang, forms the basis of the Chinese concept of balance. The intention is to balance yin and yang and to balance the energies of the five elements.

Yin is earthy, female, dark, passive, receptive, and absorbing. It is represented by the moon, the tiger, the color orange, a broken line, and the shady side of a hill. Yin is cool, inward, still, and soft.

Yang is represented by the sun, the dragon, the color blue, an unbroken line, and the sunny side of a hill. Yang is hot, outward, moving, aggressive, and bright.

Because yin and yang are intertwined halves of the same whole, all things, and all people, contain elements of both, although at any one time, one or the other will be predominant. Thus, a baby or young child is more yin; an older child more yang. When your child asserts herself, it is her yang that is coming to the fore.

The sun is yang, the moon is yin. We awaken in the morning and greet the sun. It is natural to be active and moving throughout the daylight. As twilight descends into night, we become more passive and quiet. Nighttime expresses the qualities of yin.

Chinese medical theory teaches that the two branches of the body's nervous system, the sympathetic and parasympathetic, correspond to the two halves of the yin-yang circle. The sympathetic branch is the part of the nervous system that mobilizes our bodies to respond to stress. It initiates the fight-or-flight response, a more yang part of the cycle. The parasympathetic branch replenishes and supports the body during rest, the yin part of the cycle. These two branches oppose and balance each other to create stability and health. When the yin and yang are balanced within the body, all the body's functions are healthy. Illness is caused by an imbalance between yin and yang.

Conventional Western medicine typically pinpoints and directly treats only the affected part of the body. Chinese medical philosophy encompasses the entire universe. Everything that affects the patient is considered, including emotion, environment, and diet.

Chinese philosophy proposes a way of life based on living in accordance with the laws of nature. This profound connection with nature is reflected in the language used to describe illness. For example, a patient may be diagnosed with a "wind invasion" or "excess

The Five Elements and Their Correspondences in Nature and the Human Body

In traditional Chinese philosophy, all matter is considered to be composed of five elements (wood, fire, earth, metal, and water). The elements in turn have correspondences in various aspects of the natural world, including the human body. According to this philosophy, health is achieved when yin and yang, and the energies of the five elements, are all in proper balance. The elements and some of their corresponding characteristics and parts of the body are illustrated in the chart below.

ELEMENT	THINGS IN NATURE					THE HUMAN BODY				
	Direc-tion	Taste	Color	Growth Cycle	Environ-mental Factor	Season	Organs	Sense Organ	Tissue	Emotion
Wood	East	Sour	Green	Germina-tion	Wind	Spring	Liver, gallbladder	Eye	Tendon	Anger
Fire	South	Bitter	Red	Growth	Heat	Summer	Heart, small intestine	Tongue	Vessel	Joy
Earth	Middle	Sweet	Yellow	Ripening	Dampness	Late summer	Spleen, stomach	Mouth	Muscle	Meditation
Metal	West	Pungent	White	Harvest	Dryness	Autumn	Lung, large intestine	Nose	Skin and hair	Grief and melancholy
Water	North	Salty	Black	Storing	Cold	Winter	Kidney, bladder	Ear	Bone	Fright and fear

heat." Acupuncture (or acupressure) points may be chosen to "disperse wind," "remove summer damp," or "disperse rising fire."

In traditional Chinese medicine, every aspect of health is described in terms of a balance between yin and yang. For example, yin illnesses are caused by excessive expansion (overweight as a result of eating too much sugar, for example), while yang illnesses are caused by excessive contraction (sunstroke or fever). An imbalance of yin and yang factors can be demonstrated by showing how red blood cells respond to different substances. When red blood cells are placed in water (yin), they absorb the water, expand, and finally burst. When red blood cells are placed in a concentrated saline (salt) solution (yang), they contract, shrink, and shrivel. In a solution of normal saline (0.9 percent salt), the yin and yang are perfectly balanced and the cells remain virtually unchanged. An example of how the ancient yin-yang theory can be used to describe concepts in conventional medicine can be found in the treatment of breast and prostate cancer: Female hormones (yin) help control prostate cancer (yang); male hormones (yang) help control breast cancer (yin). The interplay of the yin and yang—as one increases, the other decreases—describes the process of the universe and everything in it. In more familiar Western terms, as modern physical

science teaches, "For every action, there is an equal and opposite reaction."

In Chinese philosophy, the energy that pulses through all things, animate and inanimate, is called *chi*. Health exists when there is a harmonious balance under heaven of both internal and external forces. Each bodily organ must have the right amount of *chi* to function. Too much or too little *chi* causes an imbalance, resulting in illness or disease. *Chi* flows through all things, enters and passes through the body, creating harmony or disharmony.

Chinese medicine works directly with the natural, vital energy—or *chi*—of the body. The goal of acupuncture and acupressure is to normalize the body's energies. *Chi* can be tapped at specific points along channels known as meridians. Activating one key point sets up a predictable reaction in another area. By tonifying (increasing energy in) a specific area, the yin-yang balance is treated. Moving an excess of *chi* from one area and directing it to another, weaker area, corrects the yin-yang balance.

Acupuncture is an ancient protocol. As a component of Oriental medicine, it has been practiced for centuries. The *Huangdi Neijing* (Canon of Medicine), written about 500–300 B.C., is the oldest surviving medical text. Among other medical practices, it describes the use of acupuncture.

ACUPRESSURE TODAY

Acupressure is a form of body work in which pressure is applied to specific acupuncture points to balance internal function. Acupressure is practiced around the world.

The Chinese have a very descriptive term for taking advantage of a combination of two or more healing systems—a practice this book advocates. They say the patient is "walking on two legs." A two-year study conducted jointly by the Northwestern University Medical School and Evanston Hospital in Evanston, Illinois, employed a combination of acupuncture and acupressure. In this study, patients suffering from chronic headaches of all types, including migraine, cluster, whiplash, and tension, were first treated with acupuncture. The patients were then individually instructed in specific acupressure techniques to use when a headache seemed imminent. The researchers reported that the need for prescription painkillers and other drugs was eliminated entirely in most patients—thus verifying the effectiveness of "walking on two legs."

WORKING WITH AN ACUPRESSURIST

There are professionally trained and college-educated acupressurists, just as there are acupuncturists. If you wish to consult a trained acupressurist, check the yellow pages of your telephone book. You'll find this category listed in most large cities.

For the most part, though, the gentle form of acupressure recommended in the Treatment and Care entries in Part Two of this book is something you can do yourself, at home, to ease a hurting or ailing child.

TREATING YOUR CHILD WITH ACUPRESSURE

In *The Chinese Art of Healing* (Bantam, 1972), author Stephan Palos identifies the hand as "man's original medical tool." We instinctively use our hands to alleviate pain. When we suffer a bump or bruise, have a cramp, or hurt anywhere inside, we rub, knead, or massage the painful spot.

When your child is ill, gently working the acupressure points recommended in the appropriate entry in Part Two will probably be beneficial (the illustrations in Part Three provide guidelines for locating all of the acupressure points recommended). Your child will very likely love receiving an acupressure treatment.

Massaging a particular point will help relieve symptoms as well as strengthen and balance the yin-yang in your child's body. For example, applying acupressure to the point identified as "Large Intestine 11" helps relax the intestine, thus relieving constipation. Another related point is Stomach 36; massaging Stomach 36 helps tone an upset digestive tract. When your child is ill, the appropriate acupressure points, as well as other areas of your child's body, will be tender. Use your intuitive sense. Ask what feels good.

Common Acupressure Points

In acupressure, there are twelve lines called meridians that run along each side of the body. Each pair of meridians corresponds to a specific organ. For example, there is a pair of Lung meridians, Spleen meridians, Stomach meridians, and Liver meridians. Acupressure points are named for the meridian they lie on, and each is given a number according to where along the meridian it falls. Thus, Spleen 6 is the sixth point on the Spleen meridian. The table on page 38 lists some of the acupressure points most often recommended in the entries in Part Two of this book.

Administering Acupressure

When you give your child an acupressure treatment, your tools are your hands, notably your thumbs and fingers, and occasionally your palms. For the most part, you will be using the balls of your thumbs and fingers, never the nails. Before administering acupressure, make sure your fingernails are clipped short, so that you do not inadvertently scratch your child.

Choose a time of day when your child is most relaxed, perhaps after a warm bath and just before bedtime. Have her take a few deep breaths. This aids relaxation and will automatically focus your child's attention inward on her body.

You might want to start an acupressure session with a loving and comforting back rub, a treat most children welcome, especially when ill. Remain calm and unhurried. Make sure to keep your child warm throughout the treatment. You can apply pressure to the points directly onto the skin, or through a shirt or light sheet.

Work right-side and left-side acupressure points at the same time. Use your fingers or thumbs to apply *threshold pressure* to the point. Threshold pressure is firm pressure, just on the verge of becoming painful. The idea is to stimulate the point without causing the body to tighten up or retract from the pain. The pressure you exert should not hurt your child. Firm but gentle is the rule.

Apply from one to five minutes of continuous pressure. Or apply pressure for ten seconds, release for ten seconds, reapply pressure for ten seconds, release for ten seconds. Repeat this cycle five times.

Specific acupressure points helpful for different childhood conditions are included in the Treatment and

Care entries in Part Two of this book. To learn how to locate specific acupressure points, *see* ADMINISTERING AN ACUPRESSURE TREATMENT in Part Three.

When your child is ill, acupressure is a wonderful way to use your hands with a loving, nurturing touch, while also stimulating your child's body to heal. By using the acupressure points described in this book, you will be working to relieve the underlying cause of illness. At the same time, your gentle healing touch will convey your love and concern to your child.

COMMON ACUPRESSURE POINTS

Point	Effect	Indications
Bladder 23	Increases circulation to the urinary tract and reproductive organs.	Vaginitis; urinary tract infection; lower back pain.
Bladder 28	Master point for the bladder.	Urinary tract infection.
Bladder 60	Increases circulation to the urinary tract and reproductive organs.	Vaginitis; urinary tract infection.
Four Gates	Calms the nervous system.	Motion sickness; chickenpox; croup; hay fever; herpes; hyperactivity; pain; fever; poison ivy; sleeplessness; weight problems.
Kidney 3	Strengthens the bladder and kidneys; increases circulation to the reproductive organs.	Bedwetting; urinary tract infection; vaginitis.
Kidney 7	Strengthens the bladder and kidneys.	Bedwetting.
Large Intestine 4	Beneficial to the head and face; relieves congestion and headaches; removes energy blocks in the large intestine; clears heat.	Acne; common cold; headache; menstrual cramps; teething; sore throat; fever; toothache.
Large Intestine 11	Relieves itching; reduces allergic reactions.	Chickenpox; hay fever; constipation.
Large Intestine 20	Decreases sinus congestion.	Hay fever; sinusitis.
Liver 3	Quiets the nervous system; relaxes muscle cramps and spasms.	Asthma; menstrual cramps; teething; headache; eye pain.
Lung 7	Clears the lungs; moistens the throat.	Asthma; common cold; sore throat.
Neck and Shoulder Release	Relaxes the muscles of the neck and shoulders; relaxes the body.	Headache; weight problems.
Pericardium 6	Relaxes the chest; relieves nausea; relaxes the mind.	Asthma; motion sickness; croup; sleeplessness; stomachache; vomiting.
Points Along Either Side of the Spine	Improves circulation; relaxes the nervous system; balances the respiratory system; relaxes the spine.	Anxiety; colic; common cold; menstrual cramps; nervousness; insomnia.
Spleen 6	Reduces uterine cramping.	Menstrual cramps.
Spleen 10	Detoxifies the blood.	Acne; herpes; impetigo; poison ivy; boils; vaginitis.
Stomach 36	Tones the digestive system; strengthens overall well-being.	Colic; diarrhea; chronic runny nose; vomiting; constipation; indigestion; stomachache.

Diet and Nutrition

In his 1988 Report on Nutrition and Health, then-Surgeon General of the United States C. Everett Koop wrote, "Your choice of diet can influence your long-term health prospects more than any other action you might take." Let us rephrase this a bit: Your choice of diet *for your child* can influence *your child's* long-term health prospects more than any other action you might take *as a parent.*

Food provides the energy your child needs to grow, learn, jump, stretch, and play. It provides the nutrient base necessary for building a strong and healthy body. Food also provides immediate information to the body. It can make your child feel full and re-energized, or tired, jumpy, and irritable. The breakfasts you give your child, the lunches eaten at school, the snacks you provide, the dinners you prepare—all provide the building blocks for every cell in your child's body.

THE HISTORICAL USES OF DIET

Hippocrates, the "Father of Medicine," wrote, "Let food be your medicine. Let your medicine be your food." This recommendation is as important for us today as it was in ancient Greece. Food was a primary form of medicine in ancient cultures and has continued to be used as such through the ages. Warm teas and soups for colds, prune juice for constipation, toast and crackers for diarrhea—all are well-known and time-tested "medicines."

Food is important not only for curing illness, but for preventing it. Today, the importance of diet in maintaining health—and conversely, in contributing to the development of disease—is increasingly evident. A proper diet is therefore useful in treating acute and chronic childhood illness as well as in promoting and enhancing optimal health.

THE AMERICAN DIET TODAY

A hundred years ago, food was prepared in a very different way than it generally is today. Most importantly, food was prepared and served more simply. In the last several decades, thanks to food-processing technology, we have seen the development of a vast selection of "quick-fix" packaged, canned, frozen, boil-in-a-bag, and microwavable foods that get us in and out of the kitchen fast. Few people cook in the traditional sense of the word, at least on a regular basis. It's easier and more convenient to stir water into the contents of a package, open a can, heat up a frozen dinner, or "nuke" a prepackaged serving in the microwave.

Highly processed junk food is a billion-dollar-a-year industry. The shelves of American supermarkets are weighted down with candy, cookies, and all kinds of packaged baked goods; snacks loaded with sugar, fat, and salt; sodas, colas, "juices," and punches made with more chemicals and additives than fruit; and artificially flavored and colored cereals.

The typical American diet is in need of an overhaul. Most of us eat too much fat, too few complex carbohydrates, and too many empty calories, and are deficient in trace minerals and vitamins. The typical American gets about 42 percent of total calories from fat, with 16 percent coming from saturated fats and 26 percent from unsaturated fats. Compare this to the recommended amounts: a maximum of 30 percent of total daily calories from fat, with 10 percent from saturated fats (such as meat and dairy products), 10 percent from monounsaturated fats (such as olive oil), and 10 percent from polyunsaturated fats (such as corn, safflower, and soybean oils).

The typical American gets about 22 percent of total calories from complex carbohydrates (such as those in grains and legumes), 6 percent of calories from naturally occurring sugars (such as those found in fruits and honey), and 18 percent of calories from refined and processed sugars (such as those found in sodas, candy bars, and many processed foods). Yet it is recommended that at least 48 percent of the calories we consume should come from complex carbohydrates and naturally occurring sugars, and no more than 10 percent from refined and processed sugars.

The Influence of Television

Food manufacturers and the experts who design their advertising are doing a good job of "programming" your child. Television exerts a tremendous influence on children. Clever commercials aimed squarely at the child in the family instill a desire for many unhealthy manufactured foods loaded with sugar, additives, artificial flavors and dyes, and fats.

In early 1991, a study revealed that children watching cartoon shows for a four-hour period on a typical Saturday morning were bombarded with a total of 222 junk-food commercials. The networks monitored were ABC, NBC, CBS, Fox, and the Nickelodeon cable channel. The products advertised were dominated by sugar-coated cereals, candy, cookies, chips, fruit-flavored drinks, chocolate syrup, fast-food meals, and pizza.

Even if children know how to use the remote control, few "zap" out the commercials. Most sit passively with their eyes glued to the screen. Also, many of these junk-food ads feature colorful cartoonlike creatures. A child often cannot differentiate between the cartoon entertainment and the commercials.

Michael Jacobson, Ph.D., executive director of the Center for Science in the Public Interest, which conducted the study, sees a correlation between the reported 54-percent increase in obesity among elementary school children and a 39-percent increase in junk-food ads.

If your child coaxes you to put certain items on your grocery shopping list, you know that all that child-oriented advertising is working. A study by Texas A and M University showed that children develop brand loyalty at a very early age. Young people independently spend more than $2 billion a year on food, and influence $75 billion of the total amount spent on foods by adults.

If your child begs for certain manufactured food products that you prefer he not eat, you might want to do some "counter-programming" of your own. Even a very young child can understand a simple explanation of *why* a product is undesirable—that chemical additives are "bad" things that can hurt the body, that sugar rots the teeth, or that rancid fats can make a young body unhealthy. You might close your explanation by gently telling your child, "My saying 'no' means I love you too much to let you have something that can hurt you."

Another impact that television (and its close relative, the video game) has had on many children is to decrease their level of physical activity. Time spent getting exercise—something that should come naturally to most children—is being replaced by hours spent indoors, just sitting and watching. The healthy benefits of exercise are many, and, like a good diet, regular exercise is a habit best developed early in life. It is important for parents to insist that their children get some physical activity each day. Better yet, exercise with with your child. Consider such activities as taking a walk, bicycle riding, or playing whatever sport or game you and your child like best. You will be setting a good example, both of you will get exercise, and perhaps most important of all, you will be spending time together in a way that is pleasurable to both of you.

You can make a good start toward a better diet by focusing on five of the dietary goals determined by the Senate Select Committee on Nutrition and Human Services to optimize the health of Americans through improved nutrition:

1. Increase your intake of complex carbohydrates.
2. Decrease your intake of refined and processed sugars.
3. Decrease fat consumption.
4. Decrease cholesterol consumption.
5. Limit salt intake.

In addition, encourage your child to avoid the routine consumption of products containing refined and processed sugars, saving them instead for *occasional* treats. Base your family's diet on grains, vegetables, fruits, clean, lean proteins, and legumes. Don't depend on processed, packaged foods for your nutrition—it is a disservice to your family's health.

FOOD ADDITIVES AND OTHER CHEMICALS

Too much of what passes for food in the United States contains chemicals such as manufactured sweeteners, processed fats and/or fat substitutes, artificial flavorings and colorings, plus vast quantities of preservatives. Preservatives are nothing new. Salting down and pickling meat and vegetables were common practices centuries ago, as was the drying (dehydrating) of various foodstuffs. Foods preserved this way lasted a very long time, which was important in an era before refrigeration and efficient transport of fresh foods. But these natural methods took so much time and care that they were not easily adaptable to mass production. As the prepared-food industry grew by leaps and bounds, other time-saving and more cost-effective—if less healthy—methods of preserving foods were developed by the major food manufacturers.

Food additives and preservatives undergo exhaustive testing, on an individual basis. During the testing phase, laboratory animals are given megadoses of a single additive at a time. It's easy enough for manufacturers to explain away any adverse reactions by pointing out that a human will ingest only a tiny bit of a particular additive per serving. But few studies have been conducted on how different food additives interact with each other or what they do to the human body, even

though it's impossible to find a manufactured food product that contains only one additive. A small-scale study reported in the *Journal of Food Science* in 1976 tested three common food additives, with alarming results. When laboratory rats were given a single additive in their food, no adverse effects were noted. When two additives were combined, the rats sickened. When all three additives were given, all of the animals died within two weeks.

And what about the effects over the long term? Current scientific research can't tell us what the cumulative effects of ingesting a single food additive will be—let alone what the ever-present chemical combinations of multiple additives may do over a period of many years.

Today's food products often contain more chemical

Cholesterol and Your Child

Children raised on a diet high in animal fat are at risk for excessive blood cholesterol (for children, this is defined as anything over 170 milligrams per deciliter [mg/dL] of blood), and all the health problems associated with it. This phenomenon first came to public attention following the Korean War. Autopsies of men in their late teens and early twenties killed in battle revealed a marked narrowing of the arteries. These young men had a buildup of cholesterol-related plaque usually associated with adults in their late forties, fifties, and sixties, the age group targeted as at risk of heart attack.

It has become apparent that the children in many American families are in the very early stages of what might escalate into heart disease. A study of school-age children conducted in the early 1990s showed many with dangerously high levels of cholesterol in their blood. This was the first scientifically documented indication of the diet-related harm many American children are suffering. The problem appears to be so widespread and serious that many authorities are recommending that children be routinely tested for blood serum cholesterol levels.

Cholesterol is a primary building block for Vitamin D and for hormones from the adrenal gland and reproductive organs. It is actually a necessary nutrient. It is present in the blood, brain, liver, kidneys, adrenal glands, and the covering surrounding nerve fibers. If you don't eat any foods containing cholesterol, your liver will make it. Cholesterol becomes a problem, however, when there is too much of it in the body, which is likely to happen when a person's diet contains excessive amounts of cholesterol and fat.

The United States government, the American Heart Association, and the American Cancer Society all recommend a reduction in the total amount of fat consumed, cholesterol-containing foods included. And just because a product label says "no cholesterol," you cannot automatically assume the product is good for you; the fat content may still be detrimental to your health. In fact, highly saturated tropical oils, such as palm oil, may actually have a *worse* effect on cholesterol levels than foods that contain cholesterol.

It is recommended that only 20 to 30 percent of our total daily calories come from fat. Since each gram of fat yields approximately 9 calories of energy, to find the number of calories that come from fat in a particular food, simply multiply the number of grams of fat it contains by 9. For example, two tablespoons of peanut butter contain approximately 15 grams of fat and 200 calories. Multiply the number of fat grams (15) by 9, and you find that the number of calories from fat is 135. This means that 135 of the 200 calories the peanut butter contains are due to fat. Do this arithmetic with all of the foods in your child's diet to determine the total number of fat calories he consumes. Then figure out what percentage of his total calories that number equals. If you find it comes to 30 percent or more, you need to cut down on fat in the diet.

Dietary cholesterol is present only in animal foods such as meats, eggs, and dairy products. Plants contain no cholesterol. Food products derived from plants, such as vegetable or seed oils, peanut butter, almond butter, or tahini, contain no cholesterol. Decreasing consumption of foods high in cholesterol and fat will improve your family's long-term health and vitality.

Food Safety and the FDA

In the early 1900s, Dr. Harvey W. Wiley tested some commonly used early chemical preservatives, including deadly formaldehyde, and demonstrated their toxicity. The Federal Pure Food and Drug Act, pioneered by Dr. Wiley, became law in 1906, creating the first real protection for the commercial food consumer. In 1928, Congress authorized the creation of the Federal Food, Drug, and Insecticide Administration. Three years later the organization's name was changed to the Food and Drug Administration (FDA), as we know it today.

In 1958, the Federal Food, Drugs, and Cosmetics Act was passed. The Food Additives Amendment to this law required food and chemical manufacturers to demonstrate the safety of their products by running extensive tests on additives before they were marketed. Test results had to be submitted to the FDA, which made rulings on particular substances based on the data supplied by the manufacturers. This marked a significant change; previously, the agency had not been permitted to ban the use of a food additive on the grounds that it had been inadequately tested, or even because it was suspected of being unsafe for human consumption. In addition, the Delaney clause, written by Representative James Delaney, was part of the 1958 law. This clause specifically prohibits the use of any food additive that has been shown to cause cancer.

These developments would seem to justify consumer confidence in the safety of the foods we buy. However, since it was enacted, the Delaney clause has been repeatedly attacked and circumvented. Consider the case of saccharin, an artificial chemical sweetener in use since 1879. In 1977, researchers demonstrated that saccharin caused cancer in laboratory animals. The FDA responded by announcing a ban on the use of the substance in foods and beverages. In the six months following the FDA announcement, industry lobbyists such as the Calorie Control Council spent over $1 million fighting the ban. As a result of their efforts, people from all over the country bombarded their congressional representatives with requests to keep saccharin on the market.

In response to this overwhelming pressure, and despite the research implicating saccharin as carcinogenic, the FDA has continually postponed imposing its ban on this substance. And even though saccharin has now largely been superseded by the proliferation of aspartame, another questionable artificial sweetener (it is suspected of causing nervous system problems, including migraine headaches and seizures, may break down into toxic compounds when heated, and is potentially disastrous for children with PKU, a relatively common genetic disorder), saccharin is still around today, thirteen years after it was identified as carcinogenic. And the American Medical Association recently published a medical encyclopedia that identifies saccharin only as a "sugar substitute." The book gives no mention of its cancer-causing potential.

additives than basic food ingredients. Always read the labels! Trying to find additive-free products can be an exercise in frustration. Preparing fresh, whole foods is a good beginning and a way to avoid the frustration. Even so, farmers often use pesticides and chemicals in their fields that contaminate even what look like healthy fresh foods. Since the 1940s, the use of chemicals by the food growers of America has increased tenfold. In the last twenty years alone, the number of pesticides, herbicides, insecticides, fungicides, rodenticides, chemical fertilizers, and soil conditioners has doubled. These toxic chemicals do not disperse and decay harmlessly. They contaminate the food we eat, pollute the air we breathe, and seep into the water we drink. And these chemicals are all pervasive, often mysteriously traveling far from the areas where they were actually used.

DDT (dichlorodiphenyltrichloroethane) is a case in point. It was banned in 1972, yet nearly every American still carries traces of DDT in his or her body. DDT has even been detected in wild animals roaming free in the Antarctic, a place once thought free of man-made chemical contamination.

Each year more than 2.5 billion pounds of chemicals are sprayed or dumped on agricultural crops, spread in forests, and used to treat ponds and lakes or "green" lawns and parks. In the mid-1980s, farmers, pest-control companies, and homeowners spent over $6.5 billion on chemicals.

A 1987 study released by the National Cancer Institute showed that children living in homes where pesticides are routinely used are seven times more likely to develop childhood leukemia than are children who live in chemical-free households. In 1989, the Natural Resources Defense Council (NRDC) reported on a comprehensive two-year study of the impact on children of pesticide residues in food. It showed that, compared to adults, the average child receives four times more exposure to eight cancer-causing pesticides in food. Apples, apple products, peanut butter, and processed cherries that have been treated with the chemical growth regulator daminozide (better known as Alar) were named as foods posing the greatest potential risk to children. The average exposure of a child under six to daminozide and to UMDH, the carcinogenic compound it forms in the body, is 240 times the cancer risk that the Environmental Protection Agency (EPA) calls "acceptable" after a lifetime of exposure to this toxic chemical.

The study determined that children consume proportionally more fruits and vegetables—and thus more pesticides—than adults. Fruits are especially susceptible to pesticide contamination. On average, produce accounts for about one-third of a child's diet, with fruits predominating. The average preschool child consumes six times more fruit and fruit products, and drinks eighteen times more apple juice, than his parents do. During infancy, the average baby consumes thirty-one times more apple juice than adults in the household.

The NRDC study targeted only eight widely used chemicals. But you should be aware that the EPA has identified *sixty-six* different carcinogenic pesticides that turn up in the average child's diet. To date, the EPA has not acted to restrict the use of these chemicals.

Only about 1 percent of the produce, domestic or imported, in your supermarket has been tested for pesticide residues, and tests currently used can detect only around 40 percent of the possible chemical contaminants. Many dangerous metabolites (chemical compounds that form as the source chemicals break down in the body) cannot be detected at all.

The General Accounting Office (GAO) reports that it takes the FDA close to a month, on average, to complete a laboratory analysis of a food sample. During that time, a suspect food stays on the market. In more than 50 percent of the instances where the FDA has found violations, the GAO says, the contaminated food was not recovered. By the time the FDA had completed lab testing, unsuspecting families had eaten the "evidence."

CHOOSING FOOD AND WATER FOR YOUR CHILD

As a parent, you have an important and powerful influence on your child's eating habits. Children will learn to eat what a parent eats and serves. Children will eat what you stock in the refrigerator and cupboards. Children will learn to eat the way their parents do, whether that is slowly or quickly, to satisfy hunger or to ease or avoid feelings, at mealtimes or while sitting in front of

the television. We need to be conscious of what we are passing on to our children.

Following are some guidelines to help you provide a healthy, balanced, nutrient-rich diet for your child (and for yourself!).

Whenever possible, buy organically grown produce and grains. Buy meat from animals raised without hormones or antibiotics. Buying organically grown foods is the one way to avoid the danger of pesticides and chemical fertilizers. Organic foods are grown without the use of synthetic chemicals. They are absolutely the healthiest choice for our children, our families, and the earth and air.

Contaminants in the air, food, and drinking water of the nation are a major concern. By testing rainwater samples from twenty-three states, a recent study by the U.S. Geological Survey found that agricultural chemicals end up in the atmosphere. Along with eliminating the pesticide residues that linger on commercially farmed foods, organic farming spares the earth from these unnecessary and destructive toxins. If you have difficulty finding a source of organic foods, ask your local grocery to carry certified organic produce and grains. Certified organic farms are periodically inspected by state agencies (at present, there is no federal law or organization that oversees organic farming practices). The California law has set the standard for regulating and certifying organic farming methods. It states that in order for a farm to be certified organic, the ground must have been worked without the use of chemical sprays or fertilizers for at least four years. The soil of a farm is tested each year to determine compliance. You may also see produce marked as coming from transitional farms, meaning that the farm has not yet made the four-year mark, but is in the process of transition into farming without sprays or fertilizers.

If you cannot buy organic fruits, vegetables, and grains, wash everything thoroughly. Use a mixture of warm water and vinegar (¼ cup of vinegar for each gallon of water); vinegar accelerates the breakdown of some pesticides. When serving vegetables like cabbage and lettuce, always remove the outer leaves, which often contain many times more chemical residue than the inner leaves do. Root vegetables (carrots, potatoes, turnips, etc.) should be scrubbed and peeled. Any fruit or vegetable that has been waxed (this is often done to apples, cucumbers, eggplants, peppers, tomatoes, and citrus fruits to make them look shinier and more attractive) should be peeled as well. Even with these precautions, however, you should be aware that there will probably be some residue in the foods you eat. Some chemicals can be washed away and some cannot. Some chemicals can be peeled away, some cannot.

Offer a diet of 50 to 65 percent complex carbohydrates, 15 to 25 percent proteins, and 20 to 25 percent fats. Complex carbohydrates include whole grains (wheat, rye, barley, rice, oats, millet), vegetables, legumes (dried beans, peas), and whole fruits. The sugars found in complex carbohydrates are more gradually absorbed into the bloodstream than those from processed refined sugars. A diet rich in complex carbohydrates will help the whole family feel more alert and energetic during the day.

Complete proteins are found in milk, cheese, eggs, meat, fish, poultry, nuts, and most legumes. Combining grains and vegetables will also provide a complete protein. Proteins are essential for the growth and repair of all body tissues, including organs, muscles, bone, skin, blood, and nerves. Each cell in the body requires protein.

Fats are essential for metabolizing fat-soluble vitamins (A, D, E, and K), for normal growth and development, and for maintaining healthy skin, hair, and nails. Fats regulate digestion, influence blood pressure, and are needed for the production of prostaglandins, chemical "messengers" that are present throughout the body. It is important to remember, however, that all fats are not created equal. We recommend using unrefined, minimally processed, cold-pressed organic oils. Use flaxseed, linseed, pumpkinseed, soybean, and walnut oils in order to get important essential fatty acids. Safflower, sunflower, canola, and olive oils are also acceptable sources of fat. Polyunsaturated oils should be kept refrigerated after opening. Try to avoid animal fats and the so-called tropical oils (including palm oil and coconut oil), and steer clear of any and all products containing hydrogenated and partially hydrogenated oils. Margarine and solid shortenings are manufactured with partially hydrogenated oils (see The Hydrogenation Process, page 45). In fact, even though animal fats are not generally recommended, a small amount of butter is healthier for your child than any amount of margarine.

Offer a variety of foods. Along with the fun of trying new and different foods, variety ensures that your child will get the full range of nutrients his growing body needs. Next time you shop, buy something new. Include a vegetable and grain with each lunch and dinner.

Prepare foods simply. Foods that are steamed, baked, or broiled are easily digested. Use water, lemon juice, broths, flavorful herbs, and fruit juices to steam, bake, or broil. Avoid frying foods. Fried foods are more difficult to digest, heated oils and fats turn rancid quickly, and oils and fats add calories.

Give your child three meals a day, with wholesome snacks as necessary (see page 46). To supply the fuel your child

needs, make breakfast and lunch the larger meals; offer lighter foods at dinner to support your child's body as he slows down and prepares to rest for the night. Allow at least two hours between dinner and bedtime. Sleeping on an overly full stomach can cause restless sleep and a groggy feeling in the morning.

Reduce or eliminate refined sugars. The sugar issue may be the greatest dietary challenge a parent faces. Food advertising targeted at children often promotes products that are laden with refined sugars—breakfast cereals, candy, and cookies, among others. Even foods that don't seem like sweets, such as peanut butter, often contain sugar. Refined sugars, including glucose, fructose, and sucrose, are simple, fast-acting sugars. They cause a rapid rise in blood sugar, followed by a rapid drop. Children may react to these changes in blood sugar with hyperactive, excitable behavior and an inability to concentrate, followed by tiredness and irritability. And we all know the association of sugar with tooth decay and obesity.

There are alternatives to refined sugar. Honey, rice syrup, molasses, barley malt, and maple syrup are fair substitutes. But these too should be used sparingly, as in excess they add little to the diet except calories.

Processed foods can contain a surprisingly large amount of sugar. Thus, decreasing consumption of processed foods can significantly decrease refined sugar consumption. It is important to read food labels carefully so you know exactly what you are feeding your child.

If you can't eliminate sugar entirely, limit it to early in the day. When your child eats sugary sweets before bed, he may have difficulty settling down for sleep and may wake up groggy and tired the next morning.

Give your child lots of clean water. The only way to be absolutely certain the water your family drinks is safe is to buy clean and pure spring water from a reputable source. If you opt for purified bottled water or a water filter in your house, choose a water purification system that uses reverse osmosis. In reverse osmosis, water passes through a semipermeable membrane. The tiny water molecules pass through the membrane easily. The molecules of many pollutants, chemicals, and heavy metals (such as lead, chlorine, and fluoride), as well as bacteria and viruses, are all too large to pass through the special membrane. The undesirables are caught and flushed away.

BASIC NUTRIENTS YOUR CHILD NEEDS

The four basic building blocks of your child's diet are water, complex carbohydrates, proteins, and fats. A proper balance of these essentials is necessary for optimum health. The table on page 48 provides a brief introduction to your child's fundamental dietary requirements, as well as a guide to the functions and food sources of these four dietary elements. A diet based on a wide variety of simply prepared whole foods is most likely to meet your child's basic nutritional needs.

Parents who raise their children as vegetarians must take special care not only to provide adequate protein for healthy growth, but also to teach their children about a nutrient-rich and protein-adequate diet. Many plant foods do not contain the full spectrum of eight amino acids that make up a complete protein. At one time it was thought that to provide a complete protein, certain foods—such as rice and beans—had to be combined and eaten at the same time. Now we know that a diet based on a variety of vegetables, legumes, and grains will provide adequate protein for a child. However, it is important that vegetarian children eat a varied, balanced diet in order to get the full spectrum of amino acids, and therefore complete protein.

Also necessary for good health are nutrients that together are classified as *micronutrients*, which include vitamins and minerals.

Vitamins

Vitamins are essential to normal body function. They are not a form of energy or fuel, as foods are. But they play an indispensable role in the normal metabolism, growth, and development of your child's body.

Vitamins are classified as either water-soluble or fat-soluble, depending upon which type of molecule (fat- or water-based) transports them in the bloodstream. Water-soluble vitamins include all of the B complex and vitamin C. These vitamins are quickly used by the body or excreted in urine, so they must be replenished daily. Water-soluble vitamins may leach out of foods during cooking, be damaged by overprocessing, or be destroyed when foods are overcooked.

The fat-soluble vitamins—A, D, E, and K—are fairly stable during low-temperature cooking. However, antibiotics, mineral oil, and certain drugs (steroids, for example) interfere with their absorption from the digestive tract. Frying foods alters the fat-soluble vitamins in them as well.

For a review of the vitamins your child needs every day, as well as their respective functions and food sources, see the table on page 50.

Minerals

Minerals are part of all body tissues and fluids. They are essential in nerve responses, muscle contractions, maintaining proper fluid balance, and the internal processing of nutrients. Minerals influence the manufacture of hormones and regulate electrolyte balance throughout the body. The term *electrolyte* refers to the form in which various minerals circulate in the body. Calcium, potassium, and sodium are examples of important electrolytes. Calcium, for example, is not only an important constituent of bones and teeth; it is also involved in the

The Hydrogenation Process

Hydrogenated and partially hydrogenated fats are vegetable or seed oils that have been subjected to elaborate processing. Hydrogenating an oil means saturating its carbon molecules with hydrogen. This is accomplished under tremendous pressure at temperatures of up to 410°F in the presence of a metal catalyst (nickel, platinum, copper) for as long as eight hours.

A liquid oil can be transformed into a solid or semisolid fat by adjusting the length of the hydrogenation process. When the desired degree of hardness is attained, the process is stopped. Margarines, "soft" margarines, and solid shortenings are manufactured with partially hydrogenated oils.

Hydrogenation destroys the nutritional value of the oil. A hydrogenated product doesn't spoil, because it is a completely inert (dead) substance. It can be heated for cooking without decomposing. However, it contains chemically altered metabolites—some of which may be harmful—plus traces of the metal catalyst.

Even though logic might suggest otherwise, partially hydrogenated products are in some ways worse than completely hydrogenated products. The molecules in oil being bombarded with hydrogen become saturated (hydrogenated) erratically, and when the process is stopped a proliferation of strangely altered molecules called "trans" fatty acids are left behind. Many of these chemically altered elements are harmful because they interfere with the body's normal metabolism. Others have not been scientifically researched. There is little documentation showing how they affect the body once ingested.

Healthy Snack Ideas

Midmorning and midafternoon are likely snacktimes—times your child will need refueling in order to continue being attentive in school or active on the playing field. In keeping with your wholesome meal offerings, prepare snacks that are nutritious and based on grains, fruits, vegetables, and small amounts of protein. Avoid highly refined, sugar-laden foods that don't provide necessary nutrients.

The following are some ideas for healthful snacks to offer your child:

- Almond butter and celery
- Vegetables and onion dip
- Jicama and peanut butter or almond butter
- Tofu or chicken dogs with beans, wrapped in a whole-wheat or corn tortilla
- Rice pudding
- Rice cakes with sesame-seed butter
- Rice cakes with peanut or almond butter and fruit-sweetened jelly
- Low-fat or nonfat granola and skim or low-fat milk
- Millet or rice toast and fruit-sweetened jelly
- Low-fat cheese (made from skim milk or soy-based) and crackers
- Low-fat cream cheese and celery with raisins on top
- Nonfat plain yogurt with fresh fruit and nuts
- Baked apples
- Carrot sticks
- Fruit sticks or fruit kabobs
- Corn on the cob
- Mini-pizzas (whole-wheat English muffin topped with tomato sauce, vegetables, and part-skim mozzarella cheese)
- Cookies made with honey, maple syrup, or barley malt
- Smoothies (plain yogurt, fruit, and a dab of honey mixed in a blender) or fruit freezes (fruit, ice, and a dab of honey mixed in a blender)
- Homemade applesauce
- Almond butter on a whole-wheat tortilla
- Hummus and crackers

transmission of nerve impulses, the transmission of energy from cell to cell, and the contraction and relaxation of muscles, including the heart. Calcium, potassium, and magnesium together control the continuous cycle of contraction and relaxation of the heart muscle and blood vessels. If these electrolytes are out of balance, resulting fluid shifts may cause swelling or dehydration, the neuromuscular system may become irritable, or an irregular heart rhythm may develop.

Minerals are excreted daily and must be replaced either through the diet or in supplement form. Of all the vitamins and minerals, calcium and iron are probably the most important for children, and may be valuable to take as supplements. For a quick review of the minerals your child needs every day, as well as their functions and food sources, see the table on page 52.

Diet and nutrition comprise a huge subject that deserves your time and attention. Read more, experiment with new and different foods, use cookbooks devoted to whole-foods cooking, and ask lots of questions. The more you understand about food and nutrition, the more committed you will be to providing a healthy, wholesome diet for your child.

WORKING WITH A NUTRITIONAL COUNSELOR

There are many different kinds of professionals, with varied educational backgrounds and philosophies, who can recommend dietary programs and nutritional supplements. Registered dietitians, nutritionists, naturopathic physicians, chiropractors, medical doctors, and nurses—to name only a few—may all practice nutritional medicine. When interviewing a nutritional counselor, whether the person is a medical doctor or macrobiotic counselor, find out about his or her educational background, work experience, and nutritional philosophy.

Nutrition is a broad and constantly changing field. Providing a healthy, well-balanced, allergen-free diet, along with nutritional supplements when needed, may be the most important thing you can do to support your child's health. You may need assistance planning the optimum diet. Choose a counselor you feel you can work with, a person who believes in the fundamental importance of a healthy diet. As with any health care practitioner, choose a person who knows the current research, who is compassionate, and who will work with you as a partner to create the healthiest, most manageable plan possible.

NUTRITIONAL SUPPLEMENTS

Unless a child or teenager has a chronic illness or is unable to eat a varied, healthy diet, he is unlikely to need nutritional supplements on a daily basis. If you are unable to provide a nutritionally complete diet of wholesome, organic foods for your child, you may want to talk to your physician about supplementing your child's diet with a good multivitamin and mineral formula.

Nutritional supplements can be helpful in supporting your child's body during illness. For example, in many of the entries in Part Two we suggest boosting your child's infection-fighting capability with three specific vitamins. Vitamin C is a well-documented anti-inflammatory that eases the common cold. Bioflavonoids help fight infection, reduce inflammation, and decrease allergic reactions. Beta-carotene, which the body uses to manufacture vitamin A, helps mucous membranes to heal.

In addition to vitamins and minerals, a number of different food supplements are often recommended, including lactobacilli (*Lactobacillus acidophilus or bifidus*) and chlorophyll. When your child is taking a prescribed course of antibiotics, supplementing his diet with yogurt is helpful, and taking lactobacilli for at least ten days after the treatment is very important. Antibiotics are indiscriminate in their choice of targets. They destroy the necessary "friendly" bacteria in the gastrointestinal tract right along with the harmful bacteria they are designed to eliminate. *Lactobacillus acidophilus* and *bifidus* restore healthy flora to the intestines and bowel. Chlorophyll, the green pigment found in plant tissue, is a natural deodorizer and contains many useful trace nutrients, especially magnesium. It is helpful when treating ailments as varied as bad breath, canker sores, chronic constipation, impetigo, menstrual cramps, vaginitis, and mononucleosis, as well as in rebuilding blood after a major bleed or in rebuilding bone tissue after a break.

The Danger of Lead

Close to fifty cancer-causing chemicals and other substances, including lead, have been detected in the ground water of twenty-six states. According to the United States Senate Environment and Public Works Subcommittee on Toxic Substances, as many as 3 million American children may be exposed to excessive levels of lead.

Children are particularly susceptible to lead poisoning. A pregnant woman who has consumed excessive lead will likely give birth to a premature, underweight infant. Babies exposed to excessive lead can suffer delayed physical and mental development, even retardation. Older children can suffer impaired mental faculties, retardation, kidney damage, anemia, and hearing loss. Even a minute concentration of lead absorbed by the body can cause serious health problems.

The Senate Subcommittee's study identified drinking water contaminated by lead from antiquated lead pipes as the source of 20 percent of lead-related health problems in the United States. The Environmental Protection Agency estimates that as many as 30 million people who are served by municipal water systems may be affected. New EPA guidelines reduce the current allowable standard of 50 parts of lead per billion parts of water to 15 parts per billion coming through the tap. However, cities have until the year 2014 to comply.

To guard against lead in your drinking water, buy pure bottled water or install a good filter system. At the very least, you should let your tap run for two full minutes before using the water for drinking or cooking. Keep your child away from other potential sources of lead exposure as well, including peeling or chipping paint, pottery that may not have been glazed properly, broken plaster board, colored newsprint, and lead soldering.

Lead crystal is another source of concern. Lead from lead-crystal containers will leach into any liquid they hold. The FDA recently cautioned against storing food or beverages, especially acidic ones like orange, grapefruit, or cranberry juice, and any alcoholic beverages, in lead crystal. Pregnant women in particular must not consume food or beverages that have been kept in lead crystal. Ingested lead may injure the developing fetus. If your baby was given a lead-crystal baby bottle, use it for decorative purposes only. Because lead from crystal will migrate into an infant's formula, Waterford has now discontinued the manufacture of these once-treasured baby bottles.

GIVING NUTRITIONAL SUPPLEMENTS TO YOUR CHILD

Vitamin and mineral supplements are either isolated from food sources or manufactured synthetically. Synthetic and natural vitamins and minerals have identical chemical structures and supposedly do the same work within the body, although there is some controversy over which are more effectively absorbed and used.

Whether you select a natural or synthetic formula, be aware that the contents of any supplement have to be altered in some way to put them into pill, powder, or capsule form. A nutritious, varied diet remains the best source of both vitamins and minerals.

Many vitamin and mineral formulas designed to appeal to children contain refined sugars or artificial sweeteners, such as sucrose, mannose, xylitol, and aspartame (NutraSweet). Some health care practitioners

question whether artificial sweeteners are carcinogenic. To be safe, select a formula that does not include them. A health food store will likely carry a child-pleasing vitamin and mineral formula sweetened with honey or rice syrup. Such a formula is a better choice.

To avoid upsetting your child's stomach, it's best to give vitamins and minerals with food. Minerals are best administered at the beginning of a meal. Vitamins are best administered at the end of the meal, when your child's stomach is full. If you are giving a combination vitamin and mineral supplement, give it to your child after a meal.

Age-appropriate therapeutic dosages of nutritional supplements may be found in the beginning of Part Two. When treating your child with nutritional supplements, you should be aware that if a formula appears to be helping support your child's body, it does

BASIC NUTRIENTS

Nutrient	Function	Requirements
WATER/FLUIDS		
The body is two-thirds water by weight. Water is a primary need and essential nutrient.	Water is involved in every bodily function. It transports nutrients in and out of cells, removes toxins, and is necessary for all digestive, absorption, circulatory, and excretory functions. Water is necessary for the utilization of water-soluble B-complex and C vitamins, and for maintaining proper body temperature.	Infants: $\frac{1}{2}$–$1\frac{3}{4}$ ounces per hour or 11–43 ounces in 24 hours (requirements increase with a baby's age and body weight). School-age children: 2–$2\frac{1}{2}$ ounces per hour or 48–60 ounces in 24 hours. Adolescents: 3–$3\frac{3}{4}$ ounces per hour or 73–90 ounces in 24 hours.
COMPLEX CARBOHYDRATES		
Complex carbohydrates contain many vitamins, plus healthy fiber.	Complex carbohydrates provide the body with energy. They are needed for digestion and assimilation of food.	50 to 65 percent of total calories.
PROTEINS		
Proteins are comprised of amino acids, 22 of which are essential for normal development. The body can make 14 of them; the other 8 must be obtained in the diet.	Protein is essential for growth and development. It provides the body with energy and heat, and is needed for the manufacture of hormones, antibodies, and enzymes. It also maintains the acid/alkali balance.	15 to 25 percent of total calories.
FATTY ACIDS		
The body does require fat, but it must be the right kind. The typical American diet is top-heavy in fats but deficient in the essential fatty acids required for normal function.	Fatty acids carry fat-soluble A, D, E, and K vitamins. The essential fatty acids (EFAs) are linoleic, linolenic, and arachidonic. They help manage cholesterol, regulate body temperature, and help control blood pressure. EFAs are essential for growth and development and healthy skin, hair, and nails.	Infants: 40–50 percent of total calories (nearly half the calories in breast milk come from monounsaturated fats). Children: 20–25 percent of total calories.

not follow that "more is better." A toxic overdose of a vitamin or mineral is rare, but it can occur, especially with products containing iron. Although a reaction to an age-specific dose of a vitamin and mineral supplement is likewise rare in childhood, be responsible and careful in administering them. If your child should develop an upset stomach or any adverse reaction, decrease the dosage or stop giving him the supplement.

Follow the storage instructions on product labels. In general, you should store vitamin and mineral supplements away from heat, tightly capped, and out of reach of your child. Keep vitamins A and E in the refrigerator. These two vitamins are usually oil-based and will keep longer in a cool environment. Check expiration dates on formulas. A vitamin or mineral formula that has passed its expiration date will not have full potency.

Paying attention to diet and nutrition is perhaps the single most important supportive measure you can offer your family's health. A good diet will optimize health, just as a poor diet will chip away at your overall health and well-being. A healthy, nutritious diet based on whole grains, fresh fruits and vegetables, legumes, and moderate amounts of clean, lean protein will increase energy, strength, and vitality—and will help your child's body to resist illness. Bring home food from the produce section; limit your use of prepared foods that come in boxes, cans, or frozen packages. Discover if there are organic farmers in your area and support them, or ask your grocer to stock organic produce (or, if you can, grow your own!). Take the time to learn about preparing foods that are life enhancing—abundant in essential vitamins, minerals, and trace elements.

Signs of Deficiency	Food Sources
Pale yellow urine shows a healthy state of hydration. Dark or scanty urine, thirst, and dry mouth are early signs of dehydration. Rapid loss of body fluids as a result of fever, diarrhea, or vomiting is of particular concern in babies and children. Severe dehydration can cause serious health problems. If you cannot keep your child well hydrated, hospitalization may be necessary.	Best: Pure and clean spring water; breast milk for babies. Next best: Purified bottled water. Good: Herbal teas, diluted fruit juices, soups, homemade juice popsicles. Avoid: Beverages containing caffeine, soda, cola, prepackaged punches, and colored drinks. Packaged gelatin products are not recommended.
Lack of energy; exhaustion; mineral imbalances; breakdown of proteins in tissues.	Whole grains; vegetables; legumes (dried beans, peas); fruits.
Stunted growth; diarrhea; vomiting; lack of appetite; edema (buildup of fluids in tissues).	Complete protein: Milk, eggs, cheese, fish, meat, poultry. Good protein: Whole grains, nuts, beans, peas.
Retarded growth; skin, hair, and nail disorders; impaired metabolism of fats and fat-soluble vitamins. Infant eczema is often associated with EFA deficiency.	Best: Cold-expeller-pressed safflower, sunflower, canola, olive, flax, pumpkin, walnut oils. Acceptable: Butter. In moderation only: Saturated fats found in animal products such as meat and dairy products, tropical oils such as palm and coconut oil. Not recommended: Margarine, hydrogenated or partially hydrogenated oils or products containing them.

VITAMINS

Vitamin	Function	Recommended Daily Intake	Signs of Deficiency	Food Sources
FAT-SOLUBLE VITAMINS				
Vitamin A (Beta-carotene)	Strengthens mucous membranes, the immune system, adrenal glands, and eyes.	Birth–1 Year: 375 mcg (125 IU) 1–3 Years: 400 mcg (133 IU) 4–6 Years: 500 mcg (166 IU) 7–10 Years: 700 mcg (233 IU) 11 Years–Adult: Females, 800 mcg (266 IU); Males, 1,000 mcg (333 IU)	Night blindness; eye problems; increased susceptibility to infection; impaired growth.	Fish liver oil; dark green leafy vegetables; yellow fruits and vegetables; vitamin A-fortified milk; butter; egg yolks.
Vitamin D	Supports bone and tooth formation and muscle function. Necessary for proper absorption of calcium, phosphorus, magnesium, and zinc. Supports the healthy functioning of the thyroid gland.	Birth–6 Months: 7.5 mcg (300 IU) 6 Months–18 Years: 10 mcg (400 IU)	Bone and tooth problems.	Fish liver oil; fortified milk; salmon; herring; sardines; butter; eggs. Sunshine is the best source.
Vitamin E	Aids in tissue healing. Essential for normal cell structure. Helps maintain normal enzyme function; involved in the formation of red blood cells. Believed to slow the aging of cells. Helps protect tissues from damage by pollutants.	Birth–1 Year: 3–4 mg (3–4 IU) 1–3 Years: 6 mg (6 IU) 4–10 Years: 7 mg (7 IU) 11 Years–Adult: Females, 8 mg (8 IU); Males, 10 mg (10 IU)	Dry skin.	Wheat germ oil; wheat germ; egg yolks; butter; most vegetable oils; liver; nuts; whole wheat flour; green leafy vegetables.
Vitamin K	Essential for blood clotting. Necessary for bone formation.	Birth–1 Year: 5–10 mcg 1–3 Years: 15 mcg 4–6 Years: 20 mcg 7–10 Years: 30 mcg 11–14 Years: 45 mcg 15–18 Years: Females, 55 mcg; Males, 65 mcg	Blood clotting difficulty.	Liver; dark green leafy vegetables; vegetable oils.
WATER-SOLUBLE VITAMINS				
Vitamin B₁ (Thiamine)	Supports healthy functioning of the heart, muscles, and nerves. Plays a role in the breakdown of carbohydrates. Helps maintain normal enzyme function.	Birth–1 Year: 0.3–0.4 mg 1–3 Years: 0.7 mg 4–6 Years: 0.9 mg 7–10 Years: 1.0 mg 11–14 Years: Females, 1.1 mg; Males, 1.3 mg 15–18 Years: Females, 1.1 mg; Males 1.5 mg	Fatigue; memory loss; irritability; depression.	Brewer's yeast; kidney; liver; wheat germ; peas; peanuts; whole grains; nuts; rice bran; brown rice.
Vitamin B₂ (Riboflavin)	Plays a role in the breakdown and use of carbohydrates, fats, and proteins; involved in cell energy production; supports the production of adrenal hormones; helps the body utilize other vitamins; supports the eyes.	Birth–1 Year: 0.4–0.5 mg 1–3 Years: 0.8 mg 4–6 Years: 1.1 mg 7–10 Years: 1.2 mg 11–14 Years: Females, 1.3 mg; Males, 1.5 mg 15–18 Years: Females, 1.3 mg; Males, 1.8 mg	Light-sensitivity; reddening of the eyes; dry skin; depression; cracks at the corners of the mouth.	Brewer's yeast; kidney; liver; heart; milk; broccoli; Brussels sprouts; asparagus; green leafy vegetables; wheat germ; almonds; cottage cheese; yogurt; eggs; tuna; salmon.

Vitamin	Function	Recommended Daily Intake	Signs of Deficiency	Food Sources
WATER-SOLUBLE VITAMINS (continued)				
Vitamin B$_3$ (Niacin)	Involved in the breakdown of carbohydrates and fats, healthy functioning of the nervous and digestive systems, and the production of sex hormones; helps maintain healthy skin.	Birth–1 Year: 5–6 mg 1–3 Years: 9 mg 4–6 Years: 12 mg 7–10 Years: 13 mg 11–14 Years: Females, 15 mg; Males, 17 mg 15–18 Years: Females, 15 mg; Males, 20 mg	Fatigue; irritability; insomnia; emotional instability; blood sugar fluctuations; arthritis.	Brewer's yeast; liver; poultry; fish; peanuts; eggs; milk; whole grains.
Vitamin B$_5$ (Pantothenic Acid)	Involved in the breakdown and use of carbohydrates and fats; supports normal growth and development; involved in production of adrenal and sex hormones; helps the body use other vitamins; supports sinuses.	Birth–1 Year: 2–3 mg 1–3 Years: 3 mg 4–6 Years: 3–4 mg 7–10 Years: 4–5 mg 11 Years–Adult: 4–7 mg	None known for vitamin B$_5$ alone, but deficiency of any B vitamin usually means deficiency of others.	Liver; kidney; heart; fish; egg yolks; cheese; bran; whole-grain cereals; cauliflower; sweet potatoes; beans; nuts; brewer's yeast.
Vitamin B$_6$ (Pyridoxine)	Involved in the breakdown of proteins, carbohydrates, and fats; involved in healthy functioning of the nervous and digestive systems; involved in the production of red blood cells and antibodies; helps maintain healthy skin.	Birth–1 Year: 0.3–0.6 mg 1–3 Years: 1.0 mg 4–6 Years: 1.1 mg 7–10 Years: 1.4 mg 11–14 Years: Females, 1.4 mg; Males, 1.7 mg 15–18 Years: Females, 1.5 mg; Males, 2.0 mg	Premenstrual tension; irritability; depression.	Soybeans; liver; kidney; poultry; tuna; fish; bananas; legumes; potatoes; oatmeal; wheat germ.
Vitamin B$_{12}$ (Cobalamin)	Involved in growth and development; involved in production of red blood cells; helps the body use folic acid; supports healthy functioning of the nervous system.	Birth–1 Year: 0.3–0.5 mcg 1–3 Years: 0.7 mcg 4–6 Years: 1.0 mcg 7–10 Years: 1.4 mcg 11 Years–Adult: 2.0 mcg	Megaloblastic anemia; irritability; loss of coordination.	Liver; oysters; poultry; fish; clams; eggs; dairy products.
Biotin	Involved in metabolism of fatty acids, carbohydrates, and protein; involved in maintaining health of skin, hair, sweat glands, nerves, and bone marrow.	Birth–1 Year: 10–15 mcg 1–3 Years: 20 mcg 4–6 Years: 25 mcg 7–10 Years: 30 mcg 11 Years–Adult: 30–100 mcg	High cholesterol; skin problems; muscle cramps.	Liver; kidney; egg yolks; milk; yeast; whole grains; cauliflower; nuts; legumes.
Folic Acid	Involved in growth, development, and reproduction; involved in production of red blood cells; supports healthy functioning of the nervous system; supports hair and skin.	Birth–1 Year: 25–35 mcg 1–3 Years: 50 mcg 4–6 Years: 75 mcg 7–10 Years: 100 mcg 11–14 Years: 150 mcg 15–18 Years: Females, 180 mcg; Males, 200 mcg	Anemia; digestive problems; fatigue.	Liver; salmon; eggs; asparagus; green leafy vegetables; broccoli; sweet potatoes; beans; whole wheat.
Vitamin C	Helps maintain normal enzyme function; important for healthy growth of teeth, bones, gums, ligaments, and blood vessels; involved in production of neurotransmitters and adrenal gland hormones; plays an important role in immune response to infection and in supporting wound healing; helps in absorption of iron from the digestive tract.	Birth–1 Year: 30–35 mg 1–3 Years: 40 mg 4–10 Years: 45 mg 11–14 Years: 50 mg 15–18 Years: 60 mg	Slow wound healing; bleeding gums; recurrent infections; allergies.	Rose hips; sweet peppers; broccoli; cauliflower; kale; asparagus; spinach; tomatoes; lemons; strawberries; papayas; cantaloupe; oranges; grapefruit; kiwis; liver.

MINERALS

Mineral	Function	Recommended Daily Intake	Signs of Deficiency	Food Sources
BULK MINERALS				
Calcium	Plays a role in bone and tooth formation, blood clotting, heart rhythm, nerve transmission, muscle growth and contraction, proper functioning of cell membranes.	Birth–6 Months: 400 mg 6 Months–1 Year: 600 mg 1–10 Years: 800 mg 11–18 Years: 1,000 mg	Muscle cramps; irritability; insomnia.	Collards; turnip greens; broccoli; kale; yogurt; milk and dairy products; tempeh; tofu.
Magnesium	Involved in blood sugar metabolism and energy maintenance; plays a role in metabolism of calcium and vitamin C; involved in structuring of basic genetic material (DNA and RNA).	Birth–6 Months: 40 mg 6 Months–1 Year: 60 mg 1–3 years: 80 mg 4–6 Years: 120 mg 7–10 Years: 170 mg 11–14 years: Males, 270 mg; Females, 280 mg 15–18 Years: Females, 300 mg; Males, 400 mg	Depression; muscle tension; irritability; nervousness and hyperactivity; constipation; premenstrual tension; fatigue; muscle cramps.	Soybeans; whole grains; shellfish; salmon; liver; almonds; cashews; molasses; bananas; potatoes; milk; green vegetables; honey.
Phosphorus	Involved in bone and tooth formation, cell growth and repair, energy maintenance, heart contraction, kidney function, healthy activity of nerves and muscles, the body's use of vitamins.	Birth–6 Months: 300 mg 6 Months–1 Year: 500 mg 1–10 Years: 800 mg 11–14 Years: 1,400 mg	Muscle cramps; dizziness; bone problems.	Fish; poultry; eggs; whole grains; yellow cheese.
Potassium	Involved in healthy, steady functioning of the nervous system; supports the heart, muscles, kidneys, blood.	0–5 Months: 500 mg 6–11 Months: 700 mg 1 Year: 1,000 mg 2–5 Years: 1,400 mg 6–9 Years: 1,600 mg 10–18 Years: 2,000 mg	Muscle fatigue; general fatigue; swelling in extremities; irregular heartbeat.	Dried apricots; cantaloupe; bananas; citrus fruit; lima beans; potatoes; avocados; broccoli; liver; milk; peanut butter.
Sodium	Helps maintain normal fluid levels in the body; involved in healthy muscle functioning; supports blood and lymph system.	0–5 Months: 120 mg 6–11 Months: 200 mg 1 Year: 225 mg 2–5 Years: 300 mg 6–9 Years: 400 mg 10–18 Years: 500 mg	Fainting; intolerance to heat; muscle cramps; swelling in extremities.	Most foods and water, especially salt; salted foods; soy sauce; cheese; milk; seafood.
TRACE ELEMENTS				
Chromium	Involved in maintaining blood sugar level and in healthy functioning of the circulatory system.	Birth–6 Months: 10–40 mcg 6 Months–1 Year: 20–60 mcg 1–3 Years: 20–80 mcg 4–6 Years: 30–120 mcg 7–18 Years: 50–200 mcg	Blood sugar fluctuations; high cholesterol level.	Brewer's yeast; liver; cheese; legumes; peas; whole grains; black pepper; molasses.
Cobalt	Involved in healthy functioning of red blood cells.	Cobalt is an essential trace element, but the minimum required amount is not established.	Pernicious anemia; weakness; nausea; loss of appetite; bleeding gums.	Organ meats; milk; beet greens; spinach; cabbage.

Mineral	Function	Recommended Daily Intake	Signs of Deficiency	Food Sources
TRACE ELEMENTS (continued)				
Copper	Plays a role in bone formation, hair and skin color, healing processes, red blood cell production, and mental and emotional processes.	Birth–1 Year: 0.4–0.7 mg 1–3 Years: 0.7–1.0 mg 4–6 Years: 1.0–1.5 mg 7–10 Years: 1.0–2.0 mg 11–18 Years: 1.5–2.5 mg	Anemia; inflammation; arthritis.	Shellfish; liver; poultry; cherries; nuts; cocoa; gelatin; whole grains; eggs; legumes; peas; avocados.
Iron	Supports growth and development in children; involved in the production of hemoglobin; helps build resistance to disease.	Birth–6 Months: 6 mg 6 Months–10 Years: 10 mg 11–18 Years: Males, 12 mg; Females, 15 mg	Fatigue; anemia; intolerance to cold; intellectual impairment.	Blackstrap molasses; liver; eggs; fish; spinach; asparagus; prunes; raisins; sea vegetables.
Selenium	Involved in healthy functioning of cell membranes; may be involved in increasing resistance to cancer; supports pancreatic functioning; helps the body use vitamin E effectively.	Birth–1 Year: 10–15 mcg 1–6 Years: 20 mcg 7–10 Years: 30 mcg 11–14 Years: 40–45 mcg 15–18 Years: 50 mcg	Poor growth; dry flaky scalp; skin problems; cancer.	Whole grains; soybeans; tuna; seafood; Brazil nuts; brown rice; pineapples.
Silicon	Involved in bone formation; supports skin, major blood vessels, connective tissue, and thymus gland.	Silicon is an essential trace element, but the minimum required amount is not established.	Bone deformities; connective tissue disorders; muscle cramps; irritability; insomnia.	Foods high in fiber (apples, celery, etc.).
Zinc	Promotes burn and wound healing; supports the immune system; involved in carbohydrate and protein digestion; plays a role in reproductive organ growth and development.	Birth–1 Year: 5 mg 1–10 Years: 10 mg 11–18 Years: Females, 12 mg; Males, 15 mg	White spots on fingernails; stretch marks on skin; loss of sense of smell or taste; joint pains; poor sexual development; menstrual irregularities; slow wound healing; recurrent infections; acne.	Brewer's yeast; liver; seafood; wheat germ; bran; oatmeal; nuts; peas; carrots; spinach; sunflower seeds.

Pregnancy and Your Newborn

Pregnancy and the newborn period are unique times with special sets of concerns and challenges. To give your baby the healthiest possible start in life, you should learn as much as possible about what to expect and develop an understanding of your newborn's special needs. In this chapter, we will review the care your newborn will receive immediately after birth, plus the benefits of parent-child bonding during the hour after birth, take a look at your baby's body, and discuss the care of your new infant.

PRENATAL SAFEGUARDS

Caring for your child's health starts when you become pregnant. What you take into your body will create the environment for your developing new baby. Smoking, poor nutrition, alcohol, and certain illnesses during pregnancy will adversely affect your child's health. Each of these dangers can be avoided if you make certain right choices.

Tobacco and Alcohol

Poor maternal nutrition, smoking, and maternal alcohol intake are among the factors that can lead to birth defects. Cigarette smoking has not only been identified as a cause of many forms of cancer, but it has also been linked to negative effects on a developing fetus. Cigarette smoking during pregnancy has been related to low birth weight, increased incidence of spontaneous abortion (miscarriage), stillbirth, and infant mortality. For your health, and the health of your baby, don't smoke while you are pregnant. Better yet, don't smoke at all.

If you are a pregnant woman looking forward to the birth of a normal, healthy child, please don't drink alcoholic beverages, including wine and beer. Women who drink during pregnancy risk having a child with severe birth defects. Studies show that consuming more than two drinks per day (the equivalent of two ounces of hard liquor, eight ounces of wine, or sixteen ounces of beer) increases the possibility that your child will be

born with fetal alcohol syndrome. This amount of alcohol also adds to the risk of miscarriage. Occasional "binge drinking" can also cause problems, even if a woman drinks very little during most of the nine months she is pregnant. A portion of the alcohol from any alcoholic beverage a woman drinks while carrying a fetus will reach the child in the womb. Even very small amounts of alcohol taken only occasionally can give rise to problems such as low birth weight and delayed development.

Fetal alcohol syndrome is a documented danger to your baby. This disorder causes serious abnormalities, which can include heart defects, abnormal limb development, and lower-than-average intelligence. A baby who is severely affected may be abnormally short and have small eyes, a small jaw, and a cleft lip and palate. Such a child may be unable to suck normally, will sleep badly, and will be understandably irritable and difficult to care for. Fortunately, alcohol-related birth defects are completely preventable. To give your baby a healthy start in life, don't drink.

Cats

A pregnant woman should not tend a cat's litter box. If a mother-to-be becomes infected with the parasite that causes toxoplasmosis through contact with an infected cat's feces, there is a possibility that the parasite may migrate through the placenta to the fetus. A toxoplasmosis infection in early pregnancy can cause miscarriage. If an infected fetus is not spontaneously aborted, severe malformation of the unborn child becomes a frightening possibility. A parasite infestation in later pregnancy can cause a nervous system disorder. A child infected with toxoplasmosis as a fetus may suffer blindness in early childhood.

Genetic Counseling and Fetal Screening

If either prospective parent has family members with a hereditary condition or genetic abnormality such

The Development of the Fetus

From conception to birth, a baby grows and develops at an amazingly fast pace. All the major organs and structures of the infant are present in rudimentary form by the time a woman has missed her second menstrual cycle. By this time, the embryo has changed shape so that major features of the external body are noticeable. The second four weeks are developmentally very important. This is the time that congenital malformations most often occur. From weeks nine through forty, the embryo is called a fetus. This is a time of more specific development and differentiation. The fetus grows into a full-sized baby and begins to use its organs and structures to take care of some of its needs. Although a full-term baby is born after forty weeks in utero, by thirty-two weeks the fetus is essentially fully formed and may be able to live outside the womb.

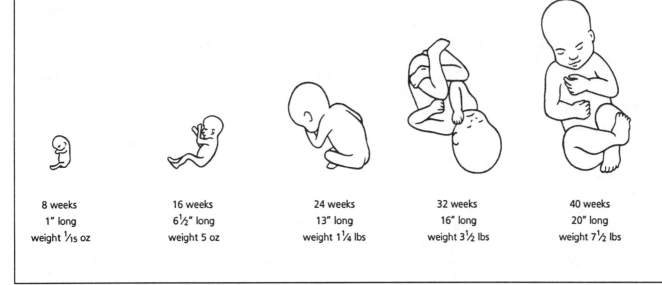

8 weeks	16 weeks	24 weeks	32 weeks	40 weeks
1" long	6½" long	13" long	16" long	20" long
weight 1/15 oz	weight 5 oz	weight 1¼ lbs	weight 3½ lbs	weight 7½ lbs

as sickle cell disease, Tay-Sachs disease, or hemophilia, you may wish to seek genetic counseling to understand the risk of giving birth to an affected child. When there is a possibility a fetus may be at risk for some abnormality, various medical tests may be used to determine whether the child has certain defects. These tests include amniocentesis, chorionic villus sampling, and ultrasound scanning. If you have fears about your unborn child, discuss these procedures with your doctor.

PREPARING TO WELCOME YOUR BABY

From the moment of conception through birth, your baby's body goes through wonderful changes. As your newborn greets the world outside the womb, she may appear uncoordinated during the early weeks. However, your infant is actually quite capable and prepared for the tasks ahead. Your baby can move, feel, see, hear, eat, and communicate with you. She even has a highly developed sense of smell. From this strong foundation, your newborn will grow and develop at a tremendous rate.

The Breast Versus the Bottle

One of the most important decisions you will make for your newborn child concerns the method of feeding. Most parents decide well in advance of birth whether their newborn child will be breastfed or bottlefed. A frank and open discussion between mother and father should be initiated on this subject. Because father's love and support is necessary in either case, it is vital that both parents agree on the choice between breast and bottle. (If your baby had a voice in the decision, she would undoubtedly choose the breast.) For help in thinking about your decision, *see* The Breast or the Bottle? on page 57 for a comparison between the two.

It is true that there are many documented benefits for the breastfed baby. But by far the greatest gift you can give your new baby is happy parents. If you cannot breastfeed, or simply decide that breastfeeding is not for you, be comfortable with the situation. Give your baby plenty of play time with good eye-to-eye contact and cuddling at feeding time. Then relax and enjoy each other. One crooked smile from your newborn will melt your heart and assure you that you're on the right track.

If you do want to nurse your child, we recommend you contact La Leche League. This organization is formed of nursing mothers, some of whom have nursed "special" babies with various illnesses and conditions. These people know everything there is to know about getting past the rough spots and making nursing a happy and rewarding experience. La Leche League has over 8,500 active leaders and operates in forty-seven countries. Each chapter meets monthly. Topics related to breastfeeding are discussed at each meeting. If you are considering nursing your newborn, plan to attend meetings prior to the birth of your baby. After your baby is born, she will be welcome at meetings. To locate a La Leche League chapter near you, contact La Leche League International, 9616 Minneapolis Avenue, Franklin Park, Illinois 60131; telephone 708–455–7730. In addition, *The Nursing Mother's Companion* by Kathleen Huggins (The Harvard Common Press, 1990) is an excellent reference for breastfeeding mothers.

Most mothers are able to nurse their babies with a minimum of problems. Our preference is for breastfeeding. However, there are some women who do not produce enough milk, and a few who are physically unable to nurse. If you are one of these women, you should know that there are millions of happy, healthy adults who were bottlefed. You can support and nurture your bottlefed child well by giving her adequate nutrition and plenty of love and cuddling.

Circumcision

Another decision you will want to make prior to birth involves the circumcision of a baby boy. The United States is one of the few countries where male children are routinely circumcised. The American Academy of Pediatrics reports that there is no medical reason for this operation, however. Studies have shown that circumcision is not necessary for cleanliness or good health. An uncircumcised male is not at greater risk for cancer or other diseases later in life.

Of course, many people make the decision to circumcise on religious grounds. But apart from that, more and more parents are deciding against the procedure. If you choose not to have your baby boy circumcised, it is increasingly unlikely that he will grow up looking "different" from the majority of his peers.

If you do opt for circumcision, talk with your doctor about the advisability of using a local anesthetic before the procedure. Surprisingly, not all doctors will agree to this. But it may be worthwhile to expend extra effort to find one who will, because circumcision can be a traumatic and painful experience for your baby boy, especially if no anesthetics are employed. Also, if you are having your son circumcised, delay the operation for at least twenty-four hours to give him time to adjust to life outside the womb. This delay is important if your little boy is to fully enjoy his first meeting with you.

CONVENTIONAL TREATMENT FOR YOUR NEWBORN

At birth, your newborn will be given standard care to help her adjust to life outside the protection of your body. This section addresses routine procedures surrounding birth in a hospital. The authors realize that many parents choose to have their babies at home with midwives and friends attending them. Many families, even those who choose a hospital birth, are wary of medical interventions. These are all personal choices. What you decide will depend primarily on your comfort level and the mother's medical history, especially her past birth experiences. No matter where you give birth, it is possible to work toward having the birth experience you want. We advise you to learn in advance about all the procedures and interventions that may be possible (and, in some environments, required). Speak with your doctor or midwife about his or her perspective and requirements. Then make your own choices about which interventions or support measures you want. If you have questions about your newborn, nurses in your doctor's office or in the hospital nursery are good first resources. They can answer most questions. If the situation seems serious or questionable, the nurse will refer you to your doctor.

As your baby's head emerges, her throat and mouth may be cleansed to remove excess mucus and ensure that her first breath is easy. Even before the umbilical cord is cut, your baby will be placed on your stomach and covered with a warm blanket. The amount of blood present on newborns varies widely. The blood is coming not from a wound to the baby, but from your womb. This is perfectly normal and not a cause for concern.

From the moment your baby leaves the comfort of your womb, she must be kept warm. Because bacteria thrive in warmth, however, the temperature of a delivery room is usually twenty degrees below body temperature. When your newborn is taken from you for routine post-birth procedures, she will be kept cozy under a warming light.

The umbilical cord will be cut and tied. Once the cord is cut, a wonderful phenomenon occurs. Because the internal blood vessels that carried blood through the umbilical cord to your baby's circulatory system

THE BREAST OR THE BOTTLE?

How will you feed your new baby? This is one of the first and most important child-rearing decisions parents make. Mothers and fathers should consider the choice from all the angles, and discuss their feelings openly before making up their minds. Below are some key points of comparison.

Point of Comparison	The Breast	The Bottle
Quality Control	Rests with the nursing mother. Mother's milk cannot become contaminated accidentally. As long as a breastfeeding mother abstains from drugs and alcohol, breast milk is never toxic. Mother's milk is always fresh, always the right temperature, always ready, always nutritionally perfect.	In the hands of companies selling prepared formulas, and various problems are possible. In 1950, babies given SMA, a cow's-milk-based product, suffered cerebral palsy and seizures because it lacked vitamin B6. In 1979 and 1980, two soy-based formulas (Neo-mull-soy and Cho-free) were manufactured without sufficient chloride. Infants fed these products suffered metabolic acidosis, and were at risk for mental retardation and other problems later in life. There have been two reported cases of an infant formula becoming contaminated and causing some illness in infants. Although these examples are the exception rather than the rule, if you are bottlefeeding your newborn, be very careful about the source of your child's prepared formula. Seek your physician's guidance in evaluating products.
Nutritive Value	Breast milk is nutritionally perfect for your newborn. Mother's milk keeps pace with your infant's changing requirements. It begins as colostrum, a sticky yellowish fluid that confers important immunity factors and has a high protein content, both necessary to start your baby off right. It also cleanses your baby's intestinal tract and helps rid her body of mucus. Mother's milk gradually changes into a thin white or bluish liquid with the perfect combination of water, fat, proteins, sugar, minerals, and vitamins. It is biochemically designed to foster brain function, growth, and development. Human milk has a relatively high carbohydrate content (7 percent, compared to 4.8 percent for cow's milk), which is thought to help the intestines develop healthy flora and to aid in the absorption of essential minerals such as calcium and magnesium. After five to six months you may want to talk to your doctor about the possible need for iron supplementation.	Animal milk lacks protective antibodies, special enzymes, hormones, vitamins, and many other important factors that are present in human milk. Cow's milk is designed to promote fast muscle growth in a newborn calf. Fully half of the protein in cow's milk is excreted unused by a human baby. A bottlefed baby will probably not need nutritional supplementation during the first four months. After that time, talk to your doctor about your infant's nutritional needs, especially for iron.
Baby's Health	Mother's milk contains special antibodies designed to boost your infant's immune defenses. Breastfed babies have fewer and milder colds, as well as fewer problems with colic, ear infections, diaper rash, and skin conditions. If there is a family history of allergies, breastfeeding becomes even more important. A child born into an "allergic" family will benefit greatly from being fed only breast milk for the first six months of life.	Because prepared formulas lack the antibodies and protective factors present in mother's milk, bottlefed infants have a higher incidence of health problems. One of the most common allergic reactions suffered by babies is an allergy to cow's milk. Most tolerate a soy-based formula fairly well, although the potential for allergic reactions still exists. A few babies cannot handle any prepared formulas at all. If such a child is initially bottlefed, it may be necessary to resort to a wet nurse until the mother can reactivate lactation and provide milk.

Point of Comparison	The Breast	The Bottle
Digestion	Because of its perfect nutrition, mother's milk is almost completely utilized. Breast milk increases the growth of friendly flora in baby's intestines. A breastfed infant is rarely constipated, seldom has bowel upsets, and rarely gets diarrhea. The stools of a breastfed baby are yellowish, rather loose, and easy to pass (greenish or foul-smelling stools are a sign that something is wrong).	Prepared formulas are not fully utilized by an infant's digestive tract. Half the protein is excreted unused. The form of iron in most formulas may be constipating and is difficult to absorb. Bottlefed babies may slow down to one stool a day, usually during or right after a feeding.
Jaw and Tooth Development	Because nursing works the facial muscles in the way nature intended, breastfed babies have better muscle and jaw development as well as healthier teeth. Studies show that children who are breastfed for three months or longer have 45 to 59 percent fewer cavities than other children.	Many experts call bottlefeeding a major cause of malocclusions and other facial and dental problems in children. They say the force that is needed to suck on a rubber nipple is insufficient for healthy jaw and tooth development. Bottlefeeding uses different muscles than those worked in breastfeeding.
Long-Term Effects	Mother's milk confers lifetime health benefits. A university study showed that children who were breastfed only for six months or longer had fewer ear infections, colds, throat and tonsil infections, intestinal infections, and allergic reactions. A British study showed that breastfed infants were unlikely to develop ulcerative colitis later in life.	A university study showed that bottlefed children had 4 times as many ear infections and colds, 11 times as many infected tonsils resulting in tonsillectomies, 20 times as many intestinal infections, and 8 to 27 times as many allergic reactions as children who who were breastfed. According to a British study, ulcerative colitis in adults is is twice as common in people who were not breastfed past two weeks of age.
Cost	Mother's milk is free. After all, mother must eat, whether breastfeeding or not.	During the first six months of your baby's life, you can expect to spend from $300 to as much as $800 on prepared formulas, bottles, nipples, and sterilizing equipment.
Benefits to Mom	Nursing stimulates the uterus to shrink and contract, and stimulates caloric burn. Nursing moms use up an extra 1040 calories daily, and will gradually lose weight. Once a rhythm is established, breastfeeding is easy and convenient. Breastfeeding may also protect a woman against breast cancer and osteoporosis.	Bottlefeeding moms can "take a break." Without the need to be ready with the breast when baby is hungry, a night out or weekend away with father becomes a possibility.
Benefits to Dad	If father opts not to share this time, middle-of-the-night feedings won't disturb dad's sleep. Many fathers say it's extremely pleasant to find a sleepy mom with babe-at-breast cuddled in bed beside them.	Father can give a baby formula as well as mother. Feeding a warm and cuddly infant is a rich nurturing and bonding experience for both dad and baby.

are no longer needed, they eventually are transformed into ligaments.

Using the Apgar method (named after its creator, Dr. Virginia Apgar), your newborn will be evaluated one minute after birth and again five minutes later. The doctor looks at the general overall condition of your infant and checks five key characteristics: color, respiration, heart rate, muscle tone, and reflexes (see inset, page 60). Your baby's first Apgar score shows the doctor how your newborn came through labor and delivery. The number of points your baby receives also gives an indication of how she will handle the postpartum pe-

riod. A score of eight to ten means your newborn's condition is good. A low rating alerts the medical staff that your child needs extra care. After five minutes has passed, your baby will be rated again. This additional test shows the doctor how your newborn is adjusting to life outside the womb. If you ask, the doctor or nurse will tell you the Apgar score your baby was given.

Your newborn will be weighed and measured. At birth, most babies tip the scales at seven to eight pounds, and measure from nineteen to twenty-one inches long. Many factors influence these "average" figures. If your baby weighs less or more, or is shorter or longer, it does not mean your child is less than perfection. There's no such thing as an "average" baby—each is a unique little person in her own right.

Shortly after birth, your fingerprints and your newborn's footprints will be recorded. The nurse will also put your baby's footprints in her baby book, if you have it with you. While you are still in the delivery room, you and your baby will each receive an identification bracelet.

Because all newborns are deficient in vitamin K, which is necessary for proper blood clotting, your baby will probably be given an injection of vitamin K. It may be given in the delivery room or in the nursery. Once your infant's gastrointestinal tract is functioning on its own, her body will begin manufacturing vitamin K. If you have strong feelings about this shot, you may want to talk with your doctor before delivery about eliminating the vitamin K injection.

In most states, newborn babies' eyes are treated with an antibiotic ointment. This procedure prevents many bacterial eye infections. If the mother has gonorrhea, the drops will prevent blindness. Although the time frame varies from state to state, the drops may be applied any time within one hour after birth. Because this procedure results in blurred vision, however, you may wish to ask your doctor to delay it until you, your spouse, and your infant have had some quiet bonding time together. (You may also decide to eliminate this procedure altogether.) More and more medical facilities are aware of the need for immediate bonding between parents and the newborn child.

Jaundice is seen fairly frequently in newborns, usually beginning the third day of life. This condition occurs because a new baby's liver is limited in its ability to process excess bilirubin, a product of the breakdown of red blood cells. To prevent complications, some hospitals treat jaundiced infants with ultraviolet light. Pathological or abnormal jaundice, a result of blood incompatibility between mother and infant (caused by a difference in either blood type or Rh factor) is cause for concern.

Most often jaundice will clear by itself as the baby feeds and eliminates the bilirubin through the stool. However, if you notice that your baby is not feeding well, is not passing one or more stools daily, is lethargic, or is jaundiced from her head to her bellybutton, or that the whites of her eyes look creamy or yellow in color, call your doctor. It may be advisable to check your baby's bilirubin level. In rare cases, treatment may include a blood transfusion to prevent brain damage.

The third day after birth, a genetic blood screen is performed, including testing for phenylketonuria (PKU). In rare cases, a child can lack the enzyme needed to convert the amino acid phenylalanine into another amino acid, tyrosine, in the course of protein metabolism. Because excess phenylalanine harms brain tissue, undiagnosed PKU can cause mental retardation. People affected by PKU have to be put on a diet that is free of phenylalanine to control the condition. If a child is found to have PKU, complications from the disorder are preventable.

If your baby boy is circumcised, be sure to call to your doctor's attention any bleeding, infection, or obvious discomfort at the site. To keep the diaper from sticking to the wound, a little petroleum jelly will be applied and the area will be covered with a sterile gauze pad. After initial healing and with your doctor's okay, you can apply a natural antibiotic salve to aid healing. A little boy who has been circumcised will be more comfortable lying on his side, rather than on his stomach.

BONDING

Bonding between baby and parents actually begins before birth. It is exciting to feel an infant move in the womb. Knowing that a new little person is in there and feeling her move around is an experience both mothers and fathers delight in and cherish.

From the beginning of time, new mothers have reached instinctively for their just-born infants, anxious to touch, soothe, cuddle, inspect, and take in the wondrous sight of their newborn children. Extensive research now shows that a mother and father who hold and fondle their child immediately after birth develop a strong bond. Bonding at birth fosters strong, healthy emotional and physical growth in babies, and builds strong, healthy parenting instincts in mothers and fathers.

Experts recommend that infants and parents spend from thirty to sixty minutes alone together as soon as immediate medical care and assessment have been completed. During your newborn's first hour of life, she is in what is medically termed a quiet-alert state. During this period, your baby will be awake and responsive.

Yes, your baby can see. A newborn's vision, while not perfect, is perfectly adequate. Your newborn starts life curious and ready to get acquainted with the most important people in her life—her parents. Your infant will intently look deep into mother's and father's eyes, will inspect and get to know your faces. Your baby sees best between twelve and fifteen inches past her little nose. (Not surprisingly, this is the approximate distance between mother's eyes and the breast.) During this warm and happy time, father can hold his newborn child in the nursing position.

Following birth, your baby will remain in the quiet-alert state for about an hour. She will then sleep deeply for three or four hours. Thereafter, the quiet-alert state will come and go, sometimes lasting for as little as a few seconds at a time.

To encourage family togetherness, many neonatal nurseries now invite family members to visit the newborn, even to participate in the care of the infant. In the case of a premature birth or other problem that requires an extended hospital stay, research shows that recovery is faster when mothers and fathers touch and soothe a newborn who requires intensive care.

During a mother's time in the hospital, both mother and child benefit from spending as much time together as the mother desires. Studies show that mothers who bond at birth with their babies and spend extra time with them while in the hospital have happier, healthier babies.

The process of bonding is strengthened immediately after birth. However, it is important to realize that the bonding process and connection between parents and child continues throughout infancy and childhood. If for some reason you are unable to be with your newborn immediately after delivery, do not be discouraged. Recognize the ongoing nature of your relationship. One way to support bonding over time is with infant massage. Feeding, cooing, eye contact, bathing, and cuddling also contribute to this important foundation.

Research shows that when their babies are one month of age, bonded mothers fondle and soothe their crying infants, talk, play, and seek strong eye-to-eye contact with their little ones. At one year, well-bonded toddlers smile and laugh more, and cry, whine, and fuss less. Bonded parents receive more cooperation during the "terrible twos," because they typically explain rather than command and punish. At age five, a child with a deep bond with her parents usually exhibits advanced speech development and better adjustment to the world outside the home, almost certainly because she feels secure and well loved.

A LOOK AT YOUR BABY'S BODY

The first thing new parents want to do is inspect the new arrival. If you are expecting a "picture-book" baby, you will almost certainly be disappointed. Your infant has just left the cozy nest where she spent nine comfortable months. Immediately after birth, your baby's skin will have a grayish or bluish cast. In the womb, your baby received oxygen from your red blood cells. When your newborn cries and begins to breathe, healthy red oxygenated blood will rush through the newly activated lungs and pump throughout the body. You will actually see your infant become pink and rosy-cheeked before your eyes, although her hands and feet may stay bluish for a few hours and may feel cold.

Cutting the umbilical cord initiates breathing. Your newborn's first breaths and cries expand her lungs and start the process of respiration. While in the womb, your baby's lungs were filled with amniotic fluid. Some fluid is squeezed out during delivery. The rest is reabsorbed in the first few hours of life.

Babies normally breathe more quickly than adults. When you take your newborn home from the hospital, her respiratory rate will be from forty to sixty breaths per minute, compared to an adult rate of between ten and twenty. Babies pant and can stop breathing for three or four seconds at a time. This range of respiration is normal. When your baby comes home, if she is taking

Apgar Scoring Chart

Characteristic	0 Points	1 point	2 Points
Color	Blue, pale	Body pink, extremities blue	Body completely pink
Respiratory Effort	Absent	Slow, irregular, weak cry	Strong cry
Heart Rate	Absent	Less than 100 beats per minute	More than 100 beats per minute
Muscle Tone	Limp	Some flexing of extremities	Active motion
Reflexes	Absent	Grimace, some motion	Cry

more than eighty or ninety breaths per minute, has frequent pauses in breathing, does not have good color, or simply doesn't look alert to you, call your physician immediately.

Your newborn has a small heart and a thin chest wall. There is not much tissue between the heart muscle and the skin covering her little chest. You may be able to see and feel your baby's heartbeat over the entire chest area. When your infant is excited or agitated, her pulse rate can become as high as 200 beats per minute. When your baby is sleeping, her heartbeat will be around 100 beats per minute. By comparison, the average adult pulse rate is between 60 and 80 beats per minute.

Your newborn's body may be coated with *vernix caseosa*, or "baby cold cream." This cheeselike coating protected your baby's body while she was floating in the amniotic fluid of the womb. The nearer to term your baby is delivered, the less vernix will be present. If your child was born after a full nine months in the womb, vernix may not be noticeable. If your child is premature, her skin may still retain considerable vernix. Some mothers massage this natural "skin conditioner" into their babies' skin, rather than having it washed off.

A premature baby may be covered with lanugo, a very fine downy hair. Lanugo disappears within a few weeks. In babies born close to term, lanugo may be present on the shoulders and over the shoulder blades. Your newborn's skin may appear dry and scaly. Some peeling may occur during the week or two after birth. Your baby may have some "angel kisses"—small clusters of capillaries appearing on the nape of the neck, the eyelids, or the bridge of the nose. These markings fade away and disappear on their own, usually within nine months.

Boy or girl, your newborn's genitals may appear swollen or puffy. The breasts may appear enlarged, and your newborn may even secrete a little milk for as long as two weeks. A baby girl may experience "false menstruation," a bit of vaginal bleeding. These effects occur as a result of the hormones your baby received from you in the womb. As the little body adjusts to the outside world, these harmless signs will disappear.

Your Baby's Proportions

Your newborn's head may look too large for her body. From the top of the head to the bottom of the chin, your baby's head takes up about one-fourth of her length. The average head of a newborn measures thirteen to fourteen inches around.

Your baby's arms and legs are proportionally short for her torso. Your newborn's arms will usually be bent at the elbow. She will hold them close to her body, with the hands curled in tiny fists. Your infant's legs will be bent at the knees and will appear bowed.

Your newborn's rib cage feels like a small version of your own. The breastbone is in three parts, the top, middle, and the xiphoid, that pointy arrow-shaped piece at the bottom. Your baby's tummy is round, protruding, and soft, although you will see the muscles tighten and harden when your child cries. A newborn's stomach is about the size of a large walnut. It holds about three ounces of fluid or food at a time. Because that tiny tummy empties quickly to make room for more nutrients, your baby needs to be fed frequently. She will let you know when it's time, usually every two to three hours for the first few weeks.

A round abdomen is normal in a newborn. Your infant's intestines are surprisingly long. They snake back and forth in a sideways "S" to fit into that tiny space. No matter how active your baby was in utero, she wasn't doing sit-ups. Her abdominal muscles lack the toning that comes with exercise.

Your Baby's Skin

You may notice little bumps or "whiteheads" scattered over your newborn's forehead, nose, and cheeks. Medically termed *milia*, these are immature oil glands. As your baby's glandular system starts to function, the bumps will fade away. Don't pick or squeeze them.

"Baby acne" is an acnelike rash that may appear on your baby's face and chest. This is related to the hormonal changes your newborn is experiencing. Although this rash has been known to last for six to eight weeks, it will go away on its own, and requires no treatment. To help hasten healing, you may rub a little breast milk on the area. (Breast milk has antibiotic properties.)

During your baby's first three to four days of life, she may have a red, splotchy, wandering rash scattered with small white dots. This is called *erythema toxicum*, but there is nothing toxic about it. It is not dangerous, requires no treatment, and is common in newborns. Erythema toxicum may appear in many places on your infant's body. It can disappear and reappear throughout the first week following birth.

A more serious rash caused by a staphylococcus infection has a similar appearance but does not fade away. If your newborn has a persistent rash answering the description of erythema toxicum, but that lasts longer than seven to ten days, it may be cause for concern. Have a nurse help identify your child's condition. Call your doctor if you think your child's rash may be serious, or if your child's rash is peeling or has open lesions, pustules, or hard bumps. A newborn with a rash accompanied by fever and lethargy also needs medical attention.

Your Baby's Face and Head

Your baby's face may be puffy. Her little nose may be flattened, and her ears may may be pressed tight to the head. Her head may look misshapen. It will probably be elongated. Within a day or two, perhaps three, your baby's head will assume its normal shape. Elongation and swelling of the skull occur as a result of molding during passage through the birth canal.

When you caress your newborn's head, the skull will feel as if it is made of several parts. Your newborn is equipped with *fontanels*, or soft spots. These are gaps between the bones of your child's skull. During passage through the birth canal, the fontanels permit molding of the bones of the skull. The bones overlap as they squeeze together. Without this wonderful arrangement, your baby's head wouldn't be able to pass through the birth canal.

The anterior fontanel is the large diamond-shaped soft spot at the top of your newborn's head. There is also a smaller soft spot, the posterior fontanel, at the back of your infant's skull. These gaps between the bones are covered with a tough, fibrous material. You may see your baby's soft spots pulse with each heartbeat. When your baby is lying down or crying, it's normal for the shape of the fontanels to change. In spite of unsettling warnings from well-meaning relatives, your baby's soft spots are not delicate. They can be touched, rubbed, and washed without hurting or harming your baby.

The bones of your baby's skull may not grow together completely until she is about two years old. The posterior fontanel closes first, usually two to fifteen weeks after birth. The anterior fontanel, the large soft spot on the top of your baby's head, usually closes when a child is between nine and eighteen months of age. These soft and flexible spots not only facilitate birth, but also give room for your child's brain to grow. The growth rate of the brain is tremendous during baby's first year.

If you have any doubts about the size and condition of your baby's soft spots after your newborn comes home, call your doctor or discuss it with his or her nurse. A depressed or "scooped-out" soft spot may be a sign of very advanced dehydration. A bulging soft spot may be a sign of a serious illness, such as meningitis, and requires medical evaluation.

Your Baby's Neck

Your newborn's head and neck muscles are not well developed. When you are holding, bathing, or carrying your newborn, be sure her neck and head are well supported.

Babies sometimes seem comfortable with their necks bent and heads resting at funny angles. You needn't get fanatic about it, but it is possible for a baby to obstruct her airway when her head is in an odd position. Use common sense. Remember that your newborn does not have the ability to hold her head up. If your baby is scrunched down with her head and neck at an awkward angle, check to make sure she is breathing easily.

Your Baby's Mouth

Your newborn's mouth has a "suckling pad," a layer of tissue lining the lower lip. To help your baby fasten onto your breast when nursing, the suckling pad becomes swollen and hard.

Your baby may have little white dots resembling pearls inside her mouth. They are called Ebstein's pearls, or inclusion cysts. These are normal and do not require any intervention. They will disappear on their own.

Your Baby's Hair

Babies are born with different amounts of hair. Some are born shiny-skulled and bald. Some are born with a sparse "monk's fringe." Others emerge from the womb with a full head of hair.

It is not unusual for an infant to lose all of her hair by three months of age, to be bald for a while, or to regrow hair so quickly you might barely notice it was once missing. Some babies create a bald band around the backs of their heads from rubbing their delicate newborn hair against the bed.

As your child grows older, her hair will probably darken. For example, a platinum-blonde toddler will usually turn honey-haired by puberty, then dark blonde by the time she reaches the age of twenty.

Your Baby's Eyes

Most babies are born with blue eyes. By six months of age, your baby's eye color will probably be established, although changes in color can occur throughout the first year.

Your newborn's eyes may be swollen, or there may be small hemorrhages in the whites of the eyes due to pressure in the birth canal. It may take several weeks until your baby's eyes are completely clear. If an antibiotic ointment has been administered, there may be a slight discharge caused by irritation (silver nitrate, once used routinely in babies' eyes, is rarely used today because of its tendency to create irritation).

It commonly takes several weeks for a newborn's tear ducts to function. Although it's a sure bet you'll hear your baby cry, don't expect real tears immediately.

The Five Senses

Your baby can see at birth. Some old folk wisdom still insists a newborn will not see until she is several weeks old, but research has shown that this is not true. Your newborn will look at you and at her surroundings. Bright light shining in your baby's eyes will cause her to blink, to look away. Because the muscles controlling eye movement are not fully developed at birth, most newborns' eyes cross. As your baby looks around and struggles to focus, expect her to appear cross-eyed at times. Your baby will respond with cooing and smiling to colors, shapes, and movement. You'll enjoy watching your infant "talk" to a bright mobile hung over her crib. When choosing a mobile, look at it from underneath, as your baby will. Stuffed animals, bright toys that rattle or ring, or a polished steel mirror at eye level all provide positive stimulation. By the time your child reaches six months of age, her eye muscles should be fully functional. If your little one is still having trouble focusing, consult your doctor.

Your baby's senses of taste and smell are well developed at birth. Interestingly, some scientific studies show that a newborn can tell the difference between the appetizing taste and appetite-stimulating aroma of her mother's breast milk and any other mother's milk. Don't be surprised if your child reacts with distaste to someone who smokes, or someone who wears perfume or cologne with a strong or heavy scent.

Even before your newborn arrived, she was aware of sound. As amniotic fluid is absorbed during the several days following birth, hearing becomes more efficient. Sharp, loud sounds will disturb a newborn and startle her awake. Soft sounds, like your gentle and loving voice, are soothing to a newborn. Some experts say that a newborn is already familiar with the voices of family members. Talking, singing, and reading to your baby will positively stimulate her development. Once your newborn comes home, it's not necessary to tiptoe around and maintain strict silence when she is sleeping. You will, of course, want to guard against sudden loud or sharp noises. But the hum of a busy, happy household may actually soothe and reassure a sleepy infant and lull her off to dreamland. After all, these are the noises she has become accustomed to over the past nine months.

During the first few weeks of life, amniotic fluid in the middle ear lessens sound vibrations transmitted by the eardrums. The ability to hear is important in the development of your child's language skills. The easiest way to test your baby's hearing is to clap your hands sharply and watch to see if your infant blinks or grimaces. If at first your newborn does not seem to react, try the test another time or two, spaced out over a few minutes. If you have any doubts about your baby's hearing, call your physician. Be persistent. Some hospitals now perform a routine screen for hearing for all newborns, but the diagnosis of congenital deafness or a hearing deficit is still almost always made by the parents. Any concern over your baby's ability to hear needs to be investigated.

The structure of the inner ear is different in infants and young children than it is in adults, predisposing babies and toddlers to ear infections (*see* EAR INFECTION in Part Two). An unusually shaped or abnormally placed ear should be brought to your doctor's attention. In some babies, there is a correlation between an abnormally placed ear and a kidney defect.

As you gently examine your newborn, notice the wonder and pleasure she experiences at your loving touch. Your baby will like clutching your fingers within a tiny fist. She will enjoy a "massage" of gentle stroking. Conversely, touching your baby roughly or crossly will disturb and distress her.

YOUR NEWBORN'S "STANDARD OPERATING PROCEDURE"

During the first few days, your baby is one of nature's ultimate conservationists. This is a time of transition. Your baby's body is busy reabsorbing leftover amniotic fluid, as well as getting rid of waste products resulting from building an entire human being.

Your baby's tiny body conserves water and nutrients and uses them very efficiently. Six to eight wet diapers in a twenty-four hour period indicates that your baby is getting enough fluid and is adequately hydrated.

When colostrum decreases and your infant begins receiving breast milk, expect that the number of wet diapers may increase from six a day to ten or twenty. If this doesn't happen, consult your physician or nurse. The initial urine your newborn puts out will be dark and strong. Babies sometimes excrete a pinkish-orange crystalline substance in their urine that resembles blood. It probably is not blood, however. It usually means the child needs more fluid. By day three or four, your baby's urine should be clear or pale yellow. If it has not cleared by this time, call your nurse or physician.

During your newborn's first two days of life, she will pass *meconium*, a thick, tarry, dark-green stool. This substance filled the intestines during fetal growth and is quickly excreted. By day five or six, expect normal stools.

A new baby can become dehydrated very quickly. If your infant's stool becomes persistently watery, or increases dramatically in quantity, check with your doctor. If your newborn has diarrhea or a viral infection (evidenced by a possible fever and a stool that increases in frequency, is loose and runny, yellow/orange/brown or even greenish in color, and has a foul odor), call your doctor or nurse promptly.

Your baby may have a bowel movement every time she is fed. As your newborn's intestines mature, the number of bowel movements will taper off. Because breast milk is so perfectly formulated, and a baby's body is so efficient in utilizing everything she takes in, it's not unusual for a breastfed baby between six and eight weeks of age to skip days in between bowel movements. A breastfed infant's stool is mostly mucus, a little bile, and a few curds left over from the breast milk.

Cord Care

You will undoubtedly be instructed in the care of your newborn's severed umbilical cord in the hospital, but here's a quick review.

To keep the area dry and free of urine, fold your baby's diaper down. Until the cord has fallen off and the area has healed completely, give only sponge baths.

While this small wound is healing, clean the stump and entire area with rubbing alcohol a few times each day. Using a cotton swab dipped in rubbing alcohol or calendula tincture, clean the stump, around the cord, at the base of the cord, and between the skin and the cord.

The stump will fall off some time between one and three weeks after you take your baby home. The area may ooze and drip a small amount of blood for a few days after the stump has come off. The area will scab over. Don't pick at or remove the scab. Allow it to fall off naturally.

During this entire period, watch for any signs of infection. If the area becomes red, swollen, oozes pus, or becomes tender, call your doctor.

Your Baby's Reflexes

When you touch your newborn's cheek, she will automatically turn her head in that direction and "root" around looking for your breast. To nurse your baby, allow your breast to touch a rosy cheek, or tap your nipple against your baby's lower lip. Your newborn will instinctively open her mouth and root around very enthusiastically until she finds the nipple. This is called the *rooting reflex*.

The *suckling reflex*, the instinct to suck, is also inborn. Even while in the womb, your newborn practiced the suckling reflex, a primary survival skill. She may even have sucked on a thumb. Your newborn baby may suck a thumb or a finger, or even try to stuff an entire tiny fist in her mouth.

When your newborn suckles, she will instinctively swallow as needed. The *swallowing reflex* is another survival skill learned in the womb, where your baby swallowed and excreted amniotic fluid.

Newborns come equipped with the *gag reflex* and the *cough reflex*, two other important survival devices. If something gets in your newborn's mouth that shouldn't be there, she will gag to expel it. The gagging reflex helps protect against choking. The coughing reflex helps your infant get rid of an accumulation of mucus.

Nature has equipped your newborn with several *protective reflexes* as well. For example, it is rare for a little one to smother in her covers. If something covers her face, your baby will move her head about and thrash her arms to get away from the obstruction. If one of your infant's arms or legs becomes uncovered and she feels chilled, that limb will quickly be drawn up close to the body to warm it. And when your baby is poked or hurt by something—perhaps pricked accidentally with a diaper pin—expect her to pull back quickly and cry. These actions call you to come to the rescue.

Baby's other reflexes include the *grasp reflex*, the *stepping reflex*, the *tonic neck reflex*, and the *Moro reflex*. When you place a finger or two in your newborn's palm, expect a firm, instinctive grip. Your baby will grasp so tightly you may be tempted to test her strength by raising your child's body. This is not a good idea. Your baby may let go suddenly and fall back. Even landing on a cushioned surface will startle your newborn and cause her to cry. The grasp reflex, which supports the newborn's social interactions, may actually be an evolutionary remnant from our primate ancestors. If you observe some of our nearer relatives, such as gorillas, you will notice that babies cling to their mothers so that they can be carried as their mothers move about; without the ability to grasp firmly from a very young age, a baby gorilla would be in serious trouble.

When you hold your baby upright, supporting her under her arms, she will "step out" in a walking motion. Scientists theorize that this "walking practice" helps strengthen the necessary muscles in preparation for learning to walk later. The tonic neck reflex describes the typical "fencing position" a baby often assumes. Your newborn may lie on her back, the head turned to one side, with the arm and leg on that side extended, while the other arm and leg are flexed. If her neck is rotated quickly, she will respond by extending the opposite arm and leg, while the previously extended limbs will flex. Finally, when your newborn is startled, she will typically thrust both arms out with a sudden, jerky motion, as if asking for a hug. This "parachute" gesture is the Moro reflex, and helps protect an infant in the event of a fall.

Height and Weight Development

In the first few days after birth, your baby will lose 5 to 10 percent of her birth weight. This weight will gradually be gained back over a period of two or three weeks.

Your infant will gain about two pounds each month during the first three months of life, and about one pound each month thereafter until age one. You can expect your baby to double her weight by six months, and triple her weight by the end of the first year.

Your baby will grow about one inch each month during her first six months, after which growth gradually slows. At twelve months, your baby will be about fifty percent longer than she was at birth.

In the first twelve to eighteen months, your baby's weight will triple and she will grow into a walking, talking, running, and exploring toddler. Your baby will be able to drink from a cup, eat, and play. She will become more and more sophisticated with sounds and words. One of the greatest joys of parenthood comes as you share the wonders that accompany the bursts of growth and learning as your baby grows and develops.

Bathing Your Baby

Never, not even for an instant, leave a newborn or a young child alone in the bath. If you must leave the room for any reason, wrap your child in a warm towel and take her with you.

Your newborn is not "dirty," so you need not bathe your baby every day. In fact, a daily bath can strip away your baby's natural protective oils and dry out her skin. When giving your newborn a sponge bath, heat the room or keep her swathed in a warm towel to prevent chilling. Uncover a small area at a time. Wash, pat dry, and cover up again as you go.

The diaper area is what needs your constant care and attention. Thoroughly clean your baby's buttocks with water after every bowel movement. Use a warm-water wash to cleanse away urine. Dry the area well, especially in the creases. Prevention and treatment of diaper rash are discussed in Part Two of this book.

If your baby boy has not been circumcised, just wash, rinse, and dry his penis along with the rest of him. *Never* pull the foreskin back over the head of the penis. In newborns, the foreskin is almost always attached to the head. Pulling it back may cause irritation or damage. It can take months, even years, before the foreskin is fully separated from the head. You may gently check for separation by pushing the foreskin back only as far as it will easily go. Don't use force.

Once the foreskin is fully separated and retractable, pull it back gently when washing the penis, then replace it. When the time comes to teach your son to bathe himself, show him how to keep the area clean by doing this himself.

When your baby is ready for a full bath, look into getting one of the hammock devices that fits into a large sink or the family tub. These hammocks cradle baby securely, leaving both of your hands free for washing, gentle laving with rinse water, and splashing. Most babies love bathtime and delight in thrashing their hands in the water.

Your Baby's Emotional Needs

The first rule in the treatment and care of your newborn is to be liberal—even extravagant—in the application of love and laughter. Your love is the basic foundation your baby needs to grow into a healthy, happy adult. Give your new baby plenty of interactive touching time, during both feeding and playtime. Cradle your baby and sing a lullaby. She will quiet and respond by intently watching your eyes and mouth.

It simply is not possible to give too much love or touching to a newborn. A baby who knows that her needs will be met grows into a secure and happy adult, capable of dealing with whatever life offers. You can't "spoil" a newborn baby.

Communication

Your little bundle communicates primarily by crying. When you soothe your crying infant, you are responding to a bulletin alerting you to a problem. Your infant may be telling you she is hungry, wet, too cold, too warm, in an uncomfortable position, or just plain lonesome for your welcoming arms. When you respond to your baby's communication with your best level of response, you are honoring and respecting your infant's needs. Your prompt response creates a safe and loving environment for your child.

Babies do cry, but it is not normal for an infant to experience inconsolable crying fits. Feeding, cuddling, changing a diaper, bouncing, walking, and feeding (yes, again) should give both you and your baby relief. If nothing helps, call your nurse, midwife, or physician and describe the situation. Persistent, inconsolable crying can be caused by colic, may signal a reaction to a vaccination, or may indicate pain or illness. For help in distinguishing what is troubling your child, it may be necessary to call your health care provider.

Feeding

During your newborn's first few weeks of life, crying usually signals hunger. Babies really do need to eat often. The number of calories per pound of body weight that your new baby needs to grow is greater than it will be at any other time in her life. Your infant's blood sugar level bounces up and down like a yo-yo. To maintain adequate blood sugar, your newborn may nurse avidly, and then need to eat again just ten minutes later. Sometimes it may seem as if playing, resting, and sleeping are just interruptions in your baby's continual quest for calories. Always answer your baby's hunger cry promptly.

Sleeping

Your baby will spend about 80 percent of her resting/sleeping time in shallow sleep, and only about 20 percent of the time in deep sleep. When your newborn seems to be sleeping, she is usually very close to awakening. If you transfer your seemingly sleeping infant from your warm and loving arms to crib or cradle, she will probably awaken.

Some babies sleep easily. Others do not. In utero, your baby was together with her mother 100 percent of the time. It may be difficult for her to give up this intimate contact. Both you and your newborn may have your best sleep with the baby resting on your chest or in your bed with you. This position will help satisfy your baby's deep need for round-the-clock attention or cuddling. Modern Western nations have the only cultures in the world with a taboo against babies sleeping with their parents. Resting or sleeping with your child in the crook of your arm will comfort your newborn, and can relax and soothe a sleepy, lonely toddler as well.

Recent research appears to indicate that sleeping in the prone (stomach down) position may be a factor in sudden infant death syndrome (SIDS), especially when a baby lies on a very soft surface, such as sheepskin.

This can cause a dangerous buildup of carbon dioxide in the blood, which may cause the baby to stop breathing. The current recommendation is that an infant sleep either on her back (supine) or on her side. After a feeding, it is best to keep your baby on her side, with her back supported by a pillow. If she should spit up in this position, the milk will drain out of her mouth and there will be no risk of choking.

Skin Care

During your newborn's first few weeks of life, she will shed every last bit of her "birthday suit." Beginning at the feet and ankles, the dry, cracked, and flaky skin typical of the newborn will gradually peel away.

No matter how good they smell to you, do not apply any scented lotions or potions to your newborn's delicate skin. Don't use preparations containing mineral oil or perfumes. The chemicals they contain can be irritating. Remember, too, that anything you put on your baby's skin may be absorbed into her body.

If you have questions as you care for your new baby, most newborn nurseries have well-trained nurses who can answer routine questions. If you want to know about such things as a rash, constipation, feeding, or daily care, ask a nurse first. Many common newborn problems can be treated easily and gently at home with natural medicine. However, if your baby develops a fever or difficulty breathing, or seems seriously ill, call your doctor immediately. Newborns can get sick very quickly, so you do not want to waste time.

The neonatal period, the time during which your baby is characterized as a "newborn," lasts from birth to twenty-eight days of age. This getting-acquainted period is an exciting and hectic time for you and for your baby. By the end of your infant's newborn days, the household will be a little calmer and more settled. Your baby will be exhibiting real personality and showing delight in little attentions. Relaxed laughter and love should replace your frantic need to jump up anxiously every other moment to check on your new arrival. After this four-week period, your newborn graduates to "baby."

Home Safety

Accidents are the leading cause of injury and death among children ages one to fourteen years. It makes sense to do everything you can to childproof your home against accidents. You may have thought of many of the suggestions contained in this chapter already, but some of them may surprise you.

Your child's age and developmental level will determine the kinds of hazards he is likely to encounter. Infants are attracted to bright and shiny objects. They are curious about everything, and everything they touch goes into their mouths, creating a risk of choking or poisoning. As a baby learns to roll over, sit, crawl, and reach, he can tumble off a bed or changing table, pull a piece of filmy plastic over his face, or slip under water in the bathtub.

Toddlers also are extremely curious. They are attracted to bright packaging, and are learning to open things. Often, they succeed. They are learning to walk and will venture out of sight from time to time.

Because the "terrible twos" are a time when little ones typically start to assert their independence by saying "no," it can be difficult to enforce limits. Toddlers are especially at risk for poisoning, choking, and burns.

Older children are mastering new skills, such as biking and swimming. They are likely to be off exploring in secret places with friends, heedless of dangers. Bicycle accidents, near-drownings, poisoning from berries and outdoor plants, and getting lost are among the potential hazards for this age group. Many authorities recommend gentle but persistent warnings against accepting gifts or other enticements from strangers, as young children tend to be trusting of anyone who acts nice to them.

Teenagers typically feel invincible and immortal. In their desire for independence, they often push parents to the limit. Teenagers are under intense peer pressure to experiment with dangerous substances, to flirt with danger, to dare anything. This age group is at risk for car accidents, bicycle and motorcycle accidents, sports injuries, and toxic ingestion of drugs and alcohol.

Children of any age who are hyperactive, visually or hearing impaired, or physically or mentally handicapped tend to suffer more accidents than other children do. In addition, some children are simply more curious and more adventuresome than others. Some constantly rebel against authority of any kind and continually test their parents' resolve. Such children can be exhausting, but it is your responsibility as a parent to persevere. Remember that children need appropriate limits; without them, a child will feel lost and insecure, even unloved.

The goal is to create a safe environment, and to continually be aware of your child's activities, while maintaining an atmosphere that promotes fun, exploration, learning, and creativity. Most accidents happen when parents are too busy, too tired, or too short of time to be aware of what the kids are getting into. Whether you are simultaneously bustling around getting dressed, worrying about getting breakfast on the table, and readying your child for the day's activities, or in the midst of dinner preparation after a long, exhausting day, try to keep aware of where your child is and what he is doing.

Talk to your child. Using language and explanations your child understands, teach safety considerations both inside and outside of the home. It's much more effective to explain to your child how he could get hurt in a given circumstance than it is to say crossly, "Don't do it because I say so."

Be especially patient with a very young child. Young children have short attention spans and may not have the ability to rationalize and retain information. A young child may be unable to follow directions or understand the consequences of certain actions. Repetition is effective. Even if you have to go over a problem again and again, keep at it until your child understands.

Keep in mind also that children are natural mimics; they imitate the adults around them. It's up to you to set a safe example. As you teach your child to fasten his seat belt, you must also fasten yours. Obey street crossing signals. Don't walk your child across a street against the light. Don't drink and drive.

Try to scan your home carefully with the curious eyes of a child. Get down on your hands and knees and crawl around. Notice that the electrical sockets are at a crawling child's eye level, easily within reach and tempting to poke at. Look for bright, shiny objects, items a child might pop into his mouth. Spot the things your child might grab or pull on with disastrous results. For example, tugging on the trailing edge of a table cover or the loop of an electrical cord could bring a tableful of dishes or a heavy lamp crashing to the floor. At a child's eye level, you'll be able to spot potential hazards more easily.

Be prepared. Not all accidents can be prevented, so knowing how to handle emergencies is an important safety precaution. Learn cardiopulmonary resuscitation (CPR) and first aid. The Red Cross offers courses in first aid, as do many hospitals. The important thing is to learn these procedures *before* you need to use them. Make sure any course you take includes a thorough grounding in infant and child CPR, and take a refresher course every year.

Assemble and keep, in a convenient but secure location, a home health kit stocked with the basics for dealing with illness and injury (see page 73). Check expiration dates periodically and replace any outdated products promptly.

SAFETY CHECKLIST

The safety checklist that follows will help you limit injuries and childproof your home.

Throughout Your Home

☐ Make sure that every room in your home has a working smoke detector. If detectors are wired in, it's a good idea to have a battery-operated backup in case of loss of electricity. Check and replace batteries as required.

☐ Close off electrical outlets with safety devices. These are available in most hardware stores.

☐ Keep floors clean of pins, buttons, food, and any other small objects a child could pick up and put in his mouth.

☐ Put colorful stickers on picture windows and glass doors at your child's eye level, so that he can see them and will not accidentally run into them.

☐ Remove heavy or sharp objects, such as picture frames, vases, and lamps, from tables, or move them away from the edges so that your child cannot pull them over.

☐ Remove tablecloths that might be grabbed and pulled off.

☐ Keep securely closed safety gates at the tops and bottoms of stairs.

☐ Secure windows so that your child cannot reach an open window and fall out. Open windows from the top; keep screens secure. Do not put furniture in front of a window; that offers a path up to the sill.

☐ Tie dangling curtain, drapery, and blind cords out of reach, especially any located near a crib or bed. Children can become entangled in such cords and suffocate.

☐ Keep plastic bags, which can cause suffocation, out of reach of your child at all times.

☐ If any work is being done in your home, talk to the workers about safety considerations for your child. Keep them aware of your child and your safety concerns. Ask them about special child hazards that might be involved in their work. Keep dirty drop cloths away from your child's sleeping and playing areas; be sure tools are properly stored, out of reach, at the end of the work day; keep lids on cans of paints, varnishes, solvents, and other products at all times; and create a safe place for your child, away from dust, nails, tools, splinters, paints, and fumes.

☐ Use only nontoxic and lead-free paints in your home.

☐ Keep all cleaning products, paints, gardening and hobby supplies, and any other dangerous substances out of reach of your child in a locked cabinet.

☐ When using any potentially harmful item, such as a cleaning product, do not let it out of your sight. If you need to leave a room to answer the door or the phone, take the product with you.

☐ Call your local Poison Control Center for information on preventing poisoning. Most centers will send you free literature with detailed instructions on how to poison-proof your home, as well as on what to do (and what *not* to do) in case of poisoning.

☐ Keep all fireplaces securely screened and free of ashes and soot, which can be inhaled by a curious child.

☐ All children are fascinated by fire, and most will eventually want to experiment with matches. Keep matches well hidden and securely out of reach.

☐ Set the temperature for the hot water heater in your home no higher than 120°F. It takes only five seconds for 140°F water to cause a severe third-degree burn, but it takes a full three minutes to get a third-degree burn from 120°F water. Those extra minutes may provide enough time for you to snatch your child out of harm's way and prevent a nasty scald.

Mealtimes

☐ Do not let an infant or young child eat alone. Always keep a watchful eye out to prevent choking.

☐ Eat slowly and chew food thoroughly, and teach your child to do the same. Sit down to eat. Make mealtime a relaxed, happy time.

☐ Cut food into small, bite-sized pieces for your child. Teach him to take small bites from crackers or cookies.

☐ Do not give a young child hot dogs, nuts, raisins, popcorn, or other similar foods. Young children may not chew finger foods sufficiently to prevent choking.

☐ Don't permit your toddler to eat while he is engaged in play activity. It's too easy for a bite to go down wrong if he takes a tumble.

In the Kitchen

☐ Keep all knives and other sharp objects out of reach.

☐ Never store any potentially harmful object in food jars or food storage containers.

☐ When cooking, use the back burners whenever possible, and be sure to keep pot handles turned toward the stove so that your child cannot reach or bump a hot pot.

☐ Keep appliances, such as the toaster, food processor, and blender, unplugged and well away from counter edges.

☐ Cover the garbage disposal.

☐ Place secure plastic fasteners (available in most hardware stores) on cabinet doors to keep your child out of cupboards holding glass, china, cleaning products, and other potentially harmful substances.

☐ Keep a fire extinguisher in a handy location near the stove, but make sure it is out of your child's reach.

In the Bathroom

☐ Apply nonslip surfaces to the bottom of the bathtub.

☐ *Never* leave an infant or young child in the bathtub alone. If you must leave the room to answer the phone or door, wrap your little one in a towel and take him with you.

☐ Keep all medicines and supplements out of reach. Throw away old medicines and prescriptions.

☐ Do not leave medicines or cleaning products on a counter within reach of your child.

☐ If you store potentially harmful products in a cupboard under your bathroom sink, secure the cabinet with a plastic fastener.

☐ Do not leave a razor within reach.

☐ Keep the toilet lid down.

In Your Child's Play Area

☐ Do not give your infant toys that are small enough to fit into his mouth.

☐ Do not give your child any toy that has small parts that could break off.

☐ A teething infant should never be permitted to play with a toy filled with liquid or gel.

☐ Check your child's playthings regularly for breakage and keep them in good repair. If repainting is necessary, use only nontoxic and lead-free paints.

☐ Choose age-appropriate toys carefully. Follow the age guidelines on the packaging. Be aware that these guidelines refer primarily to the ages a child must be to use a toy safely. Thus, if a toy is recommended for children ages two through six, it may not be safe for a child under two, even if the child seems old enough for it in other ways. Also keep an eye out for sharp edges, small parts that could loosen (glass eyes, for example), parts that could break, or any electrical wiring that might not be perfect.

☐ Choose toys made from nontoxic materials.

In the Bedroom

☐ If your baby sleeps in a crib, make sure to use one that meets current federal safety standards. It is possible for an infant to strangle if his head becomes wedged between the bars of a crib.

☐ Protect a sleeping child by making sure he wears flame-retardant clothing.

☐ Never leave your infant alone on a changing table; always keep one hand on your baby. Kicking and wriggling can propel him off the edge.

☐ Keep bureau and table tops clean and clear of sharp objects that could cut your child.

☐ Small objects, such as jewelry and safety pins, can cause choking. Keep them securely out of reach of your child.

Other Areas

☐ Prevent cuts and choking by making sure your sewing area is clean and clear of buttons, pins, needles, and scissors. Such objects are enticing to children.

Pets and Your Child

One of the most delightful aspects of childhood is interacting with pets. For the most part, a domestic animal in the household brings a unique type of unconditional love to every family member.

But there can be trouble in paradise. A once-fussed-over pet who has been in the family for a long time can become jealous of the attention paid to a new baby. Fido or Fluffy may express his dismay at being replaced in your affections by hiding or sulking—or by growling, snarling, even nipping or clawing at a newborn. Introducing a pet to a new baby takes patience and love, as well as watchfulness whenever pet and child are together.

There are also a number of diseases that can be transmitted from a pet to family members. Infectious and parasitic diseases in humans can be caused by viruses, bacteria, fungi, protozoa, worms, insects, or mites living on or in an animal. Diseases contracted from family pets—especially the more serious ones—are rare, but they do occur.

Animals usually transmit diseases or parasites to humans through saliva or by direct contact. Ticks, mites, and fungi living in an animal's fur can be transferred to a child who hugs or strokes an animal. Fleas will jump from an infested area onto a human if no animal host is available. Worm eggs or parasites infesting contaminated animal feces can be accidentally transmitted to humans by fingers or food.

The transmission of serious diseases from animals to humans can be prevented by practicing good hygiene and by keeping a watchful eye as children play with animals.

Any interaction between a pet and an infant should be closely supervised. Babies can't defend themselves against being scratched or bitten, or even against a wet tongue giving a "kiss."

Young children should be taught never to approach a strange animal, and they should be monitored when playing with family pets. It can take only a moment for play to turn rough. After they play with pets, children should have their hands washed thoroughly, with special attention to the fingernails.

To make sure that your child does not come in contact with animal feces, which may be contaminated, designate a separate, fenced outdoor area as your dog's toilet facilities, and "scoop" the area regularly to keep it clean so that he doesn't bring bits of fecal matter into the house on his feet. For cats, put the litter box in a place to which your child does not have access. Be inventive. Cats can squeeze through a tiny space, such as a cupboard or closet door that has been left ajar but secured against curious little fingers. Keep a cat's litter box scrupulously clean; sift out feces regularly and sweep up and carefully dispose of any litter that spills outside the box. This task should *not* be performed by a woman who is, or plans to become, pregnant (*see* Toxoplasmosis, page 71).

Make sure your pets get good routine health care, including regular worming and flea treatment. Keep your child away from any animal that is obviously ill, and take sick pets to the veterinarian promptly for treatment.

Following is a discussion of some of the diseases that children can contract through contact with animals.

DISEASES TRANSMITTED BY DOGS

- **Hookworms.** Hookworms typically infect the lower intestine, but can also cause pneumonia. Children who are permitted to play barefoot in areas where worm-contaminated dog feces have been dropped are particularly at risk of a hookworm infestation. Symptoms include a red and intensely itchy rash that develops around the site where the larvae penetrate the skin, typically on the feet. Treatment consists of drugs that rid the body of the worms. If a child becomes anemic, he may require supplemental iron. In an extremely serious, long-lasting infestation, a blood transfusion may become necessary.

- **Ticks.** A tick is a blood-sucking arachnid. Barbs on its proboscis, or feeding snout, enable a tick to attach itself to the skin of its victim to feed. Ticks are extremely tenacious. Even when fully engorged with blood, they seldom let go spontaneously. Because the barbs are deeply embedded, it is useless to try to pull a tick off with your fingers. Even if you manage to pinch off the body completely, the head and feeding proboscis can remain attached. The most effective way to remove a tick is to use a pair of tweezers. Grasp the tick's head as close to your child's skin as you can, then pull back slowly and firmly until the tick pulls free. Once the tick is removed, thoroughly wash and rinse the site of the injury. To reduce the risk of infection, apply rubbing alcohol or calendula tincture, followed by an antibiotic ointment, such as bacitracin, Betadine, or goldenseal.

DISEASES TRANSMITTED BY CATS

- **Cat scratch disease.** Cat scratch disease (also known as cat scratch fever) begins with a scratch or a claw puncture that becomes infected and resembles a small boil. The scratch may be deep and obvious, or it may not leave a mark at all. Cat scratch disease is most commonly reported in children under ten years of age. The suspected cause is a microbe called *Rochalimaea henselae*, which may be transmitted from cat to cat by fleas. Symptoms include swollen lymph nodes, weakness, nausea, chills, loss of appetite, headache, and low-grade fever. Some children run a fever of over 101°F for about a week; others break out in a measles-like rash. The symptoms can last for months and, in rare cases, can progress to encephalitis, an inflammation of the brain. Conventional antibiotics show varying but limited effectiveness against cat scratch disease, although trimethoprim-sulfa (Bactrim or Septra) and erythromycin are sometimes tried in complicated cases. Standard treatment includes washing the site of a cat scratch well, applying a disinfectant promptly, and keeping the area clean. Natural treatments (such as those recommended under SURGERY, RECOVERY FROM in Part Two of this book) can help support your child's body as it fights off the infection.

- **Toxoplasmosis.** A central nervous system disease, toxoplasmosis is caused by a single-celled organism, the protozoan *Toxoplasma gondii*, which is particularly fond of cats. Symptoms can include fever, blurred vision, swollen lymph nodes, muscle aches, and an enlarged spleen. It is usually transmitted to humans through infected cat feces, although inadequately cooked meat may also be a source. Toxoplasmosis is especially dangerous to children *before* they are born. If a mother-to-be becomes infected with toxoplasmosis, there is a possibility the parasite may migrate through the placenta to the fetus. A toxoplasmosis infection in early pregnancy can cause a miscarriage or severe malformation of the unborn child; in later pregnancy, it can result in serious damage to the developing child's nervous system. A child infected with toxoplasmosis as a fetus may become blind in early childhood.

  Treatment of toxoplasmosis is complicated and involves multiple medications. Care of an affected child should be handled by a medical doctor with expertise in this condition. To prevent fetal infection, a pregnant woman should never change a cat's litter box.

DISEASES TRANSMITTED BY BOTH DOGS AND CATS

- **Fleas.** Flea bites are usually more of a nuisance than a serious health problem, although they do itch and may become infected when they are scratched—especially if unwashed little fingers do the scratching. Fleas prefer animal hosts. But if any fleas get left behind when the family pet is out, they will feed on whatever human is handy. Treatment for flea bites begins with thorough cleansing of the site. To reduce the itching that can prompt a child to scratch, use calamine or Caladryl lotion, or witch hazel.

- **Rabies.** On the opposite end of the scale, rabies is a deadly disease. Any animal bite can cause bleeding and shock, but a child who is bitten by a rabid animal requires immediate vaccination (*see* BITES, ANIMAL AND HUMAN in Part Two of this book). The most commonly affected animals are dogs, cats, skunks, raccoons, and bats. Rats, mice, chipmunks, squirrels, hamsters, guinea pigs, gerbils, and rabbits are rarely implicated. Any animal suspected of carrying rabies should be quarantined for at least ten days.

- **Ringworm.** A surprising number of childhood ringworm infections come from family pets, especially cats. Unlike infected dogs, which are afflicted with hair loss and bare patches, cats rarely show obvious signs when carrying this infection. To check a cat for ringworm, examine its coat closely under ultraviolet (UV) light. UV rays cause the fungus to glow, making it visible on infected skin and hair (*see* RINGWORM in Part Two of this book).

- **Toxocariasis.** This is a serious parasitic disease. Children can contract toxocariasis through accidental ingestion of worm eggs, which are present in infested dog or cat feces. Children, especially the few who eat dirt, are particularly at risk. As the worm passes through the body, it can cause asthma-like and other allergic symptoms, respiratory difficulties, an enlarged liver, and skin rashes. Drug therapy is not very useful in fighting this disease, but recovery usually occurs spontaneously. In rare cases, a worm egg can infect an eye, causing deteriorating vision or even blindness. This manifestation of toxocariasis is most likely to occur in children who frequently play in soil or sand that has been contaminated by infected dog or cat feces. It must be treated by an ophthalmologist.

☐ Keep your sewing machine unplugged when not in use, and the cord securely out of reach.

☐ Garages, tool sheds, and workshops should be securely locked and off-limits to young children.

Outside Your Home

☐ When your child is a passenger in an automobile, keep him securely buckled up in an appropriate safety restraint at all times. Consumer magazines, the United States Department of Transportation, and the National Child Passenger Safety Association (located in Ardmore, Pennsylvania) can provide information on approved child restraint systems.

☐ Make sure your child wears appropriate protective gear when engaging in sports activities. A helmet should be worn for bicycling, horseback riding, skiing, skateboarding, and roller blading, as well as organized sports like baseball, football, hockey, and lacrosse. Eye protection is recommended for children who play baseball, hockey, racquet sports, football, basketball, and golf. Goggles are useful for protecting a child from chlorine and other chemicals while swimming. Other types of protective gear that may be appropriate include knee pads, elbow pads, shin guards, mouth guards, and padded gloves.

☐ Teach your child to cross streets safely. Young children should be taught to cross a street only in the company of an adult, never alone.

☐ Teach children to swim and teach them water safety.

☐ Never leave a child alone near a swimming pool, lake, pond, or any other body of water. Every summer, there are many instances of drowning and near-drowning that occur because young children are left unsupervised. Swimming pools should be securely fenced.

☐ When your child is riding in a boat, make sure he is wearing a life jacket.

☐ Before allowing your child to skate on a frozen pond, check with local authorities to make sure the ice is safe.

☐ Keep your child's playground equipment in good repair. Put a cushioning layer of sand under slides, swings, and jungle gyms to soften a possible fall.

☐ Always supervise a young child when he is playing outside. Be sure to keep him well away from the street. Teach your child never to chase a ball, another child, or a pet into the street.

☐ Children should never be permitted to play with fireworks. Most states prohibit the sale of fireworks to individuals, but people still manage to obtain them. Every year, some children suffer severe burns—or worse—from accidents connected with fireworks.

☐ Insist that your teenager take a driver's education course before getting his driver's license. This shouldn't be difficult; most high schools provide driving instruction. "Driver's Ed" classes are an eagerly anticipated milestone for most teenagers.

☐ Never drink and drive. Teach your teenager about the consequences and very real dangers of drinking and driving, or accepting a ride from anyone who has been drinking.

☐ Do not grow poisonous plants either inside or outside your home. The ivy and the split-leaf philodendron that look so pretty on your end tables, as well as the flowering azaleas and daffodils that brighten your yard, can be lethal if ingested. Some common plants that should be avoided are apricot, azalea, Boston ivy, caladium, castor bean, chokeberry, daffodil (jonquil, narcissus), dumb cane (dieffenbachia), emerald duke, English ivy, foxglove, hen and chicks (lantana), hydrangea, jimsonweed, lily of the valley, mistletoe, morning glory, nightshade, oleander, parlor ivy (philodendron), poison ivy, poison oak, poison sumac, rhododendron, rhubarb, split-leaf philodendron, sweet pea, tulip, and wisteria.

Not all accidents are preventable, of course, but many are. Thinking ahead is the key. Stay one step ahead of your child. By childproofing your home, you can protect against many home accidents, and also keep to a minimum the hazards your child will encounter outside.

EMERGENCY PREPAREDNESS

No matter how careful and loving parents are, they cannot prevent all of the accidents and emergencies that can arise while their children are growing up. But you can and should take measures so that you will be prepared to act quickly and effectively should an emergency arise.

Emergency Telephone Numbers

Post emergency telephone numbers near every telephone in your home. This can save precious time in any emergency, for you or for anyone else who is caring for your child. We urge you to take this precaution now, while you are thinking about it. If there is no 911 emergency service in your area, these numbers should include that of your local hospital for ambulance/paramedic service. Also post numbers for your local fire department, Poison Control Center, police, and your child's doctor and dentist.

If your telephone is the type that allows you to program numbers for automatic dialing, enter these emergency numbers into the phone as well, and label the appropriate keys clearly. Some telephone models come with keys already labeled for police, fire, and other emergency numbers, which makes this even easier. However, you should not consider this a substitute for keeping emergency numbers on hand in written form. It is possible for programmed numbers to be erased accidentally, so you should still keep a list of emergency telephone numbers in a convenient location.

Designated Surrogates

Choose and empower surrogates who can act in your stead if an emergency arises when you cannot be reached, and include their telephone numbers in the emergency list. Designate adults you trust, perhaps your child's grandparents, perhaps good friends, to make decisions in any emergency involving your child. If you have established a close and caring relationship with your child's health care provider, you might wish to empower him or her to make any necessary medical decisions involving your child. Give your surrogates written permission to act for you, such as a limited power of attorney. Your surrogates should keep this important document where it can be found easily if they must respond to an emergency, and you should give copies to your child's physician. Should an occasion ever arise when you cannot be reached immediately, your designated surrogates will be able to act. Written permission from a parent or designated guardian is sometimes required before certain life-saving measures can be taken.

Medic Alert

If you have a child with a special medical problem, obtain a Medic Alert bracelet to ensure that he will receive the right care if something happens away from home. If your child is allergic to penicillin or other medication, sulfites, or bee stings, for example, it will enable him to receive prompt and appropriate treatment for an allergic reaction. Without a Medic Alert bracelet, a diabetic teenager suffering from the typical symptoms of low blood sugar could be misdiagnosed as being intoxicated and fail to receive necessary treatment. Medic Alert information is especially important for a young child who may not be able to communicate well, or for any child who has a disorder that can cause the loss of consciousness. Without Medic Alert information, health care personnel could be working in the dark and wasting precious time. Medic Alert is the only emergency medical identification service endorsed by the American College of Emergency Physicians, the American Hospital Association, and every national pharmacy association. For more information, call Medic Alert at 800–432–5378.

First Aid Training

The primary child care provider in every household should take a good course in emergency first aid that includes infant and childhood cardiopulmonary resuscitation (CPR) procedures. We hope that you will never be called upon to use these skills, but there is simply no substitute for the hands-on training and practice in these life-saving techniques that such a course provides.

The Well-Stocked Home Health Kit

Every home should have a well-stocked home health kit. A good home health kit includes not only the bare essentials for dealing with emergencies, such as bandages, tweezers, and hydrogen peroxide, but also the basic medicines—conventional, herbal, homeopathic, and others—that are used over and over again for common illnesses (*see* Assembling a Home Health Kit on page 74). Your home health kit should be stored in a location that is convenient, but securely locked away from or out of the reach of children, and you should check it at least every three months or so to replace any products that have passed their expiration dates or that have been used up.

One of the most important things you can do for your child is to be prepared. It's impossible to create an environment so safe that there is no possibility a child will be injured, of course, just as it is impossible to prevent your child from ever becoming ill. But by scanning your home and your surroundings for potential hazards—and then eliminating them—you can prevent many of the common kinds of accidents that children are prone to suffer.

The second element of preparedness is to assemble the things you may need to treat your child should illness or injury strike. It's always stressful when your child needs your help in a hurry. But if you know that what you need is ready and on hand, you can save yourself from frantic searching and scrambling and place your focus where it belongs—on your child. This means faster treatment, as well as a less anxiety-filled experience for both parent and child. An environment that is nurturing and reassuring is an invaluable part of health and healing.

Assembling a Home Health Kit

Assembling a home health kit will give you a good base for treating the most common childhood illnesses and injuries. Begin putting it together now, so that if your child does get hurt or sick, the right treatments and remedies will be close at hand. Use the checklist that follows as a guide to some of the most important elements for a variety of different treatment approaches.

Bare Essentials

- Ace bandage.
- Adhesive bandages (Band-Aids).
- Bulb syringe.
- Hot water bottle.
- Ice bag.
- Prescription insect bite kit containing adrenaline (such as Ana-Kit or EpiPen) if your child is allergic to bites or stings.
- Rubbing alcohol, hydrogen peroxide, or witch hazel, for disinfecting wounds and sterilizing needle and tweezers.
- Scissors with rounded tips.
- Sling and safety pins.
- Sterile gauze pads and adhesive tape.
- Sterile razor blade.
- Sterilized needle.
- Syrup of ipecac.
  Caution: Syrup of ipecac should not be used except at the direction of a doctor or Poison Control Center.
- Thermometer.
- Tweezers.

Conventional Medicines

- Acetaminophen (such as Tylenol, Tempra, or the equivalent) or ibuprofen (Advil, Nuprin, Pedia-Profen, and others).
- An antihistamine (such as Benadryl or Chlor-Trimeton).
- An antiseptic ointment (such as bacitracin or Betadine).
- A decongestant (such as Sudafed).
- Emetrol syrup.
- Milk of magnesia.
- Pepto-Bismol.

Herbal Medicines

- Aloe vera gel.
- Calendula cream.
- Chamomile tea or extract.
- Echinacea tincture.
- Echinacea and goldenseal liquid combination formula.
- Flaxseed tea.
- Garlic, in capsules or fresh.
- Ginger root, in capsules or fresh.
- Licorice root extract.
- Peppermint tea or extract.
- Slippery elm powder.
- Umeboshi plum paste.
- Yin qiao tincture (liquid extract).

Homeopathic Remedies

- *Aconite.*
- *Apis mellifica.*
- *Arnica.*
- *Arnica* ointment.
- *Arsenicum album.*
- *Belladonna.*
- *Bryonia.*
- *Calcarea carbonica.*
- *Cantharis.*
- *Carbo vegetabilis.*
- *Chamomilla.*
- *Ferrum phosphoricum.*

Homeopathic Remedies (continued)

- *Gelsemium.*
- *Hepar sulphuris.*
- *Hydrastis.*
- *Hypericum.*
- *Hypericum* ointment.
- *Kali bichromicum.*
- *Kali muriaticum.*
- *Ledum.*
- *Lycopodium.*
- *Magnesia phosphorica.*
- *Mercurius dulcis.*
- *Mercurius solubilis.*
- *Nux vomica.*
- *Pulsatilla.*
- *Rhus toxicodendron.*
- *Ruta graveolens.*
- *Sulphur.*
- *Thuja.*
- *Urtica urens.*
- *Urtica urens* ointment.

Bach Flower Remedies

- Rescue Remedy.

Nutritional Supplements

- Vitamin-B complex liquid.
- Vitamin C with bioflavonoids.
- Calcium and magnesium combination formula (liquid or capsule).
- Zinc lozenges.

Miscellaneous

- Apple or grape juice, or applesauce, to mix with herbs or crushed tablets.
- Eyedropper or needleless syringe to administer liquid medicines.
- Honey, barley malt, or rice bran syrup.
- Save•A•Tooth solution (see page 396).
- Smelling salts.

PREVENTION

■ If possible, keep your child from coming into contact with plants that cause an allergic reaction, especially during their pollination seasons.

■ If animal dander causes a reaction, keep pets outside. Above all, do not let them inside an allergic child's bedroom.

■ If your child suffers from chronic allergies, look for environmental factors that may be contributing to the problem. Eliminate all possible allergens, such as dust, molds, cigarette smoke, and wood smoke. It may be necessary to eliminate feather pillows and household items that collect and hold dust, such as stuffed animals, rugs, draperies, and even upholstered furniture.

■ Check for and eliminate foods that may be the source of a hypersensitivity or allergic reaction.

■ Give your child astragalus to strengthen his immune system.

■ Visit a homeopath for a constitutional remedy for your child.

■ Provide your child with a smoke-free environment. If you smoke, please quit. Children with allergies are especially vulnerable to the effects of secondhand smoke. Wood stoves can also be a source of respiratory irritation.

Anaphylactic Shock

Anaphylactic shock is a severe and violent allergic response that may occur as a result of contact with an allergen. Possible allergens include chemicals, medicines, vaccines, particular foods or food additives—such as sulfites—and insect venom. Anaphylactic shock may cause severe breathing distress and can be life threatening.

In anaphylactic shock, the body's reaction to an allergen can cause a swelling of the air passages, with a consequent narrowing of the airway, resulting in extreme difficulty in breathing. In rare instances, your child's tongue and air passages may swell to the point where the airway closes and breathing becomes almost impossible.

Symptoms usually come on rapidly, most often within one to fifteen minutes of contact with an allergen. The more quickly a reaction begins, the more severe it is likely to be. The first signs that your child is suffering a reaction can include a sense of uneasiness, agitation, weakness, sweating, flushing, and shortness of breath, accompanied by intense fear and anxiety. Another early sign may be the presence of itchy hives that begin to spread rapidly all over the body. Other symptoms may include restlessness, falling blood pressure, shock, uneven heartbeat, wheezing, trouble swallowing, nausea, and diarrhea.

Seeing your child become terrified as she suffers this kind of an allergic reaction is frightening. But *don't panic*. As you seek treatment for your child, encourage her to calm down. Crying and screaming makes breathing even more difficult. If you become visibly upset, your child will only become more frightened. It is important that you remain calm and try to soothe her with reassuring words and your gentle touch.

EMERGENCY TREATMENT FOR ANAPHYLACTIC SHOCK

✚ At the slightest sign that your child may be having difficulty breathing due to a severe allergic reaction—especially if she has a history of such reactions—take her immediately to the emergency room of the nearest hospital. If you cannot transport your child yourself and must call for emergency help, stress the gravity of the situation. Seconds count. If an emergency adrenaline kit such as Ana-Kit or EpiPen is available, administer it immediately. Follow this with 50 milligrams of Benadryl. If Benadryl is not readily available, chlorpheniramine (Chlor-Trimeton or the equivalent) may be substituted.

✚ *Do not* give your child anything to eat or drink while she is experiencing severe breathing distress.

CONVENTIONAL TREATMENT

■ Seek emergency medical help immediately. Emergency personnel may administer epinephrine (Adrenalin or Sus-Phrine, a long-acting form), an antihistamine (such as Benadryl), intravenous steroids (hydrocortisone or prednisone), or a bronchodilator (such as Alupent or Bronkosol) to counteract the allergen, decrease inflammation, and open the airway to restore free breathing. If treatment is begun soon enough, you can expect a dramatic easing of the situation. If your child's blood pressure is extremely low, intravenous fluids may be administered as well.

HOMEOPATHY

■ Once the crisis is over and it is safe to give your child something by mouth, you may want to give your child one dose of *Aconite* 200x, 200c, or 30c to help allay the emotional distress following such an episode.

BACH FLOWER REMEDIES

■ If your child has calmed sufficiently after emergency medical personnel have administered treatment, you may give her a dose of Bach Flower Rescue Remedy on the way to the hospital. This remedy helps to ease anxiety and fright.

■ Once your child has come home from the hospital, give her one dose of Mimulus—the remedy for fear of known things—each day, for one week after the incident. (See BACH FLOWER REMEDIES in Part One.)

GENERAL RECOMMENDATIONS

■ Once the immediate crisis has passed and the source of your child's reaction has been diagnosed, *see* ALLERGIES; ASTHMA; BITES AND STINGS; or FOOD ALLERGIES, if appropriate, for natural therapies that will help support your child's full recovery from an ordeal of this nature.

PREVENTION

■ Unfortunately, there is no way to know ahead of time that your child is allergic to a particular substance. Should your child ever suffer a dangerous allergic reaction, however, it goes without saying that you should protect her from any future contact with the allergen.

■ If you have reason to suspect that your child is susceptible to anaphylaxis, based on previous reactions or family history, ask your doctor to prescribe a home emergency kit containing epinephrine, such as the Ana-Kit or EpiPen, and be sure you learn how to administer it correctly. Having a supply of epinephrine on hand may someday save your child's life.

Appendicitis

Appendicitis is an acute inflammation of the appendix, a thin, tube-shaped structure that protrudes from the first section of the large intestine. The appendix can become inflamed due either to an anatomical obstruction or a blockage of hardened feces. This inflammation can rapidly develop into an infection.

Symptoms of appendicitis usually begin with pain around the umbilicus that intensifies over several hours and moves to the lower right quadrant of the abdomen. This area will be very tender to even light pressure, and you may notice your child holding or protecting it. A decreased appetite, vomiting, and fever are frequently present. Diarrhea may be present as well, and extending the right leg may make the pain worse.

An inflamed appendix can burst, causing a life-threatening infection of the abdominal wall. If this happens, your child will rapidly become very ill, with a fever, pale color, and severe abdominal pain. Although a complaint of continuous abdominal pain is a key indicator of appendicitis, some children experience a milder onset of pain that comes and goes over several days before settling in as constant and severe. If you suspect appendicitis, seek immediate medical care.

CONVENTIONAL TREATMENT

■ In order to diagnose appendicitis, a doctor will want to know details of when the pain began and the location and quality of the pain. Your doctor will do an abdominal and rectal exam, take a sample of blood to look for signs of an infection, and might order an x-ray or ultrasound scan to look for signs of blockage or inflammation.

■ If a diagnosis of appendicitis is confirmed, surgery to remove the inflamed appendix is the recommended course of treatment. Because of the danger that the appendix may rupture, surgery is usually done soon after the diagnosis is made.

■ To lower the risk of infection, your child may be given antibiotics before and immediately after surgery. If his appendix has ruptured, your child will definitely need intravenous antibiotics, and may need to be hospitalized for one to two weeks.

■ Because of the surgery and the manipulation of your child's digestive tract, the intestines will slow down, and may even stop moving for a day or two. Your child may have a nasogastric tube, a tube placed in the nose and down into the stomach, that uses suction to pull the contents of the stomach out of the body. This prevents nausea and vomiting. Except for an occasional ice chip, your child will not be able to eat or drink anything until his intestines begin working again. He will receive intravenous fluids to prevent dehydration and pain medication to help relieve discomfort.

■ Your child will have to get up out of bed and walk the day after surgery. Even though this may seem like a daunting task, the importance of movement cannot be overemphasized. Among other things, walking helps the intestines to begin working again, and helps to prevent pneumonia from developing.

DIETARY GUIDELINES

■ Even after your doctor gives full permission for him to eat, your child may have little or no appetite. Begin slowly by offering clear liquids, such as broth, juices, and herbal teas.

■ To allow your child's gastrointestinal tract to readjust to food, gradually work

SYMPTOMS OF APPENDICITIS

The main symptom of appendicitis is abdominal pain that is characterized by one or more of the following:

● It is localized on the right side of the abdomen, or it begins around the navel and gradually moves to the lower right quadrant of the abdomen.

● It is persistent, steady, and intensifies over a period of several hours.

● It feels worse if your child sneezes, coughs, or breathes deeply. It may feel worse if your child extends his right leg.

● The painful area is very tender to the touch.

If you suspect your child may be developing appendicitis, consult your doctor or seek emergency help right away.

up to a full diet. Prepare whole, well-cooked foods that are full of the many vitamins and minerals your child's body needs to heal and regain energy.

■ Homemade applesauce and soups are excellent "starter" foods for a child who has undergone surgery. Foods high in beta-carotene, such as squash and cooked greens, are also important.

■ Try to avoid giving your child any gas-producing foods, such as nuts and legumes, for the first two weeks after surgery.

NUTRITIONAL SUPPLEMENTS

For age-appropriate dosages of some nutritional supplements, see page 81.

■ Beta-carotene, a precursor of vitamin A, helps to soothe injured mucous membranes and heal tissue. Give your child one dose of beta-carotene each day for one month.

■ *Lactobacillus acidophilus* and *bifidus* are both very good for restoring bowel health after the trauma of surgery and potent antibiotics. Follow the dosage directions on the product label and give your child one dose, twice a day, for one month. Then give your child one dose, once a day, for the second month.

■ The B vitamins help to restore strength. Give your child a liquid or capsule B-complex supplement, once a day, for one month.

■ Vitamin C and bioflavonoids aid in tissue repair and in decreasing inflammation. Give your child one dose of each, one to two times a day, for one month.

■ Vitamin E is an antioxidant nutrient and is a mild but effective natural anti-inflammatory. Give your child one dose, twice a day, for one month.

■ Zinc hastens wound and tissue healing and supports the immune system. Give your child a total of one dose of zinc each day for one month.

Note: Excessive amounts of zinc can result in nausea and vomiting. Be careful not to exceed the recommended dosage. Zinc is easiest on the stomach when taken at the beginning of a meal.

HERBAL TREATMENT

Herbal treatment for appendicitis is directed at supporting recovery from surgery. It is not meant to be a substitute for surgical treatment. If you suspect appendicitis, seek medical treatment for your child immediately. For age-appropriate dosages of herbal remedies, see page 81.

■ Once the crisis is over, follow the regimen below to help your child recover.

Days 1–3: Give your child an echinacea and goldenseal combination formula to help detoxify the chemicals remaining in his blood after anesthesia. Echinacea and goldenseal also support the immune system and can help prevent a possible infection in a surgical wound. Give your child one dose, two to three times daily.

Days 4–7: Give your child one dose of astragalus (*Astragalus membranaceous*), three times daily. With its rich concentration of trace minerals and micronutrients, astragalus helps to strengthen the immune system. Do not give this herb to a child with a fever, however. If there is fever, continue giving your child echinacea and goldenseal until the fever is gone (but not for more than ten days in a row, or it will lose its effectiveness).

Days 8–14: Give your child one dose of American ginseng, three times daily. This is another excellent source of trace minerals and micronutrients, and will help strengthen your child's internal defenses.

Note: This herb should not be given if fever or any other signs of infection are present.

Days 15–21: Give your child two to three doses of nettle and/or gotu kola daily. These herbs contain many trace minerals, are very useful for healing wounds, and are good general tonics.

Note: Neither gotu kola nor nettle should be given to a child under four years of age. Also, some children experience stomach upset as a result of taking nettle. If this happens, discontinue use of the herb.

Days 21–35: Give your child one dose of minor bupleurum formula, twice daily. This is a Chinese herbal combination that is a good tonic and will help to restore strength.

Note: Minor bupleurum should not be given to a child with a fever or any other sign of an acute infection.

■ Once the wound has closed and healing has begun, and your surgeon gives you the okay, gently rub vitamin E oil, castor oil, or evening primrose oil into the wound to minimize scarring.

HOMEOPATHY

Homeopathic treatment for appendicitis is directed at supporting recovery from surgery. It is not meant to be a substitute for surgical treatment. If you suspect appendicitis, seek professional medical treatment for your child immediately.

■ If your child seems to have had an adverse reaction to anesthesia, give him one dose of *Nux vomica* 30x or 200x to help lessen the side effects. Then follow this regimen to aid your child in his recovery from surgery.

Days 1–2: Give your child one dose of *Arnica* 30x or 9c, three or four times daily. *Arnica* helps to decrease inflammation following surgery and speeds the healing process.

Days 3–4: Give your child one dose of *Staphysagria* 30x or 15c, three times a day, to help the incision heal.

Day 4: To further hasten healing, give your child *Ledum* 12x or 6c, three times during the day.

Days 5–6: For nerve pain following surgery, give your child one dose of *Hypericum* 6x or 5c, three times a day.

ACUPRESSURE

For the locations of acupressure points on a child's body, see ADMINISTERING AN ACUPRESSURE TREATMENT in Part Three.

■ Massaging the stomach meridian, particularly Stomach 36, will help tone the digestive tract and speed recovery.

GENERAL RECOMMENDATIONS

■ To ensure a full and strong recovery after surgery, adequate rest is essential. Limit visitors and create a calm and familiar environment.

■ Once discharged from the hospital, your child will have periods of fatigue. Resuming a daily routine is probably fine, although he may need more rest than usual until his full strength is back. To help increase his energy level, you can give your child a liquid B-complex supplement for two weeks. One dose of American ginseng, given at approximately 11:00 A.M. daily, can also be helpful.

■ Contact sports, heavy lifting, and abdominal exercises must be avoided for as long as your doctor recommends, probably for six to eight weeks after surgery.

PREVENTION

■ There is no known way to prevent your child from developing appendicitis. Your best defense against the disease is to be aware of its characteristic symptoms, so that if your child develops appendicitis, he can be treated promptly and recover without complications.

Asthma

Asthma is an inflammatory respiratory illness characterized by mild to severe difficulty in breathing. This is caused by constriction and swelling of the airways, along with an increase in secretions of mucus, which plugs up the smaller passages. As a result, air cannot get into or out of the lungs as easily as it usually does. Wheezing results as air squeaks through the narrowed and inflamed air passages. An asthma attack can cause such shortness of breath and poor oxygen intake that a child may need to be hospitalized.

Asthma can be triggered by a variety of things, including exposure to pollen, dust, feathers, molds, animal dander, pollution, cigarette smoke, or cold dry air, as well as an upper respiratory infection, exercise, excitement, and stress. Sometimes a child will develop an asthma attack for no apparent reason.

A child experiencing an asthma attack will cough, wheeze, have an increased respiratory rate, have a feeling of tightness in her chest, and have difficulty breathing. Early signs of an asthma attack include an itchy throat, a change in breathing pattern, fatigue, paleness, nervousness, a runny nose, or moodiness. It is important to watch your child carefully and treat her quickly if you notice an asthma attack coming on. If you have any doubts as to your child's breathing, don't hesitate to call your doctor.

If your child suffers from asthma, one simple way you can monitor her breathing is with an instrument called a *peak flow meter*, available at many large drug stores and through medical supply catalogs. These are relatively inexpensive, simple-to-use devices that measure how much air pressure your child can exert with a full exhalation. The meter's indicator can be used to compare how your child's air flow changes from day to day. By monitoring this way, you will have a more reliable means of determining whether your child's condition is getting better or worse. Your physician will help you determine what to watch for with your child.

CONVENTIONAL TREATMENT

■ For chronic asthma, steroids are currently the conventional treatment of choice.

These medicines work by decreasing the swelling and inflammation of the airways. They can be taken orally or inhaled. Inhaled steroids (including Beclovent, Vanceril, AeroBid, and Azmacort) are more commonly used; oral steroids (such as Pediapred) are generally used only in more severe cases. All steroids potentially have significant side effects, especially when taken over the long term, that need to be understood. Talk this over with your doctor or nurse.

■ Bronchodilators, in either oral or inhaled form, may be prescribed for the relief of occasional symptoms of asthma. These medications work to open up the airways, easing breathing. Inhaled bronchodilators that may be prescribed include Alupent, Maxair, and Ventolin. Oral medications in this category (which include Alupent and theophylline-based drugs) are rarely used today because they can cause side effects such as restlessness, insomnia, headache, loss of appetite, increased heart rate, dizziness, nausea, and vomiting. Long-term use of theophylline may also be associated with behavioral problems and learning disabilities, although the evidence for this is not conclusive.

DIETARY GUIDELINES

■ A child who has asthma should eat a healthy, whole-foods diet based on lean proteins, grains, fruits, and vegetables. Avoid excessive saturated and animal fats.

■ Avoid giving your child dairy foods, which tend to increase the production of mucus.

■ Beware of foods such as nuts, citrus fruits, whole-wheat products (especially yeasted breads), seafood, and foods containing additives like preservatives or food dyes, as well as contact with animals. Any of these items can cause or exacerbate an allergy-induced asthma attack in susceptible children.

■ Following an asthma attack, encourage your child to drink plenty of fluids once her condition is stable enough for her to do so. It is important to thin secretions so that they are easily coughed out.

NUTRITIONAL SUPPLEMENTS

Nutritional supplements for asthma are directed at preventing or supporting recovery from an asthma attack, rather than treating an acute episode. In the event of an acute asthma attack, seek immediate medical care for your child. For age-appropriate dosages of nutritional supplements, see page 81.

■ Essential fatty acids (EFAs) help to regulate the inflammatory response. Good sources are evening primrose oil or EPA (fish oil). Give your child either of these supplements, one to three times a day, for two to three months, following the dosage directions on the product label. A combination of the two may be more effective in some children.

Note: Evening primrose oil should not be given to a child who has a fever.

■ Magnesium has a bronchodilating effect if taken in the proper dosage. Some doctors give magnesium sulfate by injection to treat acute asthma attacks. Try giving your child one dose of magnesium, twice a day. If she develops loose stool, reduce the dosage.

■ Pantothenic acid (vitamin B5) supports adrenal function and the nervous

EMERGENCY TREATMENT FOR ASTHMA

✚ In the event of a severe asthma attack, you need to seek immediate medical care for your child. If your child's asthma is not resolving using the treatments you know, call your physician and take your child to the emergency room.

✚ At the hospital, your child will probably be given an inhaled medication that sprays a bronchodilator (a substance that opens air passages to restore free breathing) directly into the airways. If this does not help, she may receive other drugs, such as intravenous steroids or theophylline, and may need to be hospitalized. In some cases a child will need to receive oxygen to ease the work of breathing.

✚ On the way to the hospital, you can give your child one dose of homeopathic *Aconite* to help ease her fear. Five minutes after administering the *Aconite*, give your child one dose of Bach Flower Rescue Remedy. This calming remedy will help ease the shock, anxiety, or fright your child may be experiencing.

system. Give your child one dose of pantothenic acid, two or three times a day, for two months.

Note: When giving your child supplements of any of the B vitamins, it is best to give a daily B-vitamin complex supplement as well.

■ Vitamin B$_{12}$ deficiency has been linked to some types of asthmatic conditions. Given in either oral or injectible form, this vitamin can help to prevent an asthma attack. Discuss this with a nutritionally oriented physician.

HERBAL TREATMENT

Herbal treatments for asthma are directed at preventing or supporting recovery from an asthma attack, rather than treating an acute episode. In the event of an acute asthma attack, seek immediate medical care for your child. For age-appropriate dosages of herbal remedies, see page 81.

■ Astragalus (*Astragalus membranaceous*) is a Chinese herb that helps to increase what the Chinese call *wei chi*, or a person's own protective energy. It also helps strengthen the lungs. Give your child one dose, twice a day, for two weeks out of every month, for six months following an asthma attack.

Note: This herb should not be given if a fever or any other signs of infection are present.

■ Licorice root soothes the lungs and helps to strengthen adrenal function. Give your child one dose, once a day, every other month, for six months after an asthma attack.

Note: This herb should not be given to a child with high blood pressure.

■ Minor bupleurum formula is a Chinese herbal combination that is helpful in restoring and building the immune system. Give your child one dose daily for three months following an asthma attack. Stop for three months, then repeat.

Note: Minor bupleurum should not be given to a child with a fever or any other sign of an acute infection.

HOMEOPATHY

Homeopathic treatments for asthma are directed at preventing or supporting recovery from an asthma attack, rather than treating an acute episode. In the event of an acute asthma attack, seek immediate medical care for your child.

■ If your child suffers from chronic asthma, consult a homeopath to determine an appropriate constitutional remedy.

■ *Antimonium tartaricum* is a homeopathic remedy for a child who is wheezing, with a tight feeling in her chest; there may be mucus but it is difficult to cough up. If your child's symptoms match this description, give her one dose of *Antimonium tartaricum* 12x, 30x, 6c, or 9c every hour until symptoms lessen. Then give her one dose, three times a day, for several days or until symptoms subside.

Note: Do not use this remedy in the presence of a fever.

■ *Arsenicum album* 30x, 200x, 9c, or 30c is for the tired, anxious, and cold-sensitive child with asthma, whose symptoms are often worse in the middle of the night or when she is lying down. Give this child one dose, three times a day, for several days or until symptoms subside.

■ *Chamomilla* 30x or 9c is helpful for children whose asthma is triggered or accompanied by anger and irritability. Give your child one dose, three times a day, for several days or until symptoms subside.

■ *Pulsatilla* 30x or 9c is for asthma that is often triggered by an upper respiratory tract infection. There is little or no mucus. This child has more difficulty breathing in a closed, stuffy room, and feels more comfortable outside. Give her one dose, three times a day, for several days or until symptoms subside.

ACUPRESSURE

You can massage the points listed below on a daily basis to help balance an asthmatic child's system. In the event of an acute asthma attack, seek immediate medical care for your child. (You can work these points as you are on your way to the hospital.) For the locations of acupressure points on a child's body, *see* ADMINISTERING AN ACUPRESSURE TREATMENT in Part Three.

■ Liver 3 helps to quiet the nervous system.

■ Lung 7 clears the lungs.

■ Pericardium 6 relaxes the chest.

GENERAL RECOMMENDATIONS

■ Follow the regimen prescribed by your child's physician. Be sure you understand when and how to give the medicines he or she prescribes. Taking your child off medication without careful supervision can result in a severe asthma attack and hospitalization, and should not be attempted.

■ Yoga, relaxation, and deep breathing techniques are invaluable for people with asthma, including children. In addition to building physical strength and flexibility, yoga teaches steady, controlled slow deep breathing, which helps to strengthen the respiratory system. Using relaxation and visualization exercises at the beginning of an asthma attack can help calm your child and ease her breathing (*see* RELAXATION TECHNIQUES in Part Three).

■ Encourage your child to get regular exercise to improve lung function. Swimming is particularly good, and the humidity helps to keep the mouth and air passages from drying out. (Make sure, however, that your child does not swim in an excessively chlorinated pool, since high levels of chlorine can produce allergic reactions in some people.) Depending on the severity and type of your child's asthma, she may need to take medication before an activity to prevent respiratory distress.

■ Certain food additives, especially metabisulfite, can be dangerous for the child with asthma. Sulfites are commonly found in commercially prepared foods such as dried fruits. They are also used by many restaurants to keep fruits and vegetables at salad bars looking fresh and attractive. If your child has asthma, it's best to avoid salad bars and to buy only unsulfured dried fruits. Monosodium glutamate (MSG) can also cause problems for some asthmatics, so avoid food products prepared with this additive. You should also be aware of "hidden" sources of MSG. These often show up on food labels as "hydrolyzed protein," "autolyzed yeast," "sodium caseinate," and "calcium caseinate."

■ Write to the National Asthma Center for information on programs that teach self-management skills and help children and their families learn to live with asthma. Their address is 1400 Jackson Street, Denver, CO 80206. The National

Allergy and Asthma Network is another good source of information. Their address is 3554 Chain Bridge Road, Suite 200, Fairfax, VA 22030.

PREVENTION

■ There is no known way to prevent a child from developing asthma. Obviously, however, if your child has suffered an asthmatic attack, you should keep her from coming into contact with any foods or environmental allergens that you suspect may trigger another episode.

Athlete's Foot

Athlete's foot (or *tinea pedis*) is a fungal infection caused by any of several related organisms. It is similar to the condition known as ringworm. Children commonly develop athlete's foot after prolonged exposure to warm and moist environments, such as shower floors, locker rooms, and sweaty socks. Although it is contagious, athlete's foot seems most likely to occur in predisposed individuals.

Symptoms of athlete's foot include burning, itching, scaling, cracking, sores, and tiny blisters between the toes and on the soles of the feet.

Athlete's foot can usually be treated successfully at home. However, it is possible for a bacterial infection to develop alongside a fungal infection. If your child's athlete's foot persists or gets worse after treatment, take him to the doctor for further help.

CONVENTIONAL TREATMENT

■ A number of over-the-counter antifungal creams are available that may help with athlete's foot, among them miconazole (in Micatin-Derm and Monistat-Derm), tolnaftate (Tinactin, Dr. Scholl's), undecylenic acid (Desitin), and clotrimazole (Lotrimin, Mycelex). Normally these creams are applied twice daily. They can produce results in as little three to four days, but it may be necessary to use them for up to a month in persistent cases.

■ If the infection involves a lot of inflammation (redness and swelling), your doctor may prescribe a combination antifungal/steroid preparation, such as Lotrisone. While there is little difference in potency between the over-the-counter products and most of the prescription medications used for this condition, there are individual differences in susceptibility, so if all else fails it may be worth trying a prescription cream.

■ If the skin is cracked, open, or oozing, Burow's solution is sometimes recommended as an antiseptic and astringent. This is an over-the-counter product sold as a powder and diluted for use on the skin.

DIETARY GUIDELINES

■ Avoid giving a child with athlete's foot sugary foods, including soft drinks and commercially processed foods. Sugar encourages the growth of fungus. Encourage an older child to refuse soda pop and sugary foods away from home by explaining that sugar encourages the fungal growth that is making him uncomfortable.

■ Make sure your child's menu includes plenty of fruits and vegetables.

NUTRITIONAL SUPPLEMENTS

For age-appropriate dosages of some nutritional supplements, see page 81.

■ *Lactobacillus acidophilus* helps to provide the "friendly" bacteria necessary to fight a fungal infection. If your child has been taking antibiotics, an acidophilus supplement is especially valuable. Antibiotics strip the body of beneficial bacteria that help keep fungal infections under control. Acidophilus helps to restore this friendly bacteria. Follow dosage directions on the product label.

■ Zinc helps to heal skin tissue. Give your child one-half dose, twice a day (before meals), for two weeks to one month.

Note: Excessive amounts of zinc can result in nausea and vomiting. Be careful not to exceed the recommended dosage.

HERBAL TREATMENT

■ Tea tree oil (*Melaleuca alternifolia*) is the most effective herbal treatment for athlete's foot. It speeds healing and quickly relieves the intolerable itching. Tea tree oil is considered one of the most powerful botanical antifungal remedies. Twice a day, add 10 drops of tea tree oil to 1 quart of warm water and have your child soak his feet in the treated water for ten minutes (by associating this with a game or reading a book, you may be able to avoid the inevitable impatience that younger children will display). After each soak, dry your child's feet thoroughly, especially between the toes. After drying, use a cotton swab to paint the affected area with undiluted tea tree oil. Continue these soaks for ten days. You should notice considerable improvement, marked by decreased tenderness, scaling, and blistering. Continue applying undiluted tea tree oil to the affected area for another ninety days. Although most children's athlete's foot will improve in three weeks, some cases of fungal infection are more stubborn. If your child won't sit and soak, applying the undiluted oil twice daily can be effective.

■ Let your child rub a washcloth dipped in apple cider vinegar briskly between his toes to remove the soggy skin and scales. It feels like scratching and relieves the itch. Children usually enjoy this simple treatment. A soak in warm water with a liberal amount of apple cider vinegar added also helps.

■ If your child's feet are itchy and red, try using alternate applications of aloe vera gel and calendula (in ointment form if the athlete's foot is dry, in lotion form if the skin is damp). Both of these herbs are very soothing and healing for the skin.

■ For children who are prone to infection or who protest the strong smell of tea tree oil, make a blend of equal parts of aloe vera liquid and calendula, echinacea, and goldenseal extracts. Rub the mixture well into the affected area. This liquid mixture is a good antifungal, relieves itching, and is very soothing.

■ Garlic is a powerful fungicide. Cut a few slivers of raw garlic and put them in your child's socks, or dust his shoes with garlic-based foot powder. The medicinal properties are absorbed through the skin.

■ Dust between your child's toes with an absorbent powder, such as green clay, to help keep these problem areas dry.

HOMEOPATHY

■ *Thuja* is an effective treatment for athlete's foot. Morning and evening, rub a few drops of undiluted homeopathic *Thuja* tincture (the mother tincture) directly on the affected areas of your child's feet. If you see improvement after one month, continue the treatment, as it is likely your child's infection will continue to clear. If you see no change after thirty days, it is best to try another approach.

GENERAL RECOMMENDATIONS

■ Begin with tea tree oil or *Thuja* soaks and direct applications of tea tree oil to the affected area.

■ Expose affected feet to the air as much as possible. If weather permits, this is the time for open sandals. Nonporous leather shoes and rubber-soled shoes hold in heat and moisture, creating the perfect environment for athlete's foot. When your child's feet get hot and sweaty, the healing process is inhibited. Fungi thrive in a warm, moist environment.

■ A child with athlete's foot should be taught good hygiene. Teach your child to dry his feet thoroughly, taking extra care between the toes.

■ White cotton socks allow the feet to breathe and do not contain any irritating dyes. To kill the fungus and prevent reinfection, wash your child's socks in chlorine bleach after each wearing. If your child is extremely active and sweats a lot, make sure he changes socks two or three times a day.

■ It's difficult to do, but try to prevent your child from scratching. Scratching athlete's foot breaks the blisters and spreads the fungus, making the infection worse. Applying a topical calendula gel will help reduce the itching.

PREVENTION

■ Keep your child's feet clean and dry, especially between the toes.

■ When your child will be in the type of environment where athlete's foot flourishes, such as school, camp, or public locker rooms, make sure he wears shoes or slippers. Socks alone do not provide sufficient protection.

■ Instruct your child to make sure his socks are dry before putting on shoes. Many youngsters will run around the wet floor of a locker room in stocking feet, resulting in damp—and possibly fungus-contaminated—socks. Putting on shoes over damp socks creates the perfect environment for the athlete's foot fungus to grow and thrive.

■ If you discover that your child, or one of your child's schoolmates, has athlete's foot, alert the authorities responsible for any communal area where the infected child might have contracted the fungus.

Attention Deficit Disorder

See HYPERACTIVITY.

Bad Breath

Bad breath is an embarrassing problem for a child of any age. A child with bad breath may endure ridicule and taunting, as all the advertisements for breath mints, mouthwashes, and toothpastes are so quick to point out. As a loving parent, you will want to remove any possible source of embarrassment for your child.

In some cases, an unusual breath odor may be a sign of illness, such as a herpes infection of the mouth, diabetes, postnasal drip, tonsillitis, sinusitis, dental infection, or streptococcus infection. Most of the time, however, bad breath—medically termed *halitosis*—is not the result of any major health problem. It is usually related to poor oral hygiene or poor digestion, sometimes both.

CONVENTIONAL TREATMENT

■ If you notice a bad smell on your child's breath, look first for an unused toothbrush! But if your child's breath has a persistent or unusual odor, she should be examined. Your child's physician will be able to determine whether or not her bad breath is related to an underlying infection or other illness and, if it is, to prescribe appropriate treatment. One particularly helpful diagnostic test is a comprehensive stool analysis, which can be used to determine problems with digestion and assimilation, the presence of parasites, or the overgrowth of abnormal bacteria in the digestive tract.

■ If your doctor rules out other causes, the problem is most likely related to oral care. In this case, it is best to take your child to a good pediatric dentist.

DIETARY GUIDELINES

■ If your child has a sour stomach and her bad breath is related to digestive difficulties, limit her intake of fried foods and refined sugar. Better yet, eliminate these items entirely.

NUTRITIONAL SUPPLEMENTS

■ Chlorophyll tablets help freshen the breath because of the effect they have in the intestines. Give your child a chlorophyll supplement after each meal and again at bedtime. Follow dosage directions on the product label.

■ If your child's bad breath is related to poor digestion, talk with your child's doctor about supplementing her diet with digestive enzymes. There are a number of over-the-counter products available that use natural enzymes from pineapple (bromelain) or papaya (papain), which may be helpful. Follow dosage directions on the product label.

■ Give your child a *Lactobacillus acidophilus* or *bifidus* supplement daily to establish and maintain favorable intestinal flora and healthy digestion. Follow dosage directions on the product label.

HERBAL TREATMENT

■ An herbal mouthwash can be helpful. Dissolve 400 micrograms of folic acid,

80 drops of hawthorn berry extract, 80 drops of echinacea, 10 drops of peppermint oil, and 5 drops of thyme oil in 16 ounces of spring water. Have your child swish the mixture around in her mouth after she brushes her teeth. Folic acid heals gum tissue and helps reduce plaque; hawthorn berry is astringent and helps tighten gum tissues; echinacea cleanses the mouth and kills bacteria; peppermint oil tastes great and leaves the breath smelling fresh and clean. Your child may enjoy the tingly taste of this mouthwash.

■ Choose an herbal-based toothpaste or powder formulated without sugar. Your health food store should have a selection of these products. Merfluan is a baking-soda-based tooth powder that is very popular in Europe. It comes in several different flavors.

■ Have your child chew on a small sprig of parsley to freshen her breath. Parsley is rich in the natural deodorizer chlorophyll, and also sweetens the digestive tract.

■ If your child's bad breath is an occasional problem related to poor digestion, typically accompanied by complaints of a stomachache, diarrhea, constipation, or a lot of burping, give her a cup of peppermint tea after meals to ease digestion. Or try giving your child ginger tea twice a day with meals to enhance digestion.

HOMEOPATHY

■ If your child's bad breath is related to oral herpes (cold sores), give her one dose of *Natrum muriaticum* 30x or 9c, three times daily, for three days. Follow up with one dose of *Mercurius solubilis* 12x or 6c, twice daily, for three to five days. If there is no improvement in this time, stop giving the remedy.

GENERAL RECOMMENDATIONS

■ Make sure your child practices good oral hygiene. Teach effective brushing and flossing, use a sugar- and saccharin-free toothpaste, and have your child cleanse her mouth with an herbal mouthwash at least once a day.

■ To avoid a sour stomach and improve digestion, give your child chlorophyll and acidophilus supplements. Serve peppermint tea with meals.

■ Your child should have regular appointments with a dentist and dental hygienist. It's a good idea to begin a program of regular visits to the dentist long before a cavity or other problem arises. The first checkups can begin when your child is three to four years old.

■ If simple, natural treatments do not freshen your child's breath promptly, and keep it fresh and sweet, take your child to her physician to rule out the possibility of an underlying condition.

PREVENTION

■ Bad breath is usually caused by poor oral hygiene, but that doesn't mean it shouldn't be taken seriously. It is important that children learn to take care of their teeth and gums, so they keep their bright, healthy smiles for a lifetime. Teach your child that caring for her mouth is every bit as important as bathing daily or brushing her hair.

■ Start good oral hygiene habits early. A toddler's teeth should be cleaned twice daily. Place gauze around your index or third finger and gently rub the teeth and along the gumline. If you brush your own teeth while your child can watch you, soon she will probably start imitating the brushing of teeth. Once most of your child's twenty baby teeth are in and touching each other, flossing can begin.

■ Make sure your child brushes her teeth after every meal. Ask your dentist or dental hygienist to teach you correct brushing and flossing technique, and then teach your child. Little ones may need extra help. Observe your child from time to time to make sure she is brushing correctly.

■ Limit the amount of sugar in your child's diet and serve a diet based on healthy whole foods.

Bedwetting

Bedwetting—medically termed *enuresis*—is an embarrassing and difficult problem for a child. His self-esteem may suffer. Sleepovers can be torture, and even thinking about going away to Grandma's or to summer camp can create a tremendous burden for the child who wets the bed. Bedwetting is also a distressing problem for parents concerned about their child's well-being.

It is important to understand that bedwetting is not bad behavior. It is not intentional, and it is not the child's fault. If you have a child who wets the bed, please remember that this child deserves your thoughtful attempts to help resolve the problem.

A 1987 article in *Psychiatric Clinics of North America* estimated that there are between 5 and 7 million children who wet their beds. Boys are more often affected than girls. The typical child who wets the bed has a small or immature bladder. Because he is unable to hold urine through the night, he consistently has "wet" nights.

There are also children who once had bladder control, but have lost it. This type of bedwetting is likely to be related to either emotional or organic problems. Emotional causes include stressful or scary situations, such as a move to a new house, the birth of a new baby in the family, or parental separation. Such stresses may cause a child to regress to an earlier pattern of behavior. Bedwetting due to stress is usually temporary. Organic problems include urinary tract infections, which can irritate the urethra and bladder and interfere with normal functioning; obstructive lesions of the urinary tract; and spinal disorders that interfere with sensations and voluntary control of the bladder. Children with diabetes or sickle cell disease may have difficulty concentrating their urine and typically urinate larger amounts, sometimes to the point of wetting the bed at night. A food allergy or sensitivity can also cause bedwetting, because problem foods can irritate the bladder. These problems must be diagnosed and treated by your child's physician.

The most important consideration with regard to bedwetting is to understand your child's normal growth and development so that your expectations are realistic. As your child's body grows, his bladder becomes able to hold more and more urine. Only when a child's bladder can hold about a cup and a half of urine does sleeping through the night without wetting the bed become *physically* possible.

Another requirement is the development of neuromuscular control necessary to control voiding. Because this typically occurs at around four to five years of age, it is unreasonable to expect a child younger than this to sleep through every night without wetting the bed. Moreover, every child's growth and development is unique. Full bladder control may not occur until five or six years of age.

As a child grows and learns control, it is normal to have times when he will sleep peacefully through the night without wetting, and it is equally normal to have periods of regression and bedwetting. Respect your child's individual growth and development and give him your loving support along the way.

CONVENTIONAL TREATMENT

WHEN TO CALL THE DOCTOR ABOUT BEDWETTING

• If your child begins wetting the bed consistently and also displaying symptoms of noticeably increased thirst, increased frequency and amount of urination, fatigue, increased appetite, and/or weight loss, see your physician. These can be symptoms of diabetes.

• A child who wets the bed and complains of abdominal pain should be examined by a doctor. This may be a sign of an underlying infection.

■ Once your child's doctor rules out any physical problem as the cause of bedwetting, there are prescription medications that may be helpful. DDAVP (desmopressin acetate) is a drug that is being prescribed with increasing frequency. It is a nasal spray that increases the production of antidiuretic hormone, which helps the body reabsorb water and therefore hold back urine. Some children who wet their beds at night may not produce enough of this hormone; DDAVP may be the answer for them.

■ Imipramine (Tofranil) is also prescribed for bedwetting, but less frequently than it once was. This medication may reduce the irritability of the bladder so that a child experiences less frequent and less intense bladder contractions. It can also have unpleasant side effects, including nervousness, restlessness, sleep disorders, and mild gastrointestinal disturbances. Imipramine is not recommended for children younger than six years old, and it is usually prescribed for no longer than a three-month period. And unfortunately, there is no guarantee that your child will stay dry once the medication is stopped.

■ Behavior modification is a commonly used approach. This may involve a number of different techniques, including the use of an alarm bell, hypnosis, and relaxation therapy, as well as Kegel's exercises, which help to train the bladder muscles.

DIETARY GUIDELINES

■ Many cases of bedwetting can be traced to food allergies. You may wish to try an elimination diet with your child to see if he has food allergies (*see* ELIMINATION DIET in Part Three). Milk, dairy products, citrus fruits, and wheat are the most common allergens. If you eliminate these foods, especially milk, from your child's diet, bedwetting may decrease.

■ Eliminating sugar from a child's diet, especially in the afternoon and evening, is very often helpful.

NUTRITIONAL SUPPLEMENTS

For age-appropriate dosages of nutritional supplements, see page 81.

■ A liquid calcium and magnesium combination formula is helpful for a child who wets the bed due to nervousness. This supplement helps to relax the nervous system. The liquid does not have a bad taste and can easily be given to a child either by itself or mixed with juice. Give your child one dose, twice a day, once in the morning and again at bedtime.

HERBAL TREATMENT

For age-appropriate dosages of herbal remedies, see page 81.

■ The combination of chamomile, passion flower, skullcap, and linden flower is a time-honored remedy for anxiety. These herbs relax the nervous system, which may be agitated and thus contribute to a bedwetting problem. Give your child one or two doses of tea made from a combination these herbs early in the evening (after dinner).

Note: Skullcap should not be given to a child less than six years old. If your child is under six, make a tea of chamomile, passion flower, and linden flower only.

HOMEOPATHY

Choose the symptom-specific remedy in the list below that most closely matches your child's symptoms. Give your child one dose at 3:00 P.M. and another before bed. Whichever remedy or combination of treatments you choose, allow ten days to two weeks to see a change in your child's behavior. In addition to the remedies outlined below, there are combination homeopathic remedies designed for bedwetting that are often helpful. Homeopathic pharmacies and larger health food stores will have these. You may also wish to work with a homeopathic practitioner to find a constitutional remedy for your child.

■ *Calcarea phosphorica* 30x or 9c is recommended for the restless child who often voids small amounts during the night and seldom awakens when this happens. This type of child is very difficult to awaken.

■ *Causticum* 30x or 9c will help the child who appears weak and pale, with an almost unhealthy facial appearance, usually with dark circles under his eyes. With a child of this type, bedwetting typically lessens during the summer, but worsens in the fall, winter, and spring. *Causticum* is often used very successfully for children who wet the bed when they first fall asleep.

■ *Equisetum* 30x or 9c is helpful for the child who soaks the bed. This child may complain of pain in the lower abdomen. An active dream life, with nightmares that wake him, is common for this child.

Caution: A child with abdominal pain should be checked by a physician, to rule out the possibility that it may be related to an infection.

■ *Lycopodium* 30x or 9c is indicated for difficult, intelligent children, who often look and act older than they are. Such a child will usually soak his bed late in the night.

■ *Pulsatilla* 30x or 9c is helpful for the child—often a fair-haired girl—who tends to be quite sensitive. This child exhibits a tremendous urgency to void during the day or night that is most exaggerated upon lying down.

■ *Sepia* 30x or 9c is for the darker-complected child who typically wets the bed during the first two hours of sleep.

ACUPRESSURE

For the locations of acupressure points on a child's body, *see* ADMINISTERING AN ACUPRESSURE TREATMENT in Part Three.

■ Kidney 3 strengthens the bladder and kidneys. It is the most helpful pressure point for children who wet the bed.

■ Kidney 7 also strengthens the bladder and kidneys.

■ Liver 3 is calming to the nervous system.

■ Pericardium 6 is good for relieving bedtime anxiety, as is a light back massage at bedtime.

GENERAL RECOMMENDATIONS

■ *Never* ridicule, spank, or scold a child for wetting the bed. Punishment doesn't work. Instead, praise and reward dry nights.

■ Once you are sure your child is both mentally and physically capable of dry nights, start with the following recommendations.

- Try to limit the amount of fluids your child drinks after dinner.

- Have your child urinate one hour before bedtime, again half an hour before bed, and yet again just before going to bed.

- Give your child a liquid calcium and magnesium supplement.

- Guided by your child's type, choose a homeopathic preparation. If none of the remedies seems exactly right, try a combination remedy, or consult a homeopathic practitioner for a constitutional remedy.

■ Bladder stretching exercises may be helpful. These involve encouraging your child to hold urine for as long as possible while drinking lots of fluids, in order to increase the volume capacity of his bladder. This can be done systematically, once or twice a day, by having your child wait for a short, set period of time (such as two to five minutes) past the point when he first feels the urge to urinate. You can make a game of this. Even a very young child can "dance" while watching the second hand tick around the clock. As your child develops control during short intervals, the waiting period can then gradually be extended. Patience is crucial but rewarding with this technique.

■ The stream interruption technique is another method that may be useful for helping your child develop control. This involves teaching your child to stop and start urinating several times in midstream while voiding.

■ Visualization exercises help some children. Try teaching your child to imagine going to bed, feeling a full bladder, and awakening in order to go to the bathroom.

■ Comprehensive treatment programs that use several different approaches in combination report high success rates. Bladder stretching exercises, stream interruption, counseling, and visualization can be used together.

■ Involving your child in laundering wet sheets and putting fresh, clean sheets on his bed can be effective in encouraging his participation. However, if you are feeling angry or disgusted over the need to change the bed, your child will feel it. Remain supportive and matter-of-fact.

■ Many parents need guidance and support in approaching this complex problem. Working with a counselor before implementing any of these programs is highly recommended.

■ Whatever approach you choose, it is vitally important that you—*and your child*—be involved and feel optimistic about it. For any intervention to be successful, your child must be willing to participate.

PREVENTION

■ Because of the many factors involved in the physical and mental development of your child, bedwetting is not something you can truly prevent. The passing of time may be relied upon to solve the problem in the end, though the commonsense guidelines outlined in this entry will help. Be sure you clearly realize that bedwetting is treatable by gentle means. Punishing or shaming your child is of no help. In fact, punishment often makes the problem even worse, and can actually lengthen the time it takes for your child to overcome his difficulties.

Bites, Animal and Human

Should your child suffer a bite that breaks the skin, prompt medical care is essential. This applies whether the bite is from a playmate, a wild or stray animal, or the family pet.

Biting is a natural behavior in infants that usually begins at around five to six months of age, as solid foods are introduced. Biting and chewing are among the first willful actions a baby learns (unlike suckling, which is an instinctive response). If your baby is teething, biting down on something helps relieve the pressure an emerging tooth exerts (*see* TEETHING).

Toddlers and older children may use biting to show hostility or to get attention. One child may bite another during play. Unless a child has severe emotional problems, this behavior will be outgrown. Nonetheless, it goes without saying that biting should be discouraged.

CONVENTIONAL TREATMENT

■ Your child's bite wound will be cleansed, treated with a topical antibiotic such as Betadine, bacitracin, or Neosporin, and bandaged. You will probably be instructed to change the dressing daily, with a new application of antibiotic at each change. If necessary, the wound will be stitched closed. If the wound is very deep, involves the hands or knuckles, or involves damage to tendons that requires repair, surgery may be recommended to thoroughly clean the affected tissues and close the wound before bandaging.

■ After emergency first aid has been administered, your child will be given an injection to update her immunity to tetanus if necessary. If your child was bitten by an animal and it cannot be determined that the animal is *not* infected with rabies, rabies immune globulin will be administered. A bite from a rabid animal can be fatal unless the victim receives immediate medical treatment, which consists of a series of injections into the muscles over a period of twenty-eight days and again at ninety days.

■ Once the wound is thoroughly cleansed and bandaged, and any necessary immunizations have been given, an oral antibiotic such as ampicillin, cephalexin (Keflex), clindamycin, or dicloxacillin may be prescribed to prevent infection.

■ Until it heals, your child's wound will need to be checked every few days for signs of infection, and treated accordingly.

EMERGENCY TREATMENT FOR ANIMAL AND HUMAN BITES

✚ If your child suffers a bite that breaks the skin, immediately and thoroughly disinfect the area with lots of water, soap, and hydrogen peroxide. Bite wounds that break the skin can easily become infected. This is true of human as well as animal bites. Human saliva is often alive with infectious bacteria.

✚ If your child has been bitten by an animal, try to confine the animal so it can be tested for rabies. If the animal belongs to a neighbor, be sure you can identify the owner. If you can determine that the animal is not rabid, your child can be spared the very uncomfortable (but otherwise necessary) treatment with rabies vaccine. If the animal is wild and you cannot capture it, your child will have to be treated for rabies.

✚ Call your physician or take your child to the emergency room, or call for emergency help. Any child who receives a bite wound that breaks the skin should be examined and treated by a doctor.

DIETARY GUIDELINES

■ Limit your child's consumption of sugar and fried foods while the tissue is healing.

■ Make sure your child eats plenty of dark green and yellow vegetables to increase her intake of beta-carotene.

NUTRITIONAL SUPPLEMENTS

For age-appropriate dosages of nutritional supplements, see page 81.

■ Beta-carotene helps the skin to heal. Give your child a double dose, twice daily, for two weeks.

■ Bioflavonoids fight infection and inflammation. Give your child one dose, three times daily, for two weeks.

■ Vitamin C is a mild anti-inflammatory and helps detoxify the blood. Give your child one dose, three times daily, for two weeks.

■ Zinc aids in wound healing. Give your child one dose, one to two times daily (at the start of a meal), for two weeks.

Note: Excessive amounts of zinc can result in nausea and vomiting. Be careful not to exceed the recommended dosage.

HERBAL TREATMENT

For age-appropriate dosages of herbal remedies, see page 81.

■ An echinacea and goldenseal combination formula will help detoxify the blood and prevent infection. Give your child one dose, three times daily, for three to five days.

■ To speed healing and help prevent infection, make a goldenseal and calendula compress and apply it to the bite, three times a day, until the wound has closed.

■ Garlic has antibiotic properties, and helps to detoxify the blood. Give your child one capsule of a garlic supplement, three times a day, for one week. If your child will accept it, you may give her fresh garlic instead of the capsule form. Substitute one clove of fresh garlic for each capsule.

HOMEOPATHY

■ *Arnica* 30x or 9c is useful when there is tissue damage or bruising. Give your child one dose every hour for the first three hours. Then give one dose, three times a day, for three days.

■ *Hypericum* 12x or 6c is recommended if there is nerve pain following the trauma. Give your child one dose, four times daily, for the first day or two after the injury.

■ *Ledum* 12x or 6c is good if there is bruising surrounding the bite. Give your child one dose, three times daily, for two days. *Ledum* is useful for all puncture-type wounds.

PREVENTION

■ If any of your toddler's playmates has a tendency to bite, keep a watchful eye out for a developing altercation when they are together. If two children are tugging on the same toy, for example, one of them may bite to try to get the other child to let go. Use time-out to discourage a child from biting others (*see* TIME-OUT in Part Three of this book).

■ Children who bite are often trying to express something they are unable to convey otherwise. It may be helpful to speak with a pediatric psychologist or psychiatrist to try to determine the reason behind a child's biting. There are also homeopathic remedies that may help:

- *Belladonna* can be helpful for the red-faced, furious child.
- *Stramonium* is for the child who is more hysterical and never seems to completely calm down. This is a remedy that has been used for treatment of Tourette's syndrome, for example.

■ Teach your child that it is dangerous to tease animals. Even a beloved family pet or usually-friendly neighborhood pets can become provoked.

■ Teach your child never to approach or try to touch a strange animal. Even friendly-looking kittens can have sharp teeth and claws.

■ Don't permit a young child to wander the neighborhood without supervision. If possible, get to know neighborhood pets. Identify any animals, such as guard dogs, that may jump a fence and become aggressive or dangerous.

■ Before taking your child on a camping trip, check with local authorities regarding animal life in the area where you plan to set up camp. Don't permit your child to go exploring on her own. Teach your child not to slip away from the family campsite or wander off without a responsible adult.

Bites, Snake

There are many varieties of poisonous snakes. Because a child's small body has less of a capacity for fighting a reaction to snake venom, prompt medical care for snakebite is essential.

Symptoms caused by snakebite range from mild to severe, and can include a racing pulse, with swelling and discoloration around the area of the bite. If your child is bitten by a snake, he may feel weak and be short of breath; he will probably feel nauseous and may vomit. If the venom is very strong, your child will experience severe pain and much swelling. His pupils will dilate, and shock and convulsion may occur. Your child may twitch uncontrollably and his speech may become slurred. After a severe snakebite, a child can become paralyzed and lose consciousness. If your child is bitten by a snake, act fast.

CONVENTIONAL TREATMENT

■ Seek emergency treatment (see page 116). Rely on medical personnel to take the appropriate measures. The primary treatment for snakebite is the use of intravenous antivenin. It is important to go to a hospital experienced in its use.

■ Once the wound has been treated and your child has recovered sufficiently

EMERGENCY TREATMENT FOR SNAKEBITE

✚ Take your child immediately to the emergency room of the nearest hospital, or call emergency medical personnel. *Medical intervention is essential.*

✚ If medical care is not immediately available, stay calm. Reassure your child, speaking calmly to prevent panic, and follow these steps:

1. Have your child lie down and rest quietly. Activity can spread the venom throughout the body.

2. Immobilize the affected limb. If possible, keep it at the same level as the heart.

3. If a venom extractor is available, apply suction immediately. It takes at least three minutes to begin adequate poison extraction. Continue suctioning out the venom for at least fifteen minutes, or until you can secure medical care for your child.

4. *Do not* make an incision into the bite or suck the poison out with your mouth. Both actions create more problems than they solve.

5. *Do not* use an ice pack on the wound. Cold therapy is not recommended for snake bites, as it can damage tissues.

6. Call your local Poison Control Center for instructions on how best to treat your child (*see* page 344).

7. Seek medical care as soon as possible.

from the effects of the injury to leave the hospital, medical personnel will advise you on the proper way to care for him as he recovers.

DIETARY GUIDELINES

■ Once emergency medical care has been administered and your child is well enough to leave the hospital, support his recovery by preparing a low-sugar, low-fat diet to promote a healing internal environment.

■ Increase the amount of green and yellow vegetables in your child's diet so that he gets plenty of important vitamins and minerals.

NUTRITIONAL SUPPLEMENTS

The nutritional supplements below are directed at supporting recovery from the bite once appropriate emergency medical care has been administered and your child is well enough to leave the hospital. If your child is bitten by a snake, seek emergency medical care immediately. For age-appropriate dosages of nutritional supplements, see page 81.

■ Bioflavonoids fight infection and inflammation. Give your child one dose, three or four times daily, for one week.

■ Vitamin C helps detoxify the body. Give your child one dose, four times a day, for one week.

HERBAL TREATMENT

Herbal treatments for snakebite are directed at supporting recovery from the bite once appropriate emergency medical care has been administered and your child is well enough to leave the hospital. If your child is bitten by a snake, seek emergency medical care immediately. For age-appropriate dosages of herbal remedies, see page 81.

■ Echinacea and goldenseal help to prevent or treat an infection. Both herbs have antibiotic properties and help to boost the immune system. Give your child one dose of a combination formula, three times a day, for five days. Then give one dose, twice daily, for five days.

Note: You should not give your child echinacea on a daily basis for more than ten days at a time, or it will lose its effectiveness.

■ Garlic has antibacterial properties, and helps detoxify the blood. Give your child one capsule of a garlic supplement (or one clove of fresh garlic), three times a day, for two weeks.

HOMEOPATHY

Homeopathic treatments for snakebite are directed at supporting recovery from the bite once appropriate emergency care has been administered and medical personnel advise you that your child is well enough to take something by mouth. If your child is bitten by a snake, seek emergency medical care immediately.

■ Follow these three steps, in sequence:

1. Give your child one dose of *Aconite* 30x, 200x, or 30c to ease the shock and fright.

2. Give your child one dose of *Arnica* 12x, 30x, 200x, 7c, or 30c every hour, for a total of three doses, to help the injured tissue begin to heal.

3. Give your child one dose of *Lachesis* 30x or 9c, three times a day, for two to three days. *Lachesis* will help alleviate the symptoms of the bite.

ACUPRESSURE

Acupressure treatments for snakebite are directed at supporting recovery from the bite once appropriate emergency medical care has been administered and your child is well enough to leave the hospital. If your child is bitten by a snake, seek emergency medical care immediately. For the locations of acupressure points on a child's body, *see* ADMINISTERING AN ACUPRESSURE TREATMENT in Part Three.

■ Spleen 10 helps to detoxify the body.

■ Four Gates will help to relax your child. This can be helpful immediately following emergency treatment for the bite.

GENERAL RECOMMENDATIONS

■ Make sure you know how to identify any types of venomous snakes that are indigenous to your area. Should a medical emergency arise, knowing the species of the snake that attacked your child will save precious time.

■ Along with your usual first aid supplies, keep a snakebite kit readily available, especially when camping out. We recommend The Extractor from Sawyer Products, which is available in many camping and outdoor equipment stores or directly from the company. They can be contacted at P.O. Box 188, Safety Harbor, FL 34695; telephone 813–725–1177.

PREVENTION

■ Most snake bites occur on unprotected ankles and legs. Shorts and sneakers don't provide adequate protection. Outfit your child with tough hiking boots and suitable pants, such as heavy jeans, for tramping through the woods or going on a hiking trip.

■ Teach your child not to poke sticks into inviting holes or stick his hands into underbrush.

■ When camping out, don't permit your child to go exploring alone.

Bites and Stings, Insect

Bites and stings from most common insects, such as mosquitoes, gnats, fleas, common spiders, ants, and other "creepy crawlies" can cause itchy welts on arms

EMERGENCY
TREATMENT
FOR INSECT BITES
AND STINGS

See the inset on page 119.

and legs. A bee, wasp, or hornet sting can cause swelling and stinging at the site. Usually, bites and stings are no more than an annoyance and cause only slight local swelling and irritation.

There are exceptions, however, such as a bite from a venomous insect like the brown recluse or black widow spider, or a severe allergic reaction to a bee sting. A bite from a tiny deer tick may cause a large circular lesion that progresses into a rash of small round lesions. The deer tick is the insect responsible for transmitting Lyme disease, and the characteristic rash is often the first sign of that illness (*see* LYME DISEASE).

If your child is stung by a bee, wasp, or hornet, or bitten by an insect you suspect may be poisonous (such as the black widow or brown recluse spider), she may need emergency medical treatment (see page 119).

CONVENTIONAL TREATMENT

For most insect bites and stings, home treatment is usually all that's needed. Begin with the following suggestions.

■ Remove the stinger left behind by a bee, wasp, or hornet by *gently scraping* it out with your fingernail or the back of a knife blade, rather than by pulling on it. The stingers of these insects are barbed. Pulling the stinger out directly can squeeze more venom into the wound.

■ If you find a tick on your child, *do not* try to pull it off with your fingers. The barbs on a tick's proboscis (or feeding snout) become deeply embedded in its victim, so that even if you pull off the body, the head remains. To remove a tick, use a pair of tweezers to grasp the head, as close to the spot where it is attached to your child's skin as possible. Pull back slowly and firmly until the tick pulls free. Once the tick is removed, wash, rinse, and disinfect the site of the bite thoroughly with rubbing alcohol. Then apply an antibiotic ointment, such as bacitracin or Betadine.

■ For minor insect bites, apply a cold compress to the area to reduce the spread of histamines and other body chemicals that cause itching and swelling.

■ You can give your child an oral antihistamine such as Benadryl or Chlor-Trimeton to help counteract itching and swelling. Follow the directions on the product label.

■ Witch hazel, calamine lotion, or a low-dose cortisone cream such as Lanacort or Cort-Aid may be applied to the area as needed for one or two days to relieve itching. Creams or lotions that contain Benadryl can also help relieve the itching of minor insect bites. Apply a thin layer of any of these medications to the area of the bite, but do not put them on open wounds.

DIETARY GUIDELINES

■ Give your child plenty of fluids, including pure spring water, light soups, and diluted natural juices to help her body flush out residual toxins.

NUTRITIONAL SUPPLEMENTS

For age-appropriate dosages of herbal remedies, see page 81.

■ To help relieve the pain of a bad bite or sting, give your child a liquid calcium

Emergency Treatment for Insect Bites and Stings

✚ **For venemous spider bites, get immediate help.** If you suspect that your child has been bitten by a venomous insect, such as the black widow or brown recluse spider, take her immediately to the emergency room of the nearest hospital. If you cannot transport your child, call for emergency help and explain the situation. In the very beginning stages, the only way you will know that a child has been bitten by a poisonous spider is if you see the spider in the vicinity. If possible, capture the insect and have it ready to show the doctor for quick identification.

If your child is bitten by an insect or spider you can't identify, call your local Poison Control Center for instructions on how best to treat your child (see page 344 for a complete listing of Poison Control Centers).

✚ **For black widow spider bites.** The poisonous venom of the black widow spider causes sweating, stomach cramps, nausea, headaches, and dizziness. A small child bitten by a black widow is especially endangered. Treatment for a black widow bite consists of the injection of antivenin. The antivenin itself, however, can cause an allergic reaction in some people. A known allergy to this drug or to horse serum prohibits its use. After administering the antivenin, medical personnel will monitor your child. They may also give your child muscle relaxants or intravenous calcium to relieve muscle pain and spasms.

✚ **For brown recluse spider bites.** A bite from the poisonous brown recluse spider will cause a characteristic bull's-eye marking—a blister surrounded by white and red circles. Pain, nausea, fever, and chills are common. Because a small child can have a serious reaction to this venom,

medical care is essential. If the bite is untreated, a large amount of the surrounding tissue can die, requiring surgical excision. Brown recluse spider bites may be treated with injections of steroids. A drug called Dapsone is also effective in some cases.

✚ **For bee, wasp, or hornet stings.** Should your child be stung by a bee, wasp, or hornet, remove the stinger by gently scraping it out, then wash and rinse the area thoroughly. Watch your child carefully for signs of an allergic reaction, such as redness that begins spreading rapidly outward from the area of penetration, hives, or difficulty breathing. Reactions can occur within minutes or after several hours, so keep a watchful eye on your child.

At the first sign of a severe allergic reaction, especially if your child is having difficulty breathing, take her to the emergency room of the nearest hospital. If you cannot transport your child, call for emergency help and stress the gravity of the situation. Seconds count. If an emergency adrenaline kit such as the Ana-Kit or EpiPen is available, administer it immediately. These kits, which are available by prescription only, contain a syringe filled with a premeasured dose of epinephrine, a hormone that opens the airways and restores free breathing to combat a life-threatening allergic reaction.

✚ **For common insect bites.** Monitor your child's reactions. If she should suffer a serious allergic or toxic reaction after a bite or sting from a common insect, take her to the emergency room of the nearest hospital. If your child seems listless or unlike her normal self following a bite or sting, call your physician immediately.

and magnesium combination formula to calm and soothe her nervous system. Give your child one dose of a formula containing 250 milligrams of calcium to 125 milligrams of magnesium, two to three times daily, for four days.

■ Vitamin C and bioflavonoids are helpful in relieving the toxicity of all bites and stings, and also have anti-inflammatory properties. Give your child one dose of each, four times daily, for two days. If your child develops loose stool, cut the dosage in half.

HERBAL TREATMENT

For age-appropriate dosages of herbal remedies, see page 81.

■ Aloe vera gel is very soothing for minor insect bites that are stinging and burning. Apply the gel to the area as needed.

■ Calendula tincture, gel, or cream helps to soothe and relieve the irritation of insect bites. Apply directly to the bite as needed.

■ Echinacea tincture is highly effective for wounds and stings. Give your child one dose, every two to three hours, for the first day after a bad bite or sting. Then give one dose, three or four times daily, until the swelling subsides.

Note: You should not give your child echinacea for more than ten days at a time, or it will lose its effectiveness.

■ Plantain leaves and comfrey can help draw out the poison and relieve the itching of an insect bite. Prepare and apply a poultice of plantain leaves and comfrey (*see* PREPARING HERBAL TREATMENTS in Part Three). Tobacco leaves also make a time-honored poultice for bites and stings. If these herbs are not readily available, try applying echinacea and goldenseal combination formula directly to the site.

HOMEOPATHY

■ *Natrum muriaticum* 6x, preferably in liquid form, should be applied immediately to an insect bite. This homeopathic remedy lessens itching and relieves the burning sensation. If the liquid form is unavailable, dissolve a few pellets in a small amount of distilled water and apply the resulting solution.

■ *Apis mellifica* 12x, 30x, 6c, or 9c helps decrease the swelling and stinging sensation associated with a bee sting. Give your child one dose every hour until the swelling diminishes, up to a total of four doses.

■ Homeopathic *Echinacea* 6x, 12x, or 5c helps prevent infection. Give your child one dose, twice daily, for four days.

■ *Ledum* 12x, 30x, 6c, or 9c reduces the bruising, swelling, and general discomfort of an insect bite. Give your child one dose, three times daily. Or apply homeopathic *Ledum* ointment directly to the bite.

GENERAL RECOMMENDATIONS

■ If your child has a severe allergy to bites or stings, make sure she wears a Medic Alert bracelet. The information the bracelet carries will alert those around your child to her needs in the event of an allergic reaction. Contact Medic Alert at 2323 Colorado Avenue, Turlock, CA 95380; telephone 800–432–5378.

■ If your child is stung by a bee and you know she is allergic to bee venom, seek immediate medical care. Should your child develop respiratory symptoms, such as wheezing or difficulty breathing, take her to the emergency room of the nearest hospital. A child rarely has a problem with her first bee sting. However, if there is a family history of allergies, or if your child exhibits a strong reaction to her first bee sting, a life-threatening allergy may develop.

■ If you know that your child could suffer a severe allergic reaction to a bite or sting, ask your doctor about the possibility of prescribing emergency medication for quick administration. Epinephrine, which can open your child's airways and restore free breathing in a crisis, is available for home use as the Ana-Kit or EpiPen, which contain a syringe with a premeasured dose of medication.

■ If your child is stung by a bee, wasp, or hornet, remove the stinger by gently scraping it out, not by pulling. Watch your child closely for any allergic reaction.

■ If your child is prone to stings, it may be worthwhile to invest in The Extractor, a device that can be used to extract venom from a bite or sting. It is available in many camping and outdoor equipment stores or directly through the manufacturer, Sawyer Products. Their address is P.O. Box 188, Safety Harbor, FL 34695; telephone 813–725–1177.

■ Treat minor insect bites, stings, and itches with a cold compress or ice to help stop the spread of histamine, the chemical that causes itching.

■ Apply calendula lotion to soothe and cool minor bites and stings and select an appropriate homeopathic remedy.

■ Sweating increases the discomfort of most skin irritations. Try to keep your child's skin cool and dry.

PREVENTION

■ There are many commercial insect repellents sold over the counter. These formulas may not be safe for children, however. The chemical ingredients they contain can be absorbed through the skin in doses that may be toxic to youngsters, causing headaches and other problems.

■ Citronella and pennyroyal are safe, natural repellents that may be applied to your child's exposed skin. Oils of citronella and pennyroyal are usually available in health food stores.

Caution: Pennyroyal should not be used by pregnant women.

■ Deet (diethyl toluamide) is a very effective insect repellent, but because of its high potential toxicity, it is not usually recommended for children. However, a very low dose formulation of deet is available that is safer for children. It is called Skedaddle! and is produced by Little Point Corporation of Cambridge, MA. One application of this repellent lasts for four to six hours.

■ Garlic helps to repel insects. Give your child one or two capsules, twice daily, for three days before a wilderness outing and throughout the trip.

■ Spray permethrin (available as Nix, Permanone, or Duranon) on your child's clothes. This is a medication normally used to get rid of head lice. It is very effective and virtually nontoxic when used this way as an insect repellent. One spraying can last for up to two weeks.

Caution: Do not spray permethrin on an infant's clothing.

■ Liquid vitamin B, taken orally, is effective in preventing some insect bites. Vitamin B is excreted through the skin and is believed to leave a bad taste in the mouths of mosquitoes and fleas. Before a trip to the woods, give your child 1 teaspoon of liquid vitamin-B complex, twice daily, for three days, and continue giving it throughout the trip.

■ Teach your child not to chase bees, wasps, or hornets. If you spot a nest built by one of these stinging insects, warn your child to stay well away.

■ Don't swat at or squash a yellow jacket. Recent studies show that the body of a crushed yellow jacket exudes a chemical that attracts and stimulates other yellow jackets in the area to attack. If you're being bothered by a yellow jacket, it's better to leave the area.

■ Cologne, shiny jewelry, and even perfumed suntan lotions all attract insects, so it's best not to use or wear them when spending time outdoors.

Black Eye

See BRUISES.

Bleeding, Minor

See CUTS AND SCRAPES.

Bleeding, Nose

See NOSEBLEED.

Bleeding, Severe

EMERGENCY TREATMENT FOR SEVERE BLEEDING

See the inset on page 123.

All healthy, active children get cuts and scrapes from time to time, and for the most part these minor injuries can be treated at home (*see* CUTS AND SCRAPES). But if your child receives a severe external wound that spurts or causes a great deal of steady bleeding, it is possible that an artery or vein has been cut. Arteries carry oxygen-rich blood from the lungs and heart to the rest of the body; veins carry oxygen-poor blood back to the heart and lungs. If an artery is cut, it will bleed oxygenated blood that is bright red in color. Oxygen-poor blood coming from a cut vein is a dark, bluish red.

The body of a toddler who weighs twenty-five pounds contains only about one quart of blood. An older child has from three to six quarts of blood, depending on body size. Hundreds of miles of blood vessels run to every living organ and tissue (except for the cornea of the eye). If blood flow to any part of the body is cut off, that part will die. Brain cells die after three to four minutes without a fresh supply of blood.

If your child is bleeding heavily, emergency treatment is necessary.

CONVENTIONAL TREATMENT

■ Seek emergency medical treatment (see page 123). Rely on medical personnel to take over and do what is necessary and appropriate to stop the bleeding and stabilize your child's body. He may require a blood transfusion or the administration of intravenous saline solution to maintain fluid levels.

■ On reaching the hospital, your child may require sutures (stitches) or surgery to repair the damage that caused the bleeding.

■ Once the wound has been treated and your child is well enough to leave the

Emergency Treatment for Severe Bleeding

✚ In the case of a severe external wound, have someone call immediately for emergency help.

✚ Cover the bleeding wound with a clean cloth or gauze, and quickly apply very firm, steady pressure. If there is no clean cloth or gauze immediately available, use your bare hand to apply pressure. Even if your child complains that the pressure hurts, continue applying very firm, steady pressure. It is necessary to stop the bleeding.

✚ If there is no suspicion of a spinal injury, raise the wound above the level of the heart to help minimize the amount of blood that spurts from the wound with every heartbeat. Signs of a spinal injury include pain at the site of the injury, weakness or numbness in an extremity, inability to move an extremity, or lack of feeling in an extremity. If any of these signs are present, *do not* move your child. If you do, you may worsen the injury.

✚ If the blood soaks through the cloth pad or gauze, put more cloth or gauze over the old pad and continue applying pressure. It's best not to remove the original blood-soaked pad. Early clotting may become dislodged if you try to change the bandage.

✚ If emergency medical personnel are not on their way to you, take your child to the emergency room of the nearest hospital. If you are fortunate enough to have another adult with you, have that person see to transportation while you hold your child and continue applying pressure. If you are alone with your child and must drive him yourself, tie cloth or gauze very firmly in place to maintain pressure on the wound. If you must tie on a bandage, check for a pulse beat below it to make sure that tissues below the wound are receiving an adequate supply of blood.

✚ A tourniquet is a bandage that is tied so tightly that it cuts off the flow of blood to an area of the body, usually a portion of an arm or leg. It is a drastic measure that is appropriate only if blood loss is so severe and rapid as to be immediately life threatening, such as might occur following the partial amputation of a limb. *Do not apply a tourniquet unless it is absolutely necessary and then only as a last resort.* Because it cuts off the blood supply, a tourniquet deprives the tissues below the wound of oxygen, creating the risk of your child losing a limb. If your child is losing so much blood so rapidly that you must put on a tourniquet, be sure to mark it with the time the tourniquet was applied. Never cover a tourniquet. It is vital that medical personnel can see immediately that a tourniquet is in place.

✚ A severe loss of blood will cause shock, which can be life threatening. Try to remain calm and reassuring. Any panic you display will be transmitted to your child and make the situation worse. Your immediate task is to stem the flow of blood and secure emergency medical care for your child.

✚ Do not give your child any medicine or food, or liquid of any kind, before a doctor has assessed the situation. It is important that your child's stomach be empty, as surgery may be needed to repair the wound.

hospital, medical personnel will advise you on the proper way to care for your child as he recovers from his injury. Ask your doctor for recommendations regarding diet, activity level, special exercises, and any measures necessary to guard against complications.

DIETARY GUIDELINES

◼ If your child is recovering from a blood loss, make sure his diet includes lots of green leafy vegetables, squashes, and fresh fruits, as well as liquids, to provide necessary vitamins and minerals and restore fluid balance.

◼ If you are giving your child supplementary iron (see below), his diet should also include an increased amount of fiber and liquids to prevent constipation, which is an occasional side effect of iron supplementation.

NUTRITIONAL SUPPLEMENTS

The nutritional supplements that follow are directed at supporting recovery once appropriate emergency medical care has been administered and your child is well enough to leave the hospital. If your child is bleeding profusely, seek emergency medical care immediately. For age-appropriate dosages of nutritional supplements, see page 81.

■ Bioflavonoids are helpful for wound healing. Give your child one dose a day for two to three months.

■ Give your child a chlorophyll supplement for two to three months. Chlorophyll has trace minerals that assist the body in rebuilding blood. Follow dosage directions on the product label.

■ If your physician determines that your child's blood loss has resulted in anemia, an iron supplement may be prescribed to help build up his blood. If possible, select a chelated form (ferrous chelate). Ferrous gluconate and ferrous fumarate are also acceptable. Avoid ferrous sulfate, which can cause stomach irritation and constipation. Give your child one dose daily for two to three months.

Note: To enhance absorption, iron should be given together with vitamin C (see below).

■ The B vitamins, especially vitamin B_{12} and folic acid, are very important for restoring healthy blood. Give your child a B-complex vitamin tablet, plus an additional dose of vitamin B_{12} and folic acid, every day for two to three months.

■ Vitamin C helps the body to absorb iron. Give your child one dose of vitamin C daily for two to three months.

HERBAL TREATMENT

The herbal treatments that follow are directed at supporting recovery once appropriate emergency medical care has been administered and your child is well enough to leave the hospital. If your child is bleeding profusely, seek emergency medical care immediately. For age-appropriate dosages of herbal remedies, see page 81.

■ A child who has suffered a blood loss may become anemic. Floradix formula is an herbal iron supplement that can be used to slowly help replace some of the iron lost through bleeding. Follow dosage directions on the product label for two to three months.

Note: Floradix is best for mild anemia. If your child has an anemic condition documented by a blood test, a more concentrated nutritional iron supplement may be a better way to rebuild his blood.

■ Nettle and yellow dock help build healthy blood cells. After the crisis is over, give your child one dose of either or both herbs, twice daily, for one to two weeks.

Note: Some children experience stomach upset as a result of taking nettle. If this happens, stop giving it. Nettle should not be given to a child under four.

HOMEOPATHY

Homeopathic treatment is aimed at supporting recovery once appropriate emergency medical care has been administered and your child is well enough to leave the hospital. If your child is bleeding profusely, seek emergency medical care immediately.

■ *Ferrum phosphoricum* 12x or 6c helps the body recover from a major blood loss. Give your child one dose, three times daily, for five days.

GENERAL RECOMMENDATIONS

■ Seek emergency treatment immediately.

■ Once the crisis is over and your child is well enough to leave the hospital, ask your doctor for recommendations regarding diet, activity restrictions, and other measures to support your child's recovery.

■ Give your child additional iron, B vitamins, vitamin C, and bioflavonoids.

■ Give your child nettle and/or yellow dock.

■ For additional suggestions regarding natural therapies that aid in recovery from a major blood loss and speed healing, see SURGERY, RECOVERING FROM.

PREVENTION

■ The best way to prevent an injury that causes severe bleeding is to make sure your child's environment is as safe as possible. For advice on how to reduce the risks of an accident in and around your home, see HOME SAFETY in Part One of this book.

Boils

A boil is a bacterial infection that begins deep in a hair follicle or a sebaceous gland, one of the skin's oil-producing glands, and gradually works its way up to the surface of the skin. *Staphylococcus aureus* is the bacteria most frequently responsible for boils.

Boils most often appear on the neck, face, underarms, or buttocks. If your child complains of a red, elevated, and painful bump, watch the area closely. Should a boil be developing, a pustule will form in the center of the affected area within two to four days.

It is possible, although unusual, for a boil to spread beyond the affected area and cause a more serious systemic infection. For example, nearby lymph glands may become swollen. A boil may also be a sign of an underlying infection in your child's body that is manifesting itself through the skin. In either case, your child would need medical attention.

To determine when to call the doctor, observe your child's demeanor. To get a clear, overall sense of how your child is feeling, step away from her until you can't see the boil any longer. Is your child playing and laughing, or sweaty, tired, and pale? A child with a boil who is overtired, running a fever, not eating well, or who is just not "up to par" needs to see a physician.

CONVENTIONAL TREATMENT

■ Your child's physician may recommend that the boil be incised (cut open) and allowed to drain. This is a procedure that should be done by a medical professional. If the doctor incises the boil, or if it ruptures by itself, it will drain thick pus. A topical antibiotic, such as Betadine or bacitracin, may be prescribed to help clear the infection.

■ If your child's doctor suspects that a deeper, more dangerous infection may be developing, he or she may also prescribe an oral antibiotic, such as erythromycin, dicloxacillin (Diclox), or cephalexin (Keflex).

DIETARY GUIDELINES

■ Avoid giving your child sweets and greasy, fried foods. Keep her diet simple and clean.

■ Make sure your child eats plenty of dark green vegetables.

NUTRITIONAL SUPPLEMENTS

For age-appropriate dosages of nutritional supplements, see page 81.

■ If the boil is not an open wound, open a vitamin-A capsule and apply it directly onto the boil, twice a day, for five days, to help it heal.

■ Beta-carotene helps to heal skin tissue. Give your child one dose, twice a day, for one week or until the boil is healed.

■ Vitamin C and bioflavonoids have mild anti-inflammatory properties and help to boost the immune system. Give your child one dose of each, three or four times a day, for one week or until the boil heals.

■ Zinc helps support the immune system and heal skin tissue. Give your child one dose of zinc, twice a day, for one week or until healed.

Note: Excessive amounts of zinc can result in nausea and vomiting. Be careful not to exceed the recommended dosage.

HERBAL TREATMENT

For age-appropriate dosages of herbal remedies, see page 81.

■ Burdock root is an excellent internal cleanser. Give your child one dose, three times daily, for five days.

■ Echinacea and goldenseal stimulate the immune system and help to clear infection. Echinacea has antiviral properties; goldenseal is an antibacterial herb that also soothes the skin and mucous membranes. Give your child one dose of an echinacea and goldenseal combination formula, three times daily, until the boil improves. Goldenseal can also be applied topically to a boil for its antiseptic properties.

Note: You should not give your child echinacea on a daily basis for more than ten days at a time, or it will lose its effectiveness.

■ A ginger tea compress will help to draw out infection and bring a boil to a head. Prepare a strong ginger tea and soak a clean white cloth in it. Apply this warm, wet compress to your child's boil for ten to fifteen minutes, at least four times daily.

■ Green clay paste helps draw out and dry up infection. Mix 1 teaspoon of green clay with a small amount of water, just enough to make a pastelike consistency. After using a ginger tea compress, apply this paste to your child's boil.

■ Use tea tree oil compresses. Tea tree oil is a strong antiseptic and helps to resolve infection. Add 8 to 10 drops of tea tree oil to 1 quart of warm water and soak a clean cotton cloth or cotton ball in the mixture. Apply the warm compress to the boil for ten to fifteen minutes, four times daily.

■ Usnea moss is effective against staphylococcus bacteria. Make a strong usnea tea by boiling 3 tablespoons of the whole herb in 1 cup of water for three minutes. Remove the mixture from the heat and allow it to steep for another ten minutes. Then soak a clean washcloth in the tea and apply it to the boil for ten to fifteen minutes. Repeat this procedure three or four times daily until the boil heals.

■ Usnea is also available in ointment form. One excellent ointment for boils is a product called Super Salve, which contains chaparral, echinacea, and hops, in addition to usnea. Apply the ointment to the affected area three times daily.

■ Make an herbal poultice by adding 1 tablespoon each of plantain, marshmallow root, goldenseal, and/or Oregon grape root to 1 cup of water. Bring to a boil and simmer for twenty minutes. Soak a cloth in the mixture, and apply the poultice to the affected area for twenty to thirty minutes. Do this three times a day, for two to three days.

HOMEOPATHY

The following homeopathic remedies will help relieve your child's discomfort quickly. Please note that they are to be used in stages.

■ *Belladonna* helps bring down a boil that is large, red, and hot. When a boil first appears and is red and throbbing, give your child one dose of *Belladonna* 30x or 9c, every three to four hours, for one day.

■ When the pustular head on the on the boil appears, *Hepar sulphuris* will help promote discharge. Give your child one dose of *Hepar sulphuris* 12x or 6c, three times daily, for one day after the boil comes to a head.

■ To speed draining after pus appears, give your child one dose of *Silicea* 12x or 6c, three times daily, for two days.

■ *Myristica* encourages boils to open and drain. If your child has a stubborn boil that refuses to open, give her one dose of *Myristica* 12x or 6c, four times daily, for one day.

■ *Calcarea sulphurica* is used for a boil that is not healing readily. Once the boil does begin to drain, give your child one dose of *Calcarea sulphurica* 12x, three times daily, until the boil has emptied.

GENERAL RECOMMENDATIONS

■ If your child has a boil accompanied by fever, lack of appetite, malaise, or any other sign of a systemic infection, see your physician.

■ Do not squeeze or puncture a boil. Opening it prematurely can worsen and spread the infection.

■ Avoid using tape or an adhesive bandage to cover your child's boil. Covering a boil may increase irritation and can lead to scarring.

■ To fight infection and support the immune system, give your child an echinacea and goldenseal combination formula.

■ After assessing which phase the boil is in, give your child a suitable homeopathic remedy.

■ Apply hot ginger tea compresses, followed by an application of green clay paste.

■ Give your child burdock root as a blood purifier.

PREVENTION

■ Teach your child to keep her skin clean and dry. Good hygiene is helpful. However, your child may practice meticulous skin care and still develop a boil, especially in hot and humid environments.

■ Propolis is a natural antibiotic made by bees that can be used in tincture form. Give your child one dose, three times daily, three times a week, to prevent the recurrence of boils.

■ If your child is prone to recurrent boils, try the following three-week cycle.

Week 1: Give your child one dose of echinacea tincture, twice a day.
Week 2: Give your child one dose of nettle, twice a day.
Week 3: Give your child one dose of burdock root or red clover, twice a day.

Repeat this cycle three times, for a total of nine weeks.
Note: Some children experience stomach upset as a result of taking nettle. If this happens, stop giving it. Nettle should not be given to a child under four.

■ Give your child a garlic supplement, as directed on the product label, for two months.

■ If your child still suffers from a succession of boils after taking garlic and following the echinacea/nettle/burdock cycle for two months, take her to a physician to be examined for a possible underlying condition.

Bones, Broken

When people think of bones, they often visualize them as "dead," rather like the dry skeletons that sometimes hang in science classrooms. But bones are really living tissue, with a rich supply of blood vessels and nerves. As a result, a bone fracture is not only painful, it causes shock and trauma to the whole body.

Because a child's bones are still growing, correct treatment of a broken bone is especially important in childhood. If not treated correctly, a child may lose mobility and partial function of the bone.

If your child has suffered an accident, a bad fall, or a hard blow, he may have broken a bone. Depending on the cause of the break, there may be an open wound near the fracture. Your child may lie very still to protect himself against the pain of movement. An affected limb may appear crooked or bent. The area near a fracture will be painful or tender when moved or touched, and may appear swollen, red, and bruised.

Depending on which bone is broken, there is a possibility of additional damage, including internal bleeding (see page 217). A broken rib may puncture a lung; a broken vertebra can damage the spinal cord; a skull fracture can cause bleeding into the skull. Broken bones should be taken seriously and treated immediately.

CONVENTIONAL TREATMENT

■ On arrival at the hospital, your child will be examined. A broken bone must be assessed, x-rayed, set, and possibly placed in traction by a physician.

■ The possibility of internal damage will be considered. Should any further injury come to light, emergency room personnel will take the appropriate measures.

■ If your child is in pain, pain medication may be administered.

■ The proper setting and casting of the long bones of the arms and legs are particularly critical in a still-growing child. The doctor must take care to ensure that these bones continue to grow steadily and match the growth of their counterparts.

■ Broken fingers and toes may be splinted, or the doctor may securely tape the injured digit to adjacent fingers or toes. Either method will keep the bone immobilized while it heals.

DIETARY GUIDELINES

■ Support the healing process by providing your child with plenty of lean protein, plus bone-building foods containing calcium, phosphorus, and vitamin D. Calcium-rich foods include all the familiar dairy products, but please select the low-fat varieties. Green leafy vegetables also provide calcium and valuable trace minerals. Phosphorus is found in bananas, whole-grain breads and cereals, nuts, eggs, fish, and poultry. Vitamin D is present in fortified dairy products, eggs, and saltwater fish.

■ A child recovering from a broken bone should not consume any sodas or other foods containing phosphoric acid. This substance actually depletes calcium from the bones.

NUTRITIONAL SUPPLEMENTS

For age-appropriate dosages of some nutritional supplements, see page 81.

■ A calcium and magnesium combination formula, in either liquid or capsule form, will help to rebuild bone tissue. The ideal combination is 250 milligrams of calcium to 125 milligrams of magnesium. Give your child one dose, twice daily, for a minimum of two months.

■ Chlorophyll provides trace minerals that help rebuild bone tissue. Give your child a chlorophyll supplement, following the dosage directions on the product label, for two to three months after a bone break (until the break is healed).

■ Vitamin C helps in the process of bone healing. Give your child one dose of vitamin C, once a day, for two to three months.

■ Vitamin D improves the absorption of calcium. Give your child one dose of vitamin D every day for two to three months.

HERBAL TREATMENT

Herbal treatment for broken bones is directed at supporting recovery once appropriate emergency medical care has been administered and your child is well

EMERGENCY TREATMENT FOR BROKEN BONES

✚ If you think your child may have suffered a serious bone fracture—a broken long bone, rib, or vertebra, or a skull fracture—or a neck or back injury, *do not move him.* Movement can cause additional injury. Call for emergency help.

✚ Remain calm and reassure your child. Your soothing presence, familiar voice, and gentle touch may be the most helpful things you can offer.

✚ If you have taken a first aid course and are very confident of your ability, you can use a splint to immobilize a broken limb, including the joints above and below the fracture. This is a temporary measure, of course. A doctor's evaluation and treatment are still essential.

✚ If your child has broken a smaller bone, apply ice. Take him to the hospital emergency room or see your physician promptly.

✚ If your child fractures a finger or toe, apply ice or a cool compress to the injury and elevate it above the level of the heart. This will minimize swelling and help relieve pain. Take your child to the emergency room or to your physician.

✚ Noses are seldom actually broken. A child's still-immature nose is made primarily of cartilage, not bone. A blow to the nose can be very painful, however. A blood-filled bruise may develop inside the nose, causing a black eye on one or both sides. Apply an ice pack immediately. With the ice in place, take your child to the emergency room or to your physician for prompt attention.

enough to leave the hospital. For age-appropriate dosages of herbal remedies, see page 81.

■ Horsetail is high in silica, which helps the body absorb the calcium needed for bone tissue healing. It is not suitable for infants or younger children, however. For teenagers only, give one dose, twice daily, for two weeks.

■ Nettle is high in silica and other trace minerals. It also enhances calcium absorption. Give your child one dose daily for two to three weeks.

Note: Some children experience stomach upset as a result of taking this herb. If this happens, stop giving it. This herb should not be given to a child under four.

■ Oat straw is high in silica and is a mild relaxant. Give your child one dose, twice daily, for two weeks.

HOMEOPATHY

■ If you suspect your child has broken a bone, you can give him one dose of homeopathic *Aconite* 30x, 200x, 9c, or 30c on the way to the hospital. *Aconite* is excellent for relieving the shock and fright associated with an injury. The cold sweat, fear, dizziness, and nausea your child may be experiencing will quickly be alleviated with this remedy.

■ Five minutes after administering the initial dose of *Aconite*, give your child one dose of *Arnica* 30x, 200x, 9c, or 30c. Give him another dose of *Arnica* every thirty minutes thereafter, for a total of three doses. *Arnica* helps lessen the bruising and aching pain associated with a bone fracture. It also aids in healing the injury to the soft tissue and muscle surrounding a break.

■ After the immediate crisis has been handled and your child is home from the hospital, give him the following remedies in the sequence indicated to help the break knit quickly and to speed healing.

Days 1–2: Three times a day, give your child one dose of *Arnica* 30x or 9c.

Days 3–5: Three times a day, give your child one dose of *Ruta graveolens* 12x or 6c, to help relieve bone pain.

Days 6–8: Three times a day, give your child one dose of *Symphytum* 6x, to help the bone heal quickly.

Days 9–19: Once a day, give your child one dose of *Calcarea phosphorica* 6x, to support the healing process.

Days 20–27: Stop all administration of homeopathic remedies for one week.

Days 28–38: Once a day, give your child one dose of *Calcarea phosphorica* 6x.

GENERAL RECOMMENDATIONS

■ If your child breaks a bone, take appropriate emergency measures and rely on medical personnel to treat the injury properly. Any broken bone should be evaluated by a doctor.

■ Once the crisis is over and your child is home from the hospital, use horsetail, nettle, or oat straw to support recovery.

■ Give your child the sequence of homeopathic remedies outlined above.

■ Give your child supplemental calcium, magnesium, and chlorophyll.

■ Follow the dietary guidelines above.

PREVENTION

■ An ounce of prevention is worth three weeks in the hospital. Whenever possible, keep a watchful eye on your child. Simply being there, ready to strongly caution your child or, if necessary, snatch him out of harm's way, provides enormous protection for an infant or young child.

■ Children of all ages are naturally curious and adventurous. Teach your child to be appropriately cautious and thoughtful in all of his activities.

■ For advice on ways to reduce the risk of accidents that can lead to broken bones, *see* HOME SAFETY in Part One.

Breathing Distress

See ANAPHYLACTIC SHOCK; ASTHMA; UNCONSCIOUSNESS.

Bronchiolitis

Bronchiolitis is a lower respiratory viral infection that occurs most commonly in infants one to twelve months old. It is a widespread inflammation of the small bronchi and bronchioles, the small airways in the lungs. Because of the infection, these airways become swollen, produce mucus, and may also spasm and contract, much as they do with asthma. The condition may be accompanied by an ear infection or pneumonia. Over half of the cases of bronchiolitis are caused by a virus called respiratory syncitial virus (RSV). Incidence is highest in the winter and early spring.

Bronchiolitis typically develops after a few days of cold symptoms, beginning with a harsh cough, fever, wheezing, difficulty eating, and difficulty breathing. Two to three days after the cough and breathing difficulty start, the illness can get worse. This is often the most difficult time for the child. She may have increased difficulty breathing, more anxiety, fatigue due to an inability to sleep, and difficulty eating or drinking. Many children with bronchiolitis are hospitalized so that they can be supported and watched closely during this time. There is a danger that mucus plugs, inadequate oxygen, and exhaustion can lead to respiratory failure.

For months or even years following a bout of bronchiolitis, your child may experience wheezing when she gets a cold.

CONVENTIONAL TREATMENT

■ In order to diagnose bronchiolitis, a doctor will do a careful respiratory assessment, possibly a chest x-ray, and a culture of mucus in order to identify the virus. The amount of oxygen in the blood may be checked (painlessly) with a special device called an oximeter.

■ Because bronchiolitis is usually caused by a viral infection, antibiotics are not called for unless a secondary, bacterial infection develops.

131

■ Viral bronchiolitis is treated with oxygen, fluids, and, sometimes, bronchodilators. Oxygen is given so that the child does not have to work so hard to get an adequate amount of oxygen. Fluids help to thin secretions and prevent dehydration. Bronchodilators such as metaproterenol (in Alupent or Metaprel) or albuterol (Proventil, Ventolin) may be prescribed to relax the airways, stop the wheezing, and ease breathing.

■ A child who is hospitalized will go home once she is past the critical period, is able to breathe comfortably, and is able to maintain an adequate level of oxygen in her blood.

■ Ribavirin (Virazole) is a medicine that can stop the respiratory syncitial virus from multiplying and so limit possible complications of the illness. It is generally given only to those children with a chronic lung or heart illness or an immune deficiency.

DIETARY GUIDELINES

■ Give your child plenty of fluids to help thin secretions so that they are easier to cough out.

HERBAL TREATMENT

For age-appropriate dosages of herbal remedies, see page 81.

■ Make a tea combining equal amounts (1 teaspoon or dropperful of tincture, or 1 capsule of powdered herb) of marshmallow root, slippery elm bark, licorice, and thyme. This tea is soothing to the lungs. Give your child one dose, three times a day.
   Note: Licorice should not be given to a child with high blood pressure.

■ Mix 5 drops of either thyme or eucalyptus oil in 1 cup of olive or almond oil. Rub the mixture along your child's spine, particularly in the upper back over the lungs. This will help relax your child and increase circulation to the lungs.

■ Once the infection has subsided, astragalus (*Astragalus membranaceous*) can be very useful. It has a rich concentration of trace minerals and micronutrients and helps to strengthen the immune system. Give your child one-half dose, three times a day, for two weeks.
   Note: Astragalus should not be taken until signs of acute infection (such as fever) are no longer present.

■ Like astragalus, American ginseng is an excellent source of trace minerals and micronutrients that can be beneficial to your child's recovery. It also helps to strengthen the immune system. After the infection has cleared, give your child half the recommended dose, three times a day, for two weeks.
   Note: Do not give your child American ginseng until fever and other signs of active infection have resolved.

HOMEOPATHY

■ *Antimonium tartaricum* is good for a child with a moist, rattling cough, and who is breathless and pale. Give this child *Antimonium tartaricum* 12x, 30x, 6c or 9c, three times a day, after her fever has resolved, until symptoms improve. If there is no improvement after forty-eight hours, discontinue the remedy and try another.
   Note: This remedy should not be used in the presence of a fever.

■ *Drosera* is good for a child with a dry, whooping cough. Give your child one dose of *Drosera* 12x, 30x, 6c, or 9c, three times a day, for up to forty-eight hours or until her symptoms improve.

■ *Phosphorus* should be considered for the harsh, rattling cough that is lingering. This child may have a fever. Give your child one dose of *Phosphorus* 30x or 9c, four to five times daily, until symptoms improve. If there is no improvement after forty-eight hours, discontinue the remedy.

BACH FLOWER REMEDIES

■ Aspen and Mimulus are good for relieving the anxiety of a child who has bronchiolitis. Aspen is good for a child who is afraid of unknown things; Mimulus is for a child who can name her fears. Place a few drops of the mother tincture in water and have your child sip it. (See BACH FLOWER REMEDIES in Part One.)

■ If your child is feeling irritable, whiny, and impatient, give her Impatiens. Place a few drops of the mother tincture in a glass or bottle of water and have your child sip it throughout the day.

ACUPRESSURE

For the locations of acupressure points on a child's body, *see* ADMINISTERING AN ACUPRESSURE TREATMENT in Part Three.

■ Pericardium 6 helps to relax the chest and ease breathing.

■ Massaging along the spine relaxes the nervous system and will make your child more comfortable.

GENERAL RECOMMENDATIONS

■ Cool humidity helps to thin secretions so that they are easier to cough or sneeze out. Use a cool mist humidifier in your child's room.

■ Raising the head of the bed, using additional pillows, or putting your child in an infant seat can ease breathing.

■ Offer your child small, frequent meals to maintain adequate nutrition.

■ Help your child rest. Hug, cuddle, and talk reassuringly to your child to lessen her anxiety.

PREVENTION

■ It may not be possible to prevent your child from developing bronchiolitis. However, it goes without saying that you should keep your child from contact with sick playmates and others as much as possible.

Bronchitis

Bronchitis is an inflammation of the trachea (windpipe) and the large bronchi of the respiratory tract. Bronchitis can be caused by a bacterial or viral infection, or it can be triggered by an allergic reaction to molds, pollens, dander, or dust.

Bronchitis begins with a runny nose, fever, a dry cough, and possibly wheezing. The cough eventually becomes productive, with clear sputum at first and later thick, yellow sputum. Symptoms of allergic bronchitis include a cough that is often worse at night, malaise, loss of appetite, and wheezing. Chronic bronchitis is characterized by a persistent dry cough without other symptoms. A lingering or chronic cough can be debilitating.

CONVENTIONAL TREATMENT

■ In general, a dry cough need not be encouraged and can be treated with a cough suppressant. Dextromethorphan is a common and relatively safe ingredient found in many over-the-counter cough preparations. It can usually be identified by the initials DM on the label. It is almost as effective as codeine at suppressing coughs, and has few side effects. Follow dosage directions on the product label.

■ A wet cough indicates that the body is attempting to eliminate excess mucus. In this case, an expectorant, such as guaifenesin (found in Anti-Tuss and Robitussin, among others) may be helpful. Expectorants help to thin secretions so that they are easier to cough out. These medications are not recommended for children less than two years old, however. Follow dosage directions on the product label.

■ Bronchodilators, such as metaproterenol (in Alupent or Metaprel) or albuterol (Proventil, Ventolin), may be prescribed to relax the airways, stop wheezing, and ease breathing. These medicines also have a tendency to speed up the heart rate and make a child feel anxious. Follow the prescription directions.

■ If your doctor determines that the bronchitis is caused by a bacterial infection, an antibiotic will be prescribed. Bacterial bronchitis is relatively rare, however, so if your doctor prescribes an antibiotic, be sure to ask why he or she believes that this is an important part of your child's treatment.

DIETARY GUIDELINES

■ With the onset of bronchitis, eliminate any potentially mucus-forming foods (such as dairy products, sweets, and fried foods) from your child's diet until the bronchitis is resolved.

■ Encourage your child to take plenty of fluids. Hydration helps to thin secretions so that they are easier to cough out.

■ Chicken or vegetable soup made with lots of vegetables (especially carrots, parsley, string beans, and zucchini), and the herbs ginger and garlic, is healing. Chicken soup has been shown to contain an ingredient that helps to thin mucus so that it is easier to eliminate. If you have a vegetable-resistant child, you may wish to strain the vegetables out before serving the soup. Broth and noodles are more appetizing to some children than a soup full of vegetables.

NUTRITIONAL SUPPLEMENTS

For age-appropriate dosages of nutritional supplements, see page 81.

■ Beta-carotene helps to heal mucus membranes. Give your child one dose, one to two times a day, until he recovers.

■ Vitamin C and bioflavonoids have anti-inflammatory properties. Give your child one dose of each, three times a day, until he is better.

■ Zinc helps to boost the immune system and speed recovery. It is easily taken in lozenge form. A sugar-free formula is preferred. Give your child a total of one to two doses of zinc a day for as long as symptoms last.

Note: Excessive amounts of zinc can result in nausea and vomiting. Be careful not to exceed the recommended dosage.

HERBAL TREATMENT

For age-appropriate dosages of herbal remedies, see page 81.

■ Make a cough syrup containing slippery elm, licorice, marshmallow root, and osha root. Simmer equal parts of each (40 drops of tincture or 1 tablespoon of whole herb) in 1 quart of water for twenty minutes. If your child is over one year old, you can sweeten the mixture with honey. Give your child 1 teaspoon every hour or two the first day, for a total of 8 teaspoons. Then continue giving your child 1 teaspoon, four to six times a day, until the cough subsides. Each of the herbs in this mixture is soothing to the throat and respiratory tract. If possible, have your child breathe in the vapor while the mixture is cooking.

Note: Licorice should not be given to a child with high blood pressure.

■ Thyme has a mild antimicrobial action and helps to reduce the spasmodic nature of a cough. Try giving your child one dose, three times a day. This herb has a strong taste, however. If your child finds it impossible to drink, try giving him a bath made with thyme, chamomile, or rosemary.

■ Itsiao Keh Chuan is a Chinese herbal cough medicine. It may be too strong-tasting for some children, but it is very effective in resolving a cough. Follow dosage directions on the product label.

HOMEOPATHY

Choose the most appropriate symptom-specific homeopathic remedy from the list below and give your child one dose, three times a day, until his symptoms improve. If there is no improvement in forty-eight hours, it is unlikely that the remedy will do anything more; discontinue it and try another.

■ If your child has a moist, rattling cough, and is breathless and pale, give him *Antimonium tartaricum* 12x or 6c.

Note: This remedy should not be used in the presence of a fever.

■ *Bryonia* 12x or 6c is recommended for the child whose cough is worse at night and who complains of pain in his chest or throat. This child asks for cold drinks, and is probably constipated.

■ *Drosera* 12x or 6c is for the child with a whooping-type cough that is dry and accompanied by wheezing.

■ *Kali bichromicum* 12x or 6c is for the child who has a cough accompanied by thick, stringy mucus.

■ *Phosphorus* 30x or 9c should be considered for the child with a harsh cough that is lingering. This child is usually quite sensitive.

■ *Pulsatilla* 30x or 9c is for the child with a cough, a runny nose, and thin yellow phlegm. This child is emotionally vulnerable and cries easily.

■ Give *Rumex crispus* 12x or 6c to the child with a cough and a lot of mucus. This child feels worse at night, and may wake at around 11:00 P.M. His lymph glands may be swollen.

■ *Spongia* 12x or 6c is for the child who has a crouplike cough that is worse with excitement, and who feels better with hot drinks.

ACUPRESSURE

For the locations of acupressure points on a child's body, *see* ADMINISTERING AN ACUPRESSURE TREATMENT in Part Three.

■ Pericardium 6 relaxes the chest.

■ Liver 3 relaxes the nervous system.

■ Massaging along the spine is soothing and relaxing, especially for the chest and nervous system.

GENERAL RECOMMENDATIONS

■ Rest interspersed with periods of moderate activity is important in treating bronchitis. The moderate activity is helpful in keeping secretions from settling and causing the development of pneumonia.

■ In addition to giving your your child plenty of fluids, use a humidifier to help thin secretions and soothe the respiratory tract.

■ Place a hot-water bottle on your child's chest or back for twenty minutes every day. This helps to ease breathing, especially when used in combination with a humidifier.

PREVENTION

■ If your child suffers from respiratory allergies, try to prevent exposure to those things that provoke a reaction, and try to keep any allergic reactions that do occur from escalating into bronchitis (*see* ALLERGIES).

■ When your child catches a cold, begin appropriate treatment promptly (*see* COMMON COLD). This may help decrease his chances of developing bronchitis.

■ As much as possible, keep your child from contact with sick playmates and others.

Bruises

When your child develops a bruise, a "black-and-blue mark," or a black eye, it is because an injury to a blood vessel has caused blood to leak into the surrounding tissue. Bruises are usually related to an injury to the small capillaries located near the surface of the skin. These tiny blood vessels heal fairly quickly. As the body reabsorbs the blood, the characteristic mark disappears.

Because there are many blood vessels in the head, when a child falls and hits her head, there can be a lot of bleeding into surrounding tissue, causing the classic "goose egg." A blow to the forehead or nose can cause blood to accumulate in the surrounding loose tissues, resulting in the condition commonly known as a black eye.

A new bruise will be tender to the touch and may be swollen. A bruise generally starts out as a red mark, then turns the classic black-and-blue or purple color. As the bruise fades, it becomes lighter and sometimes a bit yellow or brown from residual iron left over after the blood fluids are reabsorbed.

CONVENTIONAL TREATMENT

■ Immediately after an injury, elevate the affected area. Put ice on the bruise for five to ten minutes (if you can persuade your child to sit still long enough). Then take the ice off for fifteen to twenty minutes. Repeat this cycle at least three to five times immediately following the injury, and as much as possible for the first day or two afterward. To avoid causing frostbite damage to the tissues, place a towel or washcloth between the ice and the skin, and be careful not to leave the ice in place too long.

NUTRITIONAL SUPPLEMENTS

For age-appropriate dosages of nutritional supplements, see page 81.

■ To help restore the integrity of blood vessel walls, give your child a vitamin-C formula that contains bioflavonoids. Give your child one-half dose of vitamin C and an equal amount of bioflavonoids, three times daily, for five to seven days. Then give one dose daily for one month. If your child's bruising seems excessive, continue to give one dose daily for two to three more months.

HOMEOPATHY

■ *Arnica* is the classic homeopathic remedy for bruises. To ease the pain and prevent a bruise from becoming larger, give your child one dose of *Arnica* 30x or 9c immediately after an injury. Then give her one dose, three to four times daily, for the first twenty-four hours. After two or three doses, your child should feel less pain.

■ If the skin is *not* broken, apply a topical *Arnica* tincture, oil, or gel directly to your child's bruise. If the skin is broken, a topical homeopathic *Calendula* tincture, oil, or gel will soothe the hurt and help speed healing.

■ If the bruise is still apparent after forty-eight hours, *Ledum* 12x, 30x, 6c, or 9c, taken orally, will help resolve the discoloration. Give your child three to four doses daily for two to three days.

GENERAL RECOMMENDATIONS

■ Apply ice or a cold compress to the area, as described above.

■ If your child suffers a blow that results in a black eye, be alert for any signs that her vision has been affected. If you suspect any vision impairment, consult an ophthalmologist.

■ Administer a suitable homeopathic remedy.

■ Give your child vitamin C with bioflavonoids.

PREVENTION

■ Parents can't be everywhere, and children will inevitably take a fall from time to time. Bruises are one of the unpreventable minor hurts of childhood. There are a number of things you can do, however, to protect your child against the kinds of accidents that cause bruising. For suggestions, *see* HOME SAFETY in Part One.

Burns

EMERGENCY TREATMENT FOR BURNS

See the inset on page 139.

Your child may suffer a burn from dry heat (fire or sun); moist heat (steam or hot liquids); corrosive chemicals; or electricity.

An encounter with electricity can be particularly dangerous. A severe electrical shock may knock your child unconscious, and he may stop breathing. There may be deep burns at the point where the current entered the body, as well as internal damage.

Depending on the location, extent, and cause of the burn, your child may need immediate medical care. A burn can cause scarring, which may limit functioning of the burned area. Regardless of their size and severity, burns on the face, the palms of the hands, the soles of the feet, or on or near a joint can have serious implications. Burns in these areas should always be checked by a doctor and watched with special care. Any burn should be watched for signs of a possible infection.

When evaluating your child's burn, here's what to look for.

• A *first-degree burn* involves only the epidermis, the upper layer of the skin. The area is hot, red, and painful, but without swelling or blistering. Sunburn is usually a first-degree burn. (*See* SUNBURN.)

• A *second-degree burn* involves the epidermis and part of the underlying skin layers. The pain is severe. The area is pink or red and mottled, and is usually moist and seeping, moderately swollen, and blistered.

• Because it involves injury to all layers of the skin, a *third-degree burn* is also called a *full-thickness burn*. This severe burn destroys the nerves and blood vessels in the skin. Because the nerves are damaged, there is little or no pain at first. The affected area may be white, yellow, black, or cherry red. The skin may appear dry and leathery.

• A *fourth-degree burn* extends through the skin and penetrates into underlying structures, such as muscle and bone. It looks and feels like a third-degree burn, but it does greater damage to the body.

Emergency Treatment for Burns

✚ **Remove the cause.** All burns should be treated first by removing the cause—putting out flames, washing off chemicals, or breaking electrical contact. If your child's clothing is on fire, douse him with water or wrap him in a blanket and place him on the ground to put out the flames.

✚ **For electrical burns.** In the case of electrical shock, your inclination will probably be to snatch your child out of harm's way. *Don't.* You may receive a severe shock yourself and become unable to help your child. To break electrical contact safely, first switch off the current. If that is not possible (as in the case of a live wire) use a nonconductive item, such as a wooden broom handle, to lift or push the source of the current away from your child. Always take your child to the emergency room for medical evaluation after an electrical burn, even if he seems to have suffered only a minor burn.

✚ **For chemical burns.** If your child suffers a chemical burn from a corrosive liquid, immediately flood the area with cool running water to dilute and wash away the chemical.

✚ **Assess your child's condition.** Once the cause of the burn has been removed, check your child's breathing and pulse. *If your child's breathing or pulse has stopped, turn to* CARDIOPULMONARY RESUSCITATION (CPR) *on page 426.* Start CPR at once. Have someone call for emergency help.

✚ **For third- or fourth-degree burns.** If the burn is deep and severe, your child will require immediate medical attention. Do not remove any clothing that is stuck to the burn, but lightly cover the area with a clean white cloth. Call for emergency medical assistance or take your child immediately to the emergency room of the nearest hospital. Do not attempt to treat a severe third- or fourth-degree burn at home.

✚ **For first- or second-degree burns.** To minimize damage from a   first- or second-degree burn, cool the burn as rapidly as possible. Immerse the affected area in cool running water until the stinging and burning sensations lessen. This may take ten minutes or even longer. Do not stop prematurely.

If the burn occurs through clothing (as in a spill of hot liquid), don't wait to strip the clothes from your child. Immediately immerse the area in cool, running water. Remove the wet clothes from your child while cooling the burn.

While cooling the burn, remove any watches, bracelets, rings, belts or other constricting items from the area before the burn swells.

✚ **For burns in sensitive areas.** The thin, tender skin of a child is particularly susceptible to burns. Take your child to the emergency room if a burn appears severe or extensive, or if the burned area is on the face, the palms of the hands, the soles of the feet, or on or near a joint.

✚ **Avoid worsening the injury.** *Do not* apply butter, oil, grease, lotions, or creams to burns. *Do not* cover burns with adhesive dressings or fluffy materials.

CONVENTIONAL TREATMENT

■ A deep or extensive burn may need to be debrided, a process that cleanses the area and removes dead skin. This is procedure that must be done by a medical professional.

■ Depending on the depth and extent of the burn, your doctor may recommend that your child be given a tetanus shot and/or an antibiotic, such as penicillin, to guard against infection.

■ The physician may dress the area with a bandage that contains a film of a topical antibiotic, such as silver sulfadiazine (Silvadene).

■ Your doctor may prescribe an antibiotic ointment for dressing your child's burn at home. Antibiotic ointments such as Silvadene, povidone-iodine (Betadine), gentamicin sulfate, and bacitracin are used to treat an existing infection or to prevent one from developing. Your doctor will instruct you to apply a thin layer of ointment over the burned area, and to cover it with sterile gauze. There are also a number of new "high-tech" dressings available that can be left on for days at a time. These are especially suitable for milder burns. Ask your doctor about this.

■ Any burn that affects the mouth should be treated promptly by a doctor or pediatric dentist to ensure that it heals properly, without inflicting permanent damage. In some cases, a special appliance may be necessary to prevent the wound from contracting as it heals, leaving a child with a condition known as *microsomia* (literally, small mouth).

DIETARY GUIDELINES

■ If your child has sustained a deep, extensive burn, encourage him to drink lots of liquids to replace fluids that may have been lost through the burn.

■ After any trauma to the body, a diet high in protein helps promote healing.

■ Give your child a diet high in green and yellow vegetables to provide ample beta-carotene and vitamin C.

NUTRITIONAL SUPPLEMENTS

For age-appropriate dosages of nutritional supplements, see page 81.

■ Beta-carotene, a precursor to vitamin A, helps burned skin to heal. Give your child a double dose of beta-carotene, twice a day, until healing is complete.

■ To support the body during the healing process, give your child one-half dose of vitamin C with bioflavonoids, four times daily, for one to two weeks.

■ Vitamin C can also be applied topically in a liquid spray. To make a vitamin-C spray, combine 2 tablespoons of powdered vitamin C and ½ cup of aloe vera gel in a 16-ounce spray bottle. Apply this mixture twice a day until the burn heals.

■ Zinc aids in wound healing. Give your child one dose daily for one to two weeks.
   Note: Excessive amounts of zinc can result in nausea and vomiting. Be careful not to exceed the recommended dosage.

HERBAL TREATMENT

For age-appropriate dosages of herbal remedies, see page 81.

■ Apply aloe vera pulp, gel, or liquid to the burned area to remove the heat and sting from the burn. The pulp of the aloe vera plant has a long history of use as a soothing, cooling, and healing treatment for burns. It works quickly, and is remarkably effective. It is even used in the burn units of some hospitals.

■ Once the stinging sensation associated with a burn has subsided, apply a calendula preparation topically to help prevent infection. Select either an herbal or homeopathic preparation.

■ Apply a comfrey root salve or cream to the affected area. Comfrey root contains allantoin, which promotes tissue growth and is very healing to the skin.

■ Give your child an echinacea and goldenseal combination formula to stimulate the immune system, which is important in preventing and fighting infection. Echinacea is antiviral; goldenseal is antibacterial. Give your child one dose, three times daily, for one week to ten days following a burn.
   Note: You should not give your child echinacea on a daily basis for more than ten days at a time, or it will lose its effectiveness.

■ Gotu kola helps to speed healing of skin tissue. Give your child one dose, three times a day, for one to two weeks following a burn.
   Note: This herb should not be given to a child under four years of age.

HOMEOPATHY

■ The following thirty-minute regimen is of tremendous help following a minor burn. After completing this procedure, your child should feel considerably better.

1. Begin the process while still running cool water over the burn. Give your child one dose of *Urtica urens* 12x or 6c.

2. Five minutes after administering the *Urtica urens*, give your child one dose of Bach Flower Rescue Remedy to help ease his anxiety and fear.

3. After you have run cool water over your child's burn for ten minutes, turn off the water and apply aloe vera gel to the wound, as directed under Herbal Treatment, above.

4. Five minutes after applying the aloe vera, apply a second soothing coat of aloe vera to the wound and give your child a second dose of *Urtica urens* 12x or 6c.

5. After ten minutes have passed, apply a third coat of aloe vera to the burn and give your child a third dose of *Urtica urens* 12x or 6c. If the burn is simple, your child will feel better after the first application of aloe vera and the first dose of *Urtica urens*. If your child does not feel considerably better after the third application of aloe vera and the third dose of *Urtica urens*, consult your physician.

■ To help reduce blistering, crush a *Kali muriaticum* 6x pellet in a little distilled water. Apply the mixture topically to the wound one hour after completing the procedure outlined above. Apply the mixture again at bedtime.

■ Give your child one dose of *Kali muriaticum* 6x by mouth, three times a day, for the first two days after a burn.

■ To help lessen stinging and promote fast healing, apply homeopathic *Urtica urens* ointment or gel to the burn.

■ If your child's burn isn't healing as quickly as it should, evaluate the condition of the injury. Choose and administer the appropriate symptom-specific homeopathic remedy:

- *Apis mellifica* 12x or 6c helps to heal a burn that bubbles and resembles a bee sting. Give your child one dose every thirty minutes, for a total of three doses.

- If your child's burn remains red and throbbing and isn't calmed by the aloe vera and *Urtica urens* regimen, give him one dose of *Belladonna* 30x or 9c every thirty minutes, for a total of three doses, to help reduce the redness and throbbing pain.

- If the burn appears as if it is becoming infected, call your physician and report a possible infection. Begin giving your child *Mercurius solubilis* 12x or 6c to help ward off infection. Give one dose, three times daily, for two days.

GENERAL RECOMMENDATIONS

■ If your child suffers a serious burn, take appropriate emergency measures. Rely on medical personnel to treat the injury properly.

■ If your child suffers a minor burn, promptly cool the area under cool running water to minimize damage.

■ Give your child homeopathic *Urtica urens*.

- Apply aloe vera to the burn.

- Give your child Bach Flower Rescue Remedy.

- *Do not* use ice water directly on a burn. Doing so can deepen and worsen the burn. Instead, use cool compresses or running water.

- Never apply butter, petroleum jelly, ointment, or cream to a burn. A greasy substance will trap the heat and can cause a burn to deepen.

- *Do not* bandage or cover the affected area tightly. A tight covering traps the heat and can cause a burn to deepen.

- *Do not* burst any blisters. They form a natural bandage that aids healing.

PREVENTION

- Keep all flammable substances—including lighter fluid, gasoline, kerosene, and especially matches and lighters—well hidden and out of your child's reach, preferably in a locked storage area.

- Make sure that all heat-producing appliances are kept out of your child's reach and well away from potentially flammable items such as curtains or upholstery. This includes devices such as irons, toasters, and space heaters, as well as coffeemakers, curling irons, and halogen lamps—anything that generates heat when turned on. Always exercise special care when using such appliances if children are present. These devices should also be unplugged and their cords tucked away when not in use.

- Avoid using extension cords, and keep all electrical cords out of the reach of small children. Babies who are teething, particularly ones whose molars are erupting, are always looking for things to bite on, and electrical cords can be tempting to them. Biting on the cord of anything that is plugged in can cause a serious burn at the corners of the mouth.

- Children love to play with water. Sooner or later, your child will manage to turn on a faucet. Keep the temperature of your hot water heater set at no higher 120°F. It takes three minutes for 120°F water to cause a third-degree burn, long enough for you to hear your child scream and intervene. At 140°F, water can cause a third-degree burn in *five seconds*.

- Teach your child the basic rules of fire safety (see margin inset).

- For additional suggestions on ways to reduce your child's risk of being burned, *see* HOME SAFETY in Part One.

Cancer

Cancer is not a single disease, but rather a broad category of illnesses caused by an uncontrolled growth of certain cells in the body. A thorough discussion of the causes, physiology, and treatments of different types of cancer is far beyond the scope of this book. It is important, however, to be aware of certain symptoms, especially lingering symptoms that do not seem to get better with treatment, so that if a malignancy develops, it can be diagnosed promptly.

A cancerous tumor begins in what is called a *primary site*. Cancerous cells can invade and damage surrounding tissue, and then break off from the primary tumor to spread, through the circulatory and lymphatic systems, to other parts of the body. These secondary tumors can also be harmful.

A cancerous tumor can develop in any part of the body. Leukemia, a cancer of the blood and lymph system, is the most common cancer in children. Cancers of the brain and its lining (the *meninges*) and lymphomas (cancers of the lymph system) are the next most common childhood cancers.

Depending on the location, type, and severity of the illness, each cancer will have its own set of symptoms. Fatigue, abnormal bruising, infection, fever, bleeding gums, and paleness are common symptoms of leukemia. Swollen and tender lymph nodes, decreased appetite, fever, night sweats, and malaise are common symptoms of lymphoma. Headaches and vomiting, loss of coordination, changes in vision, and seizures can be symptoms of a brain tumor (although they may not show up until the tumor is large and pressing against brain tissue).

Tremendous amounts of time, energy, and money have been focused on researching the causes and treatment of childhood cancers. Although the exact causes of most cancers are still unknown, several factors have been identified as probable contributors. Exposure to electromagnetic radiation (especially through nearby power lines and transformers), radioactivity, certain medications (particularly diethystilbestrol, or DES), pesticides, food additives, and cigarette smoke have all been linked with cancer. Dietary choices, such as the consumption of saturated fats, are another important focus of research. An inherited predisposition or genetic condition may also increase a child's likelihood of developing cancer. For example, children born with Down's syndrome have a greater risk of developing leukemia than other children do.

Parents of a child diagnosed with cancer often experience overwhelming feelings of guilt and responsibility, and wonder if they might have done something to cause the illness, if they could have prevented it, or if they missed the signs of the developing disease. If your child has cancer, it is important—for your own sake and for your child's—that you do not blame yourself, but instead reassure yourself that you responded to your child's symptoms in the best way you knew how.

The prognosis for a child diagnosed with cancer depends on the type of cancer found, its location, the child's response to treatment, and her overall health at the time of diagnosis.

In the event that your child is diagnosed as having cancer, we urge you to seek out a pediatric oncologist—a medical doctor who specializes in childhood cancers—as well as a natural health care provider, to help maximize your child's ability to activate her healing potential. Herbs, homeopathy, acupressure, diet, and nutritional supplements can all be used to help boost your child's immune system and ease the discomforts of cancer therapies. Because your child is unique, and because her response to the disease and treatment are unique, it is best to work closely with qualified health care practitioners. We advise you to choose a medical doctor who is willing to work with a natural health care practitioner (and vice versa). Each of these professionals needs to know what the other is doing, as the interventions of one can affect the treatments prescribed by the other.

TYPES OF CANCER

Different medical terms are used to describe different types of cancers. Most of these terms end in the syllable *oma*, which means "mass" or "tumor." The basic categories of cancer include:

- **Carcinoma.** Cancers of the skin, mucous membranes, glands, and internal organs are often classified as carcinomas.

- **Leukemia.** Leukemias are cancers of the tissues that produce blood cells. Because leukemia results in abnormal blood cell formation, it is often referred to as blood cancer.

- **Lymphoma.** Lymphomas are cancers of the lymph nodes and other lymphatic tissue.

- **Sarcoma.** Sarcomas are primarily cancers of the bones, muscles, and connective tissues.

CONVENTIONAL TREATMENT

■ Diagnosis of cancer is based on the history of the illness, symptoms, a physical examination, blood tests, x-rays, magnetic resonance imaging (MRI) scans, and other specialized tests, such as tissue biopsy, that look more closely at the bone marrow, spinal fluid, or other body tissues. The physician will look for primary and secondary tumors, as well as for the specific type of cancer that has developed. Once an accurate diagnosis is made, a treatment plan will be recommended. Depending on the type and location of the cancer, and whether it is in an earlier or later stage of development, treatment options may include chemotherapy, surgery, and/or radiation.

■ Chemotherapy is medication given by mouth or by injection into the veins or muscles. It works by either killing the cancer cells or preventing them from reproducing. There are many types of chemotherapy agents. All of them are powerful medicines that cause significant side effects, including nausea, vomiting, hair loss, mouth sores, bleeding, and an inability to fight infection.

■ If a tumor is localized and can be removed without seriously damaging the body, surgery will probably be recommended.

■ Radiation treatment involves aiming a concentrated form of x-rays directly at a tumor to kill the cancerous cells. Side effects of radiation include fever, headache, nausea, vomiting, irritability, and loss of appetite. Also, the area of the skin that is exposed to radiation may become red, sore, and easily irritated.

■ The treatment of cancer is a complicated and long-term process. Once treatment is completed and tests show that no evidence of cancer remains in your child's body, it is said that your child is in remission. It is vital that you keep follow-up appointments as frequently and for as long as your doctor suggests. Cancer can reappear and treatment may need to be reinitiated.

NUTRITIONAL SUPPLEMENTS

For age-appropriate dosages of nutritional supplements, see page 81.

■ The B vitamins help to support adrenal function and strengthen the immune system. Give your child one dose of a liquid vitamin-B complex supplement twice a day. Choose a formula that contains 25 milligrams of each B vitamin per dose.

■ Vitamin C boosts the immune system and aids healing. Give your child one dose of vitamin C, preferably in mineral ascorbate form, three to four times a day, for one week following chemotherapy or radiation threatment, and once a day at all other times.

■ Zinc also helps to stimulate the immune system. Give your child one dose, twice a day (at the beginning of a meal).
   Note: Excessive amounts of zinc can result in nausea and vomiting. Give zinc supplements with food, and be careful not to exceed the recommended dosage.

HERBAL TREATMENT

For age-appropriate dosages of herbal remedies, see page 81.

■ If your child is undergoing chemotherapy, astragalus (*Astragalus membranaceous*) can be used to support her immune system. It has been shown to diminish some of the side effects of chemotherapy, including poor appetite, hair loss, and depression. Give your child one dose, two to three times a day, as needed.
   Note: This herb should not be given if a fever or any other signs of infection are present.

■ A tea of ginger or peppermint, or a combination of the two, helps to lessen the nausea that may be caused by chemotherapy or radiation treatment for cancer. Give your child one dose of tea as needed.

Note: If you are giving your child a tea containing peppermint as well as a homeopathic preparation, allow one hour between the two. Otherwise, the strong smell of the mint may interfere with the action of the homeopathic remedy.

■ Siberian ginseng is useful for a child whose main difficulty is fatigue. It improves energy and also acts to protect the liver from being damaged by chemotherapy and/or radiation treatment. Give your child one dose daily, as needed.

■ Some studies have found that shiitake mushrooms have antitumor properties. The whole mushrooms can be added to foods, such as soups. Shiitake is also available in capsule form. Follow dosage directions on the product label.

HOMEOPATHY

■ The first chemotherapy treatment is always a shock, both physically and mentally. It is helpful for both child and parents to take one dose of *Aconite* 200x or 30c after the first treatment.

■ *Arnica* can help to lessen the achiness associated with chemotherapy treatments. Give your child one dose of *Arnica* 200x or 30c after each treatment.

■ *Nux vomica* is helpful in lessening the nausea associated with chemotherapy. Give your child one dose of *Nux vomica* 30x or 6c as needed.

GENERAL RECOMMENDATIONS

■ It is imperative that parents of a child diagnosed with cancer seek out appropriate support. You need friends and family to listen and to help with daily tasks. It is also highly beneficial to find professional support, whether through a social worker, a counselor, a member of the clergy, and/or a support group. Regardless of how strong and stable you feel at the time of diagnosis, you should expect to have feelings of deep grief, confusion, anger, exhaustion, and isolation at times. This is natural. Build up a support network early so that you have a place to express and work with these feelings.

■ Childhood cancer can put a great deal of stress on a marriage. If your child is diagnosed as having cancer, we recommend that you seek marital counseling or a support group early so that conflicts and feelings of separation can be avoided. Do what you need to do to stay as physically and emotionally healthy as possible.

■ A diagnosis of cancer can also be stressful for a child's siblings. Feelings of resentment ("Why does my sister always get all the attention?"), loneliness ("I wish I didn't always have to spend the night at Grandma's. I miss my mom and dad"), guilt ("This happened because I wished my brother weren't around"), and sadness can come up. Help your children tell their stories in school, talk to their teachers, find a counselor, and look for a support group specifically for siblings of children with cancer.

■ Finally, seek out emotional support for the child with cancer. Art therapy, talk therapy, and play therapy are ways in which your child can work through her feelings. Counseling and/or a support group for children with cancer can be invaluable. Help your child talk to friends, teachers, and classmates to get the support she needs.

Resource Organizations for Families Dealing With Cancer

There are a number of organizations that offer help to families dealing with childhood cancer. They can help you to find information about your child's illness, as well as offer referrals to physicians, medical centers, support groups, and other families who are facing similar challenges. If your child is diagnosed as having cancer, consider contacting one or more of the organizations listed below.

American Cancer Society
777 Third Avenue
New York, NY 10019
212-371-2900

The Candlelighters Foundation
2025 I Street NW, Suite 1011
Washington, DC 20006
202-659-5136

Center for Medical Consumers
237 Thompson Street
New York, NY 10012
212-674-7105

Children's Hospice International
1800 Diagonal Road, Suite 600
Alexandria, VA 22314
703-684-0330

The Compassionate Friends, Inc.
P.O. Box 1347
Oak Brook, IL 60521
312-323-5010

National Hospice Organization
1901 North Moore Street
Arlington, VA 22209
703-243-5900

People Against Cancer
P.O. Box 10
Otho, IA 50569
515-972-4444

Ronald McDonald House
Kroc Drive
Oak Brook, IL 60521
708-575-7418

PREVENTION

The processes that lead to the development of many types of cancer are not well understood, and for that reason cancer, especially childhood cancers, cannot be considered preventable. However, there are measures you can take to help safeguard your child (and yourself) from known risks that might lead to the development of cancer in the future.

■ Do not smoke around your child (better yet, don't smoke at all!). Avoid secondhand smoke. Recent evidence suggests that secondhand smoke may be even more dangerous than the smoke the smoker breathes.

■ If possible, buy organically grown foods (or grow your own). The herbicides and pesticides used on commercially grown produce may be carcinogenic. Always wash produce thoroughly before eating it.

■ Keep the amount of fat in the family diet to no more than 20 percent of total calories consumed, and offer a diet that is high in fiber. A lifetime of eating too much fat and too little fiber may contribute to the development of colorectal and other cancers. It's best to start your child off with healthy eating habits.

■ Have your house and water tested for the presence of radon. Radon is a naturally occurring radioactive gas that can seep into your home from the surrounding soil. It is believed to be a common cause of lung cancer as well as of stomach cancer. You can't see or smell it, so the only way to know whether it is present is to use a radon test kit. These are available at many hardware stores. If you find that there is radon in your home, you can usually correct the problem by sealing cracks and improving ventilation in the basement.

■ Keep your child from becoming sunburned. Even a single severe sunburn in childhood increases a person's risk of developing malignant melanoma, a dangerous form of skin cancer, later in life. (*See* SUNBURN.)

■ Protect your child from breathing in fumes from paints, solvents, gasoline, pesticides, herbicides, and even such items as nail polish remover, oven cleaner, glues, and other household chemicals. Many of these substances are known to cause, or are suspected of causing, cancer.

Candida Infection

See DIAPER RASH; THRUSH; VAGINITIS, YEAST.

Canker Sores

Canker sores are small, swollen, painful ulcers that occur on the lips or in the mouth. Canker sores hurt. If your child develops a canker sore, it is possible that he won't want to eat. Acidic foods sting. Even the act of chewing can cause irritation in the area.

A canker sore begins as a small red dot on the lip or the inside of the mouth, which then develops into a vesicle with a white head. Eventually the head will rupture, leaving an open ulcer that can become secondarily infected by yeast or bacteria.

The cause of the original ulcer may be difficult to pinpoint, although food allergies, vitamin deficiencies (especially low levels of vitamin B_{12}), acidic conditions, and small cuts are probable causes. There is also some research that indicates an autoimmune phenomenon may be at work.

Canker sores and cold sores look very much alike. Cold sores, however, are caused by the herpes virus, which is highly contagious. Typically, herpes sores appear on the hard part of the gums or the "dry" part of the lips, while canker sores occur on the loose part of the gums, the insides of the cheeks, or the inner lip. Also, cold sores tend to recur at exactly the same place every time, while canker sores can occur anywhere in the mouth.

CONVENTIONAL TREATMENT

■ There is no drug that will cure a canker sore, although there are over-the-counter medicines that can be dabbed on the sore to numb the pain. These include Campho-Phenique, Carmex, Anbesol, Zilactin, and Gly-Oxide. Follow directions on the product label.

■ A mouthwash made from equal parts of hydrogen peroxide and water can decrease the superinfection of the ulcer.

■ Acetaminophen (in Tylenol, Tempra, and others) may be given to help lessen the pain of canker sores.

Note: In excessive amounts, this drug can cause liver damage. Read package directions carefully so as not to exceed the proper dosage for your child's age and size.

■ If your child is in much distress from canker sores, consult your physician. A mouthwash or paste made from triamcinolone (a prescription steroid sold as Kenalog in Orabase) has been shown to be effective in relieving canker sores.

■ For severe pain, an anesthetic called lidocaine is sometimes prescribed.

DIETARY GUIDELINES

■ If your child has canker sores, avoid giving him acidic foods, such as sugar, citrus fruits and juices, chocolate, and foods containing caffeine. Acidic foods are very irritating to canker sores.

■ Soft foods, such as steamed vegetables or warm soups, will be easier for your child to eat.

■ Try having your child drink with a straw if his tongue or lips are sensitive.

NUTRITIONAL SUPPLEMENTS

For age-appropriate dosages of nutritional supplements, see page 81.

■ Chlorophyll is a blood detoxifier and is high in micronutrients. Follow dosage directions on the product label.

■ Give your child 200 micrograms of folic acid (half of a 400-microgram tablet) to chew, twice a day, until symptoms are relieved.

■ Give your child one dose of mineral ascorbate vitamin C with bioflavonoids, two to three times daily (between meals), for five days. Choose a formula made without sugar.

■ To help boost your child's immune system, give him one dose of zinc, in chewable tablet or lozenge form, three times a week, for two months. Give this mineral during a meal or directly after eating. Zinc lozenges containing 5 milligrams of zinc, given several times daily, are very soothing and will help heal the lesion.

   Note: Excessive amounts of zinc can result in nausea and vomiting. Be careful not to exceed the recommended dosage.

HERBAL TREATMENT

For age-appropriate dosages of herbal remedies, see page 81.

■ Have your child swish aloe vera juice around in his mouth to soothe the inflamed area. Be sure to use a food-grade product for this purpose.

■ To help clear the infection and stimulate the immune system, give your child one dose of echinacea and goldenseal herbal combination formula, three times a day, until the canker sore improves.

   Note: You should not give your child echinacea on a daily basis for more than ten days at a time, or it will lose its effectiveness.

■ Make licorice root tea and have your child swish it around in his mouth twice a day. Licorice root has antiviral and antibacterial properties, and is very soothing to canker sores. The tea can be used either cool or warm. You can also cover the ulcer with a paste or a small "plug" made from licorice root powder. Even chewing on a piece of a licorice root is helpful.

Note: This herb should not be given to a child with high blood pressure.

■ Propolis lozenges can be used to help fight infection and promote healing.

■ A wet tea bag placed against the sore can be soothing. Use ordinary black tea, which contains tannic acid, an effective astringent.

HOMEOPATHY

■ Give your child one dose of *Natrum muriaticum* 12x, three times daily, for up to forty-eight hours. If there is no improvement in that time, discontinue the remedy.

GENERAL RECOMMENDATIONS

■ If your child complains of a tiny red sore, suspect a canker sore and begin treating it.

■ Mix 1 teaspoon of baking soda in 8 ounces of pure spring water and have your child swish the mixture around in his mouth. Baking soda reduces the acidity of the mouth and also promotes healing of irritated tissues.

■ Give your child folic acid tablets to chew, as well as zinc and mineral ascorbate vitamin C with bioflavonoids.

■ Give your child an echinacea and goldenseal combination formula.

■ Have your child chew a licorice root, or cover the sores with a paste made from powdered licorice root.

■ Give your child homeopathic *Natrum muriaticum*.

PREVENTION

■ Keep a diet diary that records what your child eats and tracks his responses, to help identify foods that may aggravate canker sores. Eliminate those foods from your child's diet.

■ If your child is prone to canker sores, give him five milligrams of chewable zinc, in lozenge or tablet form, once daily, for two months.

■ Have your child avoid sugary sweets.

■ Including yogurt in your child's diet may help to prevent canker sores.

Carsickness

See MOTION SICKNESS.

Cavities

See TOOTH DECAY.

Cat Scratch Disease

See Pets and Your Child in HOME SAFETY in Part One.

Celiac Disease

Celiac disease is an illness caused by an intolerance to gluten, a protein found in wheat, rye, barley, and oats. When a person with this intolerance eats these foods, it causes damage to the intestinal wall, which leads to an inability to absorb most nutrients and eventually to malnutrition. Early symptoms include changes in behavior, weight loss, abdominal distention, and diarrhea. If the condition is not identified and treated, other symptoms will develop, including vomiting, abdominal pain, loss of fat and muscle, and swelling of the legs and feet. Severe growth retardation and softening of the bones can develop in the later stages of this illness.

Celiac disease is usually diagnosed before a child is two years of age, and a diet free of gluten is the primary treatment. Your child may need a lot of support, however, in sticking to this diet. She won't be able to eat what her friends are eating, which poses a great challenge to a child. Celiac disease is a chronic problem and so must be cared for throughout your child's lifetime. Deviating from the restricted diet at any time can cause a relapse. Counseling and support groups can help parents and children deal with the emotional issues that arise with a chronic illness.

CONVENTIONAL TREATMENT

■ Treatment is based on diet. Foods containing gluten—anything made from wheat, rye, barley, or oats—must be eliminated or severely restricted.

■ A child who is severely malnourished as a result of celiac disease may need to receive intravenous nutrition to help build her body. Vitamin and mineral supplements may also be prescribed if a child is unable to absorb nutrients from foods.

■ Once a child starts to follow a gluten-free diet, her symptoms should improve quickly and she will begin gaining weight and growing appropriately. Generally, this diet must be maintained for life, as eating gluten can trigger symptoms and, eventually, malnutrition again. It is possible that once your child is symptom-free and tests show that her intestines have healed, she may be able to eat small amounts of gluten on occasion. This should be done only with medical supervision, however.

DIETARY GUIDELINES

■ As discussed under Conventional Treatment on page 150, a restricted diet is the primary form of treatment for celiac disease.

■ Nutritionists and dietitians are good sources of information about which foods have gluten in them, as well as of ideas for gluten-free cooking. Gluten is often a hidden ingredient in food products. For example, products that list "cereal fillers" or "hydrolyzed protein" on the labels contain gluten, and so must be avoided.

NUTRITIONAL SUPPLEMENTS

■ Digestive enzymes can be helpful for breaking down complex carbohydrates before they reach the intestines. These are generally made from cow pancreas and need to be concentrated to be effective. Give your child one to three capsules with each meal, as directed on the product label.

HERBAL TREATMENT

For age-appropriate dosages of herbal remedies, see page 81.

■ Aloe vera, taken in small amounts, can help decrease inflammation in the intestines. Be sure to buy the edible (food-grade) form of this plant. Give your child ½ teaspoon, twice a day, as needed.

■ Slippery elm is soothing to the digestive tract. It can be taken in capsule or tea form, or made into a paste with water and added to food. Slippery elm has a mild taste. Give your child one dose, once or twice a day, as needed.

HOMEOPATHY

■ A valuable approach when dealing with this chronic illness is to visit a homeopath who can prescribe a constitutional remedy for your child. Often a constitutional remedy can enhance digestion and ease the course of this illness.

■ For relief of acute, diffuse abdominal gas and difficulty digesting food, give your child *China* 12x or 5c, three times a day, for three days.

■ For short-term relief of low-bowel gas, give your child *Lycopodium* 12x or 5c, three times a day, for three days.

GENERAL RECOMMENDATIONS

■ Be aware of your child's reactions to the different foods in her diet. If you suspect she may be reacting to foods that contain gluten, consult your physician.

■ If your child is diagnosed with celiac disease, help her to stick to her restricted diet. Experiment with gluten-free recipes and try to find gluten-free foods she likes. Help her to understand why she must eat different foods than her friends do. Discuss ways to deal with temptation and to decline offers of forbidden foods graciously but firmly.

■ For relief of acute digestive distress, select and administer an appropriate herbal or homeopathic remedy.

■ Give your child digestive enzymes with meals.

■ Seek counseling or a support group to help your child deal with the emotional stresses of chronic illness.

PREVENTION

■ Celiac disease is hereditary and is present from birth on, although symptoms do not appear until a child begins to eat foods containing gluten. There is no known way to prevent your child from developing this illness. Your only defense against the disease is to be aware of the characteristic signs and symptoms, so that your child can begin treatment promptly if necessary, and to help your child follow the required diet and cope with the emotional issues involved in dealing with chronic illness.

Chickenpox

Chickenpox is a highly contagious childhood disease that is caused by the varicella-zoster virus, a member of the herpes family. Very few children escape chickenpox infection. It spreads quickly. Coughing and sneezing—even laughing and talking—spread the illness.

A child with developing chickenpox will be contagious for one or two days before any symptoms show. A child who plays with an infected child during this period will almost certainly catch the disease. An infected child is contagious from a few days before symptoms develop until all of the blisters are dry and have formed scabs.

The more intimate and more frequent the exposure to chickenpox, the more severe the case will be. This fact has very important implications, especially if you have more than one child. Children in different stages of the disease should be separated to minimize their exposure to each other. With minimal exposure, the second child to become ill is likely to have a less severe case of chickenpox, with less discomfort.

Chickenpox typically begins with a headache, fatigue, loss of appetite, and fever, much like any other viral illness. A day or two after these early symptoms, a rash of flat, red, splotchy dots erupts, usually beginning on the chest, stomach, and back, and spreading a day or so later to the face and scalp.

The red dots of the rash soon come together to form clusters of tiny pimples, which then progress to small, delicate, clear blisters. Some children develop 3 lesions; some develop 300. Once the rash erupts, expect new crops of blisters over the next three to five days. Scabs, which are the last phase of the pox, form five to six days after the blisters develop. These scabs last for one to two weeks before falling off, exposing tender, freshly healed skin.

Over the course of the disease, the rash shows signs of all the different phases of chickenpox, with some areas that are splotchy and red, some areas of new blisters, areas where sores are crusting over and scabbing, and areas of healing. From eruption through healing, each and every pock is *very, very itchy*. It is the extreme itchiness of chickenpox that causes the greatest torment.

Chickenpox can be contracted at any age. Because infected adults tend to feel much sicker and more miserable with this disease than youngsters do, it's probably best to have it as a child. Once you have had chickenpox, it is highly unlikely that you will ever suffer through it again.

SYMPTOMS OF CHICKENPOX

The first signs that a child is coming down with chickenpox usually include some combination of the following:

- Moderate fever.
- Headache.
- Fatigue.
- Achiness.
- Sore throat.

A day or two after these first symptoms appear, a child with chickenpox will develop the telltale rash, usually characterized by the following:

- It starts out flat and reddish, centered on the trunk of the body.
- A day or so after it first appears, it spreads to the extremities, neck, and face, and turns from red splotches into masses of tiny pimples.
- It is intensely itchy.

CONVENTIONAL TREATMENT

■ Acetaminophen (in Tylenol, Tempra, and other medications) is helpful in relieving pain and bringing down fever.

Note: In excessive amounts, this drug can cause liver damage. Read package directions carefully so as not to exceed the proper dosage for your child's age and size.

■ *Do not* give your child any product that contains aspirin. A child or teenager who has the symptoms of any viral disease, including chickenpox, should never be given aspirin, because the combination of aspirin and viral disease has been linked to the development of Reye's syndrome, a dangerous complication (see REYE'S SYNDROME).

■ The antihistamine diphenhydramine (found in Benadryl) or chlorpheniramine (Chlor-Trimeton) can help relieve the awful itching a child with chickenpox experiences. Benadryl is available in pill form as well as in a spray. The pill form is generally more effective at relieving the itching of chickenpox. An antihistamine can also help an uncomfortable child to fall asleep.

■ Viscous Xylocaine is a local anesthetic that can be used as a mouth rinse to decrease pain and itching in the mouth. This rinse numbs mucous membranes, making it more comfortable for a child with mouth sores to eat, drink, or brush his teeth. This is a prescription drug, and it must be used in small quantities because of its potential toxicity.

■ Burow's solution is a powder available over the counter at most drug stores. Mixed with water and applied as a soak, it is very effective at drying up weeping sores.

■ Calamine lotion can help to relieve itching and dry weeping sores.

■ Acyclovir (Zovirax) is a drug that has some effectiveness against the chickenpox virus. However, it is very expensive and shortens the course of the illness by only a few days. It is therefore used primarily in severe cases that occur in children with disorders that impair immune system function, such as leukemia.

DIETARY GUIDELINES

■ Offer plenty of fluids so that your child stays well hydrated.

■ Prepare a simple, clean, whole-foods diet. Include easily digested foods high in vitamins and minerals, such as soups, well-cooked whole grains, and vegetables.

■ If your child has lost his appetite and is not eating well, try tempting him with diluted fruit juices, herbal teas, and soups. Frozen fruit-juice popsicles are usually well received.

NUTRITIONAL SUPPLEMENTS

For age-appropriate dosages of nutritional supplements, see page 81.

■ Vitamin A aids in healing skin tissue. Give your child one dose of vitamin A or its precursor, beta-carotene, once a day, for ten days.

■ Vitamin C and bioflavonoids help to stimulate the immune system and resolve a fever in the initial stages of the illness. The first week, give your child one dose of vitamin C in mineral ascorbate form, and an equal amount of bioflavonoids, three to four times a day. The following week, give him the same dosage, but two to three times a day. During the third week, give the same dosage, twice a day. Then continue to give one dose, once a week, for three weeks.

WHEN TO CALL THE DOCTOR ABOUT CHICKENPOX

• If your child develops vaginal or rectal lesions, or bad sores in his mouth, call your physician.

• If your child develops a fever consistently over 102°F, an earache, a very painful sore throat, a persistent cough, and/or increased difficulty breathing, seek your doctor's advice. It is possible for a child with chickenpox to develop such complications as an ear infection, strep throat, or pneumonia. If your child seems to be developing any of these conditions, seek medical attention.

■ Try giving your child one dose of zinc, twice a day, in tablet or lozenge form, for two weeks. Zinc promotes healing and stimulates the immune system.

Note: Excessive amounts of zinc can result in nausea and vomiting. Be careful not to exceed the recommended dosage.

■ If your child is restless and having difficulty sleeping, try giving him one dose of a calcium and magnesium supplement, twice during the day and once again at bedtime, for one week. Choose a formula that contains 250 milligrams of calcium to 125 milligrams of magnesium.

Note: In excessive amounts, magnesium acts as a laxative. If your child develops diarrhea, decrease the dosage.

HERBAL TREATMENT

For age-appropriate dosages of herbal remedies, see page 81.

■ Burdock root is high in many valuable trace minerals, and helps to detoxify the body and heal skin lesions. Give your child one dose, twice daily, until he recovers.

■ Echinacea and goldenseal help to clear infection, support the immune system, and soothe the skin and mucous membranes. Echinacea is a powerful antiviral. Give your child one dose of an echinacea and goldenseal combination formula, three times a day, for up to ten days or until he recovers.

Note: Echinacea should not be given on a daily basis for more than ten days at a time, or it may lose its effectiveness.

■ If your child is feeling very restless, give him a cup of chamomile tea, twice a day, as needed.

■ Red clover, like burdock root, contains many trace minerals. It helps to detoxify the body and aids in healing skin lesions. Give your child one dose, twice daily, until he feels better.

HOMEOPATHY

■ Homeopathic *Calendula*, in tincture, oil, or gel form, helps to relieve itching and promote healing. Apply the preparation topically in the morning, in the afternoon, and at bedtime.

■ *Grindelia* tincture, applied topically to the pocks, helps to relieve itching. Apply the undiluted mother tincture in the morning, in the afternoon, and again before bedtime.

■ To fight the intense itching of chickenpox, give your child one dose of *Rhus toxicodendron* 30x or 9c, three times daily, for forty-eight hours or until symptoms improve. If there is no improvement in forty-eight hours, try a different remedy.

■ *Sulphur* 30x or 9c is often useful for very red and very itchy pocks. Give your child one dose, three times a day, for up to three days.

ACUPRESSURE

For the locations of acupressure points on a child's body, *see* ADMINISTERING AN ACUPRESSURE TREATMENT in Part Three.

■ Four Gates helps to relax a restless, uncomfortable child.

- Large Intestine 11 helps relieve itching of the skin.
- Spleen 10 is a specific for taking "heat" out of the blood.
- Stomach 36 is useful for improving appetite.

GENERAL RECOMMENDATIONS

- Give your child homeopathic *Rhus toxicodendron* daily until symptoms lessen.

- To support your child's immune system and soothe mucous membranes, give him an echinacea and goldenseal combination formula.

- Apply homeopathic *Grindelia* or *Calendula* tincture or gel to your child's lesions to relieve itching.

- Children over the age of three can usually understand why scratching should be avoided. Explain to your child that scratching or picking at scabs can cause an infection, and that rubbing open a blister or pulling off a scab before the new skin has formed underneath will leave a scar, a pockmark. Keep your child's fingernails short to prevent breaking of the skin if he does begin to scratch.

- If your child is under three, it may be difficult to convince him to leave the pocks alone. Take any and all measures to relieve the itching. The more your child scratches, the greater the danger of infection and scarring. Be diligent and creative.

- Keep your child clean, quiet, and cool. A soak in bath water treated with chamomile, calendula, or grindelia will soothe and relax your child. These herbs help relieve itching, too.

- Oatmeal baths are very soothing to dry and itching skin. Tie a handful of raw oatmeal in a washcloth and swish it around in your child's bath water. You may *gently* rub the washcloth full of oatmeal over the itchy places as well, but be very careful not to break the blisters.

- Use Burow's solution soaks to dry open or draining sores.

- Occasionally, a few extra-thick scabs refuse to drop off, and skin begins to form around them. Don't try to lift these stubborn scabs off, or your child will be left with pockmarks. If you notice some tenacious scabs that seem to be clinging on too long, encourage them to separate from the skin with a soak in one of the hot treated baths suggested above.

- If your child is left with a tiny scar after his chickenpox is fully healed, apply vitamin E oil to the scar. Break open a vitamin-E capsule and rub the oil into the pockmark in the morning and at night until it clears. Rubbing castor oil into the scar will also help.

- Once the chickenpox has cleared, protect your child's skin from the sun. The areas where pocks have healed are now tender, new skin that will burn and scar easily. Apply a good sun block or high-SPF sunscreen when your child goes outside.

PREVENTION

- Keep children who have chickenpox separated from each other. This can mean a milder case for the second child who comes down with the disease.

- It is not now possible to immunize your child against chickenpox. A vaccine is currently under research, and may become available in the future.

Emergency Treatment for Choking

Have someone call for emergency help and go to your child's aid quickly. Your child's age will determine the measures you must take to relieve choking. Perform the age-appropriate procedure outlined below. *Do not stop* until the foreign material is expelled, *or* your child begins coughing, breathing, and making normal sounds on her own, *or* another person can take over for you, *or* medical help arrives.

For an Infant Under One Year Old

If your child is under one year old, perform the Heimlich maneuver as follows.

1. Hold your baby securely, resting face down on your forearm. Rest your forearm on your thigh.
2. Use the heel of your hand to give five quick, firm blows between your infant's shoulder blades (see figure A).
3. Turn your child over to face you. With your fingers, give five quick, firm compressions to the breastbone just below the nipple line (see figure B).
4. Look for foreign material in your child's mouth. If you can see any foreign material, remove it with your finger. *Do not* blindly sweep your finger through your child's mouth.
5. Repeat steps 1 through 4, alternating between five back blows and five chest thrusts and checking your child's mouth for foreign material, until the object is expelled.

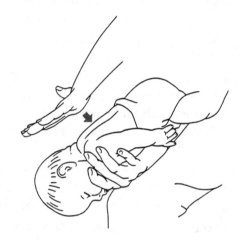

A. Back Blows for an Infant

If your baby loses consciousness at any time during this procedure, stop giving back blows and chest thrusts and open her airway as follows.

1. Look for any foreign material in your baby's mouth. If you can see anything in her mouth, remove it with your finger, but *do not* blindly sweep your finger through your infant's mouth.
2. Tip your baby's head back by pushing on her forehead. With your other hand, gently lift the bony part of the jaw (see figure C). This positioning opens the airway.
3. Cover your infant's nose and mouth with your mouth and give two gentle puffs of air, just enough to make your baby's chest rise and fall as if in normal breathing. Watch to see if your child's chest is rising and falling when you give the breaths. If it isn't, the airway is still blocked. You will have to try again to dislodge the material.
4. Turn your child face down and hold her securely on your forearm. Give her five quick blows between the shoulder blades.
5. Turn your baby face up again and give her five quick thrusts just below the nipple line.
6. Check your baby's mouth again. If you can see any foreign material, remove it with your finger. *Do not* blindly sweep your finger through your child's mouth.

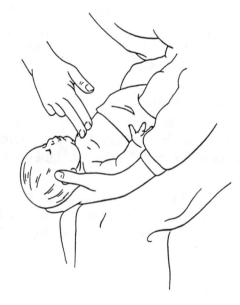

B. Chest Thrusts for an Infant

7. Continue repeating steps 2 through 6 until the material is expelled or emergency help arrives.

Even if your child seems to be fine once the material has been expelled, she should be seen by a doctor to be checked for possible damage to her windpipe or abdomen.

For a Child Over One Year Old

If your child is over one year old, perform the Heimlich maneuver as follows.

1. Stand or kneel behind your child, wrapping your arms around her waist.
2. Position the thumb side of your fist against your child's abdomen, just above the navel and below the rib cage (see figure D).
3. Use a quick, forceful, *upward* push of your fist into your child's abdomen to force air up through the windpipe.
4. Continue doing these thrusts until your child expels the foreign material.

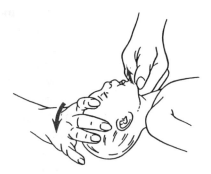

C. Opening the Airway

If your child loses consciousness at any time during this procedure, discontinue the thrusts and open her airway as follows.

1. Place your child on her back on the floor, face up. Look for any foreign material in her mouth. If you can see any foreign material, remove it with your finger. *Do not* blindly sweep your finger through your child's mouth.
2. Tip your child's head back by pushing on her forehead. With your other hand, gently lift the bony part of the jaw (see figure C). This positioning opens the airway.
3. Pinch your child's nostrils closed. Cover her mouth with yours and give two slow breaths of air. Watch to see if your child's chest is rising and falling, as in normal breathing. If it isn't, the airway is still blocked. You will have to try again to dislodge the material.
4. Straddle your child, squatting above her knees. Place the heel of your hand against her abdomen, just above the navel and below the rib cage. Place your other hand on top of the first. Use a quick, forceful *upward* push to force air up through the windpipe. Give five more thrusts to your child's abdomen.
5. Continue repeating steps 1 through 4 until the material is expelled or emergency help arrives to take over.

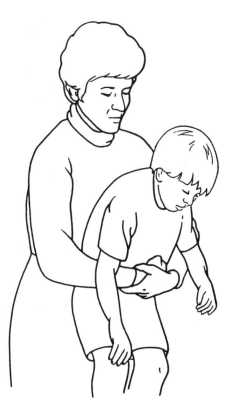

D. The Heimlich Maneuver
for a Child Over One

Even if your child seems to be fine once the material has been expelled, she should be seen by a doctor to be checked for possible damage to her windpipe or abdomen.

157

Choking

EMERGENCY TREATMENT FOR CHOKING

See the inset on page 156.

According to the American Academy of Pediatrics, children under four years of age are at the greatest risk of choking, not only on small, removable parts of toys—a danger most parents guard against—but on food as well. In 1991, the National Safety Council reported that 270 American children four years old and under died as a result of choking on food. Consumer advocates are now lobbying to have labels warning of possible choking hazards placed on certain food products popular with children.

Every parent, and everyone who cares for children regularly, should complete a course in first aid and cardiopulmonary resuscitation that includes specific instruction in coming to the aid of a child who is choking. The information in this entry cannot—and is not meant to—substitute for a class in which you can learn and practice such critical details of technique as where to place your hands and how much force to use in giving back blows or chest compressions. Rather, it is intended to serve as a refresher in case of emergency.

It's frightening to realize that your child is choking. First, make a quick assessment of the situation.

If your child is talking or coughing forcefully, you do not need to intervene. This indicates that air is getting through the windpipe. As long as your child can breathe, she may be able to expel the material on her own. Watch and wait. A child's coughing and sputtering is often enough to expel the object.

However, if your child becomes unable to speak, makes frantic, high-pitched sounds, gasps for air, turns blue, or clutches at her throat, act fast. Your child needs emergency help.

GENERAL RECOMMENDATIONS

■ Have someone call for emergency help and begin the Heimlich maneuver immediately (see page 156).

■ Once the crisis is over, give your child a dose of Bach Flower Rescue Remedy. This will help calm your child and stabilize the anxiety, shock, and fright she may be experiencing. You may also wish to take a dose of Rescue Remedy yourself. (See BACH FLOWER REMEDIES in Part One.)

PREVENTION

■ Infants and very young children explore the world around them by putting anything and everything into their mouths. Keep a close watch. Teach your child never to put any object into her mouth except for the food you provide.

■ Young children should be supervised when eating. Never allow your child to eat alone.

■ When preparing a meal or snack for a young child, cut all foods, including fruits, into very small pieces, and offer one bite at a time. Even a cookie, graham cracker, or banana can pose a risk. A young child who doesn't chew well may try to swallow a sticky, too-large "gummed" bite of food. According to the American Academy of Pediatrics, the following child-pleasing foods are particularly dangerous to children under four:

- thick "sticky" candies
- hard candies
- raw carrots
- celery
- grapes and raisins
- hot dogs
- chunks of meat
- lumps of peanut butter
- popcorn
- nuts

■ Eat slowly and chew thoroughly, and teach your child to do the same. A child in a rush to finish a meal can choke on a poorly chewed or extra-large bite.

■ Select toys that are well made and appropriate for your child's age. Examine your child's toys and playthings regularly to make sure that all small parts are secure.

■ For suggestions on how to childproof your home and minimize hazards your child may encounter outside, *see* HOME SAFETY in Part One.

Cold

See COMMON COLD.

Cold Sores

See HERPES VIRUS.

Colic

Colic has been defined as a long period of vigorous crying that persists despite all efforts at consolation. The term itself comes from the Greek word for the large intestine, reflecting the belief that the source of the discomfort is a digestive problem.

Most babies go through periods when they seem to be abnormally fussy or to cry for no apparent reason. Colic is most common during the first three to four months of an infant's life. It can begin within the first three weeks after birth, and usually stops around the age of three months. It is rarely experienced by a baby older than six months.

During the first six months of life, infants grow at an amazing rate. In that time, a newborn doubles his birth weight. Because of the amount of food they must take in to support this growth spurt, babies often suffer from indigestion and gas. Also, a baby may swallow air either when feeding or during a prolonged crying spell. Swallowing air increases gas pain. When an infant experiences a gas pain, it may be the worst pain his small body has ever felt.

The thing that differentiates colic from other problems is that no matter what you do, the crying doesn't stop. Certain body postures that occur with a gas attack may also occur with colic. For example, your baby may have a tense, distended tummy, with knees pulled up to the chest, clenched fists, and flailing arms and legs, or an arched back.

Suspect true colic if your baby has sudden, severe bouts of loud crying that last for several hours at a time; if the crying occurs at the same time each day, often in the evening or at night; if crying episodes happen over and over, beginning suddenly and ending abruptly; if your baby seems inconsolable and nothing you do brings comfort; if your infant seems angry and struggles when held; and if there doesn't seem to be any explanation for these outbreaks of crying.

If your baby has colic, the months of crying and seemingly unrelenting distress your child is experiencing can leave you feeling frustrated, anxious, confused, exhausted, guilty, and inadequate. One of the key concerns in dealing with a colicky baby, in addition to finding ways to comfort your child, is being confident of your ability to maintain and build a loving relationship with your newborn.

WHAT CAUSES COLIC?

Although it has long been assumed that colic is a sign of gas pain, it has never actually been proved that all, or even most, colicky babies do indeed have abdominal gas. Certainty as to the cause of the problem continues to elude medical science. In addition to the possibility of gas pain, there are a number of other hypotheses as to what causes colic, including:

- An allergy to milk protein or formula.
- Faulty feeding techniques.
- Spasms of the colon.
- An immature, hyperactive gastrointestinal tract.
- An immature, highly sensitive nervous system.
- Temperament.
- Tension in the home.
- Parental anxiety.
- Parental misinterpretation of crying.

It is likely that a combination of some of these factors is indeed involved in most cases of infant colic.

CONVENTIONAL TREATMENT

■ Simethicone (available in Mylicon) is a compound that acts on the surface of gas bubbles to break them up, thus relieving gas pain and pressure. If large gas bubbles are the primary problem, this can be an effective treatment. Simethicone is available over the counter in a liquid form, but it should be given only if recommended by your physician.

■ In the case of unremitting colic, your physician may recommend glycerin suppositories to help your baby expel gas or feces that may be causing his discomfort.

■ Dr. Lendon Smith, the well-known pediatrician and author, reports that careful stretching of an infant's tight anus results in successful treatment of colic. This is a procedure that must be performed by a doctor.

■ Other drugs, including antiflatulents, sedatives (such as phenobarbital), and antispasmodics like dicyclomine (Bentyl), are sometimes prescribed for colic and occasionally offer limited relief, but in most cases they are of little benefit. In addition, they can have serious side effects. Ask your doctor to explain all of the pros and cons of any prescription medications before giving them to a colicky baby.

DIETARY GUIDELINES

■ If you are breastfeeding and your infant suffers from colic, he may be sensitive to something you are eating. The most common offenders are dairy products, chocolate, caffeine, melons, cucumbers, peppers, citrus fruits and juices, and spicy foods. There's a good chance that you yourself may have hidden allergies to certain foods. To track down food allergies, try an elimination or rotation diet (see the appropriate entries in Part Three). Following these diets may seem like an overwhelming task, but the results can be very worthwhile. An alternative is to keep an ongoing food diary to help you identify correspondences between the foods you eat and symptoms, both your baby's and your own. If you discover a hidden sensitivity that you hadn't suspected, simply avoiding that food will likely help you feel better and alleviate your baby's colic as well.

■ If you are nursing a colicky baby, try deleting all gas-forming foods from your diet, including cauliflower, broccoli, Brussels sprouts, cucumbers, red and green peppers, onions, beans, and legumes. Other foods in a nursing mother's diet that can contribute to colic include cow's milk, bananas, berries, and anything that contains caffeine.

■ A mother nursing a colicky baby should minimize the amount of raw foods in her diet. A breastfeeding mother's diet should consist of 70 to 80 percent cooked foods, and only 20 to 30 percent raw foods. Keep your diet simple.

■ If your colicky infant is bottlefed, his formula may be causing the problem. Ask your doctor about the advisability of changing to a different formula.

NUTRITIONAL SUPPLEMENTS

■ *Lactobacillus acidophilus* provides the bowel with friendly intestinal flora, which will ease digestion and may help resolve colic. A breastfeeding mother should take ½ teaspoon, twice a day. Give a bottlefed baby ⅛ teaspoon of acidophilus powder dissolved in formula, twice a day.

■ *Lactobacillus bifidus* is another friendly bacteria that helps improve digestion. Some experts think bifidus may be more effective than acidophilus in young infants. A nursing mother should take one dose, twice a day. Give a bottlefed baby ⅛ teaspoon dissolved in formula, twice daily.

HERBAL TREATMENT

■ Chamomile tea is a well-known soother and relaxant. A breastfed baby's mother should drink 1 cup, twice a day. Give a bottlefed infant 1 teaspoon of tea, three times daily, in formula or water, for three to four days. Then reduce the dosage to twice daily.

■ Fennel can also be helpful in relieving colic. The nursing mother can drink 1 cup of fennel tea, three times a day. Or dilute 1 cup of fennel tea in 2 cups of water, and give your baby 1 teaspoon of the diluted tea, four times a day.

■ A nursing mother can drink 1 cup of ginger tea, three times a day, to help relieve her baby's colic.

■ Peppermint tea helps to speed the emptying time of the stomach, enhances digestion, and acts as an antiflatulent. Give your child 1 teaspoon of peppermint tea, four to five times a day.

Note: If you are giving your child peppermint tea as well as a homeopathic preparation, allow one hour between the two. Otherwise, the strong smell of the mint may interfere with the action of the homeopathic remedy.

■ Try giving your baby a combination herbal tea. Israeli researchers gave a daily dose of about ½ cup of a tea made from chamomile, licorice, fennel, and balm-mint to babies who were experiencing episodes of colic, and found that symptoms were eased in more than half the children studied.

HOMEOPATHY

Like most homeopathic formulas, the remedies listed here are symptom-specific. Based on your knowledge of your colicky baby, select a suitable remedy.

■ *Colocynthis* and *Magnesia phosphorica*, two abdominal relaxants, are the most commonly prescribed homeopathics for colic. They are especially effective when used together. Dissolve one dose of *Colocynthis* 12x or 6c and one dose of *Magnesia phosphorica* 12x or 6c in a small amount of spring or distilled water at room temperature. With an eyedropper, squeeze a dropperful into your baby's mouth, three times daily, as needed. This combination remedy should bring relief within two days. If your infant's colic has not eased after two days, stop giving the remedy. It is unlikely that it will be helpful.

■ *Carbo vegetabilis* is a homeopathic remedy for the colicky infant with a pale face and distended upper abdomen. His legs may be cold from the foot to the knee. This baby is restless and cries even when nursing or being fed, and burps for a long time after feeding. He seems to feel better when being held and worse when put down. Give this child *Carbo vegetabilis* 12x, 30x, or 9c by dissolving one dose in 8 ounces of spring water and squeezing a few drops into his mouth, three times daily, for two days or until symptoms improve.

■ If your baby has a flushed, red face that feels hot, and has a loud, demanding cry but stops crying for a short time if he is carried, give him *Chamomilla* 12x, 30x, 9c, or 15c. Dissolve one dose in 8 ounces of spring water and squeeze a few drops into his mouth, three times a day, for two days or until symptoms improve.

■ Homeopathic colic combination formulas are available that may offer relief for your baby. Follow dosage directions on the product label.

ACUPRESSURE

For the locations of acupressure points on a child's body, *see* ADMINISTERING AN ACUPRESSURE TREATMENT in Part Three.

■ Stomach 36 helps to activate the digestive system.

■ Massaging the points along either side of the spine improves circulation and relaxes the nervous system.

GENERAL RECOMMENDATIONS

If you have a colicky baby, try to keep from becoming frantic. Stress and tension— both yours and your baby's—can contribute to colic and make the problem worse. If you feel your frustration is getting out of hand, talk to your health care practitioner. Seek emotional support and counseling. In the midst of an episode of colic-related crying, try one or all of the following suggestions. Some babies respond to one; some (unfortunately) to none.

■ To help relax muscle cramps and calm your baby, place your infant over your knees or against your chest with a warm water bottle between you and your baby's stomach.

■ If your baby loves water, try a warm, soothing splash in the bath.

■ Massage your baby's stomach with a non-alcohol-based lotion or oil. Following the natural path of the intestines, gently rub from the lower right "corner" of the abdomen up across the bottom of the rib cage, down to the lower left "corner," and around again (see margin illustration).

■ Some babies respond to cuddling and rocking. Many infants will quiet down when being carried around.

■ Some babies prefer the security of being closely swaddled in a blanket; some

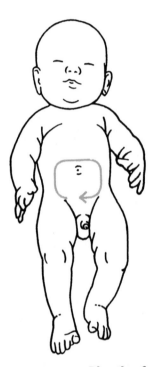

Direction for Abdominal Massage

For a colicky baby, try doing a gentle massage following the path of the intestines, as shown.

prefer loose coverings that permit free movement. Experiment to find what suits your child best.

■ Babies with sensitive nervous systems may respond better to a decrease in external stimulation. Try soft lighting, less touching, and a quiet atmosphere.

■ Some babies respond to soft, comforting music; some to recordings of a heartbeat; some to recordings of the sounds they lived with for nine months in the womb, which include both the mother's heartbeat and the steady "whoosh" of mother's blood traveling through her body. Interestingly, the sound of a washing machine often seems to have the same effect.

■ Vigorous movement distracts some babies with colic. Putting on some lively music and bebopping around with babe in arms may not be your favorite 3:00 A.M. activity, but it's been known to work.

■ Do "the bicycle" with your baby. With your baby lying on his back on the floor, gently move his legs in a bicycle-pedaling motion. Practice this exercise several times daily. These passive leg movements can be very comforting to your baby's digestive system.

■ Take an infant massage class to learn how massage supports your baby's overall growth and development. Your instructor can also teach you specific strokes and techniques for resolving colic.

PREVENTION

■ Keep a record of your child's bouts of irritability and crying, and look for a common denominator. See whether your child cries around the same time every day. Try to determine whether certain foods or activities trigger crying. If you discover a link, eliminate the food or activity that you think may be responsible.

■ Create a calm environment during feeding, and enjoy this time with your child. Play relaxing music. Make sure both you and baby are physically comfortable. Dress yourself and your baby warmly and comfortably. Be sure your baby's diaper is not too tight.

■ When feeding your infant, try holding him in an upright position so that the air stays above the milk in his stomach. This will make it easier for your baby to expel the air when he burps.

■ If you are bottlefeeding, check the size of the nipple hole. Milk should drip out slowly when the bottle is held upside down. If the hole is too small or too large, your baby may ingest too much air while feeding.

■ To control the amount of air your baby swallows when feeding, limit actual drinking time to about ten minutes. After each two ounces of fluid, try to burp your baby (but don't be discouraged if he doesn't burp).

■ At the end of each full feeding, burp your baby for ten minutes. Remain calm. Taking extra time now may prevent a bout of colic later.

■ If your baby just can't get out a burp after ten or fifteen minutes, prop him in an upright position for about half an hour, then try again.

■ If you are breastfeeding, eliminate the foods listed under Dietary Guidelines, page 160, and investigate the possibility of food allergies.

■ A nursing mother should take an acidophilus or bifidus supplement. If you are bottlefeeding your baby, administer the supplement dissolved in formula.

■ Try to avoid overfeeding or underfeeding your baby. Spitting up after feedings may indicate overfeeding; crying or continued suckling after feeding may indicate underfeeding. Follow your child's lead. As long as your baby is gaining weight and developing normally, you are probably doing just fine.

Common Cold

The common cold is a viral infection of the upper respiratory tract, caused by one of the many contagious viruses that intrude into the nose, throat, sinuses, or ears. The virus travels either from hand to mouth and nose, or through the air on minute droplets carrying infected secretions from one sneezing, wheezing, coughing child to another. On arrival, the virus settles in and multiplies, causing a multiplicity of problems.

Because your child's immune system is in the process of developing, it is not unusual for a child to seem to catch a cold week after week. As your child grows, her immune defenses evolve from an uncoordinated series of safeguards to an intricate set of responses designed to defend the body against foreign substances. In the meantime, boosting your child's immune system with diet and herbs can lessen the frequency of illness.

Doctors often say that children under six years of age have an average of seven colds a year, and older children tend to have an average of four or five colds a year. Some experts say these figures underestimate the incidence of colds in children, however. Your child can catch a cold at any time of the year, but most colds occur during the winter months, from October through February.

The well-known symptoms include a stuffy or runny nose, sneezing, headache, sore throat, coughing, loss of appetite, watery or burning eyes, ear congestion or infection, low-grade fever, and aching muscles and joints. When your child has a cold, she may suffer one, some, or all of these annoying symptoms.

As the cold virus multiplies in the body, the mucous membranes in the respiratory tract swell. Mucus production increases. The swelling causes the air passages to narrow, making breathing difficult. The sinuses become congested. The nose runs. Sneezing, a sense of fullness or achiness in the head, and tearing or burning eyes are all part of the process.

The initial phase of a cold, with nasal congestion, low-grade fever, and cough, usually lasts for two to five days. At the most contagious phase of a cold, the nasal secretions are thin, watery mucus that is almost entirely composed of viral discharge. When the secretions turn thick and yellowish or greenish, that means the discharge is full of dead white blood (immune system) cells, dead viral particles, and dead bacteria. This is a sign of healing and the least contagious stage of a cold.

From start to finish, a common cold, if uncomplicated, lasts about five to ten days. Because there are so many different viruses that cause cold symptoms, a child who is sick for more than fourteen days in a row has probably contracted a series of viruses. While your child's immature immune system is busy fighting the first virus, another can settle in more easily. If your child's temperature goes above approximately 102°F, it is likely that she is suffering from a flu, not a cold. A child with the flu is also likely to feel worse all over than a child with a cold. (*See* INFLUENZA.)

CONVENTIONAL TREATMENT

■ As we all know, there is no cure for the common cold. Antibiotics are ineffective against viruses, and therefore useless in treating colds. Unless your child develops another infection, like an ear or sinus infection, in addition to her cold, antibiotics are not given. In fact, a virus will have more room to multiply if an antibiotic destroys the bacteria normally present in the respiratory tract, so antibiotics can actually inhibit the body in its fight against the common cold.

■ Treatment of colds is aimed at providing symptomatic relief. Acetaminophen (found in Tylenol, Tempra, and other over-the-counter medications) helps to bring down fever and relieve the aches and pains of the common cold. Ibuprofen (Advil, Nuprin, and others) can be used for the same purpose.

Note: In excessive amounts, acetaminophen can cause liver damage. Read package directions carefully so as not to exceed the proper dosage for your child's age and size. Ibuprofen is best given with food to lessen the chance of stomach upset.

■ *Do not* give aspirin to a child or teenager with a cold or other viral illness. The combination of aspirin with a virus is associated with the development of Reye's syndrome, a dangerous liver disease (*see* REYE'S SYNDROME).

■ Decongestants, such as oxymetazoline (found in Dristan), phenylephrine (Neo-Synephrine), phenylpropanolamine (Congespirin, Triaminic), and pseudoephedrine (Sudafed) help decrease swelling and inflammation in the nasal cavity. As the term implies, they can provide relief from a stuffy and runny nose. Decongestants are available in pill and liquid form and as nose drops and sprays. However, if the spray forms are used for more than three days, they become irritating to nasal membranes, resulting in "rebound congestion" that can be worse than the initial symptoms. These drugs can also cause restlessness and insomnia. Because they can increase the heart rate, they are not recommended for infants.

■ Because the sneezing and discomfort of a cold can resemble that of an allergic reaction, many people try using antihistamines, such as brompheniramine (Dimetane), chlorpheniramine (Chlor-Trimeton), pyrilamine (Triaminic), and diphenhydramine (Benadryl), for colds. These medications dry up secretions in the respiratory tract. They have not been shown to be effective for the relief of cold symptoms, however. They are designed to counteract allergic responses, not viruses, and they are best reserved for their intended purpose. Antihistamines also commonly cause side effects, including drowsiness and dry mouth, and they are not recommended for children under two years of age.

■ There are many over-the-counter medicines that promise relief of the common cold. Most of these are combinations of some of the drugs listed above. In general, they are not the most effective treatment. It usually works best to give medications individually, as called for by your child's symptoms. Before giving any medication to your child, talk to your doctor about it, read the label, and consider the side effects. Always follow age-specific directions carefully.

DIETARY GUIDELINES

■ If your child doesn't feel like eating, it's best not to force food. When children are ill, they seem to instinctively know what they should eat, and usually choose simple, healthy foods. Suggest juice, applesauce, broth, soups (especially vegetable or chicken soup), and herbal teas.

WHEN TO CALL THE DOCTOR ABOUT A COLD

● If your child has a chronic stuffy nose with thick discharge, you should see your physician. A thick, greenish nasal discharge during the final stage of a cold indicates healing, but if it doesn't go away, it may be a sign of a chronic infection, such as a sinus infection.

● If your child's fever persists, or if it returns after three days, she may have developed a bacterial infection, such as an ear or sinus infection. By themselves, colds do not usually cause significant fever.

● If your child's cold does not clear up within a week, if the symptoms get worse, or if your child develops a rash or a honking cough, she may have a different viral illness. The early symptoms of many viral diseases, such as measles and whooping cough, often resemble those of the common cold.

● If at any time your child shows signs of respiratory distress, such as rapid breathing, gasping, wheezing, nasal flaring, or a pale or bluish skin color, or if your child develops a high fever or unusual lethargy, she may be coming down with a more serious infection, such as pneumonia. A child who develops pneumonia needs medical attention.

■ A child with a cold and fever is easily dehydrated and can become constipated. Flush your child's body with as much fluid as she will accept. If she becomes constipated, this condition will most likely correct itself once she begins to feel better and resumes her normal diet.

■ All fluids, including soups, help alleviate respiratory illnesses. Fluids help to thin secretions, making it easier for the body to clear them. If the secretions are thick and dry, they are more difficult to expel. Offer diluted fruit juices, homemade sugarless lemonade (use a bit of honey for sweetening, and serve either warm or cold), and lots of nourishing broth and homemade soup.

■ Limit refined sugars. Sweets can make your child feel first energized, then agitated and irritable. They also create acids in the body that can cause a cold to linger. If your child insists, give her a little bit of honey or a *tiny* bite of something sweet.

Caution: Never give honey to a child less than one year old. Honey has been associated with infant botulism, which can be life threatening.

■ Avoid dairy foods, which have a tendency to increase and thicken mucus.

■ Eliminate fats as much as possible. Fats are difficult to digest under normal circumstances, and are even harder to digest when the digestive system is weakened by the low-grade infection of a cold. Undigested fats contribute to an increase in mucus and a toxic internal environment.

NUTRITIONAL SUPPLEMENTS

For age-appropriate dosages of nutritional supplements, see page 81.

■ The body uses beta-carotene to manufacture vitamin A, which helps heal mucous membranes. Give your child a double dose of beta-carotene, twice daily, for five to seven days.

■ Vitamin C has anti-inflammatory properties and will help ease the course of a cold. Give your child one dose of vitamin C, three times daily, for three days. Choose a formula made without sugar. Avoid chewable forms, which can erode tooth enamel.

■ To help boost your child's immune system, give her a total of one dose of zinc, in chewable tablet or lozenge form, each day, for three days. Choose a lozenge made without refined sugar.

Note: Excessive amounts of zinc can result in nausea and vomiting. Be careful not to exceed the recommended dosage.

HERBAL TREATMENT

For age-appropriate dosages of herbal remedies, see page 81.

■ Yin qiao is a Chinese botanical formula that can be taken at the very first sign of a cold. This remedy usually is not helpful after the third day of symptoms. Give your child one dose, every two hours, during the acute phase of the cold. After the symptoms start to ease, reduce the dosage to one dose, three times daily, for one week.

Note: The liquid extract is the preferred form, because it contains no aspirin. The tablet form should not be given to a child under four years of age.

■ To help your child rest and relax, give her one dose of chamomile tea, twice daily, as needed.

■ To calm a restless, fussy child, prepare a soothing herbal bath with chamomile, calendula, rosemary, and/or lavender. Keep the water comfortably warm and encourage a long, lazy soak.

■ Echinacea and goldenseal both stimulate the immune system. Echinacea is antibacterial and antiviral; goldenseal is an antibacterial noted for healing irritated mucous membranes. Give your child one dose of an echinacea and goldenseal combination formula, three times a day, for five days to one week.

■ Garlic has antibacterial properties and helps detoxify the body. Give your child one capsule, two to three times a day, for one week. You can substitute one clove of fresh garlic for each capsule, but most children are more willing to accept garlic in the odorless capsule form.

■ Give your child ginger tea to increase perspiration. This helps to cleanse the body and reduce the intensity of a cold. Give one dose, every four hours, during the acute phase of a cold.

■ Sage tea helps to break up congestion and bring down a fever. Give your child one dose of sage tea, up to three times daily, for three to five days.

HOMEOPATHY

At the very first sign of a cold, give your child ⅓ tube of *Anas barbariae* (sold under various brand names, including Oscillococcinum), three times daily, for one day. Then, during the acute phase of your child's cold, give her one dose of one of the symptom-specific homeopathic remedies below, three to four times daily, for three days. If there is no improvement at all after three doses of a remedy, however, it is unlikely that it will do anything more. Switch to another that matches your child's symptoms and temperament. If your child feels better before three days have passed, stop giving the remedy.

■ For the child with a very runny nose and a great deal of irritating, watery nasal secretions that cause inflammation, as well as teary (but not burning) eyes and a lot of sneezing, give *Allium cepa* 12x or 6c. This is homeopathic red onion. It is recommended for the child who feels worse than you do when you are chopping a strong onion.

■ For the child who feels chilly, restless, and weak, give *Arsenicum album* 30x or 9c. This remedy is for the child who, paradoxically, feels worse in a cold room but wants something cold to drink. She has a red nose, with runny nasal secretions that burn the nose and upper lip. When this child is ill, she wants to sit in bed with books, magazines, and a television. This child wants to be left alone, but will demand attention and reassurance every once in a while. When she is comforted and cuddled, she will quiet down and go to sleep.

■ If the eyes are the main focus of the cold, give your child *Euphrasia* 12x. This is for a child whose symptoms are the opposite of those calling for *Allium cepa*. Her nose runs a lot, especially in the morning, but without irritation; she complains of burning eyes and stinging tears, winks frequently, and wipes and rubs her eyes. She yawns a lot, and prefers to be inside, away from sunlight and bright lights.

■ *Eupatorium* 12x or 6c is helpful for the child who complains of a severe aching deep in her bones, and says she feels sore "everywhere."

■ Give *Gelsemium* 30x or 9c to the child who has heavy, droopy eyes, who feels weak and tired, with aches and chills up and down her back, and who wants to be alone.

■ Give *Pulsatilla* 30x or 9c to the child with a stuffy nose and thick yellow discharge. This child feels worse at night and when indoors; she prefers to be outdoors and wants comfort and attention.

ACUPRESSURE

For the locations of acupressure points on a child's body, *see* ADMINISTERING AN ACUPRESSURE TREATMENT in **Part Three**.

■ Bladder 11, 12, 13, and 14 clear and balance a distressed respiratory system.

■ Large Intestine 4 relieves congestion and headaches.

■ Lung 7 clears upper respiratory tract infections.

GENERAL RECOMMENDATIONS

■ Begin treating your child's cold as soon as you notice the first symptom.

■ At the first sign that your child may be developing a cold, begin giving her an echinacea and goldenseal combination formula.

■ Select and administer an appropriate homeopathic remedy.

■ Most children instinctively sleep and rest when suffering through a cold, thus conserving energy to fight the virus. A cozy bed and an open window bringing in fresh air (when weather permits) usually help. Be sure your child doesn't get chilled.

■ Encourage your child to drink plenty of liquids, especially chamomile tea, chicken soup, and soup made with astragalus and vegetables (*see* THERAPEUTIC RECIPES in Part Three).

Note: Astragalus should not be used in the presence of a fever. If your child has a fever, omit the astragalus root from the recipe.

■ Use a cool mist humidifier in your child's room. Humidified air may help to thin secretions, helping to break up a cold and easing the discomfort of a congested head. To avoid having a lot of particles in the air, use distilled, demineralized water. Be sure the humidifier is very clean, so that bacteria do not collect and spread through it into the air.

■ Because babies tend to breathe through their noses, an infant may have particular difficulty breathing with a congested nose. To ease your baby's breathing, use a very small rubber bulb to gently suction out mucus. You can get these at most drug stores.

■ A nasal saline irrigation, followed by the suctioning out of mucus with a bulb syringe, can be very effective for loosening and removing thick mucus. This is especially important for infants, who may have a hard time getting mucus out of their noses or throats. (*See* NASAL SALINE FLUSH in Part Three).

■ *See also* COUGH; FEVER; SINUSITIS; or SORE THROAT if your child's cold is accompanied by any of these symptoms.

PREVENTION

■ Because there are so many different viruses that cause colds, it is unlikely that medical science will ever develop a vaccine that can protect against all of them. There are, however, measures that you can take to strengthen your child's resistance to illness. Although your child can suffer a cold at any time, colds are most common during early fall, midwinter, and early spring, so these are the times it makes most sense to work actively to boost immunity. Try one or several of the following suggestions:

- American ginseng helps to build the immune system and strengthens the body. Give your child one dose, once or twice weekly, during the winter months.

  Note: American ginseng should not be used if fever or any other signs of acute infection are present.

- Give your child one dose of beta-carotene daily during the cold and flu season.

- Echinacea and goldenseal stimulate the immune system and help keep the body clear of infections. A liquid extract is the preferred form. Give your child one dose of an echinacea and goldenseal combination formula, twice weekly, during the cold and flu season.

  Note: You should not give your child echinacea on a daily basis for more than ten days at a time or it may lose its effectiveness.

- Vitamin C with bioflavonoids is an effective preventive combination. If your child resists eating fruits and vegetables, supplement her diet with 150 milligrams of each daily during the cold season.

- Give your child one dose of *Anas barbariae*, once a week, during the cold and flu season.

- Make it a rule to give your child a low-sweet diet and no fried foods. During the cold season, prepare soups of chicken and vegetables, and add the herb astragalus in dried or tincture form to the soup to help boost her immune system.

■ A child under emotional distress will fall ill more easily. Emotional upset may be caused by the birth of a sibling, fear over starting school, grief or anger over parental separation, moving, or any other stresses. Try to be aware of and talk out problems, and be supportive of your child during emotional crises. (*See* EMOTIONAL UPSET.)

■ Physical stress can create a bodily imbalance that makes a child more vulnerable to illness. Exposure to dust and chemicals, too much sugar and fat in the diet, even the kind of sudden and extreme temperature change that occurs when you leave a sunny beach and enter an air-conditioned room, all can potentially make your child more susceptible to illness.

■ Practice good hygiene, especially careful and frequent hand-washing, and teach your child to do the same. This is especially important if one member of the household already has a cold. Many viruses are spread via the hands.

Concussion (Head Injury)

EMERGENCY TREATMENT FOR CONCUSSION

✚ After any injury to the head, it is wise to call your physician or take your child to the emergency room of the nearest hospital. It is important to seek the advice of a qualified medical professional. The severity of head injuries is difficult for the layperson to evaluate, and head injuries are one of the most common causes of death in children.

Any injury to your child's head, whether from falling off a swing, getting banged on the monkey bars, being hit by a flying object, or being jarred or shaken violently, may result in concussion. It is rare for a child to reach adulthood without ever experiencing a hard knock on the head from one cause or another. The severity of your child's symptoms will depend on the extent of injury to the brain.

After a simple concussion, your child may seem disoriented or lose consciousness briefly. She may have no memory of events just prior to and immediately following the injury. Headaches, dizziness, and drowsiness are all common immediately after awakening. Such symptoms usually disappear within a few weeks, but can last as long as several months.

If your child suffers a head injury, watch her closely afterward. If any of the following symptoms occurs, even as much as four weeks after a seemingly mild bang on the head, seek medical attention immediately, as these can be signs of bleeding in the brain:

- Loss of consciousness.
- Unusually widened pupils.
- Severe headache.
- Drowsiness.
- Personality changes.
- Confusion; loss of memory; speech difficulties.
- Loss of coordination; paralysis.

CONVENTIONAL TREATMENT

■ Seek medical help immediately. The doctor will examine your child and possibly order an x-ray of her skull to check for fracture, or a magnetic resonance imaging (MRI) scan to look for bleeding or swelling in the brain. Be prepared to answer questions about your child's reaction right after the accident, including any unusual behavior. The doctor will evaluate your child's condition and provide appropriate treatment.

■ Your doctor will probably recommend that you keep close watch on your child for a minimum of twenty-four hours after returning home.

HOMEOPATHY

■ If your child is fully conscious and able to swallow, give her one dose of *Aconite* 200x immediately after an accident to alleviate some of the initial shock. Wait ten minutes. Then give your child one dose of *Arnica* 30x, 200x, 15c, or 30c. *Arnica* helps to decrease bruising and aching. Continue giving your child one dose of *Arnica*, three times a day, for two days following an accident.

■ On the third day after an injury, give your child one dose of *Natrum muriaticum* 30x or 9c as needed to help resolve dizziness, forehead pain, throbbing pain in the temples, or a headache at the base of the skull. Give this remedy three times daily until the pain is alleviated. If there is no improvement after forty-eight hours, discontinue the remedy.

PREVENTION

■ There are some head injuries a parent cannot prevent; you can't always be in the right place at the right time to cushion a fall. You can, however, avoid two actions that can cause concussion:

- When playing with your child, never toss her into the air and catch her as she falls. That tender neck can snap back and forth, causing a brain stem injury or concussion.
- For the same reason, *never* punish a child by shaking her.

■ Insist that your child wear a helmet when engaging in such activities as bicycle riding, skiing, or playing football or hockey.

■ For ways to reduce the possibility that your child will suffer a head injury at home, *see* HOME SAFETY in Part One.

Conjunctivitis

Conjunctivitis, also known by the descriptive name *pinkeye*, is an inflammation of the conjunctiva, or the white of the eye, which is the transparent membrane that lines the eyeball. If your child's eye becomes inflamed, prompt treatment is essential.

Conjunctivitis can be caused by a viral or bacterial infection, an injury to the eye, or a reaction to fumes, smoke, or pollution. Though the causes may be different, the symptoms are identical. Allergic conjunctivitis is most often caused by pollen, and is therefore usually a seasonal reaction (unless it is the result of exposure to a pet, dust, mold, or some other nonseasonal allergen).

In infants less than a week old, plugged tear ducts are not uncommon. Tear ducts drain tears out of the eye. Although the situation usually resolves on its own by the time a baby is six months old, in some cases a doctor may recommend surgery to open a clogged duct. This is because a plugged tear duct can cause a backup and accumulation of fluid in the eye, creating fertile soil for an infection. If silver nitrite drops are put in a newborn baby's eyes, this also can cause a reaction.

The overwhelming majority of cases of conjunctivitis in older children are caused by viruses, although in rare cases a bacterial infection may be responsible. Viruses and bacteria may be rubbed into the eye, or may travel from an infection in the nose up through a tear duct and into the eye. The infection can be transmitted from one child to another.

Suspect conjunctivitis if the white of your child's eye shows bright pink or red coloration. In the early stages, your child may complain of burning or itching eyes and may feel as if there's something in them. His eyelid may be swollen, and there can be a sticky, yellowish discharge from the eye. The eyes may be "glued" shut in the morning when your child awakens.

Most cases of simple conjunctivitis last from five to seven days. If you are treating your child for conjunctivitis at home and notice no improvement in that time, take your child to a doctor.

CONVENTIONAL TREATMENT

WHEN TO CALL THE DOCTOR ABOUT CONJUNCTIVITIS

• If you are treating your child for conjunctivitis and notice no improvement in four to five days, or if the infection is painful, draining heavily, interfering with vision, or seems to be affecting the tissues around the eyes, take your child to a doctor for professional evaluation.

• If the infection seems to be getting worse, if there is a thick, green discharge from the eye, if the eye looks cloudy, if the eye continues swelling or shutting, or if your child is becoming increasingly sensitive to light, call your doctor. These are all signs of a worsening infection, or a possible herpes infection. A herpes infection in the eye is a serious and dangerous infection that can lead to blindness.

• Red, itchy, and tearing eyes can also be an early sign of measles. If your child develops a rash, fever, malaise, and/or cough, he may be coming down with measles. Call your doctor if you suspect measles (*see* MEASLES).

■ Warm-water compresses are the treatment of choice. Many of the microorganisms that cause conjunctivitis are exquisitely heat sensitive. The heat also loosens up debris and increases blood flow through the area, which helps the body's natural defense mechanisms. You can use either a clean cloth or a cotton ball as a compress. Your doctor is likely to recommend that compresses be applied for ten minutes, four to six times daily. Clean the eyes with warm water after applying the compresses, and wash your hands both before and after the treatment. If you use a cotton ball, throw it away after removing the compress; if you use cloth, wash the compress in detergent and hot water (with chlorine bleach added if possible), separately from all other laundry, before using it again. Always be very cautious when using warm liquids around your child's eyes. The skin of the eyelid is thin and tender and can burn easily.

■ If you can see no improvement in your child's condition in four to five days, or if the infection seems to be growing worse, you should consult a doctor to determine if it might be bacterial in origin. You may need to consult an eye specialist. If conjunctivitis is caused by bacteria, a prescription for antibiotic eye ointment or eye drops may be appropriate (antibiotics are useless against viral or allergic conjunctivitis). Many children rebel against the stinging sensation caused by some medications, so if your doctor determines that an antibiotic is in order, ask for a formula that is nonirritating, like Polysporin (which contains polymyxin), Tobrex (tobramycin), Ciloxan (ciprofloxacin), or Ilotycin (erythromycin).

■ If your child has a definite case of allergic conjunctivitis, the doctor may prescribe steroid drops to help decrease inflammation and relieve itching.

Caution: If there is *even a suspicion* of a herpes infection, steroid drops should not be used. This can be very dangerous.

■ Your doctor may recommend a topical antihistamine and decongestant, such as phenylephrine, in a form specifically designed for use in the eyes, to help reduce itching, swelling, and redness in cases of allergic conjunctivitis. Cool compresses may also be comforting in this situation.

DIETARY GUIDELINES

■ Eliminate refined sugars from your child's diet. Sugar makes the body more acidic, which inhibits healing. In addition, bacterial infections thrive in the presence of sugar.

■ Encourage your child to eat green and yellow vegetables and fruits, which are high in fiber and rich in vitamins A and C. Both of these vitamins support the immune system. In addition, vitamin A protects and heals mucous membranes, and vitamin C fosters healing and is mildly anti-inflammatory.

NUTRITIONAL SUPPLEMENTS

For age-appropriate dosages of nutritional supplements, see page 81.

■ Give your child one dose of beta-carotene, twice a day, for five to seven days.

■ Three times a day, for five to seven days, give your child one dose of vitamin C with bioflavonoids.

■ Give your child one-half dose of zinc, twice a day, for five to seven days.

   Note: Excessive amounts of zinc can result in nausea and vomiting. Be careful not to exceed the recommended dosage.

HERBAL TREATMENT

For age-appropriate dosages of herbal remedies, see page 81.

■ Echinacea and goldenseal stimulate the immune system, so an echinacea and goldenseal combination formula is important in clearing any infection. Echinacea fights viral infections; goldenseal fights bacteria and soothes mucous membranes. Give your child one dose, every two hours, during the first day. After that, give him one dose, three times daily, until the condition improves, for up to one week.

   Note: You should not give your child echinacea on a daily basis for more than ten days at a time, or it will lose its effectiveness.

■ A warm eyebright compress will help to increase the blood flow to the eye and wash discharge away. Eyebright, a most appropriately named herb, helps relieve redness and swelling of the eye, and will help clear an eye infection. To prepare an eyebright compress, simmer 1 teaspoon of the dried herb in 1 pint of water for ten minutes. Cool the resulting tea to a comfortably warm temperature. Moisten a thin white cotton cloth with the warm eyebright tea and place it over your child's eyes. Encourage him to keep the compress in place for fifteen minutes (admittedly a challenge for some children). Then wipe the eyelids and clear the softened discharge from around the eyes with the compress. Always be very cautious when using warm liquids around your child's eyes. The skin of the eyelid is thin and tender and can burn easily. Wash your hands before and after the treatment, and either throw away the compress after using it or wash it separately in detergent and hot water with chlorine bleach added before using it again.

■ If you are unable to find the herb eyebright, you can use goldenseal root or simply a compress made with warm spring water, as described under Conventional Treatment, above.

HOMEOPATHY

■ *Euphrasia* is a homeopathic preparation made from eyebright. When your child's eyes are burning, itching, and tearing, give him one dose of *Euphrasia* 12x or 6c, three times daily, for two days.

■ If your child has a thick, yellowish discharge and his eyes are matted tightly closed in the morning, give him one dose of *Pulsatilla* 12x, 30x, 6c, or 9c, three times daily, for two days. This is good for a child who experiences burning and itching so intensely that there is a constant urge to rub the eyes.

ACUPRESSURE

For the locations of acupressure points on a child's body, *see* ADMINISTERING AN ACUPRESSURE TREATMENT in Part Three.

■ In Chinese medicine, the liver "rules" the eyes. Pressure on Liver 3 will help to take the "heat" out of the eyes.

■ Spleen 10 removes "heat" from the blood.

■ Gallbladder 20 improves circulation to the head.

■ Gallbladder 21 takes excessive energy away and down from the infection.

GENERAL RECOMMENDATIONS

■ Apply a warm and soothing eyebright compress every two to three hours.

■ If your child's symptoms don't respond within four to five days, see your doctor.

■ Give your child an echinacea and goldenseal combination formula orally.

■ Select and administer a suitable homeopathic remedy.

■ So that your child does not continually reinfect his eyes, teach him not to touch them. Given the discomfort he is experiencing, however, that's asking a lot. You may have to settle for making sure that your child keeps his hands very clean.

■ A nursing mother has a natural antibiotic in her breast milk that is useful for all sorts of infant problems. For a cleansing and soothing antibiotic eyewash for your newborn, put a drop or two of breast milk in his eyes.

■ If your newborn's tear ducts are clogged, massage them with five or six gentle strokes, six to eight times daily, to help them drain.

■ If your child's conjunctivitis is related to exposure to chemicals, such as sprays, fumes, smoke, or pollution, gently wash his eyes with warm water. If the condition worsens, call your physician.

■ A child who has been diagnosed as having bacterial conjunctivitis should not be permitted to go swimming until the infection has cleared.

PREVENTION

■ Both viral and bacterial conjunctivitis are highly contagious. To avoid passing an existing case of conjunctivitis around the entire family, teach children to use only their own washcloths, towels, and pillows.

■ To prevent your child from introducing bacteria or viruses into his eyes in the future, teach him to wash his hands carefully and frequently. Teach him to avoid scratching or rubbing his eyes.

■ Keep your child from being exposed to known eye irritants, such as cigarette smoke, dust, fumes, sprays, pollution, household cleaning products, and excessively chlorinated swimming pools.

■ Your child's daily diet should include lots of green and yellow vegetables and fruits, which are high in vitamins A and C.

Consciousness, Loss of

See FAINTING; UNCONSCIOUSNESS.

Constipation

The term constipation refers to a change in daily bowel habits, particularly a decrease in the number or consistency of bowel movements, or pain or difficulty passing stools. By the end of their first year, most children have one comfortable bowel movement every day. If a usually regular child goes two or more days without a bowel movement, and then has pain or difficulty passing a large, hard stool, he is constipated.

Breastfed babies have fewer bowel movements than bottlefed babies. Because just about every drop of breast milk is very efficiently used, a breastfed infant has less waste to excrete. It's not unusual for a breastfed baby of two, three, or four months of age to have no bowel movements for several days in a row. If the child has a good appetite and is not uncomfortable, there's no need to worry. However, if your baby doesn't want to nurse, is vomiting, or has discomfort, consult your physician immediately.

Constipation is commonly caused by insufficient fluids and too little fiber in the diet. Without enough fluids and bulk, stool becomes hard and develops rough edges. These rough edges can cause a rectal fissure, a painful microscopic tear in the rectum. Too much emphasis on toilet training, emotional stress (such as a move to a new location), the introduction of new foods, or too much fat in the diet may also contribute to constipation, as can a lack of proper exercise.

Children can also become constipated as a result of holding back stool. An active child may not want to take the time to interrupt his play to have a bowel movement. When that happens, the retained stool becomes dehydrated and hard and is painful to pass. A painful passing in turn makes the child want to hold back as long as possible the next time, to avoid the pain.

Even babies learn to hold back stool to avoid pain. A diaper rash that burns and hurts when a bowel movement occurs can make an infant reluctant to go.

The most important factor in determining whether your child is constipated is his level of comfort when passing a stool. Even if your child has a bowel movement every day, a hard-to-pass stool may indicate constipation. Another indication is a stomachache. A constipated child's stomach may be firm and tender to the touch.

CONVENTIONAL TREATMENT

■ Increasing the amount of fiber and fluid in your child's diet is the best place to start when treating constipation (*see* Dietary Guidelines, page 176).

■ A stool softener, such as docusate sodium, may be prescribed to soften the stool and help it pass through the intestines more easily.

■ A bulk-forming laxative such as Maltsupex or psyllium seed increases the amount of bulk in the intestines, softens the stool to make it easier to pass, and initiates peristalsis (the contraction of the intestines that pushes waste along). Either of these products should be taken with plenty of water.

■ Magnesium hydroxide (found in milk of magnesia), magnesium citrate (Evac-Q-Kwik), and phosphosoda (Phospho-soda, Sal-Hepatica) are bulk-forming laxatives that work by drawing fluids from the body into the intestine, increasing the contents of the intestines and thereby initiating a bowel movement. Magnesium hydroxide and magnesium citrate should not be given to a child under two years

WHEN TO CALL THE DOCTOR ABOUT CONSTIPATION

• A constipated infant who is vomiting or uncomfortable, and/or who doesn't want to nurse should be examined by a doctor.

• If your child experiences severe pain when passing a stool, if there is blood in the stools, or if you notice a cut or tear near your child's rectum, consult your physician.

• If your child develops chronic or persistent constipation, he should be examined by a doctor. In some cases, constipation may be a sign of an internal problem, such as an intestinal obstruction. Certain serious health problems, including lead poisoning and hypothyroidism, can also cause chronic constipation. Even if unrelated to an underlying problem, chronic constipation should be taken seriously because it can lead to a loss of muscle tone in the bowel, setting the stage for a lifelong problem.

of age. Phosphosoda should not be given to children under six. No laxative should be used on a regular basis. Do not give your child any medication without discussing it with your doctor.

■ Stimulant laxatives, such as bisacodyl (found in Ducolax), castor oil, phenolphthalein (Modane), and senna leaf extract, work by irritating the intestinal wall, thus stimulating peristalsis. Stimulant laxatives are harsh and can cause cramping. If you use these medications at all, do so sparingly. Bulk-forming laxatives are preferable to stimulant types. No laxative should be used on a regular basis, as dependency can develop. Do not give your child any medication without discussing it with your doctor.

■ Lubricants, such as glycerin and mineral oil, coat the stool and help it slip more easily through the rectum. However, prolonged use of mineral oil can cause inflammation of the liver, spleen, and abdominal lymph nodes, and interfere with the body's absorption of vitamins A and D. Also, a lubricant can be dangerous if it accidentally goes down the windpipe and enters the lungs.

DIETARY GUIDELINES

■ Because dehydration can lead to constipation, increase the amount of fluids in your child's diet. Have spring water, herbal teas, juices, and soups readily available, and encourage your child to take them often.

■ Increase the amount of fiber in your child's diet. Simply eating a piece of fruit, such as banana, apple, orange, or prune, may help resolve constipation. The whole fruit provides the most fiber. Serve your child a piece of fruit one-half to one hour before a meal or about one hour after a meal. A prune soaked overnight in a glass of water contains extra moisture and is easier to digest. For a toddler, a teaspoon of syrup from a soaked or cooked prune may be easier to take, and will help resolve constipation. Vegetables and whole grains are also rich sources of fiber.

■ Serving warm liquids or hot cereal such as oatmeal every morning acts gently to stimulate the intestinal tract, in addition to providing fiber.

■ Foods high in magnesium, such as dark green, leafy vegetables, are very helpful for the constipated child (the trick may be getting your child to eat them often).

■ For overnight relief of constipation, mix ½ cup of prune juice and 1 tablespoon of lemon juice with 1 cup of spring water. Have your child drink this before bedtime. This mixture is too strong for babies, however, and may cause diarrhea in a tiny body.

NUTRITIONAL SUPPLEMENTS

■ *Lactobacillus acidophilus* or *bifidus* helps to establish favorable intestinal flora, which is very helpful in relieving constipation. For a child with chronic or recurrent constipation, lactobacilli are strongly indicated. Give your child one dose daily, as directed on the product label.

■ If your child's stool has an exceptionally foul odor, consider giving him chlorophyll supplements. Chlorophyll is high in trace minerals, especially magnesium, and has natural antibacterial properties. Follow the dosage directions on the product label.

HERBAL TREATMENT

For age-appropriate dosages of herbal remedies, see page 81.

■ If your child is experiencing alternating constipation and diarrhea, oatmeal cooked in flaxseed tea can be very helpful. It soothes irritated intestines and relieves constipation. Prepare flaxseed tea by mixing 1 teaspoon of flaxseed in 1 quart of spring water; simmer for fifteen minutes. Use the resulting liquid instead of water to cook oatmeal. Or add ¼ to ½ cup of the tea to 4 ounces of juice and give your child one dose daily. Constipation should be relieved within forty-eight hours.

■ Licorice tea or tincture is soothing to irritated intestinal walls and helps relieve chronic constipation. Give your child one dose, once or twice daily, for three or four days.

Note: This herb should not be given to a child with high blood pressure.

■ Liquid food-grade aloe vera juice is quite helpful in resolving constipation. Make sure you purchase the edible form of aloe vera juice. Combine 1 tablespoon of the liquid with fruit juice or applesauce to make it more palatable, and give it to your child once or twice daily.

■ One to 10 drops of organic flaxseed oil, given twice daily in food, can help ease your child's bowel movements.

HOMEOPATHY

If your child is chronically constipated, it may be best to treat him with a constitutional remedy prescribed by a homeopathic physician. For an occasional constipation problem, select a remedy that matches your child's symptoms from the list that follows.

■ Use *Alumina* for a child who has stools that are small, hard, dry pellets, often covered with mucus. Elimination is very difficult for this child. Give him one dose of *Alumina* 30x or 9c, two or three times daily, for two or three days.

■ *Calcarea carbonica* is often used for constipation in small children with digestive disorders. If your child is constipated, with a hard, distended stomach, but is not cranky, crying, or complaining and seems to be feeling fine, give him one dose of *Calcarea carbonica* 30x or 9c, twice daily, for two or three days.

■ If your child has a hard, dry stool and experiences pain right before a bowel movement, give him one dose of *Lycopodium* 30x or 9c, two or three times daily, for two or three days. This remedy is also recommended for the child with lower intestinal gas that smells like rotten eggs.

■ *Natrum muriaticum* is the remedy for children who love salt—they lick salt off their plates and suck salt off pretzels and crackers—and are on the thin side, especially around the neck. These children are typically thirsty, yet have hard, dry stools. They benefit from one dose of *Natrum muriaticum* 30x or 9c, given twice daily, for two or three days.

■ *Nux vomica* is helpful for a child who may overeat and thus become constipated or gassy. If your child is impatient and agitated; craves rich, greasy, and/or spicy foods; and passes small, dark, hard stools after trying many times to have a bowel movement, give him one dose of *Nux vomica* 30x or 9c, twice daily, for two or three days.

■ *Sulphur* is for the child who often experiences anal itching and irritation, and typically has an unsuccessful urge to have a bowel movement. This child hates having a bowel movement and often holds back, because he is afraid the passing will cause pain. His stool is very odorous. Give this child one dose of *Sulphur* 30x or 9c, twice daily, for two or three days.

ACUPRESSURE

For the locations of acupressure points on a child's body, *see* ADMINISTERING AN ACUPRESSURE TREATMENT in Part Three.

■ Large Intestine 11 helps relax the large intestine.

■ Stomach 36 tones the digestive tract.

■ Massaging Bladder 20 to 25 along the lower back relaxes the nerves that stimulate the intestine.

GENERAL RECOMMENDATIONS

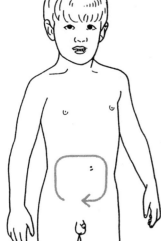

Direction for Abdominal Massage

An abdominal massage that follows the path of the intestines, as shown, can be helpful for relieving constipation.

■ Increase the amount of fiber and fluid in your child's diet.

■ To encourage normal bowel action, give your child flaxseed tea.

■ To normalize bowel flora, give your child a lactobacillus supplement.

■ Select and administer an appropriate homeopathic remedy.

■ If you feel you must give your child a laxative on occasion, use Maltsupex or psyllium powder.

■ Enemas have virtually no place in the treatment of constipation in children. The digestive tract is a "one-way street." It was not designed to be flushed from the bottom. Unless your physician prescribes an enema, your child's constipation is better treated in other ways.

■ An Epsom salts bath is relaxing and increases circulation. Epsom salts contain magnesium sulfate. An hour or two after an Epsom salts bath, a bowel movement will often occur.

■ Massaging your child's lower abdomen is comforting and helps to get things moving. Gently massage your child's abdomen, following the natural movement of the intestines. Start in the lower right "corner," move up toward the ribs, over to the left side, and then down toward the pelvis (see margin illustration).

■ Avoid using aluminum cookware. It is possible that taking in minute traces of aluminum can exacerbate constipation.

PREVENTION

■ Follow the dietary guidelines given in this section. Encourage your child to drink plenty of spring water and other fluids, and eat a high-fiber diet. Fruits, vegetables, and whole grains should figure prominently on the menu.

■ Encourage your child to be physically active. Limit television watching!

■ Give your child one dose of *Lactobacillus acidophilus* or *bifidus*, once daily, for one month, to maintain friendly flora in the intestines and bowels.

■ Encourage your child to become aware of and respond promptly to his bodily needs. Explain that holding back causes a difficult and painful bowel movement. When a young child indicates an urge, respond as soon as possible and take him to the bathroom.

Convulsion

See SEIZURE.

Cough

Coughing is a natural protective mechanism designed to clear bacteria, viruses, dust, and pollen out of the body. Coughing clears the lungs and throat of irritants and fluids. A productive cough forces sputum from the breathing tract, thereby clearing the air passages and allowing oxygen to reach the lungs.

A cough is also a common symptom of diseases of the ear, nose, and throat. Coughing may be related to a bacterial or viral infection of the respiratory tract, such as bronchitis, laryngitis, pneumonia, or croup. A cough can also be caused by inhaling irritating substances, such as dust, chemical fumes, or cigarette smoke. Food sensitivities and environmental allergies can cause a cough, as can inhaling very cold or very hot air. If your child has a persistent cough, emotional stress is another important factor to consider.

Depending on the cause, a child's cough may be loud and gasping, harsh and high-pitched, or barking. It may be dry and rasping, or moist with mucus. If asthma is involved, your child may wheeze every time she inhales or exhales.

Although coughing is a necessary and helpful physical response, it can be distressing and very tiring to your child. Continuous, uncontrollable coughing makes sleeping difficult, and may also cause your child to feel as if she aches all over. The chest and abdominal muscles can be pulled or strained by continual coughing. Coughing may also cause further irritation to an inflamed respiratory tract.

A sudden coughing fit may signal the presence of a foreign body in your child's airway. Because young children put everything in their mouths, they have been known to get objects like coins or buttons lodged in the respiratory tract. Watch your child closely. *If other signs indicate a blocking of the airway—if your child becomes unable to speak, makes high-pitched sounds with breathing, gasps for breath, turns blue, or clutches at her throat—turn to* CHOKING *on page 158.*

In some cases, a cough may indicate the onset of a more serious or chronic illness, such as asthma, a tumor, heart disease, cystic fibrosis, or epiglottitis. Epiglottitis is a dangerous condition that mainly affects children between two and seven years of age. It can cause the windpipe to close when the child swallows. It usually comes on suddenly, and rapidly worsens over a few hours. If you suspect your child may be developing epiglottitis (*see* Signs of Epiglottitis, page 180), take her to the emergency room of the nearest hospital or call for emergency medical assistance immediately.

Signs of Epiglottitis

Epiglottitis is a bacterial infection of the epiglottis, the structure that closes off the windpipe when a person swallows to keep food and liquid from entering the lungs. Often preceded by a day or two of an upper respiratory tract infection, epiglottitis can develop very quickly and cause such severe swelling in the back of the throat that the airway can be completely cut off. Needless to say, this is a medical emergency and requires immediate intervention.

Signs that epiglottitis may be developing include:

- Sudden onset of fever, usually above 101°F;
- Lethargy;
- Difficulty in breathing;
- Drooling and refusing to eat because of very severe throat pain;
- Restlessness;
- The need to sit up and lean forward in order to breathe;
- A wheezing sound when inhaling;
- A snoring sound when exhaling;
- A muffled-sounding voice.

If you suspect that your child may be developing epiglottitis, call for emergency medical assistance or take her to the emergency room of the nearest hospital immediately.

Even an ordinary cough should never be ignored. An untreated cough can lead to pneumonia, and the constant irritation coughing causes may result in damage to the respiratory tract.

CONVENTIONAL TREATMENT

If your child's sleep is interrupted by continual coughing, your doctor may recommend a cough suppressant, because fatigue inhibits healing. There are different types of cough medicines, some available by prescription and others over the counter.

■ Codeine is a narcotic cough suppressant that may be prescribed for a cough in severe cases. It works by "turning off" the part of the brain that controls the coughing response. Codeine is a powerful drug and can have side effects, including nausea, sleepiness, and constipation. It can also be highly addictive.

■ Dextromethorphan is a common cough suppressant found in many popular over-the-counter medications, usually signified by the initials DM on the label. It is almost as effective as codeine, but is nonnarcotic and reportedly has few side effects. Follow age-specific label directions carefully when using this drug.

■ Benzonatate (Tessalon) is a prescription cough suppressant that works by anesthetizing the respiratory tract. Unlike other cough medicines, it comes in capsule rather than liquid form, and is a safer alternative to codeine. The capsules should be swallowed whole, never chewed.

■ Expectorants are medications that work by increasing the production of fluids in the respiratory tract, helping to thin and loosen mucus so that it is easier to cough out. Guaifenesin is an expectorant found in many over-the-counter cough formulas. It can cause drowsiness, so if you give your child this drug, follow label directions carefully.

■ Throat lozenges, such as Chloraseptic lozenges, coat and soothe a sore, irritated throat, and may give your child temporary relief. Many over-the-counter lozenges contain food colorings and sugar, however, which a sick child should not ingest. Read the ingredients list and label directions carefully before purchasing throat lozenges.

DIETARY GUIDELINES

■ When your child has a cough, or any other respiratory condition, eliminate potentially mucus-forming foods, especially dairy products.

■ Encourage your child to drink plenty of fluids, preferably at room temperature or warmer. Fluids help to thin mucus and make it easier for your child to cough up. Hot soups and broths are particularly good.

NUTRITIONAL SUPPLEMENTS

■ Give your child sugar-free lozenges boosted with vitamin C. Vitamin C has anti-inflammatory properties, combats infection, and is soothing and healing to an irritated throat. Give your child one lozenge an hour, as needed.

■ Give your child zinc-based lozenges to improve immune response and help reduce infection and inflammation. Choose sugar-free zinc-based lozenges. Give your child one lozenge, one to three times daily, as needed.

Note: Excessive amounts of zinc can result in nausea and vomiting. Be careful not to exceed the recommended dosage.

HERBAL TREATMENT

For age-appropriate dosages of herbal remedies, see page 81.

■ The herb coltsfoot helps to clear congestion from the lungs. Make a tea and give your child one dose, three times a day, for two days.

■ Licorice tea or tincture has antibacterial properties, soothes the throat and respiratory tract, and tastes sweet. For a cough, licorice works best when taken warm. Give your child one dose, three times daily, for two to three days. A combination of coltsfoot and licorice can also be used.

Note: Licorice should not be given to a child with high blood pressure.

■ If your child has a cough with diarrhea, lungwort is the herbal medicine of choice. Lungwort is high in vitamin C, has astringent properties, and is known for its ability to help clear a cough. Give your child one dose, two to three times daily, for two to three days.

■ Marshmallow root is soothing to the throat and respiratory tract. Make a tea and give your child one dose, three times daily, for two days.

■ Menthol lozenges contain a purified and refined form of peppermint oil, which is recognized by the Food and Drug Administration as an effective cough suppressant. Menthol lozenges made without sugar are preferable. Give your child one lozenge each hour, as needed.

■ When your child first begins to cough, give her mullein tea. This is a very effective herb known to be highly beneficial to the throat and lungs. It is particularly good in the early stages of a cough, before an expectorant is needed. Give your child one dose, two to three times daily, for two to three days.

■ Osha root, in tea or tincture form, is highly aromatic and helps to clear the lungs. It is especially good for a dry cough. Give your child one dose, three times a day, for three to four days.

■ A tea made from sage and thyme helps to clear mucus out of the lungs. Give your child one dose, three times daily, for two days.

■ Slippery elm bark makes a soothing lozenge or tea. Give your child one dose, three times a day, for three to four days.

■ Many Native Americans used wild cherry bark, a flavorful and effective herb, in a tea or syrup for coughs, colds, and bronchitis. Give one dose, twice a day, for three days.

Caution: Wild cherry bark can be toxic in large amounts. It should not be taken by children under four, nor by pregnant women.

■ Try using an herbal rub. Take 4 tablespoons of olive oil and add 2 drops of one or all of the following: eucalyptus, sage, rosemary, and peppermint oil. To ease your child's coughing and soothe her respiratory tract, rub this mixture onto her chest.

■ Prepare an herbal bath by putting a few drops of eucalyptus, sage, or thyme oil into a warm bath for your child. Breathing in the herbal vapors will soothe an irritated throat.

HOMEOPATHY

Choose an appropriate symptom-specific homeopathic remedy from the list below. Please note that if you are also treating your child with an aromatic herbal treatment (such as menthol lozenges, osha root tea, or an herbal rub with eucalyptus and/or peppermint), you should allow one hour between the two. Otherwise, the strong smell of the herbal treatment may interfere with the action of the homeopathic remedy.

■ Use *Antimonium tartaricum* if your child is pale and tired and complains of a tight, burning sensation in her chest and of feeling "breathless." She has a rattling cough, due to a respiratory tract filled with thick mucus that is difficult to cough up. To loosen the congestion, give her one dose of *Antimonium tartaricum* 30x or 9c, three times daily, for twenty-four to thirty-six hours.

Note: Antimonium tartaricum should not be used in the presence of fever. If your child has a fever, select a different remedy.

■ If your child has a high fever with her cough and is sweating copiously, give her one dose of *Belladonna* 30x or 9c, three times daily, for one day.

■ If your child has a dry, painful cough and feels better resting and worse with activity, give her one dose of *Bryonia* 30x or 9c, three times daily, for two days.

■ Give a child with a dry and spasmodic cough *Drosera* 12x or 6c. This is for a child who usually feels worse at night and when lying down. Give one dose, three times daily, for two days.

■ If your child has a loose, rattling cough, has a yellow-green nasal discharge, and is tearful, give her one dose of *Pulsatilla* 30x or 9c, three times a day, for two days.

■ *Spongia* is for the child with a dry, barking cough. The *Spongia* child typically feels better sipping a hot drink. One dose of *Spongia* 12x or 6c, given three times daily, for two days, will help. If your child has this type of cough, she should also be examined for croup (*see* CROUP).

■ If none of the remedies above seems right for your child, a homeopathic combination cough remedy, available in homeopathic pharmacies and larger health food stores, may be helpful.

GENERAL RECOMMENDATIONS

■ Make a tea from osha root, slippery elm bark, coltsfoot, and/or marshmallow root, and give it to your child three to four times daily.

■ Choose and administer a suitable homeopathic remedy.

■ Give your child menthol or zinc and herbal lozenges.

■ Prepare an herbal bath or herbal chest rub for your child.

■ Avoid exposing your child to cold winds and changes in temperature, which can aggravate a cough.

■ To help moisten the respiratory tract and thin mucus, use a cool mist humidifier in your child's room. Be sure to keep this equipment scrupulously clean so that bacteria do not collect in it.

■ *See also* FEVER and/or SORE THROAT if your child's cough is accompanied by either of these symptoms.

■ Coughing is not so much an illness as a symptom of illness. Many coughs are caused by allergies, colds, and the flu (*see* ALLERGIES; COMMON COLD; INFLUENZA). Less frequently, a cough may be a sign of a more serious problem. A cough that comes on rapidly and is accompanied by wheezing, a feeling of tightness in the chest, and difficulty breathing may be caused by asthma (*see* ASTHMA). A persistent, lingering cough may be a sign of bronchitis (*see* BRONCHITIS). A child whose cough has a "barking" sound may be suffering from croup (*see* CROUP). A harsh cough that comes on after a cold and is accompanied by fever, fatigue, and difficulty breathing may be a sign of bronchiolitis or pneumonia (*see* BRONCHIOLITIS; PNEUMONIA). In very rare cases, a chronic cough may be a sign of tuberculosis (*see* TUBERCULOSIS).

PREVENTION

■ Help your child avoid respiratory irritants and allergens, including environmental pollutants and foods to which she is sensitive. Wood-burning fireplaces and stoves can also be a source of lung irritation.

■ Do not expose your child to cigarette smoke. Teach your child at an early age about the dangers of smoking.

Cradle Cap

Cradle cap is a form of seborrheic dermatitis, an inflammatory skin disease. It is common in infancy. Cradle cap usually occurs on the scalp, but it can also appear on the eyebrows, eyelids, behind and in the ears, on the sides of the nose, and in the groin area. Cradle cap can occur anytime between two and twelve weeks of age, and usually clears by the time a child reaches eight to twelve months.

Cradle cap is characterized by thick yellow, greasy scales, which are caused by overactive sebaceous (oil) glands. When the oil from these glands dries and flakes, plugging up the ducts, the glands promptly secrete even more oil in an attempt to force out the plugs and open passageways to the surface. The result is the development of even deeper, heavier plugs and more thick yellow, greasy scales with patches of dry, yellowish crust. Although this condition may look itchy, it is not.

Cradle cap can occur even if you wash your baby's head and hair during his bath every day. Although an infant's skin and skull may seem fragile, they are actually quite strong and can tolerate a thorough washing. Rubbing too gently can fail to clear the scalp of excess oil.

If your infant has cradle cap, it is important to care for the lesions. Like other skin disorders, cradle cap can set the stage for a bacterial or fungal infection.

CONVENTIONAL TREATMENT

WHEN TO CALL THE DOCTOR ABOUT CRADLE CAP

When shampooing or combing the scales from your baby's hair, always check for signs of a local infection. If you notice that the area is warm and red, or is developing an infected-looking discharge, consult your pediatrician.

■ For severe cases of cradle cap, an antiseborrheic shampoo such as Sebulex, Ionil, or tar shampoo may be recommended.

■ If your infant's condition persists or becomes itchy and flaky, your doctor may recommend a steroid cream or ointment such as triamcinolone or hydrocortisone.

■ If a bacterial infection develops, your child's physician may prescribe an antibiotic, such as erythromycin. Signs of a bacterial infection include drainage, open lesions, or honey-colored crusts.

■ If a fungal (yeast) infection develops, an antifungal cream such as miconazole (Monistat) or clotrimazole (Lotrimin or Mycelex) may be prescribed.

DIETARY GUIDELINES

■ If you are nursing your child, avoid eating refined sugar. Both bacteria and yeast thrive on sugar.

■ A nursing mother should avoid saturated animal fats. Eat fish, such as salmon, for essential fatty acids, and include an evening primrose or borage oil supplement in your daily vitamin regimen for a couple of weeks. Follow dosage directions on the product label.

NUTRITIONAL SUPPLEMENTS

■ When fighting cradle cap, *Lactobacillus acidophilus* or *bifidus* is an important supplement. Both of these supplements foster healthy flora ("friendly bacteria") in the bowel and help prevent fungal infections. A breastfeeding mother should take one dose, twice daily, as directed on the product label. For a bottlefed baby, put half a capsule, or 1/8 teaspoon, of the supplement in your child's bottle, once a day.

■ For resistant cases, apply a vitamin-B_6 salve or cream to your infant's scalp, twice daily, for two to three days.

■ To rule out nutritional deficiencies that might be contributing to the problem, give your child a multiple vitamin and mineral complex formulated for infants.

HERBAL TREATMENT

■ If the skin on your baby's head is very dry, massage his scalp with calendula lotion and vitamin E oil, alternately. Almond oil can also be used. Allow the oil to remain on your infant's scalp for fifteen minutes. Then shampoo, and gently comb away the loosened scales with a fine-toothed comb. Both calendula and vitamin E are helpful for skin irritations and will moisten and help heal the lesions.

HOMEOPATHY

Like most homeopathic preparations, remedies for cradle cap are symptom-specific. Choose the remedy that most closely matches your child's symptoms.

■ *Sulphur* is a general remedy for skin conditions. Use *Sulphur* for the child who doesn't like wearing clothes and usually kicks off the bedclothes. Give one dose of *Sulphur* 30x or 9c, twice a day, for two to three days.

■ *Thuja* is for the child who is cooler and calmer and likes being snuggled. If *Sulphur* doesn't clear your infant's cradle cap, try one dose of *Thuja* 30x or 9c, twice daily, for two days.

■ If neither *Sulphur* nor *Thuja* seems right for your baby, a homeopathic combination remedy for cradle cap may be helpful.

GENERAL RECOMMENDATIONS

■ If your infant has cradle cap, do not pick at the lesions to remove scales. This can cause an infection.

■ Rub calendula lotion, vitamin-E oil, aloe vera liquid, or almond oil into your baby's scalp. Then shampoo and gently comb away the loosened scales with a fine-toothed comb.

■ Give your child homeopathic *Sulphur* or *Thuja*.

■ A nursing mother should take a lactobacillus supplement, as well as primrose or borage oil. A bottlefed baby should be given *Lactobacillus bifidus* with his formula.

■ Massage evening primrose oil lotion into your baby's scalp nightly.

PREVENTION

■ There is no sure way to prevent cradle cap, but keeping your baby's scalp clean and dry is helpful.

■ To prevent an accumulation of dead skin cells, gently but thoroughly brush or comb your baby's hair every day.

■ When shampooing your infant's hair, gently but thoroughly wash his scalp to clear away any excess oil that might otherwise accumulate.

Croup

Croup is an infection of the upper respiratory tract that results in the swelling and inflammation of the area below the vocal cords. Before the onset of croup, your child may have had an upper respiratory tract infection, such as a cold, sinus infection, or sore throat. Croup is almost always caused by a virus, which may also affect membranes above and below the larynx (the "voice box"). It is most common in children from about three months to three years of age. As with many viral infections, it occurs most frequently in late fall and winter.

Croup is distinguished by a brassy, barking cough, difficulty breathing, and a harsh, low-pitched wheezing sound with each intake of breath. These symptoms are caused by the inflammation and swelling of the vocal cords. The infection may also increase mucus production, which can block the airway. While not usually life threatening, croup is one of the nastiest and scariest of the childhood illnesses.

The symptoms of croup may be mild or severe. Breathing may become difficult or more rapid. The muscles between the ribs may pull in as your child inhales, and it may appear as if your child has to work hard just to take a breath. Because an upright position eases breathing, your child will probably prefer to sit up in bed or be held upright. Your child may also have a fever and congestion.

Children typically awaken in the middle of the night with croup. An attack can last for several hours, subside, and recur over the next few nights. Although croup does not usually last beyond three days, it is possible for it to become chronic.

There are several other conditions that can mimic this disease. For example, a child who is choking may also have a crouplike cough. However, a child with croup will be able to talk in between bouts of coughing, whereas a child who is choking because of an obstruction in the airway may make frantic, high-pitched sounds, but will not be able to talk normally (*see* CHOKING). The symptoms of viral croup are also similar to those of acute epiglottitis, a rapidly progressing bacterial infection (*see* Signs of Epiglottitis, page 180).

CONVENTIONAL TREATMENT

■ Keep your child quiet and calm, and don't panic. If you do, your child will very quickly pick up on your feelings. Anxiety makes breathing more difficult.

■ If your child has a severe case of croup, your doctor may give her racemic epinephrine (Vaponefrin) or albuterol (Proventil, Ventolin) as an inhalation treatment to help open her airways and ease breathing quickly. A child who receives inhalation treatment may be hospitalized for forty-eight hours so that she can be watched for any reaction to the medication or a "rebound" effect after she stops receiving the drug.

■ To quickly decrease inflammation and swelling of the air passages, a steroid, such as dexamethasone (Decadron) or methylprednisolone (Solu-Medrol) may be administered intravenously.

■ Unless your child develops a bacterial infection in addition to the viral infection causing her croup, antibiotics are *not* indicated. They are not effective against a viral illness.

WHEN TO CALL THE DOCTOR ABOUT CROUP

● If your child has to work very hard to take in enough air and is having serious trouble breathing, call your physician or take your child to the emergency room.

● The symptoms of croup are very like those of acute epiglottitis, a bacterial infection that comes on very quickly, with a sudden high fever (*see* Signs of Epiglottitis, page 180). Acute epiglottitis can cause an obstruction of the airway and respiratory failure. If you have any suspicion that your child may be developing epiglottitis, seek emergency medical assistance for your child.

● If your child has a croupy cough and wheezing, and you have any doubts about her condition, call your health care provider and describe the symptoms.

DIETARY GUIDELINES

■ Encourage a croupy child to take liquids. This helps to thin secretions, making it easier for her to cough up mucus.

■ Unless your child feels better sipping something cold, encourage her to drink warm teas and soups, to soothe and relax the throat and ease coughing spasms.

■ Avoid dairy products, which can thicken and increase mucus.

■ If your child's coughing fits are severe enough to cause vomiting, it may be best to stay with a liquid diet.

HERBAL TREATMENT

■ Prepare a tea of equal parts of marshmallow root, mullein, osha root, and licorice, and give your child one dose of tea, twice daily, for as long as symptoms are present. Marshmallow root lessens inflammation and coats and soothes an irritated throat; mullein helps promote expectoration and soothes the respiratory tract; osha helps to clear the lungs; and licorice has antiviral and anti-inflammatory properties and sweetens the tea.

Note: Licorice should not be given to a child with high blood pressure.

HOMEOPATHY

Select one of the symptom-specific remedies listed below and give your child one dose, every four hours, for a total of three doses. Then give the remedy three times daily for two days.

■ *Kali muriaticum* 12x or 6c is a principal homeopathic remedy for croup and is the best place to start. Give your child *Kali muriaticum* for the first forty-eight hours, or until another remedy more clearly matches your child's symptoms.

■ If your child wakes with a barking cough between 11:00 P.M. and midnight, is irritable, and is coughing up phlegm, give her *Coccus cacti* 30x or 9c.

■ A child with a spasmodic cough, who cries from fear of the intense spasm coughing brings on, will benefit from *Cuprum metallicum* 30x or 9c.

■ For the child who complains of a tickling sensation in her throat, wheezes when she inhales, and awakens around 2:00 A.M. with a dry, frequent, spasmodic cough, try *Drosera* 12x or 6c.

■ For a croupy child with a fever, give *Ferrum phosphoricum* 12x or 6c in combination with any other symptom-specific remedy.

■ If your child has a spasmodic cough accompanied by nausea and vomiting, give her *Ipecac* 30x or 9c.

Caution: Do not confuse homeopathic Ipecac with conventional syrup of ipecac. That is an entirely different product, and it should be used only at the direction of a doctor or Poison Control Center.

■ Give *Spongia* 12x to a child with a dry, rattling cough and loud breathing. This child feels worse toward evening, when inhaling, and when lying down.

BACH FLOWER REMEDIES

■ Give a child with croup Rescue Remedy to help ease her fear and anxiety. Put

187

a few drops in a bottle or glass of water and have your child sip it throughout the day. (See BACH FLOWER REMEDIES in Part One.)

ACUPRESSURE

For the locations of acupressure points on a child's body, *see* ADMINISTERING AN ACUPRESSURE TREATMENT in Part Three.

■ Four Gates helps to relax an anxious child.

■ Pericardium 6 relaxes a stressed chest.

■ Massage your child's upper back along the spine.

GENERAL RECOMMENDATIONS

■ The anxiety and fear a child experiences during a bout of croup often makes breathing even more difficult. Stay calm and quiet. Hold your child and speak reassuringly to her. Your love and emotional support are very important.

■ Select and administer a suitable homeopathic remedy.

■ Use a cool mist humidifier in your child's room.

■ Cold wet air often relieves croup. If it is a cool night, bundle up your child well and take her for a short drive with the car windows open. Cool wet air decreases inflammation and swelling, opening the respiratory tract so that air moves in and out more easily.

■ Warm wet air is second best for relieving croup. Let the steam from a hot shower fill your bathroom. Sit in the room with your child and encourage her to breathe slowly and deeply.

■ A *small* amount (no more than ¼ teaspoon) of syrup of ipecac can sometimes break the coughing cycle. However, you should not give your child syrup of ipecac unless directed to do so by a doctor.

PREVENTION

■ Keep a healthy child away from one who has croup. This is a highly infectious viral condition.

■ If your child is prone to croup, use a cool mist humidifier in her bedroom whenever she has a respiratory tract infection. The mist will moisten and soothe irritated airways and can help prevent further infection or spasm.

Cuts and Scrapes

Cuts, scrapes, and skinned knees and elbows are an inevitable part of childhood. Because any break in the skin can become infected, even minor injuries should be treated fairly aggressively. A child's skin is thin and delicate. Also, whereas an adult body has had decades to develop infection-fighting antibodies, your child has not yet developed a full storehouse of the antibodies that fight skin bacteria.

Cuts and scrapes on the head, face, hands, mouth, and feet can bleed profusely, because there are many blood vessels close to the surface of the skin in these areas. To avoid scarring, you'll want to treat a cut on your child's face especially carefully. Cuts on the face, fingers, and hands are particularly vulnerable to infection, because they are not covered with clothing. Cuts involving the lips should be inspected by a doctor. Stitches may be required to ensure that your child's mouth heals normally.

You can treat minor cuts and scrapes at home with basic first aid. However, occasions may arise when medical care is essential. If you have any doubt about your ability to care for a child's injury properly, consult your doctor.

CONVENTIONAL TREATMENT

■ The first step in treating any wound is to cleanse and disinfect the site. For a minor cut or scrape, you can do this at home. If the injury is more serious, your child's physician can do it. If a wound is severe or dirty, your doctor may administer a tetanus shot, especially if it has been more than five years since your child last had one.

■ Depending on the extent of the wound, your child's doctor may close a cut with stitches or a butterfly adhesive bandage. If you are treating a minor cut at home, cover it with an adhesive bandage. A wound that is covered is less likely to become infected.

■ To prevent infection, over-the-counter antibiotic ointments such as Neosporin, Betadine, or bacitracin are often recommended.

DIETARY GUIDELINES

■ Your child's diet should not contain refined sugars. Sugar makes the body more acidic, which slows healing. When your child's body is working to repair itself, avoiding sugar helps create a more balanced, alkaline internal environment.

NUTRITIONAL SUPPLEMENTS

For age-appropriate dosages of nutritional supplements, see page 81.

■ If your child has a tendency to develop infections, give him the following supplements for five days to one week following an injury that breaks the skin. These supplements help to heal skin tissue and support the immune system.

- One dose of beta-carotene, twice a day.
- One dose of mineral ascorbate vitamin C with an equal amount of bioflavonoids, two to three times daily.
- A double dose of vitamin E, daily.
- One dose of zinc, once or twice a day.
  Note: Excessive amounts of zinc can result in nausea and vomiting. Be careful not to exceed the recommended dosage.

HERBAL TREATMENT

For age-appropriate dosages of herbal remedies, see page 81.

■ After cleansing the wound, apply an herbal or homeopathic calendula gel or

EMERGENCY TREATMENT FOR CUTS AND SCRAPES

✚ If your child's wound is caused by a dirty or rusty object, or if there is foreign material embedded in the wound, take your child to the doctor promptly. A serious infection could result. Also, your child may require a tetanus shot.

✚ If bleeding does not stop within ten to fifteen minutes, if the edges of the skin are separated and the wound is open, or if the wound is deep or extensive, see your doctor. Your child may require stitches, which can help prevent infection, hasten healing, and make any scar that results smaller and less noticeable.

ointment topically. Calendula has antibacterial properties and helps to speed healing. It is exceptionally soothing to skin tissue.

■ Aloe vera gel has skin-soothing and calming properties.

■ Apply sage ointment to the wound for its antiseptic properties.

■ If none of the above is available, raw honey may be applied to the wound. It has natural antibiotic properties and is very effective.

■ An echinacea and goldenseal herbal combination remedy should be given internally if the wound becomes infected. It has natural antiviral and antibiotic properties, and can be taken along with any prescribed antibiotics. Give your child one dose, twice daily, for five days.

■ Goldenseal powder applied topically will work overnight to prevent infection and encourage scabbing. Break open a capsule and add just enough water to make a paste.

HOMEOPATHY

■ Homeopathic *Hypericum* ointment helps to relieve pain following injury to the fingers or toes. Apply twice a day for three days.

BACH FLOWER REMEDIES

■ Following any injury or crisis, give your child Bach Flower Rescue Remedy to calm and stabilize anxiety, shock, or fright. (See BACH FLOWER REMEDIES in Part One.)

GENERAL RECOMMENDATIONS

■ To stop bleeding, apply firm pressure to the wound with a piece of sterile gauze or a clean cloth. Putting ice on the cut will also stop bleeding, because cold constricts blood vessels and slows blood flow. If your child's mouth or tongue is cut, try using a fruit-juice popsicle.

■ Cleansing is the cornerstone of treatment for any break in the skin. Wash your child's wound with generous amounts of water. Thoroughly clean out any particles of dirt or foreign matter that may have gotten into the cut by holding the wound under running water. Be sure the wound is cleaned well immediately after the injury, and keep the area scrupulously clean while it is still open and healing.

■ If your child's cut is deeper than a scratch, cover it with gauze or an adhesive bandage. A superficial scratch can be left open to the air.

■ Keep the wound dry for at least two days, but cover it with the ointment of your choice to speed healing. In addition to the products listed above, Aquaphor and Super Salve ointments are very good.

■ Give your child Bach Flower Rescue Remedy after any injury or crisis. Many parents are very thankful for this remarkable calming and stabilizing herbal preparation.

■ Raw, unprocessed honey is a natural antiseptic that can be applied directly to a wound. It is especially helpful when no other treatments are readily available.

■ In a pinch, plain yogurt can be applied to a cut or scrape. It is soothing, prevents infection, and helps to speed healing.

PREVENTION

■ Not all cuts and scrapes can be prevented, but you can reduce the possibility that your child will receive more than his share. *See* HOME SAFETY in Part One.

■ Always make sure your child is buckled up in his seat belt or car safety seat when riding in a car. This will prevent your child from being thrown onto the floor or against the dashboard or front seat during a sudden, unavoidable stop.

Cystitis

See URINARY TRACT INFECTION.

Dental Problems

See TEETHING; THRUSH; THUMB-SUCKING; TOOTH DECAY; TOOTH, BROKEN OR KNOCKED OUT.

Diabetes Mellitus

Diabetes is a chronic condition characterized by a deficiency in the production of insulin, a hormone produced by the pancreas. Insulin plays an essential role in carbohydrate metabolism. As food goes through the digestive system, it breaks down further and further into its basic components. Glucose, a simple sugar, is one of the final breakdown products of carbohydrates. Every cell in the body needs and uses glucose as its fuel; glucose gives our cells the energy to perform their tasks. Insulin functions as the "key" that opens the door of the cells to let the glucose in. Without insulin, glucose cannot get into the cells, and without glucose, the cells do not have the energy they need to function properly.

There are two types of diabetes mellitus, Type I and Type II. Type I diabetes is usually diagnosed in childhood and involves such a severe depletion of insulin that it must be taken by injection every day. Type II diabetes is usually diagnosed in adulthood, and most often can be managed with diet and oral medication rather than insulin injections. This entry addresses Type I diabetes, also known as insulin-dependent diabetes mellitus or juvenile-onset diabetes.

Type I diabetes is thought to be an autoimmune disorder. That is, the immune system turns on the body's own tissues and attacks the specific cells of the pancreas that manufacture insulin. Why this happens is not entirely understood, although there seems to be a genetic predisposition to the disease, as well as some relationship between viral infection and the onset of diabetes.

SYMPTOMS OF DIABETES

The first signs that a child has diabetes usually develop over a period of one to three weeks. They include the following:

- A notable increase in thirst, to the point that it may seem your child's thirst simply cannot be satisfied.

- A significant increase in the frequency and amount of urination.

- Frequent and copious bedwetting, especially in a child who did not previously wet the bed.

- Increased appetite, often, paradoxically, in combination with weight loss.

- Unusual irritability or fatigue.

If your child consistently displays one or more of these symptoms, take her to your doctor for a professional evaluation.

Symptoms of diabetes include increased frequency of urination, increased and often extreme thirst, increased appetite, weight loss, irritability, and fatigue. Excessive bedwetting is a classic sign of diabetes. These symptoms usually appear over a period of about three weeks.

Short-term complications of diabetes include episodes of both very low and very high blood sugar. When blood sugar is abnormally low, a child may feel dizzy, lethargic, and irritable, may be pale and sweaty, and may have a headache and a loss of coordination. Such a mild hypoglycemic episode is treated by giving the child quick-acting sugar (such as in the form of orange juice, raisins, or honey). A more severe episode may require hospitalization and an intravenous infusion of glucose. A high blood sugar episode can lead to a condition known as diabetic ketoacidosis, which, if untreated, can cause loss of consciousness, coma, and death. Diabetic ketoacidosis is treated in the hospital with intravenous insulin, fluid, glucose, and electrolytes.

Diabetes can also lead to serious long-term complications. These include changes in vision, kidney disease, cardiovascular disease, and nerve problems. Careful treatment of diabetes, conscientious compliance with treatment, and regular doctor appointments can help to prevent complications from developing. It is important that a person with diabetes get regular eye examinations as well as special periodic blood and urine tests to screen for cholesterol and kidney changes.

Treatment of juvenile diabetes is based on insulin injections, appropriate diet, and adequate exercise. The goal is to maintain a normal blood glucose level so that the body will have enough energy to function properly.

With the help of your doctor, nurse, and nutritionist, you and your child will learn how to balance insulin injections, dietary carbohydrates, and exercise in order to achieve normal blood glucose levels. Diabetes is a lifelong challenge that must be carefully taken care of in order to avoid long-term complications. Because of the complexity and intricacies of treatment, if your child is diagnosed as having diabetes it is best to work with a physician and nurse who specialize in the treatment of this illness. A regional children's hospital or a diabetes center is a good place to start looking for information and references. In addition to conventional medical treatment and dietary modification, herbs, homeopathy, acupressure, and nutritional supplements can be used to support your child's endocrine system. Because your child and her response to this disease and treatment are unique, it is best to work closely with qualified professionals. We advise that you choose a medical doctor who is willing to work with a natural health care practitioner (and vice versa). Each of these professionals needs to know what the other is doing, as the interventions of one can affect the treatments of the other.

CONVENTIONAL TREATMENT

Conventional treatment for diabetes involves three key components: insulin, diet, and exercise. These work together to help regulate a diabetic's blood glucose levels.

■ Because her body is not producing adequate amounts of insulin, your child will need to be given injections to get this essential hormone. Your child's age will be a key factor in determining whether she can give herself the injections or whether you should give them. This is an important skill that must be taught by a clinic or hospital nurse. Within a few weeks or months of beginning insulin treatment, a child's insulin needs may decrease significantly. Some children may not need insulin at all at this point. You should be aware that while this "honeymoon period" can last for up to two years, eventually your child will need to go back to taking insulin.

■ Attention to diet is important. Too many carbohydrates can increase blood sugar; too few will lower it. Children with diabetes have the same nutritional and caloric requirements as other children do, but they need a diet that is carefully designed to give them the correct balance of carbohydrates, protein, and fats. Simply cutting out sugar is *not* enough. A successful diet plan includes all types of foods. Once a child takes a shot of insulin, she needs to eat appropriately so that her blood sugar doesn't get *too* low and cause a hypoglycemic (low blood sugar) reaction (characterized by paleness, shakiness, irritability, and loss of coordination). A child with diabetes needs to eat at the same times each day. She needs to eat a snack at midmorning and midafternoon, and she needs to eat the same amount of calories from one day to the next.

Most meal plans begin by estimating the amount of calories an individual child needs to grow and maintain a realistic weight. Then 55 to 65 percent of the total daily calories are allocated for complex carbohydrates (grains, vegetables, legumes), 20 to 30 percent for protein foods, and 15 to 25 percent for fatty foods. A diet high in fiber, especially soluble fibers, is beneficial. Encourage your child to eat plenty of fresh vegetables, whole-grain cereals, brown rice, barley, millet, and oats. Oat bran seems to be particularly helpful for maintaining a steady blood sugar level. Finally, to prevent the early onset of heart disease, it is important for a child with diabetes to limit her intake of fat. Don't fry foods; use low-fat or skim-milk dairy products; purchase canned foods packed in water rather than in oil; remove the skin from turkey, chicken, and fish; and limit or eliminate red meat. Replace sugary snacks with fresh fruits.

■ Exercise is important because it helps to lower blood glucose levels, strengthen the body, and improve glucose and insulin management. It may be recommended that your child eat a snack before exercise so that her blood sugar level is maintained throughout the activity.

■ There are many intricacies in dealing with diabetes. Making sure your child takes her injection in a different spot each day, learning about different types of insulin, and blood and urine tests are some of the many areas you will explore as you and your child learn to live with diabetes.

NUTRITIONAL SUPPLEMENTS

For age-appropriate dosages of some nutritional supplements, see page 81.

■ Chromium picolinate, or glucose tolerance factor, helps to stabilize blood sugar. Give a child who is thirteen or older 100 micrograms, once daily.

■ In general, a good multiple vitamin and mineral supplement is useful for people with diabetes. Choose a formula that provides at least the recommended daily allowance (RDA) of the included vitamins and minerals, and follow dosage directions on the product label.

■ Bioflavonoids may be useful for preventing damage to the nerves caused by excessively elevated blood sugar. Give your child one dose daily.

HERBAL TREATMENT

■ Siberian ginseng (also called *eleutherococcus*) may help to stabilize your child's blood sugar. Begin with a low dosage. Try using Siberian ginseng, every other week, for three to four months. Stop for two months, then resume.

■ Evening primrose oil, or its active component, GLA, has been shown to help prevent nerve damage due to fluctuations in blood sugar. Give a child over twelve years of age one capsule a day.

Note: Evening primrose oil should not be given to a child who has a fever.

GENERAL RECOMMENDATIONS

■ Monitor your child's insulin level carefully. It is possible that her insulin requirements may change over time.

■ Appropriate support for parents, siblings, and the child with diabetes is an essential part of successful treatment and a long and happy life. Dealing with a chronic illness is not easy, and it affects many aspects of a family's life. The American Diabetes Association (telephone 800–232–3472 or 703–549–1500) has chapters throughout the country and can help you find needed support for everyone in your family.

■ The Joslin Diabetes Center in Massachusetts sponsors a summer camp for children with diabetes. A week or two at a camp with other children and counselors who have diabetes can offer invaluable teaching, support, and fun. The address of the Joslin Center is One Joslin Place, Boston, Massachusetts 02215 (telephone 617–732–2400).

PREVENTION

■ There is no known way to prevent juvenile-onset diabetes. Your only defense against the disease is to be aware of the characteristic signs and symptoms so that, should it become necessary, your child can begin treatment promptly.

Diaper Rash

Diaper rash is an inflammation of the skin that is caused by a reaction to the strong chemicals and enzymes in feces and urine, plus the buildup of heat those substances generate. The diaper traps and holds this noxious mixture against your baby's bottom.

If your baby has a contact diaper rash—diaper rash caused by a reaction to feces, urine, soaps, disposable diapers, plastic pants, and/or diarrhea—the area will be sore and tender. The skin will be red and irritated. There may be swollen areas and superficial ulcerations. The skin may be dry and scaling, with discolored patches. If your child has a fungal diaper rash—caused by the presence of *Candida albicans* in the intestinal tract—the skin will be smooth, shiny, and bright red. The borders of the lesions and rash will be well defined, and there may be scattered spots in the inguinal (groin) area. Ask your doctor or nurse to diagnose the rash so that you can treat the problem correctly.

Diaper rash is common. Although it can occur at any time as long as your child is in diapers, the most common age for diaper rash is around nine months. Certain factors increase the risk of diaper rash. Antibiotics, dehydration, and diarrhea, for example, make skin more vulnerable to diaper rash. The use of disposable diapers, in addition to contributing to the problem of clogged landfills, has also increased the incidence of diaper rash. Children wearing disposable diapers are much more likely to suffer from diaper rash than those in laundered cotton diapers are.

CONVENTIONAL TREATMENT

With careful skin care, diaper rash should improve in two to three days, and resolve completely in several more days.

■ Apply zinc oxide ointment to the affected area at each diaper change to help dry the area and resolve the rash. Because it forms a barrier between baby's skin and the acid chemicals in urine and stool, the ointment works as a protective blanket. It has a drying effect, however, so it should not be used if your child's skin is dry and cracked.

■ If your child's diaper rash is caused by a yeast infection (*Candida albicans*), a topical antifungal medication such as nystatin, miconazole (Monistat), or clotrimazole (Lotrimin, Mycelex) may be used.

■ For chronic yeast infection, an oral antifungal, usually nystatin, may be prescribed to decrease the amount of yeast in the digestive tract.

■ If the rash is especially red, inflamed, and oozing, Burow's solution (aluminum acetate) will help. Both astringent and antiseptic, this solution is mild, but it may be diluted further if it seems irritating to your baby's skin.

■ In a particularly persistent and nasty case of diaper rash, a topical corticosteroid such as hydrocortisone (found in Vioform HC, Westcort, and others), triamcinolone (Aristocort, Kenalog), or Lotrisone may be necessary to promote healing and reduce inflammation. However, corticosteroids should never be used for longer than two to three weeks, as they can cause atrophy (thinning) of the skin.

DIETARY GUIDELINES

■ Make sure your baby is getting plenty of water. This helps dilute the irritating acids present in urine and stool.

■ A nursing mother should eliminate possible allergenic foods from her diet (*see* ELIMINATION DIET in Part Three). Potential culprits include citrus fruits and juices, dairy products, excessive amounts of yeasted breads, sugar, and caffeine. Drink plenty of spring water to dilute any offending substances that may be passing through your breast milk to your baby.

■ Diaper rash may be related to the introduction of new foods, particularly foods that cause the stool to become more acidic and irritating to your baby's skin. Some experts believe a new food that causes a reaction should be permanently eliminated from the diet. Others maintain that a new food is difficult to digest only because the body is unfamiliar with it, and once your child's body has adjusted to it, the reaction will no longer occur. A helpful rule of thumb that combines both of these perspectives is to observe your child carefully. If a rash develops every time a particular food is given, eliminate that food for the time being. You can reintroduce the food to your child when he is a little older.

■ If you believe your child's diaper rash may be related to a food allergy, you

WHEN TO CALL THE DOCTOR ABOUT DIAPER RASH

As with any skin irritation, it is possible for diaper rash to become infected. When changing your baby, watch for signs of increased redness, swelling, tenderness, and discharge. If you notice any of these symptoms, or if your child develops a fever, shows irritability, or loses his appetite, call your doctor. These can all be signs of an infection that may have to be treated with an antibiotic.

195

may wish to try an elimination diet. However, it takes time to discover food allergies this way. In the case of diaper rash, use topical and preventive measures first.

NUTRITIONAL SUPPLEMENTS

■ Lactobacillus supplements are important for an infant or nursing mother with candida. This common yeast infection yields to either *Lactobacillus acidophilus* or *bifidus*. A nursing mother can take a regular adult dose of the supplement, as directed on the product label. A bottlefed infant can be given ⅛ to ¼ teaspoon daily in formula for two to three weeks, or even longer in chronic cases.

■ If the rash is extremely dry, open a capsule of vitamin-E oil and rub it into the skin at each diaper change.

HERBAL TREATMENT

■ Warm water increases circulation and promotes healing. A full tub bath or sitz bath (in the sink) will help make your child more comfortable. To further soothe the skin, add calendula or chamomile to the water.

■ If the rash is red and irritated, apply calendula lotion, gel, or cream at each diaper change. Both are soothing and promote healing.

■ Apply evening primrose oil or lotion, a natural anti-inflammatory, at each diaper change until the rash clears.

■ If the rash is moist, lightly sprinkle kaolin clay or cornstarch onto the affected area.

HOMEOPATHY

■ If your baby's diaper rash is very red, irritated, and sore, give him one dose of *Sulphur* 30x or 9c, twice daily, until the redness begins to fade. Do not give this remedy for more than three days, however.

■ For a persistent diaper rash, one dose of *Thuja* 30x or 9c, given twice daily for two days, will be helpful.

■ If neither of the above remedies seems right for your child, a homeopathic combination diaper rash remedy may be useful.

GENERAL RECOMMENDATIONS

■ Air and sunlight are helpful in both preventing and healing a diaper rash. Let your child go without a diaper as much as possible. A child whose bottom is exposed to the air will heal more quickly and will have fewer diaper rashes than a child who is kept closely covered most of the time. In tropical cultures where few clothes are worn by children, diaper rash is almost nonexistent.

■ When a diaper is necessary, a loosely pinned cloth diaper will permit some airing, and will offer gentle protection against accidents.

■ Use nonirritating cloth diapers rather than disposables. Change your baby as soon as he voids or has a bowel movement.

■ Avoid using commercial diaper wipes. Many contain strong chemicals that can be irritating. Use diaper wipes moistened primarily with witch hazel (aqua hamamelis) or calendula, both of which are safe and gentle on an infant's delicate skin.

■ Gently clean your baby's skin with each diaper change, using a mild soap and gentle friction. Be sure to clean well between skin folds, rinse well, and pat dry. Avoid harsh detergents and vigorous scrubbing, which aggravate diaper rash.

■ After cleansing, sponge your baby's diaper area with a mixture of 1 tablespoon of baking soda dissolved in 4 ounces of spring water. The alkalinity of baking soda balances the acidity of urine and stool. Make a new batch of this mixture every two days, and keep it on the changing table.

■ If your baby's bottom is red and irritated, apply calendula lotion or ointment, then dust with kaolin clay or cornstarch.

■ If the rash is very, very dry, apply vitamin-E oil or evening primrose lotion.

■ Give your baby homeopathic *Thuja* or *Sulphur*.

■ Give your baby a *Lactobacillus acidophilus* or *Lactobacillus bifidus* supplement.

PREVENTION

■ Expose your baby's bottom to fresh air and sunlight whenever possible.

■ Use nonirritating, breathable cloth diapers, and pin them loosely to allow as much air as possible to reach the skin. Change your baby at least eight times every day.

■ Use a mild soap when washing cloth diapers, and rinse the soap out very thoroughly. If you've been using disposables because of the problem of laundering all those diapers, consider hiring a diaper service. Diaper services are making a comeback and are well worth the cost. In fact, it can cost less to use a diaper service than to buy disposables.

■ Prepare a baking-soda rinse and use it on your child's diaper area.

■ At each diaper change, rub calendula or vitamin-E lotion or cream into your baby's skin.

Diarrhea

Diarrhea, or frequent and watery stools, is the body's way of ridding itself of toxins and foreign substances. Most cases of simple diarrhea should not be suppressed too quickly. It may be healthier to allow your child's body to flush itself clean, while supporting her with adequate fluids.

There are many microorganisms that can cause diarrhea, including viruses, bacteria, fungi, and protozoa. Your child can pick up viruses, bacteria, or protozoa from other children, or from contaminated food and water. Food poisoning causes diarrhea very quickly. A milk allergy or food sensitivity, which may surface with the introduction of new foods, can also cause diarrhea.

Less common causes of diarrhea include reactions to medication, inflammatory bowel disease, hepatitis, cystic fibrosis, and pancreatitis. An anatomical deformity, such as a fistula, or a congenital defect, such as Hirschsprung's disease or short bowel syndrome, can also cause diarrhea. If your child's diarrhea arises from any of these conditions, she requires medical attention.

Most cases of simple diarrhea are caused by viruses. Viruses invade a child's intestinal tract, causing irritation and inflammation of the intestinal walls. Viruses also induce the cells lining the intestines to secrete fluids. The increase in fluid volume in turn increases peristalsis, the wavelike contractions of the intestines. The result is cramping and the loose, watery, frequent stools characteristic of diarrhea.

Vomiting and stomachache often accompany diarrhea, and abdominal cramps usually come and go, often occurring right before a bowel movement. Depending on the cause of the diarrhea, a fever may or may not be present. When a child is suffering from diarrhea, dehydration is always a serious concern, especially if her temperature is elevated. In the first two or three months of life, an infant can become dehydrated very quickly, so if your newborn develops diarrhea, call your physician.

Observe your child between episodes of diarrhea to get a sense of how sick she is. If your child is alert and not experiencing cramping between episodes, it's safe to assume her body has the situation under control. But if your child seems weak and the cramping is not relieved between episodes, call your health care provider.

WHEN TO CALL THE DOCTOR ABOUT DIARRHEA

- In newborns, diarrhea is signaled by an increase in stools, stools that are unusually loose or watery, stools that are yellowish or greenish in color, or stools with a foul odor. You should always consult a doctor about a newborn's diarrhea.

- If your child experiences severe or persistent abdominal pain with diarrhea, or has blood in the stool, call your doctor right away.

- If your child has a case of diarrhea that lasts for longer than forty-eight hours, or intermittent diarrhea that comes and goes over a period of two weeks or longer, seek the advice of your health care practitioner.

- Vomiting that accompanies gastrointestinal upsets should not last for more than twenty-four hours. Call your doctor if your child has been experiencing diarrhea with vomiting for longer than that.

CONVENTIONAL TREATMENT

■ To prevent dehydration, oral electrolyte formulas, such as Pedialyte, Lytren, Ricelyte, and Resol, are commonly recommended for children with diarrhea.

■ Loperamide (sold as Imodium AD tablets and liquid) is the most commonly used antidiarrheal, now that it is available over the counter. It acts by slowing the movement of the intestinal muscle.

Note: You should never give your child loperamide if she has a fever over 101°F or bloody stools. This drug is not recommended for children under twelve.

■ Kaolin-pectin, an over-the-counter drug better known as Kaopectate, binds substances in the intestines with excess water, thereby solidifying and drying diarrheal stools. This makes it appear as if your child is having less diarrhea and more formed stools, but she is actually still losing the same amount of water as she would be if untreated. It just looks different. Kaolin medications give a false sense of reassurance.

■ Bismuth subsalicylate (Pepto-Bismol) is an over-the-counter drug that works by attaching to the toxin or bacteria that is causing the problem in the intestines. This deactivates the foreign substance and it loses its ability to hurt the body. This medication can turn the stools black. It is not recommended for children under two years of age.

■ Antibiotics can help, but only if your child's diarrhea is due to a parasitic or bacterial infection. They should be prescribed only after a stool analysis or culture confirms this.

■ Antidiarrheal medications that contain opiates, such as paregoric and Lomotil, are not recommended for children. Like loperamide, these drugs work by slowing down intestinal action and halting bowel movements. But these are powerful drugs that contain narcotics, and are not necessarily safe.

DIETARY GUIDELINES

■ Your primary concern when caring for a child with diarrhea is to prevent dehydration. During the acute phase of diarrhea, when the stools are frequent and watery, make sure your child is taking in enough fluids. Give your child frequent small sips or drinks of water. To prevent vomiting, don't give her a big glass of water at any one time.

■ To give the intestines time to settle and heal, avoid giving your child dairy products during an episode of diarrhea and for two weeks after it is resolved.

■ If you are breastfeeding your child, continue nursing. Mother's milk does not create or exacerbate diarrhea. In fact, a diet comprised solely of breast milk and water can often help to resolve it. A nursing mother can also try adding an acidophilus or bifidus supplement to her diet, or taking one dose of Curing Pills (*see* Herbal Treatment, below) or homeopathic *Arsenicum album* 200x.

■ Children usually do not want to eat very much when they are acutely sick with diarrhea. Offer clear liquids, such as broths, diluted apple juice, and herbal teas. Avoid filling your child's stomach, so that her stomach and intestines will have time to rest and heal. An upset digestive tract is like any other injury. Do not expect it to heal overnight.

■ As your child starts to feel better, offer a simple diet so that the digestive tract can easily process and absorb nutrients. Choose familiar foods that are easily digested and absorbed, such as puréed rice, bananas, dry cereal, crackers, toast, mashed potatoes (without butter), well-cooked vegetables, and grains.

■ Eliminate foods that are difficult to digest. Proteins should be avoided for about forty-eight hours. Fats should be eliminated from the diet during any illness. They are difficult even for a healthy body to digest, and a distressed intestinal tract makes it even harder. Undigested fats contribute to a toxic internal environment.

■ Eliminate refined sugars, especially if your child's diarrhea is bacterial in origin. Bacteria thrive in the presence of sugar. Sugar also makes the body more acidic. An overly acidic internal environment slows healing.

NUTRITIONAL SUPPLEMENTS

■ *Lactobacillus acidophilus* and *bifidus* restore healthy flora to the intestines and bowel, so they are helpful in resolving diarrhea. Give a child with diarrhea one capsule of either, twice daily, for five days.

■ Pro-Bio-Plex is a globulin concentrate made from whey. It contains antibodies similar to those found in mother's milk and helps fight off an infection. Pro-Bio-Plex is available by prescription only. Ethical Nutrients, the consumer division of the company that makes it, also sells a similar product, called Inner Strength, that is available over the counter in health food stores. For Pro-Bio-Plex, follow your doctor's prescription; for Inner Strength, follow the dosage directions on the product label and give it to your child four times daily until the diarrhea resolves.

HERBAL TREATMENT

■ Powdered slippery elm bark is healing and comforting to intestines in distress. Slippery elm has little taste. Make the powder into a paste by mixing it with a little bit of water, apple juice, or applesauce. Give a child between the ages of three

199

and six 1 teaspoon, once daily; a child between the ages of seven and twelve should be given 1 teaspoon, two to three times daily.

■ Goldenseal helps to control diarrhea that is caused by a bacterial infection. Give a child between the ages of three and six 3 drops, three times daily, for two days. Give a child between the ages of seven and twelve 10 drops, three times daily, for two days.

■ Curing Pills, a Chinese herbal formula, help to resolve a wide variety of digestive problems, including diarrhea. A child between the ages of three and six should take ¼ tube, or ½ dropperful, three times daily. A child between seven and twelve should take ⅓ tube, or 1 dropperful, three times daily.

■ A cream made from kuzu root and umeboshi (salt) plum paste is helpful for easing intestinal upset (*see* THERAPEUTIC RECIPES in Part Three).

HOMEOPATHY

Select a symptom-specific remedy from the suggestions below. The right remedy should work within forty-eight hours. Unless otherwise directed, give your child one dose, three to four times a day, until symptoms are relieved. If your child gets no relief in forty-eight hours, try another remedy.

■ If your child has diarrhea after eating too much sugar, give her *Argentum nitricum* 30x or 9c.

■ *Arsenicum album* 30x or 9c helps to resolve diarrhea related to food poisoning, anxiety, or stress. This remedy is usually needed for only one or two days.

■ If your child has diarrhea after eating dairy products, or is teething with diarrhea, give her *Calcarea carbonica* 30x or 9c.

■ If your child has abdominal bloating and diarrhea after eating too much fruit, give her *China* 30x or 9c.

■ *Colocynthis* 12x or 6c is very effective against the twisting and cramping abdominal pain that often accompanies diarrhea.

■ *Magnesia phosphorica* 12x or 6c helps relax the bowel and ease cramping.

■ For any kind of abdominal pain, alternating *Colycynthis* with *Magnesia phosphorica* is excellent. You should not need to give these remedies for more than 24 hours.

■ If your child has green, foul-smelling diarrhea, use *Mercurius solubilis* 30x or 9c.

■ If your child has a tendency toward recurrent diarrhea and craves salt, give her *Natrum muriaticum* 30x or 9c.

■ If your child has diarrhea after eating fatty foods, give her *Pulsatilla* 30x or 9c.

■ If none of the above remedies seems right for your child, a homeopathic combination diarrhea remedy may be helpful.

BACH FLOWER REMEDIES

■ If you suspect that your child's diarrhea is emotionally based, try giving her Mimulus to help balance her emotions. (See BACH FLOWER REMEDIES in Part One.)

ACUPRESSURE

For the locations of acupressure points on a child's body, *see* ADMINISTERING AN ACUPRESSURE TREATMENT in Part Three.

■ Stomach 36 tones the digestive system.

GENERAL RECOMMENDATIONS

■ Be sure your child is taking adequate fluids. When a small body is losing fluids as rapidly as it does with diarrhea, dehydration is a very serious concern. If you are not comfortable with the progress your child is making, do not hesitate to consult your doctor.

■ If your child has repeated episodes of diarrhea, rest the gastrointestinal tract as much as possible. To avoid dehydration, give her repeated small sips of water, miso soup, or diluted fruit juices.

■ Make a rice or barley water formula by boiling ½ cup of brown rice or barley in 1 quart of spring water. Once the rice or barley is cooked, pour off the water and let your child drink it in small sips. This nourishing broth is widely used throughout the world.

■ If your child is vomiting in addition to having diarrhea, even a small sip of water may cause another upset. If vomiting occurs after your child takes water, wait one hour and then offer small chips of ice. If the vomiting reflex is not triggered by the ice, after an hour of calm has passed, offer more chips of ice or small sips of water. Or, as an alternative, try giving your child a teaspoon of Emetrol syrup or raw honey to settle her stomach.

Caution: Never give honey to a child less than one year old. Honey has been associated with infant botulism, which can be life threatening.

■ *Do not* offer your child food until she signals a readiness to eat. If your child is hungry, give her simple, easily digested foods.

■ Give your child slippery elm paste or umeboshi plum and kuzu root cream.

■ Give your child a *Lactobacillus acidophilus* or *bifidus* supplement.

■ Select and administer a suitable homeopathic remedy.

PREVENTION

■ To prevent bacteria and foreign substances from finding their way into your child's system, teach your child to wash her hands properly after going to the bathroom and before eating.

■ Try to eliminate any food allergies or sensitivities as a cause of diarrhea. Common allergens include citrus fruits, wheat, sugar, and dairy products.

■ If your child suffers repeated bouts of diarrhea, she may have a lactose intolerance. The absorption of lactose, or milk sugar, depends on the presence of the enzyme lactase. Most infants have adequate amounts of this enzyme, but older children and adults often don't produce enough of it to process lactose. As a result, they suffer from diarrhea, bloating, vague abdominal pain, gas, and indigestion when they consume dairy products. About 33 million people in the United States are lactose intolerant. The most effective treatment for this condition is to limit the intake of milk and dairy products, as well as processed food products that contain lactose as an ingredient.

Diphtheria

Diphtheria is a serious bacterial invasion that can infect any mucous membrane, including the skin. The onset of this illness is gradual and is characterized by a headache, malaise, low-grade fever, a throat that is sore with a yellowish-white or grayish coating, bad breath, and, in some cases, swollen lymph glands in the neck. It is usually seen in children between one and ten years of age. It is an uncommon illness in the United States, Canada, and Europe, where most children are vaccinated against it (the D in the DT and DPT vaccines stands for protection against diphtheria), but if your child travels with you to other parts of the world, the potential for exposure still exists.

Diphtheria is spread from one person to another by coughing, sneezing, or talking. Once a person is infected, the bacteria can incubate for one to six days before symptoms begin to appear. A culture taken from the nose and throat is used to diagnose the presence of *Corynebacterium diphtheriae*, the organism responsible for causing the disease.

CONVENTIONAL TREATMENT

■ A child with diphtheria may need to be hospitalized. Because there is a possibility of heart and nervous system involvement with this bacterial infection, absolute bed rest is an important part of the treatment. Also, because of the possibility of heart or breathing problems arising from this illness, patients with diphtheria must be closely monitored for any developing signs of complications.

■ A child diagnosed with diphtheria will be given an antitoxin and antibiotic, usually penicillin or erythromycin. Although this is a potentially fatal illness, if the antitoxin is given in sufficient quantity within the first three days of the onset, the child is likely to recover fully. Because timing is crucial to the success of this treatment, if diphtheria is suspected, antitoxin may be given even before a culture confirms the presence of the disease.

■ A person is no longer contagious one to two days after treatment with antibiotics and antitoxin begins. Recovery, however, is slow, and care should be taken that your child does not resume activity too soon. Follow your doctor's instructions.

GENERAL RECOMMENDATIONS

■ A child with diphtheria needs total bed rest, and must be isolated from others in order to prevent the spread of this illness. Infants and the elderly are at the greatest risk for complications and death resulting from this infection.

■ Anyone who has been exposed to a child with diphtheria should be tested for the disease. Medication may be necessary. If you suspect that your child has been exposed to diphtheria, and he has not been immunized against the disease, it is vital that you consult a physician immediately.

PREVENTION

■ A vaccine that protects against *Corynebacterium diphtheriae* is available. It is usually given in combination with the tetanus or tetanus and pertussis vaccines.

This is normally administered as a series of injections, given to children at approximately two months, four months, six months, eighteen months, four to six years, and fourteen to sixteen years of age. Thereafter, a booster may be given every ten years, or after exposure to the disease. (*See* IMMUNIZATION PROBLEMS.)

■ As much as possible, try to keep your child from contact with others who may be contagious, or who have been exposed to the disease, especially if he is not (or is not yet) immunized against diphtheria.

Drowning, Near

A child of any age, even a good swimmer, can suffer a water accident that causes a near-drowning. It can happen even in very shallow water. In fact, a 1985 article in *Emergency Medical Review* noted that 90 percent of all drownings occur within ten yards of land. The biggest danger of drowning comes from a lack of oxygen. Cardiac arrest as a result of immersion in cold water can also be a cause of death in drowning. Complications of a near-drowning can include damage to internal organs, especially the brain, due to lack of oxygen, and damage to the lungs from inhaling water, salt, sand, or bacteria.

EMERGENCY TREATMENT FOR NEAR-DROWNING

See the inset on page 204.

CONVENTIONAL TREATMENT

■ Seek emergency medical attention for your child (see page 204). Once your child has recovered sufficiently from the incident for you to take her home, medical personnel will advise you on the proper way to care for her as she completes her recovery.

HOMEOPATHY

■ Following a near-drowning incident, a child will often be traumatized and fearful of water. A dose of *Aconite* 200x, given once a week for three weeks afterward, is often helpful in recovery from such a trauma.

PREVENTION

■ Make sure your child learns to swim and learns water safety.

■ Do not permit your child to jump into deep water unless there is an easy way for her to get out again, such as a ladder on the side of a pool, or a nearby bank with a shallow slope. A child who jumps into deep water from the side of a boat, the edge of a cliff, or a steep bank may be difficult to rescue in case of an accident.

■ Always outfit your child with a suitable life jacket when she is engaged in any activity in or on the water, including boating, sailing, and windsurfing, even if she is a good swimmer.

■ Allow your child to swim in pools or at public beaches only if a lifeguard is on duty.

■ Always make sure your child is supervised by a responsible adult when she is around water, including bathtime. *Never* leave a child alone in the tub or near water.

Emergency Treatment for Near-Drowning

✚ If your child is thrashing around in a panic or is unconscious, go into the water after her (if you are not a good swimmer, take a life preserver with you). Check for breathing as soon as you reach your child, while you are still in the water.

✚ If your child is not breathing, you must breathe for her immediately. Don't waste time getting your child out of the water first, and don't worry about getting the water out of her lungs. Begin rescue breathing immediately, in the manner appropriate for your child's age, as you carry her out of the water (turn to CARDIOPULMONARY RESUSCITATION on page 426). Maintain artificial respiration continuously until emergency personnel arrive or until you can get your child to the emergency room of the nearest hospital. Don't panic, and don't become discouraged and give up prematurely. Victims of near-drowning with barely perceptible pulses have been successfully revived when artificial respiration was steadily maintained for an hour or more.

✚ Once your child is breathing and out of the water, drain as much water as possible from her lungs. Hold your child around the waist, allowing her trunk and head to hang down. Sometimes just holding a child in this position is sufficient to expel inhaled water. If your child begins coughing and sputtering, and struggles to reach an upright position, you may safely assume that the initial crisis has passed. She will still need medical attention to detect and treat any possible complications.

✚ If your child is breathing on her own, but the above procedure fails to expel water from the lungs, try the following. Place her on her stomach, with the leg and arm on one side of her body straight out, the hand palm side flat to the ground. On the other side of the body, position the leg with the knee bent and drawn up toward the body at a right angle, and the arm with elbow bent and drawn toward the chest, the hand palm side flat to the ground. Turn her head toward the side with the limbs bent, with the jaw jutting slightly forward to open the airway.

Then, with the heels of your hands, press down on the upper quadrant of the back to compress the lungs and force any inhaled water up through the windpipe, or trachea. If there is water in your child's lungs, it should gush out, initiating coughing and spluttering. If paramedics are not already on their way to you, seek medical attention immediately.

✚ After a near-drowning, even if your child seems to be fine, she should be examined by a doctor.

■ Do not permit your child to walk or slide on an iced-over pond, river, creek, or lake unless the ice has been thoroughly tested by a responsible adult.

■ When you are enjoying water sports with your child, don't drink. Alcohol impairs your reflexes and could keep you from acting quickly and surely enough to help your child if a crisis arises.

Ear Infection

Every year, over 10 million children in the United States are treated for ear infections. Chances are that by the time a child reaches the age of six, he will have suffered *otitis media*, an infection of the middle ear. Ear infections are most common in children between the ages of six months and three years.

The ear is a complex structure that consists of three sections: the outer, middle, and inner ears. The outer ear is the part we see. It is the external canal that picks up the vibrations from sound and transmits them through the eardrum to the middle ear. The middle ear contains three small bones that take these vibrations into the inner ear, which contains the nerve endings that make hearing possible. The inner ear is also involved in maintaining balance.

The middle ear is connected to the nasal cavity and the throat by means of a passageway called the *eustachian tube*. This allows excess secretions from the middle ear to drain away from the ear and into the nose and throat. If the eustachian tube is not draining properly, these secretions build up in the middle ear, with the result that pressure in the ear rises and the ear becomes painful and, often, infected.

Young children are more likely than others to develop middle ear infections because in infants, the eustachian tube is oriented more horizontally than vertically, making drainage more difficult than it is in older children. Fluids can collect and become blocked, creating an ideal environment for bacterial growth.

Most children outgrow ear infections as their bodies mature and the structure of the inner ear changes. As a child grows, the eustachian tube begins to curve downward, allowing fluids to drain more easily. When the eustachian tube develops its characteristic mature curve, fluids drain readily and infections are less of a problem. When fully mature, the eustachian tube has a pronounced downward angle (see illustrations, page 206).

Ear infections are often a complication of a common cold or other upper respiratory infection, such as infection of the adenoids, tonsils, or sinuses. They are sometimes accompanied by coughing, runny nose, sore throat, and, occasionally, vomiting and diarrhea. Depending on the cause of the infection, a fever may be present.

A child who can talk will be quick to tell you, "My ear hurts!" Babies and toddlers will "tell" you by pulling or tugging on their ears, by rubbing or hitting their ears, or by fussing and crying. A young infant may simply be irritable or run a high fever for no apparent reason.

Another common symptom of ear infection, which your child may not have the words to express, is a feeling of fullness and pressure. This is caused by the excess fluid pushing against the eardrum. Your child may have a slight hearing loss in the affected ear. In most cases, this is temporary. However, if ear infection and hearing loss occur repeatedly, they can cause long-term problems. According to the American Academy of Pediatrics, recurring ear infections with hearing impairment may slow speech and learning development, even if there is no permanent hearing loss.

After initial treatment, if your child does not improve within twenty-four hours, call your doctor again. The risk of a permanent hearing loss increases if an ear infection is not properly treated or does not respond to treatment promptly. It may be necessary to try another treatment.

CONVENTIONAL TREATMENT

■ Antibiotics, such as amoxicillin, Bactrim, Septra, Augmentin, Ceclor, Suprax, and Pediazole, are commonly prescribed for ear infections. Most children with a first-time infection feel significantly better within forty-eight to seventy-two hours after starting a course of antibiotics, but it is important for them to continue taking the medication for the full course to be certain all infection is gone. Your health care provider will want to see your child once the full course of antibiotics is completed, to make sure the infection has cleared. Because many ear infections persist even after the symptoms have eased, it's important to keep follow-up appointments.

While antibiotics are a common treatment for ear infections, parents should be

EMERGENCY TREATMENT FOR EAR INFECTION

✚ If your child experiences a sudden, severe pain, with drainage from the ear, it can mean that he has a perforated eardrum. When the buildup of pressure finally causes the drum to rupture, the relief from pressure can actually cause a dramatic lessening of the pain. Even if your child seems to be feeling better, take him to the doctor right away for an examination.

✚ If your child experiences fever, chills, dizziness, or a serious hearing loss, call your doctor. These signs indicate that the infection may have worsened or traveled to the inner ear, requiring prompt medical attention.

✚ Another potential, and extremely serious, complication is meningitis. If your child complains of a severe headache, stiff neck, and lethargy, contact your physician immediately (*see* MENINGITIS).

aware that a study done in the Netherlands compared children with ear infections who were treated with antibiotics to a control group who were given a placebo. Although the antibiotic group improved somewhat faster, it is interesting to note that there was little difference between the two groups in long-term outcome.

■ Some ear infections may not respond to the first medication prescribed. If your child doesn't seem to be improving after four or five days, talk with your doctor. Another office visit and evaluation, and possibly a change of medication, may be required.

■ An analgesic, such as acetaminophen (Tylenol, Tempra, and others) can help to relieve the pain of an ear infection and also bring down fever.

Note: In excessive amounts, this drug can cause liver damage. Read package directions carefully so as not to exceed the proper dosage for your child's age and size.

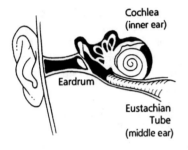

Cochlea
(inner ear)

Eardrum

Eustachian
Tube
(middle ear)

A. Infant

■ If your child's ear infection is related to sinus or nasal congestion, an antihistamine and/or a decongestant may be prescribed. Antihistamines often cause sleepiness, so if your child can't sleep because of the discomfort, your doctor may recommend one. Research has not shown these medications to be helpful in actually curing ear infections, however.

■ Frequent ear infections are the most common reason for childhood surgery. If your child has had more than three ear infections within a six-month period, with resulting documented hearing loss, surgery may be recommended. *Myringotomy* is one of the most common operations performed in the United States. In this procedure, performed under general anesthesia, a physician inserts tiny plastic tubes into the middle ear to allow drainage of the fluid that is not draining, as it should, through the eustachian tube. Once in place, the tubes do not hurt. Your child should not even be aware of them. If infected tonsils or adenoids are causing recurring ear infections, your doctor may recommend *tonsillectomy* or *adenoidectomy*. Reports of long-term outcomes for these treatments are contradictory, however.

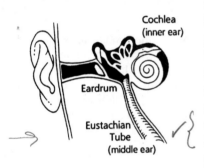

Cochlea
(inner ear)

Eardrum

Eustachian
Tube
(middle ear)

B. Older Child

Structure of the Ear

In infants, the eustachian tube extends almost horizontally from the middle ear to the nasal cavity and the throat (figure A). As a child grows, the eustachian tube develops a downward curve (figure B).

■ Some doctors prescribe a steroid, prednisone, for children with chronic ear infections. Steroids are powerful drugs with potentially serious side effects and are not suitable for long-term use. If your doctor recommends this, discuss in detail his or her reasons for thinking that this is the appropriate treatment for your child.

DIETARY GUIDELINES

■ Keep your child well hydrated. If you are breastfeeding, do so frequently. Offer an older child plenty of spring water, soups, herbal teas, and diluted fruit juices.

■ Eliminate dairy foods. Dairy foods thicken and increase mucus, making it more difficult for an infected ear to drain.

NUTRITIONAL SUPPLEMENTS

For age-appropriate dosages of some nutritional supplements, see page 81.

■ *Lactobacillus acidophilus* or *bifidus* is valuable for a child who is taking antibiotics, who has chronic ear infections, or who has an ear infection with a stomachache. In addition to killing infectious bacteria, antibiotics strip the body of necessary friendly bacteria in the intestinal tract. Replace the friendly bacteria by giving your child lactobacilli (either ¼ teaspoon of powder, 1 teaspoon of liquid, or half of the contents of a capsule), once daily, two hours after administering the antibiotic.

■ Vitamin C and bioflavonoids are helpful for an ear infection. They are both mildly anti-inflammatory. Give a child over four years old one dose, six times daily. Select a product that contains mineral-ascorbate-buffered vitamin C but no sugar. For younger children, purchase a vitamin-C supplement made specifically for infants and toddlers.

■ Zinc boosts the immune response and helps reduce infection. Give your child zinc-based lozenges, two to three times daily, as needed, for a total of one dose of zinc a day.

Note: Excessive amounts of zinc can result in nausea and vomiting. Be careful not to exceed the recommended dosage.

HERBAL TREATMENT

For age-appropriate dosages of herbal remedies, see page 81.

■ Echinacea and goldenseal herbal combination formula is important for clearing any type of infection. Echinacea is antiviral; goldenseal is antibacterial and soothes irritated mucous membranes. Both herbs stimulate the immune system. The liquid extract is the preferred form. Give your child one dose, every two hours, while the infection is acute. After his symptoms have eased, give him one dose, three times daily, for one week.

Note: You should not give your child echinacea on a daily basis for more than two weeks at a time, or it will lose its effectiveness.

■ Garlic is an antibacterial that can help heal an ear infection. Choose an odorless form of garlic capsules; with the smell missing, children don't usually object to it. Your child can either swallow the capsule whole or take it dissolved in soup or hot water. Follow the age-specific dosage directions on the product label. Or heat a fresh garlic clove in olive oil and, with your child lying on his side, put one or two drops of warm (not hot) oil into the affected ear.

■ Mullein oil is a traditional Native American remedy used to reduce swelling and inflammation. Gently heat mullein oil to slightly above body temperature and, with your child lying on his side, put one or two drops into the affected ear. The heat feels comforting, while the mullein goes to work on the problem.

HOMEOPATHY

The symptom-specific remedies listed here should work quickly. If your child's pain does not subside within twenty-four hours, call your physician.

■ If your child has a fever, a red face, dilated pupils, and hot and moist skin, give him *Belladonna*. This is for a child with a throbbing earache that is relieved by resting with the head elevated. Give this child one dose of *Belladonna* 30x or 9c, two to three times daily, for one day.

■ For an earache that occurs with teething, give *Chamomilla*. The *Chamomilla* baby is crying, angry, obstinant, whiny, and irritable, but is comforted when carried around. Often he has one red cheek and one pale cheek with hot, moist skin, and his pain is intolerable. Give him one dose of *Chamomilla* 12x, 30x, 6c, or 9c, three times daily, for one to two days.

■ If your child has a fever along with an ear infection, give him *Ferrum phosphoricum*. This homeopathic preparation can be given together with another symptom-specific remedy. Give up to four doses of *Ferrum phosphoricum* 12x or 6c, thirty minutes apart.

■ *Kali muriaticum* helps relieve nasal congestion and swollen glands. It will benefit the child with a blocked eustachian tube that has affected his hearing. Give one dose of *Kali muriaticum* 12x or 6c, three times daily, for one to two days.

■ For a child who has a moderate fever and an earache that comes on gradually, use *Pulsatilla*. An important symptom that distinguishes a *Pulsatilla* child is the desire for cold; this child wants to be in fresh air—near a window or outdoors—and feels better with a cold compress. Give this child one dose of *Pulsatilla* 30x or 9c, three times daily, for one to two days.

■ *Mercurius dulcis* often works if other remedies have failed. Give your child one dose of *Mercurius dulcis* 12x or 6c, three times daily, for two days.

■ If none of the above remedies seems right for your child, a homeopathic combination earache remedy may be helpful.

■ If your child has ear surgery with a myringotomy and tube placement, give him one dose of *Arnica* 30x or 9c, three or four times daily, for two days. *Arnica* helps reduce inflammation surrounding the tube and also helps the body adjust to the tube's presence.

GENERAL RECOMMENDATIONS

■ The pain of an earache is caused by pressure as the congested middle ear pushes on the eardrum. To promote drainage, prop your child at a 30-degree angle.

■ Prepare and use one of the herbal oil ear drops recommended under Herbal Treatment, above. A drop or two of warm oil on the eardrum helps relax and anesthetize the membrane, lessening the pain.

■ If your child cannot tolerate ear drops, apply a warm compress. If the warmth is comforting, use that knowledge to guide you in choosing an appropriate symptom-specific homeopathic remedy. Some children seem to feel better with a cold compress. Experiment with hot and cold to see what helps. If your child doesn't like the warmth, give him homeopathic *Pulsatilla*.

■ If your child has an ear infection, avoid taking him on airplane flights. A child with an earache or upper respiratory infection will be very uncomfortable traveling by air. Air travel does not necessarily injure the ear or increase your child's risk of developing an ear infection, but the change of air pressure in the cabin on takeoff and landing can greatly increase the pain. If you must fly with a child who has an ear infection, it may be worthwhile to give him nasal decongestant drops, along with acetaminophen, before takeoff.

PREVENTION

■ Do not expose your child to cigarette smoke. Studies show that children who live in households with one or more smokers suffer more ear infections than those from smoke-free households.

■ Do not give your baby a bottle to suck on while he is lying flat on his back.

This position allows fluid to drain directly into the middle ear. Instead, hold or prop your infant at a 30-degree angle.

■ Massaging your child's ear can help keep the eustachian tube open. Using gentle pressure, draw a line along the back of the ear and down the back of the jawbone. Gently push and release the flap of skin in front of the ear several times. You can also massage your child's ear by placing the fleshy part of your palm, just below your thumb, over your child's ear, and rotating the ear in all directions.

■ Use an elimination diet to determine if food allergies are contributing to the problem. Cow's milk tops the list of common troublemakers. Other common allergens worth deleting for a child with recurring ear infections include eggs, wheat, corn, oranges, and peanut butter.

■ If your child is subject to recurring ear infections, do not expose him to common irritating allergens such as pet dander. Down comforters and pillows are another possible source of trouble. Items like carpets, draperies, and stuffed toys all collect dust and are possible offenders as well.

■ Minor bupleurum is a Chinese herbal formula that helps to strengthen resistance to infection. It can be very helpful in preventing the recurrence of ear infections. Give your child 3 to 5 drops, five days a week, for one month. Discontinue it for three weeks, then resume giving 3 to 5 drops, five days a week, for another month. Discontinue it for another three weeks. Repeat this regimen for a six-month period.

Note: Minor bupleurum should be used as a preventive only. It should not be given to a child with a fever or any other sign of an acute infection.

■ If your child suffers from repeated ear infections, give him ⅓ tube of homeopathic *Anas barbariae* (available as a product called Oscillococcinum), once a week, during the month or two he is most susceptible to infection.

■ In some cases, chiropractic care and cranial-sacral work may be helpful for a child with recurrent ear infections.

■ If your child suffers from recurring earaches, your physician may recommend a daily low dose of antibiotic to suppress any possible developing infections. If your doctor advises this, discuss it thoroughly to find out why he or she considers it an appropriate treatment for your child. A child on such a regimen will need to be seen by the doctor every month or so. He will also need to take yogurt or a *lactobacillus acidophilus* or *bifidus* supplement every day to counteract the effect of the medication on his digestive system. This approach may be effective in a few particularly intractable cases, but it runs the risk of creating antibiotic-resistant organisms and inhibiting the development of the body's own natural resistance. It is better to consider and try all other options before agreeing to give your child a daily dose of antibiotics. It may not be presented as such, but this is an extreme—and not necessarily health-promoting—type of treatment.

Eating Disorders

See OBESITY.

Eczema

Eczema is an inflammatory skin disorder characterized by patches of red, dry, flaking skin and areas that are inflamed, moist, and oozing. If the condition becomes chronic, the affected skin cells may become thick and scaly and the skin may change color. Itching can be so severe that scratching is inevitable. A child with eczema may scratch until the skin cracks and bleeds, preferring the hurt caused by rubbing the skin raw to the intolerable itching.

The condition can affect any part of the body, but is most common on the face and scalp, behind the ears, and in the creases of the elbows, knees, and groin. A child with eczema usually has very dry, itchy skin that doesn't hold moisture well.

Eczema can occur at any age, but seems to be most common in young girls. It can be short-lived (acute) or last for several years with periods of remission and exacerbation (chronic). It is not contagious.

Eczema can be a result of either *atopic dermatitis* or *contact dermatitis*. Atopic dermatitis is an inherited form of the condition that usually first appears when an infant is two to three months old. Often a child with atopic dermatitis has other family members with allergies and a history of eczema. This type of eczema is often associated with other allergies. It can become worse when new foods are introduced, or when your baby is exposed to an allergen like dust or pollen. Atopic eczema may be a long-term condition.

Contact dermatitis is the more common form of the condition. In an infant, contact dermatitis is most often caused by drooling and licking the lips. This type of eczema is often an allergic response to something your child has ingested, such as food or medicine, and is more common in older children. Eczema can also be caused by something that comes in contact with your child's sensitive skin, such as soaps, bubble bath, fabric dyes, feathers, cosmetics, wool, plants, and environmental pollutants.

Both types of eczema are considered allergic responses, and it is possible that a child with eczema will develop other allergies as well, such as food sensitivities, asthma, or hay fever.

Emotional stress can exacerbate a case of eczema. Also, even though eczema is not caused by a virus or bacteria, the open lesions can become infected. When caring for a child with eczema, watch for signs of infection, and if infection develops, call your doctor.

CONVENTIONAL TREATMENT

■ Topical anti-inflammatory ointments, such as hydrocortisone, triamcinolone, or betamethasone, are the medications most commonly prescribed for eczema. Your doctor will direct you to rub a small amount into the affected area, taking care not to apply it to open lesions. In more severe cases, you may be instructed to wrap the area with an occlusive dressing, such as Saran Wrap, to increase the medication's effectiveness. Because long-term use of steroids often creates side effects, such as thin, fragile skin, these medications should be used only for a short time.

■ To counter the allergic response and help decrease the awful itching, an antihis-

tamine such as diphenhydramine (found in Benadryl), hydroxyzine hydrochloride (Atarax), or chlorpheniramine (Chlor-Trimeton) may be recommended. Antihista-
..., but this can be very helpful at bedtime, when itching is
...t difficult for your child to fall asleep.

Eczema

...are weeping, Burow's solution may be recommended.
...vailable over the counter at many drug stores.

...citrus fruits, eggs, wheat, cow's milk, shellfish, and/or
...zema. Use an elimination diet to check for any possible
...eding mother's diet or in the child's diet (*see* ELIMINATION

...otassium and vitamin A or beta-carotene in your child's
...eafy greens are excellent choices.

...for your child. You can use the recipe for Astragalus
...under THERAPEUTIC RECIPES in Part Three, with the follow-
...ate the astragalus root and add parsley and garlic to
...Chinese herb paeonia in tincture form and 80 drops of
...and onions contain sulfur and amino acids beneficial
...in calcium and magnesium, which are also beneficial
...cleanse the blood. If your child is a finicky eater, you
...the herbs and vegetables, and add noodles, rice, or
...serving it. That way, she can ingest all those beneficial
...hout having to actually fork down the vegetables.

...MENTS

...lucing the nutritional supplements that follow one at
...responds to the first nutrient you introduce, and add
...or age-appropriate dosages of nutritional supplements,

...rsor of vitamin A, promotes tissue healing. Give your
...a-carotene daily until the condition improves. Then
...our child one dose a day on an ongoing basis.

...n be taken internally (one or two capsules daily) or
...luce inflammation.
...il should not be given to a child who has a fever.

...use vitamin E effectively and supports the healthy
...es. Give your child one-half dose daily for up to one

...scorbate form and bioflavonoids have a mild anti-
...elpful for eczema. Give your child at least two doses
...nths.

■ Vitamin E is good for the skin and aids tissue healing. It can be applied topically, taken internally, or both. Give your child one dose, three times a day, for one month.

211

■ Zinc promotes the healing of wounds. Give your child one dose of zinc daily for one month.

Note: Excessive amounts of zinc can result in nausea and vomiting. Be careful not to exceed the recommended dosage.

HERBAL TREATMENT

For age-appropriate dosages of herbal remedies, see page 81.

■ For children ten years of age and older, a five-week herbal regimen can help resolve eczema. Each herb is to be given for seven days, in the order given, as follows.

Week 1: Burdock root, taken as extract or tea, acts to detoxify the blood and helps to heal the skin. Give your child one dose, twice daily.

Week 2: A combination echinacea and goldenseal formula helps detoxify the blood. Give your child one dose, twice daily.

Week 3: Red clover is a cleansing and blood-purifying herb useful in treating skin conditions. Give your child one dose, twice daily.

Week 4: Give your child one dose of nettle, twice daily. This herb is a blood builder that is full of important trace minerals.

Note: Some children experience stomach upset as a result of taking this herb. If this happens, you can try mixing it with ginger or simply stop giving it.

Week 5: To continue detoxifying the blood, give your child one dose of echinacea and goldenseal combination formula, twice daily.

■ Balsam of Peru can be useful against eczema. It can be applied to the skin alone, or diluted with oil.

■ An herbal cream made from comfrey and licorice, such as Simicort or Alticort, or a high-potency chamomile cream such as CamoCare can have a very soothing and anti-inflammatory effect. Follow the directions on the product label.

■ Dry eczema can benefit from the application of calendula ointment. Follow the directions on the product label.

HOMEOPATHY

When treating eczema with a symptom-specific homeopathic remedy, continue giving your child the remedy until you notice an improvement. Once your child's skin begins to improve, discontinue the remedy. If the eczema gets worse, stop giving the remedy.

■ Give your child *Graphites* if her patches of eczema are moist and oozing, with a clear or slightly yellow discharge. This child may have eczema anywhere on her body, but it is most likely to be on the palms of the hands, behind the ears, and on the scalp. Give her one dose of *Graphites* 30x or 9c, three times a day, for up to five days.

■ For a child whose eczema is infected, oozing, and particularly bad on the scalp, give one dose of *Mezereum* 30x or 9c, three times daily, for up to five days.

■ If your child's eczema is worse on her legs, try using *Psorinum* 30x or 9c, three times a day, for up to three days.

■ For the child with dry, red, itchy areas in the folds of the joints, often with small blisters on the surface of the skin, use *Rhus toxicodendron*. This is for the child who feels better with warmth and likes to snuggle under the covers. She enjoys warm oatmeal baths (see below). Give this child one dose of *Rhus toxicodendron* 30x or 9c, three times daily, for up to five days.

■ If your child is sweaty, dislikes being washed, throws off the covers, and wants her skin exposed to the air, choose *Sulphur*. This child feels warm and often has very red, dry, hot-looking patches of skin. Give her *Sulphur* 30x or 9c, once daily, for three days.

■ If your child's eczema is dry and scaly, apply *Urtica urens* ointment or gel, two to three times a day, until the dryness is relieved.

■ If your child's eczema is wet and weeping, apply homeopathic *Calendula* directly to the area, two to three times a day.

■ If none of the above remedies seems right for your child, a homeopathic combination eczema remedy may be helpful.

BACH FLOWER REMEDIES

■ Rescue Remedy is available in an ointment form that is soothing and helpful for dry eczema. Follow the directions on the product label.

GENERAL RECOMMENDATIONS

■ Do anything and everything you can to reduce the itching. When your child scratches, skin cells reproduce rapidly and the patches of eczema spread, making the condition difficult to control.

■ Keep your child's fingernails clipped very short so she is less likely to open a wound if she scratches.

■ Expose your child's eczema to fresh air and moderate amounts of sunshine. A thirty-minute exposure to ultraviolet rays will reduce inflammation. Monitor your child carefully, however, and don't let her stay out in the sun too long. Lengthy exposure to the sun can worsen eczema.

■ Distract your child with games that require the use of the hands. Join in, laugh a lot, and gently remind your child not to scratch.

■ To decrease the stress associated with this condition, teach your child relaxation and visualization techniques (*see* RELAXATION TECHNIQUES in Part Three). Offer support and encouragement by doing the exercises with her. Help your child visualize patches of itchy eczema being eaten up or destroyed by her favorite superhero or video-game character, for example.

■ Avoid anything that dries out your child's skin. Discourage long showers or baths, which strip natural oils from the skin.

■ To counteract itching, add a few drops of herbal oil to your child's bath water, or give your child an Aveeno or oatmeal bath. Wrap a cup of oatmeal in a clean cloth or washcloth. Put this bag under the running faucet and swish it through the bath water. Squeeze and rub the wet bag over your child's skin. Oatmeal is very soothing to dry and inflamed skin.

■ After an oatmeal bath, gently rub a very mild, non-allergenic lotion all over your child's body to lock in moisture and prevent further drying.

■ A cool, wet compress applied to the area may help decrease itching.

■ Soft, gentle, clean cotton clothes are the most comfortable for a child with eczema. Avoid skin-irritating substances, such as soap residue in just-washed clothes, and other allergens that can exacerbate the condition. Make sure that clothes, towels, and washcloths are free of soap. A second rinse cycle may be helpful.

■ Consider possible food and environmental allergies. If the affected child is breastfed, the nursing mother should consider possible allergens in her own diet.

Electric Shock

EMERGENCY TREATMENT FOR ELECTRIC SHOCK

✚ You will probably instinctively reach to snatch your child out of harm's way. *Don't*. You may receive a severe shock yourself and become unable to help your child. To break the electrical contact safely, first switch off the current. If this is not possible, as in the case of a live wire, use a nonconductive item, such as a wooden broom handle, to lift or push away the source of the current.

✚ If your child is not breathing, turn to CARDIOPULMONARY RESUSCITATION (CPR) on page 426. Start artificial respiration at once.

✚ Always take your child to the doctor or the emergency room for evaluation after a severe electric shock, even if he seems to have suffered only a minor electrical burn. There may be internal damage that is not readily visible, but which requires treatment.

A severe electric shock may knock your child unconscious, and he may stop breathing. There may be deep burns at the point where the current entered the body. There may also be internal damage.

If your child suffers a severe electrical shock, take emergency measures.

CONVENTIONAL TREATMENT

■ If your child has suffered a burn as a result of an electric shock, *see* BURNS for appropriate treatment suggestions.

DIETARY GUIDELINES

■ If your child has suffered a burn at the site of the injury, encourage him to drink plenty of liquids to replace fluids that may have been lost.

■ After any trauma to the body, a diet high in protein helps promote healing.

■ Give your child a diet high in green and yellow vegetables.

NUTRITIONAL SUPPLEMENTS

For age-appropriate dosages of nutritional supplements, see page 81.

■ Beta-carotene, a precursor to vitamin A, helps burned skin to heal. Give your child a double dose, twice a day, until healing is complete.

■ To support the body's recovery from an electric shock, give your child one dose of mineral ascorbate of vitamin C with bioflavonoids, four times daily, for one week, then twice daily for two to three weeks.

■ If your child has suffered a burn as a result of the shock, you can make a vitamin-C spray by combining 2 tablespoons of powdered vitamin C and ½ cup of aloe vera gel in a 16-ounce spray bottle, and apply this mixture to the burned area, twice a day, for two weeks or until healed.

Note: This treatment is appropriate for minor burns only. More serious burns that involve loss of skin should be treated by a physician.

■ Zinc aids in healing. Give your child one dose, once or twice a day, for two weeks or until the wound is healed.

Note: Excessive amounts of zinc can result in nausea and vomiting. Be careful not to exceed the recommended dosage.

HERBAL TREATMENT

■ Once the crisis is over, if your child has suffered a burn at the site of the injury, apply aloe vera pulp, gel, or liquid to the burned area to remove the heat and sting from the burn. Aloe vera is extremely soothing and cooling, and helps burned skin to heal.

■ Once the stinging sensation associated with a burn has subsided, apply a calendula preparation topically to help prevent infection. Select either an herbal or a homeopathic preparation.

■ Apply a comfrey root salve or cream to the affected area. Comfrey root contains allantoin, which promotes tissue growth and is very healing to the skin.

■ Three capsules of gotu kola daily, for up to ten days, will help speed healing of skin tissue.

Note: Do not give this herb to a child under four years of age.

HOMEOPATHY

■ Give your child one dose of *Aconite* 200x or 30c as soon as you can following the injury. *Aconite* helps to ease fear and shock.

■ Give your child one dose of *Arnica* 30x or 9c, every hour, for three hours. *Arnica* also helps to ease shock, as well as aiding the repair of damaged tissue.

■ Once the shock has subsided, if there is burning pain at the site of the injury, give your child one dose of *Cantharis* 12x or 6c, three times a day, for up to three days.

■ Give your child one dose of *Hypericum* 12x or 6c, three times a day, for two days. *Hypericum* is used in situations where nerve damage or nerve pain has occurred.

■ If there is nerve pain, apply a topical *Hypericum* ointment to the site, twice a day, for three days.

■ If there is burning pain at the site of the injury, apply homeopathic *Calendula* topically, twice a day, for three days.

BACH FLOWER REMEDIES

■ Give your child Bach Flower Rescue Remedy following an electric shock. Mix a few drops in a small amount of water and give it three times a day for two days.

GENERAL RECOMMENDATIONS

■ Seek emergency medical assistance if appropriate.

■ Give your child *Aconite* 200x as soon as you can following the injury. *Aconite* helps to ease fear and shock.

■ Even if your child seems to have suffered only a minor burn, always take a child who has received a severe electric shock to the doctor or the emergency room for evaluation. An electric shock can cause internal damage, which you cannot see.

■ If your child suffered a burn at the site of the injury, cool the burn by holding it under cool running water or by applying cool compresses. Then apply aloe vera to the burn.

■ *Do not* use ice water, butter, petroleum jelly, ointment, or cream on a burn. *Do not* bandage or cover a burn area tightly. *Do not* burst any blisters.

■ Give your child Bach Flower Rescue Remedy.

■ Select and administer an appropriate symptom-specific homeopathic remedy.

■ If your child's skin is burned, *see* BURNS for additional treatment suggestions.

PREVENTION

■ For suggestions on how to prevent accidents that can lead to electric shock, *see* HOME SAFETY in Part One.

Emergencies

Accidents can—and do—happen, even in the most careful and well-prepared households. Knowing what to do when the unthinkable occurs can literally mean the difference between life and death for your child.

We strongly recommend that the primary child-care provider in the family (as well as anyone else who cares for children on a regular basis) complete a good hands-on course in emergency first aid that includes infant and childhood cardiopulmonary resuscitation (CPR) procedures. There is simply no substitute for the instruction and practice you will get in a good first aid course.

The following are general guidelines to follow in responding to any emergency, no matter what its nature.

WHAT TO DO IN AN EMERGENCY

■ *Stay calm. Take a moment to assess what has happened.* It won't help your child if you scream or panic. Your child needs you to be a calm and reassuring presence.

■ *Make sure your child is breathing and check for a pulse.* For an infant under one year, check for a pulse on the brachial artery by placing the tips of your first two fingers on the infant's inner arm above the elbow. For a child older than one year, check for a pulse on the carotid artery, located at the side of the neck. Touch your first two fingers to the Adam's apple, and run your fingers across the neck to the depression between the Adam's apple and the large neck muscle. Allow five to ten seconds to feel for a pulse. If your child is not breathing or does not have a pulse, turn to CARDIOPULMONARY RESUSCITATION (CPR) on page 426. Begin performing CPR at once.

■ *Check for bleeding and for obviously broken bones.*

■ *Try to determine what has happened.* If your child can respond, ask. If not, observe the surroundings. For example, is there a bottle of pills or cleaning compounds nearby? Is the child lying on her back under a tree? If the person is unknown to you, is she wearing a Medic Alert bracelet that identifies a specific medical condition? The few moments you take to assess the situation are vitally important. After close observation, you'll have a better sense of whom to call and what to do. Without careful assessment, you are more likely to panic and do the wrong thing.

What You Should Know About Internal Bleeding

If your child has been involved in an accident and broken a bone, ruptured an internal organ, or suffered a blow to the abdomen or head, internal bleeding may result. Internal bleeding occurs when blood leaks from damaged vessels inside the body into body cavities, such as the abdomen, chest, or skull, or into other tissues.

Internal bleeding is not easily observed from outside. Signs of internal bleeding can include a rigid, tight abdomen; a tight, painful chest; blood in the vomit or stools; or a trickle of blood coming from the mouth, nose, or ear. Bright red, frothy blood tends to be coming from the lungs; dark red or black blood tends to be coming from the stomach. Internal bleeding can cause your child to go into shock.

A definitive diagnosis of internal bleeding must usually be made by a physician, who will rely on x-rays, laboratory tests, and blood measurements to assess your child's condition.

If you suspect that your child may be bleeding internally, call for emergency help and stress the urgency of the situation. As you wait for help to arrive, have your child lie down as follows:

- If your child is conscious and not vomiting, place her on her back with a small pillow under her head, which should be turned to one side.

- If your child is unconscious, or is vomiting, place her on her stomach, with her head turned to one side. Arrange the arm and leg on that side of your child's body with the elbow bent and the hand level with the jaw; the knee should be bent and the leg pulled up so that the thigh is at a right angle to the body. Pull your child's chin forward and up so that her tongue cannot block her throat. Do not use a pillow.

Cover your child lightly with a blanket and keep her still. Do not give her anything by mouth—no medicine or food, or liquid of any kind—before a doctor has assessed the situation, and do not move her. Stay with your child, and try to remain calm and reassuring. Rely on medical personnel to take the appropriate emergency steps to stabilize your child's condition and prepare her body for transport to the hospital. Be prepared for the possibility that she may require a blood transfusion or the administration of intravenous saline solution to maintain fluid levels even before reaching the hospital. Upon arrival at the hospital, a child with internal bleeding will likely need immediate surgery to repair the damage that is causing the bleeding. After surgery, your child may be put in an intensive care unit and monitored closely until her condition has stabilized and she can begin the process of recovery.

■ *If you suspect a head, neck, or spinal injury, do not pick up or move the child, even to offer comfort.* Moving someone with a possible head, neck, or back injury can worsen the damage. Unless there is a threat that the child will vomit and choke, it is best to leave her in the same position in which you found her. Rely on medical personnel to know how to stabilize the child so that transport to the hospital will be safe.

■ *Call for emergency help.* When calling for emergency help, speak distinctly. Give your name, the address you're calling from, your phone number, and your assessment of the situation. *Don't rush.* If you remain calm, you will save time in the long run. If you give clear, distinct, precise information so that the operator can route emergency help to your location quickly, you won't have to repeat your message. Try to relate enough of the problem so that the people who respond to your call will be prepared to deal with it when they arrive. You don't have to know exactly what's wrong; just convey as clearly and completely as you can what you have observed and what your assessment of the situation is.

■ *Stay with your child.* Try to stay with your child until emergency personnel arrive, or until the situation is resolved. If possible, have someone else place the call for emergency services. Your child needs to feel the reassurance of your presence. Talk to her, using simple explanations to describe what's happening. Fear of the unknown makes matters worse. If you are sure that she has not suffered an injury to her head, neck, or back, hold your child close. Otherwise, just gently touch and soothe. As you do so, carefully observe any changes in your child's condition, such as shifts in breathing or heart rate, or changes in her level of pain or consciousness. Certain emergencies will require your immediate intervention.

■ *Be alert for signs of shock.* Shock is a serious condition that results from a sudden and life-threatening drop in blood pressure, which in turn impairs circulation and threatens the brain's oxygen supply. Shock can occur after any trauma to the body, whether from near-drowning, severe injury, major blood loss, or overwhelming infection.

A child suffering from shock may become pale and sweaty, possibly drowsy, confused, and/or disoriented. Shock is usually accompanied by profound weakness, dizziness, faintness, and a cold sweat. The pulse may be weak and feeble.

If you suspect shock, lay your child down on her back and put pillows under her feet to raise her feet higher than her head. Loosen tight or constricting clothing, and cover your child with a blanket. The goal is to insure normal breathing while maintaining normal body temperature and adequate blood circulation to the brain.

If emergency personnel are not already on their way to you, seek emergency medical attention for your child immediately.

■ Depending on the nature of the emergency, *see also* ANAPHYLACTIC SHOCK; APPENDICITIS; ASTHMA; BITES, ANIMAL AND HUMAN; BITES, SNAKE; BITES AND STINGS, INSECT; BLEEDING, SEVERE; BONES, BROKEN; BURNS; CHOKING; CONCUSSION (HEAD INJURY); CUTS AND SCRAPES; DROWNING, NEAR; EAR INFECTION; ELECTRIC SHOCK; EPILEPSY; FEVER; INFLUENZA; NAIL INJURIES, FINGER AND TOE; NAUSEA AND VOMITING; POISONING; POLIOMYELITIS; SEIZURE; SHOCK; UNCONSCIOUSNESS; WHOOPING COUGH.

EMERGENCY PREPAREDNESS

Even the most careful and loving parents can't prevent all emergencies. You can and should, therefore, take measures in advance to prepare you to act quickly and effectively should an emergency arise.

■ *Have a list of emergency telephone numbers handy.* This can save precious time in any emergency, for you or for anyone else who is caring for your children. We urge you to take this precaution now, while you are thinking about it. Post emergency telephone numbers near every telephone in your home. If there is no 911 emergency service in your area, these numbers should include that of your local hospital for ambulance/paramedic service. Also post numbers for your local fire department, Poison Control Center, police, and your child's doctor and dentist. If your telephones can be programmed to automatically dial certain numbers, program these numbers into the telephones (but keep written lists handy in case a phone becomes *un*programmed).

■ *Designate surrogates who will act in your stead should an emergency arise when you cannot be reached, and include their telephone numbers in the emergency list.* Designate adults you trust, perhaps your child's grandparents, perhaps good friends, to make decisions in any emergency involving your child. If you have established a close and caring relationship with your child's health care provider, you might wish to give him or her the legal authority to make any necessary medical decisions involving your child.

■ *Empower your designated surrogates to act for your child by giving them written permission to act for you, such as a limited power of attorney.* Your surrogates should keep this important document where it can be found easily if they must respond to an emergency, and you should give copies to your child's physician. Should an occasion ever arise when you cannot be reached immediately, your designated surrogates will be able to act. Written permission from a parent or designated guardian is sometimes required before certain life-saving measures can be taken.

■ *Provide your child with a Medic Alert bracelet if she has a special medical problem, to ensure that she will receive the right care if something happens away from home.* If your child is allergic to penicillin or other medication, sulfites, or bee stings, for example, it will enable her to receive prompt and appropriate treatment for an allergic reaction. Without a Medic Alert bracelet, a teenager with diabetes who is suffering from the typical symptoms of low blood sugar could be misdiagnosed as being intoxicated and fail to receive necessary treatment. Medic Alert information is especially important for a young child who may not be able to communicate well, or for any child who has a disorder that can cause the loss of consciousness. Without Medic Alert information, health care personnel could be working in the dark and wasting precious time. Medic Alert is the only emergency medical identification service endorsed by the American College of Emergency Physicians, the American Hospital Association, and every national pharmacy association. For more information, call Medic Alert at 800–432–5378.

■ *Have the primary child-care provider in the family take a good course in emergency first aid that includes infant and childhood cardiopulmonary resuscitation (CPR) procedures.* We hope that you will never be called upon to use these skills, but there is simply no substitute for the hands-on training and practice in these life-saving techniques that such a course provides.

■ *As soon as your child is old enough to understand, teach her to respond to emergencies.* Children as young as three years old have been known to use the telephone to summon emergency help. Teach your child how to dial 911, if that service is available in your area (or, if not, how to dial 0 for operator) for emergency assistance, and have your child practice this skill. Use a toy telephone or simply hold the disconnect button down on your regular phone and practice with your child so that she becomes accustomed to the procedure. Also, make sure your child can recite her full name, address, and telephone number.

■ *Take steps to minimize the danger of accidents and injuries occurring in your home and outside.* For suggestions, *see* HOME SAFETY in Part One.

Emotional Upset

Emotional upset—whether anger, sadness, or fear—is a normal response to different stresses in a child's life. Children may not be able to express in words exactly what it is they are feeling. Instead, they may show their feelings by acting out in anger, by withdrawing, or by displaying physical symptoms such as vague abdominal pain, fatigue, or headache. Physical signs of stress can also include dizzy spells; a racing pulse; sweaty palms, feet, or face, not associated with physical activity; chronic headaches; trembling; hives; and insomnia.

The behavior or response you see may not seem to match or articulate the underlying feeling, but it is usually the best way available to the child to express himself in that situation. When a child says, "I hurt," a parent should, of course, explore the physical symptoms, but also be sure to take time to explore whether the pain is actually an emotional hurt. Instead of focusing only on the anger or physical symptom your child displays, look for the deeper emotional need that may be giving rise to it. Help your child verbalize his feelings to ask for what he is really wanting or needing. For example, by saying, "It seems that there is something that you want or need right now. Do you know what that is?" or, "What are you hurting about?" you may be able to get beyond the immediate behavior or illness to a deeper concern or need. It also helps the child know that you are available and that you care about him. Be willing to be patient, listen, and help your child express what he is feeling. Sometimes all a child needs is to feel heard and to be acknowledged. Instead of quickly "kissing and making it all better," sit with your child, hold him, and acknowledge his hurt. Tell him, "I see that you are hurting," or, "I hear that you are needing more of my time," or, "You're right, it *is* so sad that that happened." Acknowledging your child's feelings, and helping him to articulate those feelings, may be one of the greatest gifts you can offer as a parent. It helps to build a child's self-esteem.

Children thrive in an environment that feels safe and secure, and in which they receive plenty of love, support, and guidance. Any major change, instability, or ongoing conflict will have an impact (*see* Sources of Stress in Your Child's Life, page 221). Don't assume that a child doesn't know about family stresses unless you tell him. In fact, it is more realistic to assume that a child *does* know about whatever stresses there are in the family, and needs support to deal with what he is feeling. Children are like very sensitive weathervanes. They have a natural ability to pick up on feelings, conflicts, or changes in their environments. Using language your child can understand, talk about changes or conflicts in the family. Help your child to understand what is really happening so that he does not need to guess or imagine. The explanations children come up with on their own are often more frightening than the reality.

If, after you have identified a problem and addressed it in the most compassionate and complete way you know, your child's emotional upset or behavior seems unchanged or even worse, or if it is disrupting the family or his ability to function at school, it is time to seek further help. In the event of certain traumatic situations, such as a divorce or a death in the family, it is beneficial to seek counseling for your child regardless of how he seems to be handling the problem. Group or individual counseling can help your child learn to understand and express his feelings appropriately.

More long-term and complicated emotional and behavioral disorders, such as violence and aggression, drug abuse, depression, developmental disabilities, and learning disabilities, are beyond the scope of this book. Signs of a more serious problem include violent or aggressive behavior; withdrawal from the family; a drastic change in usual behavior; an unwillingness to talk; changes in eating habits; an inability to sleep or sleeping much more than usual; deteriorating school performance; continuous conflict with parents, teachers, or peers; difficulty making friends; and chronic tearfulness or apathy. If you suspect a serious or chronic emotional or behavioral problem, consult your child's teacher, school guidance counselor, or physician. Your child and/or your family may need professional help.

Children need emotional support and guidance throughout their lives as the challenges and tasks they face continue to expand and change. Part of your responsibility as a parent is to stay current and aware of your child's needs so that you can support his emotional health.

Sources of Stress in Your Child's Life

Adults are often inclined to think of childhood as a happy time, free of stresses and concerns. Children's problems may seem minor—perhaps even "cute"—in comparison with their own. Parents should always remember, however, that as far as a child is concerned, the problems of childhood are serious indeed, and that they pose real challenges to a child's emotional resources.

Below is a list of some of the possible sources of stress that may cause emotional upset and resulting behavioral changes in your child. Realizing that these situations can create upset for your child gives you the opportunity to support your child throughout the situation—in preparation for, during, and after the transition or difficulty.

- Death of a close family member.
- Death of a friend.
- Death of a pet.
- Parental fighting.
- Divorce of parents.
- Moving, even if only to a new neighborhood in the same town.
- Best friend moving away.
- Changing schools.
- Pregnancy of mother.
- Birth of a new sibling.
- Parent with a new girlfriend or boyfriend.
- Remarriage of a parent.
- Parent losing a job.

- Financial troubles in the family.
- Illness of a close friend or family member.
- Holidays.
- Bullies at school.
- First day of school.
- Going away to camp.
- Beginning a new grade.
- Spending the night away from home, especially for the first time.
- Fight with a friend.
- Peer pressures, particularly in adolescence with drugs, smoking, drinking, sexuality.
- Threat of war, including the threat of nuclear war.

CONVENTIONAL TREATMENT

■ A family physician, pediatrician, or pediatric nurse practitioner is a good resource for helping parents understand developmental stages and healthy emotional responses. These professionals can provide important information and guidance for facing the challenges that might be coming up in a child's life and helping you to support your child through these transitions. They can also help you sort out the difference between a normal response and behavior that may signal an emotional problem needing further exploration and intervention. A doctor or nurse practitioner can refer the family to a counselor, a learning specialist, or appropriate community resources. Many naturopathic physicians are also extensively trained in counseling.

DIETARY GUIDELINES

■ Limit your child's consumption of foods containing refined sugars and caffeine, both of which can cause mood swings.

Dealing With Temper Tantrums

Alexis Augustine, child therapist and author, offers the following information and advice regarding children's temper tantrums.

A temper tantrum is an outburst or violent demonstration of anger or frustration. Temper tantrums get our attention. The behavior of a child during a temper tantrum can range from crying and sobbing to screaming, shrieking, and throwing himself on the ground. Tantrums can happen in the middle of the grocery store, when you have company over, or when you really need that quiet moment to yourself. The most important thing to understand about temper tantrums is that they happen for different reasons and need to be dealt with in different ways.

There are three basic categories of temper tantrums.

1. Some tantrums occur because small children are unable to contain strong emotions, such as disappointment, frustration, or anger. They are still learning how to cope with their feelings. This type of tantrum can occur when a child gets overtired or overstimulated; children are more vulnerable at these times. Having a tantrum then is a way for a child to discharge the tension that has built up in his body. A child who is having this type of tantrum is *not* using his behavior to manipulate you; he simply cannot contain the strength of his emotions. If this is the case, it is important to maintain contact with the child at this time and help him feel safe. He is out of control, and that can feel scary. Also, children need to learn that they are loved even though their behavior is not always "nice." An effective way to support a child who is having this kind of tantrum is to hold him or sit with him while he is going through it.

2. Another type of tantrum may occur if a child is not allowed to show anger or feelings that occur naturally. Children do not have the control over their emotions that adults have. They naturally have strong feelings, and for the sake of their emotional health they must be allowed to express these feelings and learn from them. When a child is not allowed to say that he is angry, an outburst of bottled-up feelings can be the result.

3. Finally, a child may have a tantrum to try to exert control over a situation or another person, whether that means getting his way about which game to play or postponing his bedtime. Children are in the process of learning about getting their needs met. They need guidance in learning the best, most direct, and most appropriate ways to do this. If having a tantrum seems to work, a child may conclude that it is a viable way to get what he wants. If a child is having this type of tantrum, it is a good idea to acknowledge the child's feelings, but *not* to acquiesce to his demands. For example, if a child has a tantrum when his friends want to play a different game than he does, you might tell the child you understand that he wants to play something else, but then have him move to a safe place to have his tantrum. When he's finished, have him come back to join in playing. This way, he will realize that having a tantrum is a waste of time; he isn't getting what he wants, and besides, everyone else is having fun without him. A child having this type of tantrum is testing the limits on his behavior. A firm but matter-of-fact response is an effective way to deal with it.

When dealing with a child's temper tantrum, keep the following points in mind.

- Children need help in learning effective coping strategies.

- Children need to learn a variety of ways of coping, so that they don't have to rely on just one. If they know only one coping mechanism, and that one doesn't fit the situation they're in, they won't know what to do.

- Shaming or embarrassing children for their behavior undermines their confidence.

- Talking with children about their behavior is more effective once everyone has calmed down.

- Self-regulation is age related. Children get better at it as they get older. It helps to have patience.

■ Food allergies and sensitivities can cause or contribute to mental and emotional difficulties such as anxiety, depression, hyperactivity, irritability, and difficulty concentrating. Use an elimination diet or a food diary to track down food allergies and sensitivities (*see* ELIMINATION DIET in Part Three).

HERBAL TREATMENT

For age-appropriate dosages of herbal remedies, see page 81.

■ Chamomile tea helps calm and ease stress and tension. Give your child one dose of tea as needed.

■ Oat straw is nourishing and calming to the nervous system. This herb is helpful for a child who is dealing with stressful emotions over an extended period of time. Give your child one dose of oat straw tea, twice a day, as needed.

■ Skullcap is helpful for nervousness and anxiety and the headaches that often follow. Give your child one dose daily for up to two weeks.
Note: This herb should not be given to a child less than six years old.

HOMEOPATHY

When your child is distressed, the appropriate symptom-specific homeopathic remedy will likely be very helpful. Choose the remedy that matches your child's symptoms from the list that follows. Unless otherwise indicated, give your child one dose, three times a day, for up to five days.

■ Give *Aconite* to a child who is fearful and anxious, especially if the feeling came on suddenly. This child may be very restless and sensitive to noise, smell, and touch. He feels better outdoors and worse in a warm, closed room. Give one dose of *Aconite* 200x when needed.

■ *Arsenicum album* 30x or 9c will ease a child who acts restless and fussy and is afraid of being alone. This child may obsessively organize his room when feeling insecure.

■ *Chamomilla* 30x or 9c is good for an angry child who is upset, who insists on being held, and whose temper flares when you put him down.

■ *Cina* is for the angry, contrary, and ill-tempered child who does not want to be touched or hugged. This is the type of child who will ask for a toy and then toss it away in front of your nose. (He may pick his own nose constantly as well.)

■ *Colocynthis* 30x or 9c is helpful for a child who complains of a stomachache after being angry.

■ *Ignatia* 30x or 9c is especially helpful after a loss, emotional trauma, or disappointment. Grief associated with the death of a parent or grandparent, breaking up with a boyfriend or girlfriend, or moving to a new town will be eased by *Ignatia*. It is helpful for a child who is quiet and tearful. This is a child who sighs a lot.

■ *Lycopodium* 30x or 9c is for a child who gets angry as a result of his insecurity. This is helpful for the angry child living in a home filled with feelings of uncertainty. *Lycopodium* is also useful for a child who experiences fear and anxiety in any new situation. It is good for situations involving a performance, such as getting up in front of the class or trying a new sport or game.

■ Give *Natrum muriaticum* 30x or 9c to a sad child who dwells on morbid ideas in the home or in the news, rejects sympathy, is sensitive, and does not like being fussed over.

■ If a child is critical, has feelings of superiority, experiences outbursts of anger, and is short-tempered, give him *Nux vomica* 30x or 9c.

■ *Phosphorus* 30x or 9c is for the fearful, extremely sensitive child who develops feelings of anxiety over what others may be thinking or feeling about him.

■ *Pulsatilla* 30x or 9c is good for a child who is timid, sensitive, and easily frightened, and who cries easily. *Pulsatilla* is homeopathic windflower, and it is beneficial for the child whose moods change like the wind.

■ If your child voices a particular recurrent or outstanding fear, an appropriate homeopathic remedy may be very helpful. Try giving your child one dose of a remedy (use a 30x or 15c potency), three times a day, for three days. Discontinue for one week and repeat. If this seems to have a beneficial effect, wait one month and repeat the entire cycle.

The following are some remedies that may be useful to investigate for this purpose:

- For fear of aliens, try *Phosphorus* or *Arsenicum album*.
- For fear of the dark, try *Calcarea carbonica*, *Lycopodium*, or *Stramonium*.
- For fear of death, try *Calcarea carbonica*, *Arsenicum album*, *Lycopodium*, or *Phosphorus*.
- For fear of being eaten by animals, try *Stramonium*.
- For fear of insects, try *Calcarea carbonica*.
- For fear upon closing one's eyes, try *Causticum*.
- For fear of crowds, try *Lycopodium*, *Argentum nitricum*, or *Aconite*.
- For fear of going to church, try *Argentum nitricum*.
- For fear of knives, try *Arsenicum album*, *Alumina*, or *China*.
- For fear of cockroaches, try *Phosphorus*.
- For fear of doctors, try *Ignatia* or *Phosphorus*.
- For fear of dogs, try *Calcarea carbonica*, *Belladonna*, *China*, or *Tuberculinum*.
- For fear of high places, try *Argentum nitricum*, *Natrum muriaticum*, *Phosphorus*, or *Pulsatilla*.
- For fear of water, try *Lyssin*.
- For fear of everything, try *Calcarea carbonica* or *Pulsatilla*.

■ If your child's moods are extreme and highly changeable, a constitutional remedy prescribed by a homeopath may be helpful in easing and balancing emotional swings and patterns.

BACH FLOWER REMEDIES

■ Bach Flower Rescue Remedy helps to calm a child, restore his balance and confidence, and relieve apprehension. It will help a child who is upset, whether angry, crying, afraid, or tense. It is useful in many crisis situations, such as after hearing bad news, before a test, before going to the dentist, after falling and getting hurt, or upon waking up from a nightmare. Rescue Remedy is particularly good in acute situations in which the cause of the distress is not always clear—times when a child begins screaming and crying and feeling intensely and inconsolably frustrated for no apparent reason. Place a drop of the mother tincture into a small glass of noncarbonated water and have your child sip it. Ask him to swish the mixture around in his mouth before swallowing. Or mix 3 drops of the mother tincture with 2 ounces of water and give your child 2 droppersful, or 1 teaspoon, three times a day.

■ There are two Bach Flower remedies that are standards for the fearful child. If your child has fears but cannot name what they are about, give him Aspen. If he can name the source of his fear, use Mimulus.

■ Other individual Bach Flower Remedies are helpful for easing specific emotional upsets or balancing certain temperaments. To select the remedy that is most appropriate for your child's situation, *see* BACH FLOWER REMEDIES in Part One.

ACUPRESSURE

For the locations of acupressure points on a child's body, see ADMINISTERING AN ACUPRESSURE TREATMENT in Part Three.

■ Four Gates is calming and soothing to a child who is upset.

■ Neck and Shoulder Release helps release tension centered in the head, neck, and shoulder area, and will help relax your child.

GENERAL RECOMMENDATIONS

■ Make your family's emotional and physical well-being a priority. Part of that commitment is to realize that you have physical, emotional, and spiritual needs of your own that must be nurtured and cared for.

■ When you notice yourself having a strong response to your child's sadness, anger, or fear, try to explore what this can teach you about your own emotions. In *The Tao of Motherhood* (Nucleus Publishers, 1991), Vimala McClure, founder of the International Association of Infant Massage Instructors, writes, "Parenting is a spiritual path which can bring you great pain and great joy and which can have a tremendous positive impact on your personality and behavior. I believe our children, unknowingly and with innocent trickery, teach us the deeper knowledge of how to be a true human being."

■ Help your child acknowledge and name feelings. For instance, you might say, "You sound angry that your sister took your favorite toy without asking," or, "I hear your frustration about losing that game."

■ Help your child name his deeper emotional needs, and offer suggestions about how he might be able to get what he wants. What your child expresses as anger may actually be a need for your attention, for example. Once you are able to determine this, you may be able to meet that need by spending an afternoon together or having breakfast together each morning. A child who is unwilling to go to bed on time may really be afraid of the dark, something that might be relieved by a night-light or a bedtime story.

■ Put yourself in the child's place. Try to "get inside" his mind and inner world. Feel how big and scary the adult world must be at times. Imagine how hard it must be to try to explain feelings you don't have the words for or perhaps don't even understand yet. Situations that we take for granted as adults may be overwhelming and difficult for a child. Imagine the guidance and support he needs. Putting yourself in your child's place can help you to understand and guide him in a way that is supportive.

■ Help your child develop constructive ways of handling strong feelings, and, if possible, to express his feelings and wants to the specific person involved. Or, if the person is not available and the frustration is unbearable, teach your child to punch a pillow or yell at a doll and take out his anger in a way that is safe and healthy. Teach children to be respectful of themselves and of those around them. Acting out and yelling at a person or hitting a person are not acceptable behaviors. (For suggestions on how to deal with unacceptable behavior, *see* TIME-OUT in Part Three.)

■ Be clear and, above all, *consistent* in establishing guidelines and agreements.

■ Be a role model for your child. Handle your own feelings by being truthful about them and constructive and safe in how you deal with them. It is far better to say, "I am angry about my friend missing our appointment," than it is to say you feel fine while your behavior and the tone of your voice say something else. Children are confused by mixed messages. They are likely to assume that you are angry at them, as well as to learn that it is not okay to express feelings.

■ Supporting a child's emotional well-being is a responsibility parents face over many years. It requires a lot of attention. There are parent support groups, parent training opportunities, and workshops for children that help develop healthy self-esteem and healthy family dynamics. Whether or not you are facing a specific stress or emotional problem in your family, these workshops and groups can help promote emotional health for the whole family.

Epilepsy

Epilepsy is a chronic seizure disorder that affects approximately 1 to 2 percent of children in the United States. A seizure is caused by excessive and chaotic firing of *neurons* (brain cells), resulting in a sudden and temporary change in brain function. Seizures vary in severity, from a slight change in consciousness, tingling or numbness in the limbs, and apparent clumsiness, to severe, rigid, and spastic muscle jerking and loss of consciousness. Twitching, weakness, a feeling of warmth, confusion, staring, garbled speech, vomiting, or a shrill cry may be part of a seizure.

Many children experience a seizure as a result of a high fever associated with an otherwise uncomplicated viral illness such as the flu. Most of these children never have another episode and do not require long-term medication (*see* FEVER). A child with epilepsy, however, experiences chronic seizures that may be brought on by a variety of things, including fever, illness, lack of sleep, low blood sugar, certain drugs, flashing lights, and/or loud noises. Some children experience abdominal pain, nausea, dizziness, shakiness, fear, or changes in vision or hearing right before the onset of a seizure.

Although a seizure generally stops and resolves itself on its own, it is essential to stay with your child when she is having a seizure to keep her safe and to ensure that the situation resolves itself. After a seizure, it is common for a child to be sleepy and somewhat confused. She may or may not remember the episode.

It is important to consult a pediatric neurologist when treating a child who has epilepsy. In addition, herbs, homeopathy, acupressure, dietary modifications, and nutritional supplements may be helpful in alleviating symptoms. Because your child and her response to her disease are unique, it is best to seek out and work with knowledgeable and experienced health care practitioners rather than attempting to manage this illness on your own. We advise you to choose a medical doctor who is willing to work with a natural health care practitioner (and vice versa). Each of these professionals will need to know what the other is doing, as the interventions of one may affect the treatments of the other.

CONVENTIONAL TREATMENT

■ Diagnosis of epilepsy is based on the history of the illness, a description of the seizure episodes, a neurological examination, and certain blood tests. An electroencephalogram (EEG) is done to look for signs of abnormal activity in the brain. If there are signs of possible neurological damage, a magnetic resonance imaging (MRI) scan of the brain may be performed.

■ Treatment for epilepsy focuses on using medication to prevent the recurrence of seizures. The most commonly used anticonvulsant medications include phenobarbital; phenytoin (Dilantin); primidone (Mysoline); carbamazepine (Tegretol); divalproex sodium (Depakote); valproic acid (Depakene); ethosuximide (Zarontin); and clonazepam (Klonopin). Which medication is prescribed for your child will probably be determined by her age, the particular symptoms she experiences while having a seizure, and other factors. Generally, a child begins by taking a relatively low dose of seizure medication. The dosage is then gradually increased until the seizures are under control. Anticonvulsant medications can have significant side effects, including drowsiness, irritability, nausea, suppressed immune function, and liver damage. One seizure drug, Dilantin, can cause an overgrowth of gum tissue in children. If your child must take this drug, careful tooth-brushing and regular visits to the dentist are especially important. With all of these drugs, it is critical that blood levels of the drugs and specific blood tests be monitored, and follow-up appointments with your doctor kept, so that the best seizure control can be maintained with the fewest side effects.

■ In some cases, a physician may recommend a specific diet based on low but adequate amounts of protein, high levels of fats, low carbohydrates, and vitamin supplements to help control seizure activity. However, this diet is otherwise not very healthy. It should be used only when other approaches have failed.

■ In extremely rare cases, surgery may be recommended. This is reserved for cases where medication has not helped and a specialized test such as an MRI scan shows a lesion or tumor in the brain that may be causing the seizures.

NUTRITIONAL SUPPLEMENTS

For age-appropriate dosages of nutritional supplements, see page 81.

■ Magnesium has a beneficial effect on the nervous system. Give your child one dose of magnesium at bedtime.

EMERGENCY TREATMENT FOR A SEIZURE

If your child has a seizure, do the following:

✚ If this is your child's first seizure, call your doctor or get emergency help immediately.

✚ Stay with your child while she is having a seizure. Talk reassuringly to her.

✚ Watch closely for changes in breathing and color. Be sure your child's airway stays open.

✚ Clear the area around your child to prevent injury. Move back tables, chairs, or anything else your child could knock into. *Do not* try to hold her down. Restraining a child who is having a seizure can cause additional injury.

✚ *Do not* try to force anything into your child's mouth or hold down her tongue. You might cause choking or be bitten. To prevent the possibility of her choking on inhaled vomit, keep her head turned toward the side or roll her onto her side.

✚ Try placing a soft pillow or blanket under your child's head. If possible, loosen clothing to prevent injury and ease discomfort.

✚ If the seizure lasts longer than ten minutes, or if your child is having difficulty breathing, or if she is turning blue or hurting herself, call for emergency help.

■ The B-complex vitamins are crucial to healthy functioning of the central nervous system. Give your child one dose of a B-complex supplement daily.

■ Taurine is an amino acid found in eggs, fish, meat, and milk, as well as in supplement form. It has been shown in some studies to help anticonvulsant medications work more effectively, so that a lower dose of the drug may successfully control seizures. This is a complex interaction, however, so you should seek out a nutritionally oriented physician to help determine the dosage.

■ Dimethylglycine, sometimes called pangamic acid or vitamin B15 (although technically it is not a vitamin), has been reported to help reduce the frequency of seizures in people with chronic seizure disorders. Discuss this with your child's doctor.

■ The initial medical evaluation of your child should include a thorough investigation of possible nutritional deficiencies, especially deficiencies of zinc and manganese, both of which have been found to be low in patients with epilepsy.

HERBAL TREATMENT

For age-appropriate dosages of herbal remedies, see page 81.

■ Milk thistle helps detoxify the liver and can be helpful in avoiding side effects or damage from anticonvulsant medication.

■ Minor bupleurum helps to calm and strengthen the nervous system. Give your child one dose, twice a day, for three months of the year (one month each in winter, spring, and fall).

Note: Minor bupleurum should not be given to a child who has a fever or any other sign of an acute infection.

HOMEOPATHY

■ If your child has epilepsy, working with a homeopath to find a constitutional remedy for your child can be very beneficial in easing symptoms and strengthening her overall health.

■ *Cicuta virosa* 12x or 6c may be used immediately following a seizure. Give your child one dose, every five minutes, for a total of three doses.

GENERAL RECOMMENDATIONS

■ Make certain that food allergies or sensitivities are not triggering your child's seizures. Keep a diet diary and use an elimination diet if you suspect certain foods may be implicated (see ELIMINATION DIET in Part Three).

■ If your child is diagnosed as having epilepsy, be certain you understand how to administer her medication and what to do in case she experiences a seizure. Ask questions of your doctor until you feel confident in your knowledge. Follow your doctor's instructions exactly.

■ Obtain a Medic Alert bracelet or necklace and make sure your child wears it so that others will be alerted to her illness, if necessary. For information, you can write to Medic Alert at 2323 Colorado Avenue, Turlock, CA 95380; or call them at 800–432–5378.

■ Meet with your child's teachers to explain her illness, what factors may precipitate a seizure, and what to do in case of a seizure.

■ Parents of children with epilepsy are often concerned with issues surrounding the child's emotional and social development. In fact, many parents want more information about this than about managing the medical situation. Self-esteem issues can be particularly challenging for a child with epilepsy. The seizures may make her feel out of control, embarrassed, or abnormal in comparison to peers. Adolescents may have an especially difficult time as they face concerns about obtaining a job or a driver's license. Help your child to live as normal a life as possible, and try not to let your natural concern for your child turn into overprotectiveness. Seek information from nurses, child psychologists, social workers, and support groups. The Epilepsy Foundation of America is one source of information. Their address is 4351 Garden City Drive, Landover, MD 29785.

PREVENTION

■ The underlying cause or causes of the majority of cases of epilepsy are unknown, so for the most part it is not possible to prevent the disease in the true sense of that word. However, individual seizures can be triggered by a variety of physical and environmental factors. In addition to following the course of treatment recommended by your doctor, be aware of those things that seem to have set off seizures in your child in the past and help her to avoid them, much as you would identify and avoid substances that cause allergic reactions.

■ Some cases of seizure disorder are the result of trauma to the head. Take measures to protect your child from head injuries. Never toss a child, even in play, and never punish a child by shaking her. Have your child wear a helmet when engaging in such activities as bicycle or horseback riding, skiing, or playing sports like football or hockey. For ways to reduce the possibility that your child will suffer a head injury at home, *see* HOME SAFETY in Part One.

Fainting

Fainting—medically termed *syncope* (sing'-ka-pee)—is a sudden and temporary loss of consciousness that occurs as a result of a lack of blood flow to the brain. There are a number of things that can cause this to occur, including a sudden drop in blood pressure, anemia, epilepsy, extreme heat, breath-holding and hyperventilation, hunger, and hypoglycemia. Standing for a long time in a hot, stuffy room, exhaustion, emotional upset, fear, or fever may also cause a child to faint.

In the moments before a fainting episode, a child may experience dizziness, weakness, and a feeling of numbness in the hands or feet; he may suddenly turn pale and his skin may feel cold. Upon awakening, he may feel tired and develop a headache.

If a child loses consciousness apparently due to one of the factors listed above and makes a complete recovery within fifteen minutes, it is likely that he has experienced a fainting episode. A child who has fainted will usually awaken fairly readily, especially if you use smelling salts, and will be aware and oriented upon awakening.

If you find a child unconscious and have not actually seen him faint, or if he regained consciousness with difficulty and is disoriented, it is possible that he has a more serious problem. Turn to UNCONSCIOUSNESS *on page 404.*

EMERGENCY TREATMENT FOR FAINTING

See the inset on page 230.

Emergency Treatment for Fainting

✚ If you see your child lose consciousness, take the following measures immediately.

1. Check for pulse and breathing. *If pulse and/or breathing are absent, or if either stops at any time during the episode, turn to* CARDIOPULMONARY RESUSCITATION *on page 426.* Begin taking the appropriate measures at once.

2. If the child is breathing and his heart rate seems to be fine, check for signs of injury. If the child is unknown to you, look to see if he is wearing a Medic Alert bracelet that offers an explanation for the episode, such as a history of diabetes or epilepsy.

3. If there are no signs of injury, try the following, in order, to provoke a response:

    *   Call the child's name.

    *   Pat his face gently.

    *   Wave smelling salts under his nose. If smelling salts are not readily available, try using an open bottle of perfume.

    *   Apply acupressure to Gallbladder 21 (see illustration, right).

    *   *Do not* splash cold water on your child's face. *Do not* shake your child.

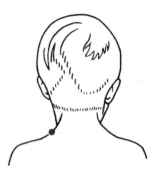

Acupressure Point
Gallbladder 21

4. If the child is still limp and unresponsive, lay him flat with his feet elevated, or head lowered, to a 45-degree angle if possible. This will increase the flow of blood to the brain. Loosen his clothing. Place him in the recovery position as follows: Roll his body as a unit (without twisting the torso) onto one side. Place his lower arm behind his back and pull the top knee up and forward slightly so that it rests on the ground. Place the upper arm under his head, which should be turned to the side (see illustration, below). This position ensures that if vomiting occurs, the child's airway will not be obstructed. Cover him with a blanket or sweater so that he stays warm. Stay with your child and continue to monitor his pulse and breathing.

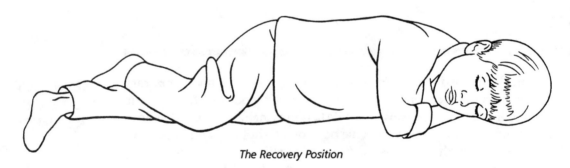

The Recovery Position

5. If he does not regain consciousness within two or three minutes, or if his pulse or breathing becomes weaker, call for emergency help.

✚ Once the child regains consciousness, help him up into a sitting position. Have him lean forward, with his head between his knees, to increase circulation to the brain.

✚ Have your child lie still for an additional ten to fifteen minutes after he has recovered from the episode, to be sure he is stable enough to walk.

✚ Call your doctor and explain the situation. A child who has experienced a fainting episode should be examined by a physician.

CONVENTIONAL TREATMENT

■ If your child faints, follow the procedure outlined under Emergency Treatment for Fainting (see inset, page 230).

■ Once your child recovers and his condition is stable, call your doctor and explain the situation. Your doctor will want to examine your child so that the cause of the problem can be determined and, if appropriate, treated. Your doctor may order blood tests, a chest x-ray, an electrocardiogram, an electroencephalogram, or other tests to see if there is any underlying health problem that may have caused your child to faint. Treatment recommendations, if any, will depend on the results of your doctor's evaluation.

DIETARY GUIDELINES

■ If you suspect low blood sugar (hypoglycemia) as the cause of your child's fainting, give him a glass of fruit juice or sweetened tea as soon as he can swallow.

HERBAL TREATMENT

For age-appropriate dosages of herbal remedies, see page 81.

■ Once your child regains consciousness, give him one dose of ginger and/or licorice tea to help increase circulation.

HOMEOPATHY

■ Give your child one dose of *Aconite* 30x or 9c as soon as he awakens to help ease the shock from fainting. Then follow the *Aconite* with one dose of one of the following symptom-specific remedies, every ten minutes, until your child feels better, up to a total of three doses.

- If the fainting episode was related to exhaustion and weakness, choose *China* 30x or 9c.

- If the fainting episode was due to emotional upset or nervousness, perhaps even bordering on hysteria, choose *Ignatia* 30x or 9c.

- If the fainting occurred as a result of extreme pain, choose *Chamomilla* 30x or 9c.

- For fainting that occurred indoors in a stuffy room, use *Pulsatilla* 30x or 9c.

BACH FLOWER REMEDIES

■ After a fainting episode, put a few drops of Bach Flower Rescue Remedy in a glass of water and have your child sip it throughout the day. (See BACH FLOWER REMEDIES in Part One.)

■ If your child fainted due to fear, give him one dose of Bach Flower Mimulus.

ACUPRESSURE

For the locations of acupressure points on a child's body, *see* ADMINISTERING AN ACUPRESSURE TREATMENT in Part Three.

■ If your child awakens with a headache, apply pressure to Large Intestine 4. This acupressure point relaxes tension in the head.

■ Four Gates helps to relax and reestablish equilibrium throughout the body.

PREVENTION

■ If your child starts to feel dizzy and faint, or shows any of the other signs that a fainting episode may be coming on, have him sit down immediately, leaning forward, with his head lowered between his legs. Encourage him to give a few deep coughs. This will increase the blood flow to the brain. Applying pressure to the acupressure point called Governing Vessel 21, located directly under the nose, can prevent a faint if done immediately (see margin illustration).

■ If your child has low blood pressure that sometimes causes momentary dizziness, teach him to go from lying down to sitting to standing slowly and gradually.

■ Avoid situations and circumstances that are conducive to fainting, such as warm, stuffy rooms, standing for too long, overexertion and exhaustion, or anything else that has been associated with fainting spells in the past. If your child becomes faint in response to his emotions, such as fear or anxiety, try teaching him relaxation or visualization techniques to help him deal with powerful feelings. Sometimes just learning to breathe regularly, deeply, and consciously is all a child needs to keep his emotions from overpowering his body. (*See* RELAXATION TECHNIQUES in Part Three.)

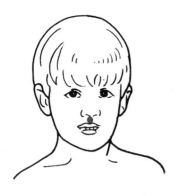

Governing Vessel 21

Applying pressure to this point at the first sign that a child is feeling faint can sometimes prevent a fainting episode.

Fatigue

Every child develops a sleep/wake cycle that gives her enough energy to learn, stay awake in school, participate in sports or after-school activities, and keep up with friends. A child who is unable to keep up with her daily activities because of fatigue, or who begins sleeping more than usual, deserves attention. While all children get "run down" from time to time, any fatigue that lasts longer than two or three weeks indicates a problem. The problem may be an unhealthy lifestyle, emotional distress, or an underlying illness. Fatigue can be the earliest sign of an illness and may appear before other symptoms, or even before a blood test or other diagnostic tool indicates that something is wrong.

Excessive fatigue can be a symptom of anemia, leukemia, and many bacterial and viral infections. Chronic fatigue syndrome is also a possibility. This syndrome is now recognized as a pediatric illness, albeit a rare one. Because there is a possibility that fatigue may be caused by an underlying illness, a child who is unusually tired should be examined by a doctor.

Excessive fatigue can also be a sign of depression. Stress in the household or at school can create emotional upset that a child may not be able to express. Instead, a child on the edge of depression will often "escape" into sleep.

CONVENTIONAL TREATMENT

■ A doctor may do a physical examination and blood tests to rule out hypothyroidism, diabetes, anemia, allergies, leukemia, or a viral or bacterial infection. Medical science is often unable to identify the cause of fatigue. If a serious underlying condition is ruled out, this is the perfect time to use natural remedies.

DIETARY GUIDELINES

■ Excessive fatigue can often be traced to diet. Give your child a wholesome, whole-foods diet based on fresh vegetables, fruits, grains, and lean proteins. Avoid processed foods and sugar. Reduce your child's intake of fat, and eliminate caffeine- and sugar-laden soft drinks. Be sure your child is eating adequate amounts of protein.

■ Use an elimination diet or diet diary to check for food allergies and sensitivities. Unsuspected food allergies can be a drain on your child's system. (*See* ELIMINATION DIET in Part Three.)

NUTRITIONAL SUPPLEMENTS

For age-appropriate dosages of nutritional supplements, see page 81.

■ Chlorophyll is filled with magnesium and other micronutrients that help to build up the blood. Give your child a chlorophyll supplement, following the dosage directions on the product label, for one month. Then discontinue the supplement for one month. Repeat this cycle three times (a total of six months).

■ Floradix, a plant-based iron supplement, may help ease fatigue related to iron deficiency. Follow the dosage directions on the product label and give it to your child for one month, then stop for one month. Repeat this cycle three times (a total of six months).

■ Green drink products, such as Green Magma and Green Essence, available in health food stores, provide many enzymes, proteins, vitamins, minerals, and other nutrients that may be helpful in eliminating fatigue related to nutritional deficiency. Follow the dosage directions on the product label for one to two months.

■ A vitamin-B complex supplement may be helpful in resolving fatigue that is caused by poor diet. Select a balanced liquid formula that contains 25 milligrams of each B vitamin per dose. Follow dosage directions on the product label for three weeks to one month.

■ Vitamin C can help with fatigue, especially if it is related to iron deficiency. Vitamin C enhances the absorption of iron. Give your child one dose of vitamin C daily for one month.

■ Try giving your child a multiple vitamin each day to help resolve any possible vitamin deficiencies that may be contributing to her fatigue.

HERBAL TREATMENT

For age-appropriate dosages of herbal remedies, see page 81.

■ Both American and Siberian ginseng contain micronutrients and trace minerals that help strengthen the overall constitution. Give a child over six years of age 10 drops of either, once daily, five times a week, for six weeks. Stop for one week, then resume giving 10 drops, once daily, five times a week, for another six weeks.

■ Echinacea and goldenseal help to treat lingering fatigue and weakness after an infection. Give your child one dose of a liquid echinacea and goldenseal combination formula, three times a day, for one week.

Note: You should not give your child echinacea on a daily basis for more than ten days at a time, or it will lose its effectiveness.

■ Licorice root helps to support the adrenal glands and ease fatigue. Give your child one dose, twice a day, for two weeks.

Note: This herb should not be given to a child with high blood pressure.

GENERAL RECOMMENDATIONS

■ Serve a healthy, whole-foods diet. Check for hidden food allergies that may be causing a drain on your child's system and eliminate suspect foods from her diet.

■ Give your child American or Siberian ginseng and nutritional supplements.

■ Maintain a regular sleep cycle. Awaken your child at the same time every day and set a regular bedtime. Support your child's need to rest when she is tired and cranky. Sleep requirements vary from one child to another. A newborn may sleep anywhere from ten to twenty-two hours a day, although the average is about sixteen hours. Most toddlers (children about eighteen months to four years) need twelve to fourteen hours of sleep, including naps. Children four to eight years old usually need about twelve hours of sleep a night. Four- to six-year-olds may also need a nap or rest time every once in a while to help them recharge. Eight- to twelve-year-olds usually need ten to eleven hours of sleep each night. A bedtime of 8:00 or 9:00 P.M. generally works well for them. And teenagers—they love to sleep! Many would stay in bed all morning if they could. And there is some evidence that sleep requirements do in fact increase in adolescence, so that a teenager may need as much sleep as a toddler does. This is probably related to the rapid rate of growth and development in those years. Help your child to take responsibility for her own sleep. Be sure that she learns to go to bed early enough to ensure that she has enough energy for the day, let her learn the consequences of her actions, and teach her about alarm clocks.

PREVENTION

■ The best way to prevent fatigue from developing is to ensure that the diet includes healthy, whole foods that provide a full range of necessary nutrients, that your child gets regular exercise, and that you follow a consistent sleep schedule, with exceptions only on special occasions. Also, make sure your child has enough time to unwind before going to bed.

■ Stress and anxiety can cause fatigue. When there are stressful problems in your household, explain them to your child calmly. A child who feels the stress but is not told the truth about what is going on will make up her own explanations, which may be more frightening or upsetting than what is really happening. Also, a child will often assume that a problem is her fault. When talking to your child, be loving, honest, and reassuring. (*See* EMOTIONAL UPSET.)

Fever

Fever has been defined as a body temperature elevated to at least 1°F above 98.6°F (37.0°C). Actually, a child's temperature normally varies by as much as 2°F, depending on his level of activity, emotional stress, the amount of clothing worn, the time of day, and the temperature of the environment, among other factors. When taken by mouth, a child's body temperature is usually between 96.8° and 99.4°F.

A fever can be caused by a wide variety of things, including dehydration, overexertion, mosquito bites, bee stings, an allergic or toxic reaction, or a viral or bacterial infection. Fever of unknown origin (FUO) is a condition defined as an elevated temperature lasting for a week or more without an identifiable cause.

In most cases, a fever is the body's reaction to an acute viral or bacterial infection. It is not necessarily a dangerous condition. Rather, it is a sign that the body is defending itself against the infectious invader. Since viruses and bacteria do not survive as well in a body with an elevated temperature, fever is actually an ally in fighting infection. It is one of the ways in which the body defends and heals itself. An elevated temperature also increases the production of infection-fighting white blood cells and even increases their speed of response and enhances their killing capacity.

In an adult, the level of fever generally reflects the severity of the illness causing it. In a child, however, this is not necessarily the case. A child with a mild cold may have a 105°F fever, while a child with a serious illness—bacterial pneumonia, for example—may have only a 100°F fever.

In a newborn, the body's temperature control is not yet well developed. As a result, signs other than a fever—poor appetite, lethargy, and irritability—may be earlier indicators of an infection and therefore more helpful than temperature in assessing your newborn's condition. However, when a newborn has a persistently elevated (or low) temperature, he should be examined by a doctor.

When assessing your child's condition, the most important thing to do is to observe how your child is acting. How sick does your child seem to you? A child with a fever may be pale or flushed, feel hot to the touch, and have dry or sweaty skin. He may feel restless, achy, unable to sleep, and unwilling to eat. Be aware of other symptoms that accompany your child's fever. If a feverish child has red spots on his skin, a runny nose, and eyes that are red and perhaps more sensitive to light than usual, he may be getting measles (*see* MEASLES). If a child has a fever and red, itchy spots on his body, he may be coming down with chickenpox (*see* CHICKENPOX). A baby with a fever in combination with a reddish-pink rash and swollen glands in his neck may have roseola (*see* ROSEOLA).

If your child has a slight fever, no intervention may be necessary. Unless your child's temperature is higher than 102°F, fever-reducing medication is generally not needed. However, a child with an elevated temperature may be very uncomfortable. A feverish child typically doesn't rest or desire food. His whole body aches. A fever raises the child's overall metabolic rate. When his metabolism is racing, your child can easily lose weight and body fluids. Gently bringing a fever down can not only help your child feel better, but can also help to prevent complications, such as dehydration.

Bringing down a fever can also help indicate the severity of your child's illness and aid in diagnosis. With a temperature of 103°F or more, a child will look and feel terrible, whether the fever is caused by a cold or a serious infection. After the fever is brought down, the child with a cold will look and feel noticeably better—a strong indication that it was the fever itself that was causing the child to look and feel ill—whereas the child with a serious infection will continue to look and feel sick, even with a lower temperature.

In some cases, a feverish child may have what is called a febrile seizure. Febrile seizures, which occur in a very small percentage of children, are frightening to see. They do not seem to be related to the height of the fever, or to the rapidity

EMERGENCY TREATMENT FOR A FEBRILE SEIZURE

Occasionally, a child with a fever will have a seizure. This is called a febrile seizure, and it demands immediate attention.

✚ If your child has a febrile seizure, he needs to see a doctor *immediately*—not tomorrow morning. Call for emergency help.

✚ While waiting for emergency help, keep your child upright and make sure he is breathing well. Stay with him and talk reassuringly to him.

✚ Watch for changes in your child's breathing and/or color. Be sure his airway stays open.

✚ Clear the area around your child to prevent injury. Do not try to hold him down. Restraining a thrashing child can cause additional injury. Try placing a soft pillow or blanket under your child's head. Loosen clothing to prevent injury and ease discomfort.

✚ *Do not* try to force anything into your child's mouth. You might cause him to choke, or suffer a bite yourself.

✚ If vomiting occurs, turn your child's head to the side so that there is no risk of his choking on inhaled vomit. If possible, keep his whole body turned on the side as well.

with which it rises, but rather to the idiosyncratic predisposition of certain children. About 50 percent of the children who suffer one febrile seizure will go on to have another one. About 33 percent will have a third one. If your child experiences a febrile seizure, there is a good chance that he could have another.

Although seeing your child experience a seizure is distressing, there is no evidence that febrile seizures cause any permanent harm, nor that this type of convulsion leads to epilepsy or any other seizure disorder. However, if your child has a febrile seizure, it is important to have your doctor examine him to rule out any underlying condition and discuss what to do to prevent a recurrence.

Some children run a fever after a day at an amusement park. Others develop a fever only in response to a serious illness. Your observation of your child's overall condition is the best indicator of its severity. If you are uneasy about your child's condition, call your health care provider for advice.

CONVENTIONAL TREATMENT

■ Acetaminophen (found in Tylenol, Tempra, and other over-the-counter medications) is a drug that helps to lower fever. Acetaminophen is also an analgesic, so it eases the discomfort and body aches that accompany a fever. It is available in liquid or pill form, as well as in suppository form for infants.

Note: In excessive amounts, this drug can cause liver damage. Be careful not to exceed the correct dosage for your child's age and size.

■ Ibuprofen (Advil, Nuprin, and others) is another fever-reducing medication that relieves mild to moderate aches and pains. When giving your child ibuprofen, be sure to give it with food to prevent an upset stomach. Ibuprofen is available in liquid or pill form. Follow dosage directions on the product label.

■ *Do not* give aspirin to a child with a fever. Many fevers are caused by viral infections, and the combination of aspirin and viral illness has been linked to the development of Reye's syndrome, a progressive and very dangerous liver disease (*see* REYE'S SYNDROME).

DIETARY GUIDELINES

■ Generous amounts of fluids are essential to prevent dehydration. Keep a feverish child well hydrated. Offer fruit-juice popsicles, spring water, herbal teas, soups, and diluted fruit juices.

NUTRITIONAL SUPPLEMENTS

For age-appropriate dosages of nutritional supplements, see page 81.

■ Vitamin C has anti-inflammatory properties and is helpful in resolving a fever associated with a minor infection. Select powdered mineral ascorbate vitamin C with bioflavonoids. For a child six years of age or older, give one dose, every two hours, for a total of four doses.

HERBAL TREATMENT

For age-appropriate dosages of herbal remedies, see page 81.

■ Brew a fever-reducing herbal tea to help decrease chills and increase perspiration.

WHEN TO CALL THE DOCTOR ABOUT A FEVER

There are certain situations in which you should always seek a doctor's advice concerning a child with a fever:

• If your child is under six months of age.

• If your child is between six months and three years old and has a temperature of 102°F or higher.

• If your child is over three years old and has a fever of 104°F or higher that does not respond to normal fever control measures within four hours.

• No matter what your child's age, if he is listless, lethargic, unusually sleepy, in pain, or extremely irritable, or if he complains of a stiff neck, is having difficulty breathing, or has a significant decrease in urine output, or if he just doesn't seem right to you.

Use equal parts of some or all of the following: lemon balm leaf, chamomile flower, peppermint leaf, licorice root, and elder flower. Lemon balm and elder flower are soothing and promote perspiration; chamomile calms and relaxes; peppermint cools a fever; licorice sweetens the tea and enhances the effects of the other herbs. To improve the flavor, you can sweeten the tea with a bit of honey. If you are using peppermint in the tea and also giving your child a homeopathic preparation, allow one hour both before and after administering the homeopathic and giving this tea. Give a child over two years of age ½ cup of tea, four times daily, for one day. For a breastfed baby, a nursing mother can take 1 cup, four times daily, for one day; the healing properties of the tea will be passed to her baby in her breast milk. The tea should be taken as hot as possible.

Caution: Never give tea with honey in it to a child less than one year old. Honey has been associated with infant botulism, which can be life threatening.

■ To help clear a possible underlying infection, give your child an echinacea and goldenseal combination formula. The immune-boosting effects of these herbs are well documented, and both of them have infection-fighting properties as well. Give your child one dose, every two hours, for eight hours. Then give him one dose, three times daily, for one week.

Note: You should not give your child echinacea on a daily basis for more than ten days at a time, or it will lose its effectiveness.

■ Garlic has documented antibacterial properties. It can help resolve an infection associated with fever. This pungent herb is more pleasant to take in odorless capsule form. Follow the age-specific dosage directions on the label. You can have your child swallow the capsules, or dissolve them in hot water or soup.

■ Ginger tea is especially effective against a fever associated with a cold, flu, or stomachache. It is most helpful for the child who tends to feel cold, especially in the hands and feet. To decrease chills and increase perspiration, snuggle your child under light covers after giving him the tea. Give your child ½ cup, four times daily, for one day. If your child finds the taste too pungent, mix the tea with fruit juice, or dilute it with water. If your child is over one year old, you can add a bit of honey to sweeten the tea.

HOMEOPATHY

When your child has a fever, select the most appropriate symptom-specific homeopathic remedy and begin administering it as soon as possible. You should notice some response within thirty minutes. After one or two doses, the temperature will usually start coming down. If the fever does not respond, try a different remedy. If you try two remedies without a response, call your doctor.

■ *Aconite* is useful at the very beginning of a fever and for a fever of sudden onset. This homeopathic is most often used during winter, when a child may have been exposed to a cold wind. It is recommended for the child who is restless, moving around and tossing in bed, difficult to calm down, hyperactive, and possibly afraid. Give this child one dose of *Aconite* 30x or 9c, every two hours, for a total of two doses. After the second dose of *Aconite*, switch to another remedy.

■ *Arsenicum album* 30x or 9c is for the child whose fever increases between midnight and 2:00 A.M. This child is anxious and fidgety, and reports pain in his legs. He wants a cold compress on his head and blankets on his legs. Give this child one dose, every two hours, up to a total of four doses.

■ *Belladonna* is also used against sudden fevers. This is for a feverish child who has chills, with a flushed and heated face and body. His pupils are typically dilated, and noise and light bother him. Give this child one dose of *Belladonna* 30x, 200x, 15c, or 30c, every hour, up to a total of four doses.

■ *Bryonia* 30x or 9c is for the irritable child with a fever, strong thirst, and possibly constipation. This child asks to be left alone. Give him one dose, every two hours, up to a total of four doses.

■ For a fever associated with teething, give *Chamomilla*. This is for a child who feels worse with any kind of heat, worse in a hot room, worse under blankets, and, unfortunately, worse at night. If your baby has one hot, red cheek, and one pale and cold cheek, and wakes up crying throughout the night, an emerging tooth may be the cause of the fever. The child may seem comforted when carried around, but the calm will last only for a short time. Give him one dose of *Chamomilla* 12x, 30x, 6c, or 9c, every two hours, up to a total of three doses. Once this infant is no longer red-cheeked and clutching at you for comfort, his fever can be further resolved with *Ferrum phosphoricum*. (*See also* TEETHING.)

■ *Ferrum phosphoricum* treats a moderate fever, including a previously high fever that has been lowered by *Aconite* or *Belladonna*. *Ferrum phosphoricum* is also useful for a fever that is not sudden, high, or rapid in onset. It is good for a child who is pale and feels weak. Give your child one dose of *Ferrum phosphoricum* 6x, 12x, 6c, or 9c, every two hours, up to a total of six doses.

■ *Gelsemium* is for the child who sustains a fever and whose whole body feels achy and flushed. His eyelids are heavy and droopy, and he has no thirst. Give this child one dose of *Gelsemium* 30x or 9c, every two hours, up to a total of four doses.

■ *Mercurius solubilis* is recommended for the feverish child with offensive-smelling breath, body odor, stool, and/or urine. Give this child one dose of *Mercurius solubilis* 12x or 6c, every two hours, up to a total of four doses.

■ *Phosphorus* 30x or 9c is useful for a child suffering from a cough or respiratory infection with fever and who craves ice-cold drinks (which, unfortunately, he may not be able to keep down for very long). Give him one dose, every two hours, up to a total of four doses.

■ If none of the above remedies seems right for your child, a homeopathic combination fever remedy may be helpful. Follow dosage directions on the product label.

ACUPRESSURE

For the locations of acupressure points on a child's body, *see* ADMINISTERING AN ACUPRESSURE TREATMENT in Part Three.

■ Large Intestine 4 clears heat in the body and promotes calm.

■ Four Gates helps to relax a feverish child.

GENERAL RECOMMENDATIONS

■ To prevent dehydration, encourage a feverish child to drink plenty of fluids. The increased metabolic rate that results from a fever causes the body to lose fluids rapidly.

■ Give your child an echinacea and goldenseal combination formula.

■ Select and administer a symptom-specific homeopathic remedy.

■ If your child is running a low temperature, encourage him to rest in cool pajamas under a light sheet. Keep a watchful eye on him, and do not let him become chilled. A chill brings on shivering, which can increase the metabolic rate and cause the fever to escalate.

■ To promote perspiration and bring down a moderate to high temperature, give your child fever-reducing herbal tea.

■ Sponging your child with warm water or having him soak in a tepid bath can help reduce a fever. Give your child a soothing herbal bath. Beneficial herbs can be absorbed through the skin. You can pour several cupfuls of fever-reducing tea into tepid bath water, or, if your child is uncomfortable and restless, prepare chamomile tea and add several cupfuls of that to the bath. Allow your child to enjoy a leisurely soak.

■ Do not sponge your child with cold water or rubbing alcohol or give him a cold bath. Cold and alcohol cause the blood vessels in the skin to constrict, making it more difficult for heat to escape from the body.

PREVENTION

■ Although it's impossible to protect your child from every illness, try to keep your child away from sick playmates. Fever-producing contagious viruses and bacterial infections travel easily from child to child.

■ Your know your child better than anyone else does. If your child runs a fever when overtired or overexcited, intervene and encourage a rest period to allow his body to slow down and recuperate.

■ If your child suffers a seizure as a result of high fever, putting him on an anticonvulsant medication, such as phenobarbital, may be recommended to prevent a recurrence. You should be aware that the usefulness of these drugs in preventing febrile seizures is a subject of ongoing controversy. Anticonvulsants can also cause grogginess and may be implicated in the development of learning deficits. These drugs should therefore be used with great caution, if at all. There is some evidence that a low dose of the tranquilizer diazepam (Valium) can help prevent febrile seizures in some children. According to one study, it is more effective than phenobarbital, and it is a milder drug. It can still cause side effects, however. Some experts believe that taking ordinary measures to reduce fever, when necessary, is at least as effective at preventing febrile seizures as giving a child more powerful drugs is. Be certain to discuss your options thoroughly with your doctor before starting your child on any such type of drug treatment. Don't hesitate to ask questions and voice your concerns.

Fever Blisters

See HERPES VIRUS.

Flu

See INFLUENZA.

Food Allergies

**EMERGENCY
TREATMENT
FOR FOOD ALLERGIES**

✚ Occasionally, an allergic reaction is so severe it can be life threatening. If your child exhibits rapidly spreading hives or has difficulty breathing, seek medical attention immediately.

✚ If there is any sign that your child is having difficulty breathing due to a severe allergic reaction, especially if she has a history of severe reactions, take her immediately to the emergency room of the nearest hospital. If you cannot transport your child yourself, call for emergency help and stress the urgency of the situation. Every second counts.

✚ If an emergency adrenaline kit, such as the Ana-Kit or Epi-Pen, is available, administer it immediately, followed by 50 milligrams of an antihistamine such as Benadryl. *Do not* give your child anything to eat or drink if she is having difficulty breathing. Even if your child responds quickly to the administration of the emergency adrenaline kit, she should still be taken to the emergency room for professional evaluation and treatment.

An allergy is a hypersensitive reaction to a normally harmless substance. About one in every six children in the United States is allergic to one or more substances. There are a variety of substances, termed allergens, that may trouble your child. Common allergens include pollen, animal dander, house dust, feathers, mites, chemicals, and a variety of foods. This section is devoted to food-related allergies.

Allergic reactions can occur immediately, or they can be delayed and take days to surface. A delayed allergic reaction can make it more difficult to pinpoint the allergen.

Common symptoms of an allergic reaction are respiratory congestion, eye inflammation, swelling, itching, hives, and stomachache and vomiting. Food allergies can contribute to chronic health problems, such as acne, asthma, bedwetting, diarrhea, ear infections, eczema, fatigue, hay fever, headache, irritability, chronic runny nose, and even difficulty maintaining concentration (attention deficit disorder, or hyperactivity). Food allergies can also cause intestinal irritation and swelling that interferes with the absorption of vitamins and minerals. Even if you are providing your child with a wholesome, nutritious diet, if she is consuming foods to which she is allergic, she may not be able to absorb food properly, and therefore may not be deriving the full benefits of all the foods she is eating.

The most common foods that cause allergic reactions in children are wheat, milk and other dairy products, eggs, fish and seafood, chocolate, citrus fruits, soy products, corn, nuts, and berries. Many children also are allergic to sulfites, which are found in some frozen foods and dried fruits, as well as in medications. Some people seem to be genetically predisposed to food allergies. If family members, especially parents, have food allergies, there is a greater chance a child will have the same difficulties.

Sometimes, if all the irritating foods are eliminated from a child's diet for several months, her body will have a chance to rest and heal, after which it will be able to handle small amounts of these foods without reacting. Sometimes, too, there is an underlying issue such as a parasitic or yeast infection in the intestine that is contributing to the allergic response. If these underlying problems are cleared up, the child's body may be less reactive to certain substances.

It has been observed that some children actively dislike the foods that produce an allergic reaction. They seem to know instinctively that certain foods will cause a problem. If your child continually refuses particular foods, it may be wise not to force the issue.

Paradoxically, however, some children seem to be particularly drawn to the very foods that cause a problem. For example, many children are allergic to peanut butter, a staple in many homes. Children who continually ask for peanut butter, or those who enthusiastically eat lots of wheat bread, wheat crackers, and wheat cereals, or who crave milk, ice cream, and other dairy products, may actually be exhibiting an allergy to those foods.

CONVENTIONAL TREATMENT

■ The most important part of treating food allergies, obviously, is to identify— and then avoid—the foods that are causing your child's reaction. There are two techniques, the elimination diet and the rotation diet, that enable you to do this (see ELIMINATION DIET and ROTATION DIET in Part Three). Once you have identified the foods or classes of foods that cause symptoms in your child, remember to read the labels on all the processed food products you buy. Many food products will contain one or more of the substances you have identified as the source of your child's allergy.

■ In cases of severe multiple food allergies, oral cromolyn sodium (Gastrocrom) may be prescribed as a preventive measure. This is the same drug that is used in inhaled form to prevent asthma attacks.

■ If your child suffers from recurrent allergic reactions, an antihistamine may be recommended.

DIETARY GUIDELINES

■ Use an elimination diet to determine which foods are causing your child's symptoms. Some of the foods that most commonly cause a reaction are dairy products, wheat, citrus fruits, nuts (including peanut butter), corn, soy products, cane sugar, and eggs. You may wish to try eliminating these first.

■ Always read product labels and be aware of the ingredients in manufactured food products, especially additives such as artificial flavorings and colorings. Processed foods often contain a surprising array of ingredients and additives. It's better to base your child's diet on whole foods that you prepare yourself.

NUTRITIONAL SUPPLEMENTS

For age-appropriate dosages of nutritional supplements, see page 81.

■ Calcium and magnesium help to reduce sensitivity and nervousness associated with allergies. Give your child a combination liquid containing 250 milligrams of calcium and 125 milligrams of magnesium, twice a day, for two to three months.

■ Give your child 50 to 100 milligrams of pantothenic acid, twice daily, at least one hour away from food, for one month to support adrenal function.

■ The B vitamins help support adrenal function. Give your child a vitamin-B complex supplement, twice a day, for two to three months.

■ Vitamin C helps to stimulate immune function. Give your child one dose of vitamin C, in mineral ascorbate form with bioflavonoids, twice a day, for two to three months.

GENERAL RECOMMENDATIONS

■ Use an elimination or rotation diet to identify the food or foods that are causing your child's allergic response.

■ Because allergic reactions can take a wide variety of forms, from headaches to bedwetting, you may want to consult other entries in this book that correspond to your child's symptoms.

PREVENTION

■ There is no way to prevent your child from developing a food allergy. It goes without saying, however, that you should make sure she is not exposed to any known allergens.

Food Poisoning

SYMPTOMS OF SALMONELLA POISONING

Salmonella is an increasingly common type of food poisoning. It is the possibility of salmonella contamination that has led to recent recommendations against eating any foods containing raw eggs, for example. Symptoms of salmonella poisoning include:

• Stomach cramps.
• Diarrhea.
• Chills.
• High fever.
• Headache.
• Nausea and vomiting.

Salmonella poisoning usually comes on fairly soon after contact with the contaminated food and runs its course in twenty-four hours or so.

Food poisoning is most commonly a reaction to toxins produced by bacteria. These organisms thrive in food that is not prepared hygienically, that is kept out of refrigeration for too long, or that is not thoroughly cooked.

Most cases of food poisoning are the result of food being handled by unclean hands or the failure to cook meat long enough and at a high enough temperature to kill microorganisms. For example, if a cook shapes hamburger patties and then cuts raw vegetables, without washing his hands in between, bacteria from the meat can migrate via his hands to contaminate the vegetables. Foods with mayonnaise-type dressings that have been left out of refrigeration for too long can also cause problems, as can cooked foods (such as pizza) that have been removed from heat and left at room temperature for too long. Other food poisonings occur as a result of a toxic reaction to poisonous plants, certain types of mushrooms, or contaminated shellfish. Eating raw fish or shellfish, foods containing raw eggs (such as homemade eggnog or Caesar salad dressing), food that was canned improperly, or food from damaged cans can also lead to food poisoning. Another possible cause is exposure to chemical contaminants such as heavy metals or pesticides.

Common symptoms of food poisoning include nausea, vomiting, diarrhea, abdominal pain and cramping, fever, and general malaise. Symptoms of food poisoning usually come on suddenly, sometimes within hours of eating the contaminated food. Because the symptoms can persist for several days, however, food poisoning is often mistaken for a case of the flu. If your child experiences a sudden bout of nausea, vomiting, and/or diarrhea a couple of hours after eating, he may be suffering from food poisoning.

If you have any suspicion of food poisoning, contact your child's physician immediately if any of the following symptoms develop:

• Fever above 102°F.
• Severe vomiting.
• Severe diarrhea, especially if it continues for more than twenty-four hours or contains blood.
• Difficulty breathing or speaking.
• Changes in vision.
• Localized abdominal pain.

CONVENTIONAL TREATMENT

■ Emetrol is a gentle over-the-counter product that is useful for relieving nausea and vomiting. Follow the dosage directions on the product label.

■ For frequent, watery diarrhea, loperamide (Imodium AD) may be helpful. This over-the-counter medication works by slowing the movement of the intestinal muscle. Follow the dosage directions on the product label.

Note: Loperamide is not recommended for children under twelve.

■ If your child's vomiting is severe and he is unable to keep anything down, your doctor may prescribe an antiemetic in suppository form. Prochlorperazine (sold under the brand name Compazine), promethazine (Phenergan), and trimethobenzamide (Tigan) are prescription drugs that are sometimes used for this purpose. Occasionally these are given in injectable form as well.

■ Dimenhydrinate (Dramamine) is sometimes useful for milder vomiting. Follow dosage directions on the product label.

Note: This medication should not be given to a child under two years old.

■ Activated charcoal, which can be given in capsule form or mixed with water, may be recommended, particularly if a drug or chemical toxin is suspected.

DIETARY GUIDELINES

■ The most important thing to remember in treating food poisoning is that an inflamed stomach tends to go into spasm when stretched, resulting in vomiting. Consequently, if you give a child who is vomiting anything by mouth, it should be in very small quantities (1 teaspoon or less), given at frequent intervals.

■ Have your child rest and offer frequent small sips of fluids. Diarrhea and vomiting can cause serious dehydration. If your child appears to be dehydrated, you can give him an oral electrolyte formula, such as Pedialyte, Lytren, Ricelyte, or Resol. These are available over the counter. Or you can make the following mixtures:

First glass: 8 ounces of orange or apple juice, ½ teaspoon honey or corn syrup, and a pinch of salt. (Do not use honey if your child is under eighteen months old.)

Second glass: 8 ounces of water and ¼ teaspoon of baking soda.

Give your child small sips of each, alternating between the two glasses.

■ Do not give your child any food until he tells you that he is hungry and wants to eat.

■ Once your child signals a readiness to eat, start slowly, with toast, broth, applesauce, mashed bananas, and diluted juices.

■ Do not give your child milk or any other dairy products during and for at least seventy-two hours after an episode of food poisoning.

NUTRITIONAL SUPPLEMENTS

■ A *Lactobacillus acidophilus* or *bifidus* supplement is useful for helping to reintroduce beneficial flora to the intestinal tract. Starting twenty-four hours after an episode of food poisoning, give your child one dose, as directed on the product label, three times daily, for one week. Then give your child one dose daily for at least one month.

SYMPTOMS OF BOTULISM

Botulism is a severe, even potentially life-threatening, form of food poisoning. Symptoms include:

- Headache and dizziness, beginning sometime between sixteen hours and five days after ingestion of contaminated food.
- Double vision.
- Muscle paralysis.
- Vomiting.
- Difficulty breathing and swallowing.

In babies, symptoms may be:

- Constipation.
- Lethargy.
- Poor muscle tone.

Any child who displays the symptoms of botulism requires immediate medical attention.

HERBAL TREATMENT

For age-appropriate dosages of herbal remedies, see page 81.

■ Ginger tea helps to stop nausea and cleanse the digestive tract, as well as providing fluids. Give your child one dose, three times a day, for the first twenty-four hours.

■ Curing Pill formula, a Chinese herbal combination, helps to resolve diarrhea, nausea, and stomach pain. Give your child one dose, three or four times a day, for the first day or two following an episode of food poisoning.

■ Goldenseal tea is useful as an antibacterial for resolving diarrhea. It has a bitter taste, however. If your child will accept it, give him one dose, three times a day, for the first twenty-four hours.

■ A paste made from the Japanese umeboshi plum is gentle and very settling for a child's upset stomach (*see* THERAPEUTIC RECIPES in Part Three). This can be diluted in warm water and drunk as a tea, or you can put a small dab (about ¼ teaspoon) on your child's tongue and have him eat it. It has a pleasing taste and is very gentle, so it can be repeated frequently.

■ Peppermint tea may help to restore appetite following a bout of food poisoning. Try giving your child one dose, three times a day, for two to three days.

HOMEOPATHY

Choose the appropriate homeopathic remedy from the list below, and give your child one dose every hour, up to a total of five doses.

■ *Arsenicum album* 30x or 9c is the premier homeopathic for food poisoning. This is for the child who has diarrhea and chills, feels anxious, and is worse between midnight and 2:00 A.M.

■ *Pulsatilla* 30x or 9c will help the child whose stools are quite varied. Any consumption of fatty foods in the seventy-two hours after the initial food poisoning episode makes the diarrhea worse. This child is emotionally vulnerable and cries easily.

■ *China* 30x or 9c is for the child who is exhausted and weak, and whose lower abdomen is very gaseous and sensitive to touch or pressure. It is a good remedy to use once the initial phase of food poisoning has been addressed because it helps the digestive tract to repair itself.

■ *Colocynthis* 12x or 6c will help a child who has stabbing pains in the lower abdomen. The poisoning episode may have occurred after he experienced overwhelming anger.

■ *Nux vomica* 30x or 9c is for food poisoning that occurs after excessive consumption of rich foods. It is helpful for a child who is predominantly irritable, and whose abdominal pain is improved with the passing of stool.

■ *Phosphorus* 30x or 9c is useful for a child who is vomiting, suffering from diarrhea with burning pain as stool passes, and complaining of anal pain. This child craves ice and iced drinks, but can't keep them down.

■ *Podophyllum* 12x or 9c is for the child with greenish-colored diarrhea that is worse in the morning and that is accompanied by abdominal cramping.

PREVENTION

■ Keep all hot foods hot and cold foods cold. Bacteria do not grow at temperatures below 40°F or above 150°F.

■ Keep the temperature in your refrigerator at 40°F or below and that in your freezer at 0°F or below. You can use a refrigerator thermometer to monitor temperature.

■ Thaw all frozen foods in the refrigerator, rather than at room temperature. If you use a microwave oven to defrost food, make sure to finish cooking it right away.

■ Keep uncooked meats, fish, and poultry in the refrigerator as briefly as possible. In any case, use red meat within three to five days, poultry within two days, and fish within twenty-four hours.

■ Keep two cutting boards in your kitchen, one for cutting meat and the other for fruits and vegetables. Wash your cutting boards with a solution of bleach and water. Contrary to what some believe, a recent study showed that wooden cutting boards are easier to clean and keep free of bacteria than plastic ones are. Wash kitchen towels in bleach and hot water as well.

■ Always wash your hands thoroughly before handling food, and make sure to keep them clean by washing as often as necessary during food preparation.

■ Cook all red meat, fish, and poultry thoroughly. Meats should be cooked to an internal temperature of at least 165°F, poultry to 180°F, and fish to 140°F. Do not allow your child to eat any meat (especially pork) raw, rare, or even medium-rare. If meat is even a little pink, it may harbor live bacteria.

■ Be careful when cooking with a microwave. If you cook meat in your microwave, always use a thermometer to verify that the internal temperature is high enough. When cooking red meat in a microwave, precook the meat on the high setting for thirty to ninety seconds and discard the juices. Then continue cooking the meat immediately.

■ Do not cook stuffing inside turkeys or other poultry. Instead, bake stuffing separately in the oven or prepare it on top of the stove.

■ Always cook eggs for at least three minutes. Never use raw eggs that are cracked.

■ Use different utensils for handling raw and cooked foods.

■ Clean any dishes and utensils that have come into contact with raw meat, poultry, eggs, or seafood. Do not put cooked foods into dishes that held them when they were raw without washing the dishes first.

■ Never eat foods containing raw meat, poultry, eggs, fish, or shellfish either before or during cooking. (This means no nibbling on raw cookie dough!)

■ Never use food from any can that is bulging, rusted, bent, or sticky, or that has a loose lid.

■ After meals, refrigerate any leftovers as soon as possible. Do not refrigerate foods in the same pots or bowls you used for cooking or serving; if you transfer them to different containers before refrigerating, the food will take less time to cool. Use any stored leftovers within five days.

■ When reheating soups, stews, sauces, and gravies, bring them to a rapid boil, if possible, and cook for at least four minutes. Be aware that microwave ovens, while convenient, do not necessarily kill bacteria when they are used to reheat food.

■ Be careful when eating out. Do not eat foods that smell odd or taste spoiled, even if you're eating in a "nice" restaurant. Avoid salad bars that do not look fresh and clean. If you are traveling in a less developed country, you may want to completely avoid foods that can spoil or become contaminated easily, such as mayonnaise and dairy products.

Gas, Intestinal

See COLIC; CONSTIPATION; NAUSEA.

German Measles

German measles (rubella) is a common childhood illness caused by a virus. It is characterized by general malaise, a rash, and swollen lymph glands. Typically the lymph glands become swollen first. Then a rash begins on the face and neck, and spreads to the trunk and extremities. The rash lasts for about three to five days, with the first lesions to appear being the first to heal. It is a pink or red raised rash that looks like small pimples. A child with German measles may also have achy and swollen joints. Her throat may appear red or pinkish, but usually will not feel sore.

German measles is spread by respiratory contact. The virus incubates for fourteen to twenty-one days before signs of illness appear. The illness itself usually lasts for about five days. A child with German measles is contagious from approximately seven days before to five days after the rash appears, so if your child comes down with German measles, you should contact anyone who has been exposed to her over the previous week. This is important because, while German measles causes a relatively mild illness in children, it poses a very serious problem for pregnant women. Every effort should be made to avoid exposing a woman who is pregnant, or who is likely to become pregnant in the very near future, to this disease. If this occurs, the virus can affect the developing fetus and cause severe deformities.

CONVENTIONAL TREATMENT

■ If necessary, a blood test can be used to confirm a diagnosis of German measles. The disease usually is relatively mild and runs its course without complications.

■ If your child is feverish or uncomfortable, you can give her acetaminophen (in Tylenol, Tempra, and other medications) or ibuprofen (Advil, Nuprin, and others) to ease symptoms.

Note: In excessive amounts, acetaminophen can cause liver damage. Read package directions carefully so as not to exceed the proper dosage for your child's age and size. Ibuprofen is usually better tolerated when given with food to prevent possible stomach upset.

■ *Do not* give your child aspirin if she has German measles. This is a viral illness, and the combination of aspirin and a viral infection has been linked to the development of Reye's syndrome, a potentially dangerous complication (*see* REYE'S SYNDROME).

DIETARY GUIDELINES

■ Offer plenty of fluids so your child stays well hydrated.

■ Prepare a simple diet including easily digested foods that are high in vitamins and minerals, such as soups, well-cooked whole grains, and vegetables.

■ Eliminate fats as much as possible. Fats are difficult to digest, and undigested fats contribute to a toxic internal environment, making it harder for the body to heal.

NUTRITIONAL SUPPLEMENTS

For age-appropriate dosages of nutritional supplements, see page 81.

■ Vitamin C and bioflavonoids help to stimulate the immune system. Three to four times a day, give your child one dose of mineral ascorbate vitamin C, and an equal amount of bioflavonoids, for one week.

■ Zinc also stimulates the immune system. Give your child one dose, once or twice a day, for one week.

Note: Excessive amounts of zinc can result in nausea and vomiting. Be careful not to exceed the recommended dosage.

HERBAL TREATMENT

■ Echinacea and goldenseal stimulate the immune system to help it fight off a viral infection. Give your child one dose of a liquid combination formula, three times daily, for up to one week.

HOMEOPATHY

■ *Ferrum phosphoricum* 12x or 6c is useful during the first twenty-four hours when there is fever. Give your child one dose, four times a day, during that period.

■ *Natrum muriaticum* 30x or 9c is for a child who has swollen glands, a sore throat, and a rash accompanied by oral canker sores. Give this child one dose, three to four times a day, for up to two days.

■ *Phytolacca* is recommended for a child with a sore throat, swollen glands, and eye pain, and whose throat feels better after cold drinks. Give this child one dose, three to four times daily, for up to two days.

■ *Pulsatilla* 30x or 9c is for the child who is clingy and cries easily. This child's rash is accompanied by a stuffy nose with a mucous discharge. Give her one dose, three to four times a day, for up to two days.

GENERAL RECOMMENDATIONS

■ German measles is usually only mildly uncomfortable for the child who has it. The principal danger lies in the possibility that an infected child may come into contact with an expectant mother. If your child comes down with German measles, keep her from coming into contact with pregnant women and make sure you tell everyone who has been in contact with her for the preceding week about her illness. Even though they may have no symptoms, her playmates may be carrying the virus and they, too, should be kept away from others, especially pregnant women.

PREVENTION

■ A vaccine that protects against German measles is usually given in combination with the mumps and measles vaccines (in the MMR vaccine) as an injection when a child is fifteen months old. A second dose is recommended either when a child is four to six years old (before entering school) or between eleven and thirteen years old (in middle school or junior high school). If a girl reaches her teens without achieving immunity (either by vaccination or by having a case of the disease), a separate rubella vaccine may be recommended.

■ As much as possible, try to keep your child from contact with contagious children, particularly if she is not (or is not yet) immunized against the disease.

Hay Fever

See ALLERGIES.

Head Injury

See CONCUSSION.

Head Lice

See LICE.

Headache

Headaches can be caused by muscle tension, an underlying illness or infection, or disturbances in the blood vessels in the head. The latter scenario produces migraine headaches, which typically recur periodically and are characterized by severe pain, often concentrated on one side of the head, that is aggravated by light, sometimes preceded by disturbances in vision, and is often associated with nausea and vomiting. Headaches can sometimes be related to disorders that warrant further investigation, such as infections of the scalp, ears, sinuses, or spinal fluid. They can also be caused by allergies, fever, high blood pressure, epilepsy, brain tumors, severe cavities or oral infections, certain drugs, or an injury to the head.

Most often, headaches are related to tension. However, if your child awakens crying and holding his head, the cause is most likely something other than tension. If your child has a headache in combination with a high fever, severe vomiting, a stiff neck, confusion, disorientation, or extreme fatigue, see your doctor immediately. This can be a sign of a serious illness, such as meningitis or encephalitis. If a child's headache is so severe that he isn't tempted by a promise of his favorite activity or a favorite food, or if the headaches are frequent and chronic, you should consult with a physician.

A young child with a limited vocabulary may be unable to describe how his head feels. A tension headache often feels like a tight band around the head. The pain may be throbbing or dull, mild or severe. Sudden movements often seem to make a tension headache worse. A headache may develop suddenly, or come on gradually. Tension headaches most often develop during the day, worsen as the day goes on, and may be relieved with sleep.

An attack of migraine, on the other hand, can last for days; sleep may or may not be helpful in easing the pain. Some children with migraines may not even complain of head pain, but rather of nausea, vomiting, and stomachache. Migraines can be triggered by a number of different factors, including emotional stress, hypoglycemia, food allergies, head injuries, oral contraceptives, or hormonal changes related to the menstrual cycle, which may be why more females than males suffer from them. The disorder also tends to run in families.

CONVENTIONAL TREATMENT

■ A mild pain reliever, such as ibuprofen (found in Advil, Nuprin, and other medications) or acetaminophen (Tylenol, Tempra, and others) can relieve a headache. These drugs are most effective when given early; headache pain becomes increasingly difficult to relieve as it becomes more severe. Ibuprofen generally works better for headaches, especially migraine headaches, than acetaminophen does.

Note: Ibuprofen is best given with food to avoid possible stomach upset. Acetaminophen can cause liver damage if taken in excessive amounts. If you give your child acetaminophen, make sure to read package directions carefully so as not to exceed the proper dosage for your child's age and size.

■ *Do not* give a child aspirin for a headache unless a viral illness has been ruled out by your doctor. The combination of aspirin and certain viral infections is associated with the development of Reye's syndrome, a dangerous liver disease (*see* REYE'S SYNDROME).

■ For extremely severe headaches, a combination of acetaminophen and codeine may be prescribed. Codeine is a powerful narcotic painkiller that can cause serious side effects, including nausea, sleepiness, and constipation, and that can also be highly addictive.

■ If your child suffers from migraines, ibuprofen or acetaminophen is likely to be suggested first, and may be all that is needed to ease the pain. The antihistamine diphenhydramine (Benadryl) may also be suggested. The reason it works is not well understood, but it may offer relief for your child.

■ If your child has migraines that are not relieved by ordinary painkillers, an

WHEN TO CALL THE DOCTOR ABOUT A HEADACHE

• If your child has a headache in combination with a high fever, extreme fatigue, a stiff neck, severe vomiting, or confusion or disorientation, call your doctor immediately or take your child to the emergency room of the nearest hospital. These can be signs of an infection affecting the brain, such as encephalitis or meningitis.

• If your child's headaches are so severe that they interfere with normal activities, or if they are frequent rather than isolated occurrences, consult with your doctor.

ergotamine preparation may be prescribed. These drugs work by constricting blood vessels. They are available in forms that can be taken orally, rectally, as a nasal spray, or placed under the tongue; some formulations contain caffeine. Ergotamine works best if it is taken as soon as possible after the pain begins, but it should be used with care because it is possible to become dependent on it. Possible side effects include stomach and/or muscle cramps, dizziness, nausea, vomiting, and diarrhea.

■ A relatively new drug, sumatriptan (sold under the brand name Imitrex), appears to be very effective in alleviating a severe attack of migraine. It works by increasing the amount of serotonin in the brain. Serotonin is involved in vasoconstriction (the constriction of blood vessels); since migraine is in part a result of a disturbance in circulation in the brain, increasing serotonin levels may help to restore balance in the tension of blood vessels. This treatment is expensive, however, and as of this writing, must be administered by injection. It can also produce unpleasant side effects, including increased heart rate, elevated blood pressure, and a feeling of tightness in the chest, jaw, or neck. An oral form may be approved in the near future, and it may be better tolerated. Although this drug may be safe for children, especially teenagers, it is not yet officially indicated for use in children.

■ There is some evidence that a daily low dose of the beta-blocker propranolol (Inderal) may help if a child suffers from recurrent, incapacitating migraine headaches. This drug should not be taken by a child with asthma or diabetes, however, and it can cause such side effects as fatigue, depression, shortness of breath, and cold hands and feet.

■ If your child's headaches are chronic and debilitating, it may be helpful to consult a pediatric neurologist to investigate the possibility of an underlying problem.

DIETARY GUIDELINES

■ Because low blood sugar can provoke a headache, see to it that a headache-prone child has three whole-foods meals and several snacks each day. Do not offer sugary foods. Sugar causes blood sugar levels to soar, then crash, making a headache worse.

■ Limit fat, which is difficult to digest and can lead to a stomachache and headache. Avoid greasy and fried foods.

■ Chocolate, monosodium glutamate (MSG), and the preservatives in hot dogs and other processed meats have been found to cause headaches, especially migraines. If your child typically gets a headache after eating one of these foods, banish the offender from the menu. Be aware of hidden MSG in processed food products. For example, if the label lists an additive called hydrolyzed protein, the product contains MSG. Other additives that contain MSG include autolyzed yeast, sodium caseinate, and calcium caseinate. Read labels carefully.

■ A food allergy or sensitivity can provoke headaches. Use an elimination diet or a diet diary to uncover hidden food allergies (see ELIMINATION DIET in Part Three).

NUTRITIONAL SUPPLEMENTS

■ Calcium and magnesium help to calm muscles and relax blood vessels. A transitory deficit of magnesium especially has been associated with the onset of migraine. Give your child one dose of a liquid combination supplement containing 250 milligrams of calcium and 125 milligrams of magnesium, twice a day, until the headache is better.

■ If your child's headache (whether tension or migraine) is centered in the front of the head—especially if you suspect it may be related to something he ate—try giving him an acidophilus supplement. Give one dose, as directed on the product label, every four hours, until the headache is gone.

■ For persistent migraines, a supplement called EPA, derived from fish oils, can help to thin the blood and block the cycle that leads to recurrent headaches. Give an older child one capsule, three times daily, for one to two months.

HERBAL TREATMENT

For age-appropriate dosages of herbal remedies, see page 81.

■ Chamomile relaxes the nervous system and can bring relief for a tension headache. Give your child one dose of chamomile tea as needed. You can also prepare a chamomile bath and encourage a long, relaxing soak. The herb's beneficial effects will be absorbed through the skin.

■ If your child suffers from migraines, try feverfew. This herb has an anti-inflammatory effect and may be taken at the onset of a migraine. Or you can give your child one dose, twice a day, over a period of several months as a preventive.

■ Ginger tea is helpful for either a tension or a migraine headache that is located in the front of the head. Give your child one dose as needed.

■ Peppermint tea is helpful for a congested and full headache. It can also help relieve a headache caused by overeating. Give your child one dose as needed.

■ Skullcap is excellent for headaches due to nervous tension. Give your child one dose as needed.

Note: This herb should not be given to a child less than six years old.

■ When used as a rub, an herbal tincture of arnica or peppermint oil can be effective in resolving a headache. Rub arnica tincture into the temple or forehead area, or peppermint oil into the temple area. Be very careful to keep tinctures away from your child's eyes and do not use them on broken skin.

■ Tiger Balm liniment works very well for tension headaches. Rub the ointment into the temple area.

HOMEOPATHY

■ For tension headaches, choose the homeopathic remedy most suited to your child's symptoms and administer it as follows: Give your child one dose of the remedy. Wait twenty minutes. If there is no relief after twenty minutes, give a second dose and wait another twenty minutes. If your child still feels no relief, wait thirty minutes and select another remedy that suits your child's symptoms and temperament.

- *Bryonia* 30x or 9c is recommended for a child who has a headache in combination with constipation and much eye pain.
- *Ferrum phosphoricum* 12x or 5c is for the child whose face may be pale and

cold, or red and flushed, and generally alternates between the two. His hands and feet are cold. This child may get a headache when he is fatigued.

- *Gelsemium* 12x or 6c is useful for the child who describes visual disturbances, such as blurring, and for the type of tension headache that is associated with performance anxiety and commonly occurs before a test, school play, or similar event.

- Give *Natrum muriaticum* 30x or 9c to a child who develops a headache after any kind of intense mental work, such as a school project or homework that has a grade riding on it. The *Natrum muriaticum* child is very ambitious, hard on himself, and eager to achieve. This child also has a craving for salt.

■ If your child has a migraine, choose one of the following and give him one dose, four times a day, for up to two days:

- *Iris* 30x or 9c is recommended for the child who complains of impaired or blurred vision. This child may also be vomiting and the pain may recur periodically—he may have a headache every Sunday, for example.

- Use *Lachesis* 30x or 9c if the pain begins or is worse on the left side of the head.

- If your child's migraine begins or is worse on the right side of the head, choose *Lycopodium* 30x or 9c.

- *Silica* 30x or 9c is for a migraine that starts at the base of the back of the head and travels into one eye.

■ Whichever remedy you choose, if you are using any form of peppermint or Tiger Balm in addition to one of the homeopathic remedies recommended here, you should give your child homeopathic remedies at least half an hour before or after. Otherwise, the strong odors of these herbal preparations may interfere with the action of the remedy.

■ If headaches are chronic, and an underlying illness has been ruled out, it may be helpful to consult a homeopathic physician for a constitutional remedy.

ACUPRESSURE

For the locations of acupressure points on a child's body, *see* ADMINISTERING AN ACUPRESSURE TREATMENT in Part Three.

■ Large Intestine 4 relaxes tension in the head. It is especially comforting to a child with a frontal headache.

■ Neck and Shoulder Release will unkink and relax the muscles most often tight and tense during a headache.

■ When your child has a headache, rub the two muscles that run along the spine to help him relax.

GENERAL RECOMMENDATIONS

■ Encourage your child to lie down in a darkened, quiet room.

■ Put a cool washcloth on his forehead.

■ A tension headache may get better on its own when you give your child the time and attention he needs to express his concerns. Be loving and supportive.

■ A very important and effective course of action for a child who suffers from migraines is to learn a relaxation exercise. As soon as the sensation of the headache appears, he can begin a relaxation or visualization exercise. This can relax the blood vessels and prevent the development of a full-blown headache.

■ Give your child chamomile tea for its calming, relaxing effect.

■ Rub Tiger Balm into your child's temples.

■ Choose a symptom-specific homeopathic remedy.

■ Use acupressure.

■ A back rub or foot rub can help release tension and make a tense or upset child feel cared for and nurtured.

■ For a child whose headache is related to constipation, give an Epsom salts bath. The salts will increase circulation and help relax tension. A bowel movement will usually occur an hour or two after the bath.

■ If headaches are due to a structural stress, chiropractic work may be helpful.

PREVENTION

■ Some children tend to get tense, depressed, or overwhelmed. By carefully observing and responding to your child's needs, you can help him deal with emotional and physical stresses and perhaps avert tension headaches.

■ To help a child release the tensions of the day, give him a warm herbal bath and a loving massage before bed. Encourage him to talk about the day, express concerns or anxieties, and ask for help.

■ Offer three good meals every day and have healthy snacks on hand. Avoid sugars, fried foods, and heavy fats. Eliminate any foods that have been shown by experience to trigger a headache.

■ Do not expose children to cigarette smoke.

■ Explore meditation or relaxation techniques with your child (*see* RELAXATION TECHNIQUES in Part Three). Massage or chiropractic adjustment may also help.

■ A variety of different drugs may be recommended as preventives for a child who suffers recurring migraines. These include beta-blockers (propranolol [Inderal] is one of the most popular of these), calcium-channel blockers, and low-dose antidepressants, among others. All of these are powerful medications that can have serious side effects, and should be used with caution, if at all.

■ If your child suffers from migraine headaches, keep a diary that records the circumstances surrounding each attack, such as foods recently eaten, exposure to possible environmental allergens, activities, emotional factors, physical environment, etc. Try to be as observant as possible. Notice the obviously unhealthy things, such as cigarette smoke or car exhaust, but don't overlook things that seem harmless or even pleasant, such as perfumes or the smell of new fabrics. Once you do this, a pattern may emerge pointing to certain factors that could be triggering your child's headaches. You can then make appropriate alterations in your child's diet or lifestyle.

■ Acupuncture and biofeedback have both been used to good effect against chronic headaches, whether from migraine or tension. If frequent headaches are making your child miserable, it may be worthwhile to consult a qualified acupuncturist or a practitioner skilled in biofeedback techniques.

Hepatitis

Symptoms of hepatitis can be mild or severe, but they usually involve a combination of the following:

- Loss of appetite.
- Flulike symptoms, including nausea, vomiting, fever, and malaise.
- Dark-colored urine.
- Stools that are clay-colored, or lighter in color than normal.
- A yellowish coloration to the skin (jaundice).

If your child displays symptoms like these, take her to your doctor for a professional evaluation.

Hepatitis is a general term that means inflammation of the liver. Located just under the breastbone and extending to just under the bottom of the rib cage on the right side, the liver is the body's largest internal organ. Its functions include the production and metabolism of bile, which is necessary to metabolize fats, and the detoxification of harmful substances that find their way into the body. When the liver isn't working at top efficiency, as occurs during hepatitis, it cannot excrete bile efficiently. Bile then accumulates in the skin, giving it the typical yellowish cast of jaundice. Excess bile also makes the urine dark. In severe hepatitis, the liver may become enlarged. Other symptoms include nausea, vomiting, loss of appetite, fever, malaise, flulike symptoms, clay-colored stools, and diarrhea.

The form of hepatitis most often seen in infants and young children is *anicteric hepatitis*, a mild form of the disease that is distinguished by the absence of jaundice. Symptoms include a loss of appetite, stomach upset, and a slight fever. Because the symptoms are so mild, anicteric hepatitis often goes undiagnosed, and is usually found only by testing the blood of children with known exposure to the disease.

Hepatitis can be caused by a wide range of viruses. In addition to the hepatitis A, B, and C viruses, Epstein-Barr virus (also responsible for infectious mononucleosis) and cytomegalovirus (CMV) can cause hepatitis. The diagnosis of which virus is involved is made based on the history of the illness and blood tests. There are also drugs, toxins, and allergic reactions that can lead to hepatitis.

There are three basic classifications of the disease. Hepatitis A, once called infectious hepatitis because of its highly contagious nature, is spread by direct contact with an infected person, or through fecal-infected food or water. Hepatitis A has a one-month incubation period—that is, it can take one month for the illness to appear after the virus enters the body—but illness can then come on very rapidly. Hepatitis B has a two- to four-month incubation period. The onset is slow, the course may be longer, and the illness is more serious. Hepatitis B is not highly contagious. It can be transmitted by the transfusion of infected blood, by the use of unsterile needles and instruments, or through sexual contact. In addition to the standard symptoms, a child with hepatitis B may also have arthritis, rashes, and very itchy skin. The C virus is the one responsible for most cases of hepatitis related to blood transfusions.

There is no cure for hepatitis, but most children recover completely without suffering permanent consequences. Recovery may take one to three months, however. A small percentage of children develop chronic hepatitis, which lasts for six months or longer. The good news is that chronic hepatitis too may clear up without inflicting permanent harm, even if the sufferer has carried the virus for years.

CONVENTIONAL TREATMENT

■ Medical treatment for hepatitis consists primarily of observation to make sure the illness resolves and that complications do not develop. Hospitalization is reserved for the most serious cases, in which nitrogen builds up in the blood because the liver cannot process it normally. This can create complications in the brain. A low-protein diet, intravenous potassium, laxatives, and medication may be prescribed to bring down blood nitrogen levels.

■ If your child is diagnosed with hepatitis, dietary modifications may be pre-scribed. If so, your doctor will tell you how to modify her diet. Antiemetics (drugs that inhibit vomiting), such as Tigan, Compazine, and Phenergan, are sometimes used, if nausea interferes with adequate nutrition.

■ During the acute and recovery phases of hepatitis, it is important to maintain close medical follow-up to make certain the inflammation clears and does not become chronic.

■ Alpha interferon is a drug that appears to have some effectiveness against chronic hepatitis B, as well as limited effectiveness against chronic hepatitis C.

DIETARY GUIDELINES

■ To rest your child's liver and allow it to heal, eliminate fats from her diet.

■ To support your child's body in the healing process, offer very small, nutri-ent-dense meals.

■ Fruits are usually well tolerated. Try applesauce, fruit-juice popsicles, or fruit juices diluted with spring water.

■ Keep a glass of fresh water by your child's bed and encourage her to sip it frequently.

NUTRITIONAL SUPPLEMENTS

For age-appropriate dosages of some nutritional supplements, see page 81.

■ Vitamin C with bioflavonoids has an anti-inflammatory effect. Give your child one dose, three times a day, during the acute phase. Then give her one dose a day for one month.

■ One particular bioflavonoid, called catechin, has been shown to be very helpful in treating the symptoms of hepatitis. Give your child one dose, four times a day, until she recovers.

■ Chlorophyll is high in vitamins and minerals, especially magnesium. It helps to restore and detoxify the blood. Follow dosage directions on the product label.

■ *Lactobacillus acidophilus* or *bifidus* helps to maintain friendly flora in the gastro-intestinal tract. Follow dosage directions on the product label.

■ Phosphatidyl choline, a component of lecithin, is beneficial to the liver. If your child is fourteen years of age or older, give her 500 milligrams a day until she recovers. Choline can also be given in the form of choline citrate.

HERBAL TREATMENT

For age-appropriate dosages of herbal remedies, see page 81.

■ Dandelion root is noted for its strengthening effect on the liver. Give your child one dose, as a tea or extract, three times a day, for up to one month.

■ To support your child's immune system and give it a boost, give her an echinacea and goldenseal combination formula. This herbal combination is both antibacterial and antiviral. Give your child one dose, twice a day, for one week. Then discontinue for one week. Repeat this cycle for up to two months.

■ Milk thistle (*Silybum marianum*) is most helpful for hepatitis caused by the ingestion of toxic mushrooms, but is also good for other types of liver inflammation. Give your child one dose, in capsule or tincture form, three times a day during the acute phase, and once a day for one month during recovery.

■ Minor bupleurum is an herbal preparation that strengthens the immune system. It is also specifically helpful to the liver. Give your child one dose, twice a day, for two weeks.

Note: Minor bupleurum should not be given to a child with a fever or any other sign of an acute infection. It should be used only during the recovery phase.

HOMEOPATHY

■ *Phosphorus* is the first homeopathic remedy to give for hepatitis. Give your child one dose of *Phosphorus* 30x or 9c, twice daily, for three days. Stop for three days. Then give her one dose, twice daily, for another three days. Then choose one of the symptom-specific remedies that follow.

■ *Chelidonium* helps to relieve pain in the upper right quadrant of the abdomen, over the liver, as well as in the right shoulder. Give your child *Chelidonium* 12x or 6c, three times a day, until the pain lessens.

■ *Taraxacum* helps relieve bitter burping and nausea. It is also helpful for pain on the left side of the abdomen. Give your child *Taraxacum* 12x or 6c, three times a day, until symptoms are relieved.

ACUPRESSURE

For the locations of acupressure points on a child's body, *see* ADMINISTERING AN ACUPRESSURE TREATMENT in Part Three.

■ Four Gates will help to calm and soothe a restless, uncomfortable child.

GENERAL RECOMMENDATIONS

■ Rest is of primary importance in the treatment of hepatitis.

■ Ask your doctor about the need to isolate your child from other children. Some doctors recommend that a child diagnosed with hepatitis not have contact with other children for at least three weeks from the beginning of the illness.

■ Give your child an echinacea and goldenseal combination formula and dandelion as a tea or extract.

■ Give your child milk thistle, three times a day, until she recovers.

■ Give your child vitamin C, vitamin E, bioflavonoids, and phosphatidyl choline.

■ If you do not have a dishwasher, wash dishes and tableware used by the infected child with hot water and soap, separately from the rest of the family's.

■ Wash the infected child's bed linens separately. Don't mix them with the family wash.

■ A child is no longer contagious seven to ten days after the onset of jaundice. Be sure to check with your doctor first, but if your child is feeling well, she may be able to return to school around this time.

PREVENTION

■ If one of your child's schoolmates contracts hepatitis, expect a note or phone call from school authorities. Should you learn that your child has been exposed to the disease, contact your physician immediately.

■ Immune globulin increases immunity against a variety of viruses, including hepatitis A. To prevent or reduce the symptoms of hepatitis, it must be given within two weeks of exposure. It is also given prior to foreign travel. Possible side effects include allergic reaction, and pain and swelling at the site of the injection.

■ If your child is exposed to a person with a known case of hepatitis B, your doctor may administer hepatitis B immune globulin (HBIG). This is given not to cure hepatitis, but rather to protect a person who has been exposed to hepatitis from getting the illness. An allergic reaction to this drug is possible.

■ Medical doctors now recommend that all children receive a series of vaccinations against hepatitis B. (*See* IMMUNIZATION-RELATED PROBLEMS.)

Hernia, Congenital Inguinal

An inguinal hernia is caused by an incomplete closing of a membrane between the abdominal cavity, which holds the abdominal organs, and the testes. The intestines or peritoneal fluid can pouch down into the inguinal canal and scrotum. If part of the intestines become trapped in this area, the problem is called a hernia; if fluid gets caught in this area, the problem is called a hydrocele. Hernias are much more common in males than females.

During the eighth month of pregnancy, the fetus's peritoneum (the membrane that lines the walls of the abdominal cavity) fuses to separate the abdominal cavity from the scrotum. In some cases, however, this fusion is incomplete. If the defect is large enough, it may permit the intestines, together with the peritoneum, to protrude into the scrotum, causing the condition known as a congenital inguinal hernia (see margin illustration, page 258).

Symptoms of a hernia include swelling and pain in the groin area. You may be able to see a mass when the child is crying, coughing, or straining. It is possible for the intestines involved in the hernia to become obstructed, causing severe pain, redness, and warmth in the area. One or both testes may become swollen.

CONVENTIONAL TREATMENT

■ Surgery is the treatment of choice for a hernia, because hernias rarely close up on their own. Surgery is done to repair the incomplete closure in the membrane and to prevent obstruction and decay of the area involved. Hernia surgery is usually done in one day on an outpatient basis.

DIETARY GUIDELINES

■ Once your child has undergone surgery, even after your doctor gives full permission for him to eat, he may have little or no appetite. When your child feels like eating, begin slowly by offering clear liquids, such as broth, apple juice, and herbal teas.

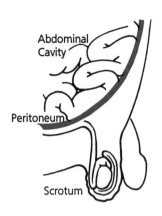

A. Peritoneum Fused Normally

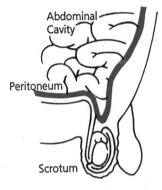

B. Incomplete Fusion of Peritoneum

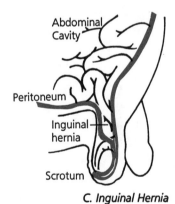

C. Inguinal Hernia

How a Hernia Develops

The peritoneum (shown in red) normally fuses before birth, separating the abdominal cavity from the scrotum (figure A). In some cases, the membrane does not fuse completely (figure B). If this happens, the intestines, together with the peritoneum, may pouch down into the scrotum, creating a hernia (figure C).

■ To allow your child's gastrointestinal tract to readjust to food, work up to a full diet gradually. Prepare whole foods full of the many vitamins and minerals your child's body needs to heal and regain energy.

■ Stick to high-fiber foods and offer plenty of liquids to help your child avoid becoming constipated. Constipation can aggravate the wound and interfere with healing.

NUTRITIONAL SUPPLEMENTS

The following nutritional supplements will help support your child's recovery from hernia surgery. For age-appropriate dosages of nutritional supplements, see page 81.

■ Beta-carotene aids in tissue healing and helps soothe mucous membranes. Give your child one dose of beta-carotene a day until healing is complete.

■ Vitamin C helps decrease inflammation and repair tissues. Give your child one dose of mineral ascorbate vitamin C with bioflavonoids, once or twice a day, for two weeks.

■ Give your child a double dose of vitamin E, twice a day, for two to three weeks. Vitamin E is an antioxidant as well as mildly anti-inflammatory.

■ To help speed tissue healing, give your child one dose of zinc, two to three times a day, for two weeks.
Note: Excessive amounts of zinc can result in nausea and vomiting. Be careful not to exceed the recommended dosage.

HERBAL TREATMENT

Herbal treatment is directed at supporting recovery once your child is home from the hospital following surgery to repair the hernia. It is not intended as a substitute for surgical treatment. For age-appropriate dosages of herbal remedies, see page 81.

■ The following two-week program is useful for a child recovering from hernia surgery.

Days 1–3: Twice a day, give your child one dose of an echinacea and goldenseal combination formula. This herbal remedy helps to detoxify the chemicals remaining in the blood after anesthesia, as well as to support the immune system and prevent a possible infection from developing in the surgical wound.

Days 4–6: Three times a day, give your child one dose of astragalus (*Astragalus membranaceous*). This healing herb, with its rich concentration of trace minerals and micronutrients, helps to strengthen the immune system.

Days 7–14: Three times a day, give your child one dose of American ginseng. This is another excellent source of trace minerals and micronutrients that will help to strengthen your child's internal defenses.
Note: Neither astragalus nor American ginseng should be given if a fever or any other signs of infection are present.

■ Gotu kola is very useful for wound healing and is a good general tonic. Give your child two to three doses daily until he is fully recovered.
Note: This herb should not be given to a child under four years of age.

HOMEOPATHY

Homeopathic treatment is directed at supporting recovery once your child is home from the hospital following surgery to repair the hernia. It is not intended as a substitute for surgical treatment. It can be combined with herbal treatment, but herbs and homeopathic remedies should be given at least one hour apart.

■ The following regimen is useful for a child recovering from hernia surgery.

Days 1–2: Give your child one dose of *Arnica* 30x, three times daily. *Arnica* helps to decrease inflammation following surgery and speed the healing process.

Days 3–4: Give your child one dose of *Staphysagria* 30x, three times a day, to aid in tissue healing.

Day 4: In addition to the *Staphysagria*, give your child one dose of *Ledum* 12x three times during the day.

Days 5–6: For nerve pain following surgery, give your child one dose of *Hypericum* 6x, three times daily.

■ If your child has been diagnosed with a hernia on the right side of the groin, accompanied by intense pain, give him one dose of *Aesculus* 12x or 6c, two to three times a day, to ease his discomfort until surgery can be scheduled to correct the problem.

GENERAL RECOMMENDATIONS

■ Following surgery, watch your child's incision for signs of a developing infection. If you notice increased redness, warmth, tenderness, or drainage, consult your physician.

■ If your child is still in diapers, change him frequently to prevent infection. If the incision does get contaminated, gently cleanse the area with a mild soap and water.

PREVENTION

■ A hernia is the result of a congenital defect, so it cannot be prevented. You should, however, be aware of characteristic signs and symptoms so that, if necessary, your child can be treated promptly and recover without complications.

Herpes Virus

Herpes viruses are a group of viruses that cause skin eruptions or blisters. The herpes simplex virus 1 (HSV1) usually causes cold sores (also known as fever blisters). Herpes simplex 2 (HSV2) involves the genitals and is usually, although not always, passed through sexual contact. The varicella-zoster virus causes chickenpox and shingles. Zoster oticus involves facial nerves. The Epstein-Barr virus causes mononucleosis.

This entry addresses the problems caused by HSV1 and HSV2. Once these viruses enter the body, they can remain dormant in the nervous system for varying amounts of time. They can then be reactivated by fever, physical or emotional

WHY DO WE CALL THEM COLD SORES?

Cold sores are not actually caused by colds, but by the herpes simplex virus. This common name for these annoying sores probably comes from the fact that a herpes-related outbreak is more likely if a person's immune system is under stress, such as when fighting off infection, and a cold is the most common type of infection. Other infectious illnesses, allergies, emotional stress, and even exposure to sun and wind can lead to outbreaks just as well as colds can.

stress, excessive exposure to sunlight, and some foods or drugs. Herpes outbreaks can recur for life, but they generally taper off after age fifty.

Herpes simplex produces small, irritating fluid-filled blisters and red, burning, itchy sores on the skin and mucous membranes. It also affects the nervous system. Symptoms of HSV generally make themselves known within one or two weeks after contraction of the virus.

The initial symptoms of HSV1 include a burning, tingling, or itching sensation around the edges of the lips or nose as a cold sore begins to form. Small red pimples develop within a few hours, followed by the formation of small fever blisters filled with fluid. The blisters itch and hurt and are very annoying. Your child may run a mild fever, and the lymph nodes in her neck may become enlarged. After about seven days, the blisters form thin yellow crusts, indicating that the virus has run its course and healing has begun.

In both males and females, initial symptoms of HSV2 include a burning, tingling, or itching sensation in the genital area, progressing to painful blisters on the skin and moist linings of the sex organs. The fluid-filled blisters turn into red and painful surface sores that itch and burn and can easily become infected. Fever and swelling of the lymph nodes in the groin are common. Members of both sexes may experience pain when urinating.

Both HSV1 and HSV2 infections are extremely common. According to some estimates, over 90 percent of the American population will be infected with the herpes virus by the year 2000. A herpes outbreak can be extremely irritating and uncomfortable. For those who have had herpes before, the early burning and tingling sensation signals an imminent outbreak. Knowing what's coming can add to the stress, which in turn may increase the severity of the outbreak. Once the blisters form into sores, healing usually occurs within seven to ten days.

An HSV2 infection in a pregnant woman poses a serious danger to the fetus. The virus can travel from infected genitalia to the fetus, or the newborn can contract the illness from contact with the lesions during the birth process. The herpes virus can attack the nervous system of a newborn, leading to seizures, mental retardation, or developmental disabilities. To avoid infecting the newborn with this serious illness, it is recommended that the infant be delivered by cesarean section if the mother has a herpes outbreak within three weeks of delivery.

CONVENTIONAL TREATMENT

■ The treatment of cold sores caused by HSV is aimed at relieving symptoms. To reduce the risk of secondary infection, the sores may be washed gently with soap and water. Application of ointments that inhibit the herpes virus (see below) may be helpful in speeding healing.

■ Viscous Xylocaine is a topical anesthetic that can be prescribed to decrease the pain of a herpes sore in the mouth.

Note: It is extremely important not to exceed the recommended dosage of this drug because of its potential toxicity.

■ To ease discomfort, you can give your child acetaminophen (in the form of Tylenol, Tempra, and other medications).

Note: In excessive amounts, this drug can cause liver damage. Read package directions carefully so as not to exceed the proper dosage for your child's age and size.

■ An astringent, such as Campho-Phenique, can help relieve symptoms and speed healing, although it may sting when first applied.

■ The antibiotic acyclovir (Zovirax) is commonly prescribed for treatment of genital and oral herpes. It is a relatively safe and well-tolerated drug that has been taken for years by some patients. The course of treatment requires that the drug be taken every four hours for up to ten days. If acyclovir is taken on a regular basis as a preventive measure, exercise caution. When the drug is stopped, outbreaks sometimes become more severe. However, studies show that the drug does prevent outbreaks in over 90 percent of patients. Acyclovir is also available in ointment form. When applied at the beginning of an outbreak, it can minimize the severity of the attack, but it is not as effective as the oral form of the drug.

DIETARY GUIDELINES

■ To help cleanse your child's system, keep her body well hydrated. Make sure she drinks six to eight glasses of pure water every day. Herbal teas (without caffeine) are highly recommended, as are vegetable soups and juices.

■ Maintain a nutritious diet of healthy whole foods, including plenty of vegetables.

■ Your child should avoid processed foods, soft drinks, alcohol, sugar, refined carbohydrates, and any beverages that contain caffeine. All of these contribute to a buildup of toxins in the body.

■ During an outbreak, or when one is imminent, reduce your child's consumption of (or eliminate) foods containing the amino acid L-arginine, which can promote the growth of the virus. Foods containing L-arginine include whole-wheat products, brown rice, raw cereals (including oatmeal), chocolate, carob, corn (including popcorn), dairy products, raisins, nuts, and seeds.

■ While the virus is active, eliminate acidic citrus fruits and juices, such as orange and grapefruit juice, from the diet. An overly acidic internal environment can slow healing.

■ Soft, cool foods may cause less discomfort to a sore mouth.

NUTRITIONAL SUPPLEMENTS

For age-appropriate dosages of some nutritional supplements, see page 81.

■ Folic acid helps to heal mucous membranes and is helpful for oral herpes. For one week, or until the outbreak subsides, have your child chew a 100-microgram tablet three times a day.

■ *Lactobacillus acidophilus* helps to balance the acidity of the body and thus speed healing. Give your child this supplement for two weeks, following dosage directions on the product label.

■ L-lysine fights the herpes virus. Give a child over twelve 250 milligrams, four times a day (on an empty stomach), for one to two weeks. Then give the same dose, twice a week, for three months. L-lysine is also available in a cream form. The application of this over-the-counter cream can help minimize an outbreak.

■ Selenium has antioxidant properties that activate the immune system. Give your child one dose daily for the duration of the outbreak.

■ Mineral ascorbate vitamin C and bioflavonoids have anti-inflammatory properties. Give your child one dose of each, three times daily, for three days. Then give one dose a day for four days, followed by one-half dose a day for one week.

■ Vitamin E is an anti-inflammatory and is helpful in treating all skin conditions. It may be applied topically once the sores close.

HERBAL TREATMENT

For age-appropriate dosages of herbal remedies, see page 81.

■ Echinacea and goldenseal combination formula has antiviral and astringent properties. It also stimulates the immune system, helps detoxify the blood, and soothes irritated mucous membranes. The liquid formula is preferable because it is more bioavailable, meaning that it is more readily used by the body. Give your child one dose, three times daily, during a herpes outbreak. This combination may also be used topically to help dry out the lesions.

Note: You should not give your child echinacea on a daily basis for more than ten days at a time, or it can lose its effectiveness.

■ Garlic has antiviral properties helpful in treating herpes. Give your child one capsule of odorless garlic, twice daily, for one week. Then give her one capsule, once daily, for one week.

■ Goldenseal root powder can be made into a paste and applied topically to dry out the lesions.

■ Grindelia tincture makes a useful topical treatment. The sticky gum from the fresh plant, if available, also works well.

■ Licorice root has antibiotic properties that are helpful in clearing an infection and detoxifying the blood. Give your child one dose, three times daily, during an outbreak.

Note: This herb should not be given to a child with high blood pressure.

HOMEOPATHY

The following homeopathic remedies are recommended for oral herpes. They are also helpful for genital herpes when the penis or testes are swollen, or when there is inflammation of the vulva. Use these remedies if a genital herpes outbreak is accompanied by a sore throat.

■ If your child's tongue and the inside of her mouth are swollen, red, and dry, and pushing the tongue against the floor of the mouth causes pain, give her *Mercurius corrosivus* or *Mercurius solubilis* 12x, 30x, 6c, or 9c. This child is likely to be subdued, with a depressed spirit. Give her one dose, three times daily, for up to three days.

■ *Natrum muriaticum* is for the child with mouth sores and an increased desire for salt. Give her one dose of *Natrum muriaticum* 12x, 30x, 6c, or 9c, three times daily, for up to three days.

■ If neither of the above remedies seems right for your child, a combination homeopathic herpes remedy may be helpful.

ACUPRESSURE

For the locations of acupressure points on a child's body, *see* ADMINISTERING AN ACUPRESSURE TREATMENT in Part Three.

■ Four Gates relaxes the nervous system.

■ Spleen 10 detoxifies the blood.

GENERAL RECOMMENDATIONS

■ Give your child an echinacea and goldenseal combination formula.

■ Follow the dietary guidelines above.

■ Give your child L-lysine, vitamins C and E, selenium, and bioflavonoids.

■ Stress can add to the possibility and severity of an outbreak. Help your child learn to manage stressful situations. Encourage her to talk about her feelings and concerns. Offer support. Teach relaxation techniques and practice them with your child. Encourage her to get plenty of rest.

■ Practice scrupulous hygiene. Keep the genital area clean.

■ To encourage air circulation, have your child wear loose-fitting cotton underwear. Boys and young men should wear boxer shorts, not briefs, which hold the genitals close to the body, creating a warm, moist environment that fosters the growth of the virus. For both sexes, bikinis are out, especially the nylon ones, which don't breathe.

PREVENTION

■ Children with cold sores are highly contagious. Try to minimize your child's contact with infected children.

■ Teach your child about sexual contact and the possibility of contracting herpes. This caution can be part of a discussion of sexuality.

Hiccups

Hiccups are sudden, involuntary spasms of the diaphragm. They are usually harmless and most go away on their own within a few minutes. Even babies in utero can have hiccups.

Hiccups have a variety of causes, including indigestion and rapid eating. When a child eats too fast, he will sometimes swallow air. With no place to go, the swallowed air can come out in hiccups. When your child gets the hiccups, he may think they are rather funny.

CONVENTIONAL TREATMENT

■ In very extreme and rare cases, a sedative is sometimes used. Otherwise, your doctor is likely to make suggestions similar to the ones listed under General Recommendations, below.

HOMEOPATHY

■ Follow these five steps to help your child get rid of hiccups.

1. Begin with one dose of *Aconite* 30x, 200x, 9c, or 30c. Wait five minutes.
2. If the hiccups are still occurring, give one dose of *Arnica* 30x or 9c. Wait another five minutes.
3. If your child is still hiccupping, try one dose of *Ignatia* 30x or 9c and wait five minutes.
4. If your child is *still* hiccupping, give him one dose of *Magnesia phosphorica* 30x or 9c. Wait five minutes.
5. Finally, you can try a dose of *Lycopodium* 30x or 9c. This remedy is especially helpful if your child has a history of low-bowel gas and repeated hiccups.

ACUPRESSURE

For the locations of acupressure points on a child's body, *see* ADMINISTERING AN ACUPRESSURE TREATMENT in Part Three.

■ Pericardium 6 helps to relax the chest.

GENERAL RECOMMENDATIONS

Every family has a favorite way of getting rid of hiccups. Many have found the following interventions helpful.

■ A baby will sometimes start hiccupping during or after feeding. Help your infant bring up air bubbles by burping.

■ Have your child slowly sip several glasses of cold water.

■ Have an older child take a deep breath and hold it for as long as possible. (Only older children should be taught this technique.)

■ Have an older child breathe into a paper bag. (Again, only older children should be taught this approach.)

■ Have your child slowly sip cold water while holding his breath.

■ Have your child gargle with water for a minute or two.

■ If your child is old enough, teach him to lean over and sip cold water from the opposite rim of the glass.

■ Give your child a glass of cold water. Close your child's ears with your thumbs. Press firmly enough to block his ears, but not hard enough to hurt. While your child's ears are blocked, have him slowly sip water while holding his breath.

PREVENTION

■ Eating slowly is probably the best way to prevent hiccups. To avoid swallowing air, eat at a leisurely pace and teach your children to do the same. Relaxed mealtimes with the family should be a pleasant time together. When meals are enjoyable, children will be less likely to rush to finish eating and resume other activities.

Hyperactivity

Hyperactivity, medically termed *attention deficit hyperactive disorder*, can affect children, adolescents, and even some adults. Symptoms range from mild to severe, and may include problems with language, memory, and motor skills. Although the hyperactive child is often of normal or above-average intelligence, the condition is characterized by learning and behavioral problems. Teachers and parents of a hyperactive child must cope with the child's short attention span, impulsiveness, emotional instability, and uncontrollable overactivity.

Hyperactive behavior may be related to a vision or hearing loss, a communication disorder such as an inability to properly process incoming symbols and ideas, emotional stress, seizures, or sleep disorders. It can also be related to cerebral palsy, lead poisoning, prenatal alcohol or drug abuse, a reaction to certain medicines or foods, and birth complications such as oxygen deprivation or injury at birth. These problems must be ruled out as the cause of the behavior before treating a child for hyperactivity.

True hyperactive behavior interferes with a child's home, school, and social life. Hyperactive children have trouble paying attention and learning. Because they are unable to screen out stimuli, they are very easily distracted. These children may talk a lot, too loudly, and at inappropriate times. Hyperactive children are in constant motion, always into something, and unable to sit still. They are impulsive. They don't stop to look or listen. Because of their amazing and seemingly endless energy, curiosity, and need to explore, they are prone to hurt themselves and to break and damage things. Hyperactive children have a low tolerance for frustration. They argue with parents, teachers, adults, and friends. They have temper tantrums and rapid mood swings. These children also tend to cling. They need lots of attention and reassurance. It is important for parents to realize that hyperactive children *understand* rules, instructions, and social expectations. The problem is that they have a difficult time following them. These behaviors are accidental, not intentional.

For a hyperactive child and his family, a trip to an amusement park or a supermarket can be a disaster. There is simply too much going on—too much simultaneous input. Because of his inability to focus and the constant bombardment of stimuli, a hyperactive child can go into overload.

A hyperactive child may carry a heavy burden. Despite the learning-disabled label, this child is usually very intelligent. He knows that certain behaviors are not acceptable. But despite wanting to please, and to be polite and restrained, the hyperactive child just isn't able to maintain control. He can become frustrated, dismayed, and ashamed. He knows that the "smarts" are there, but he isn't able to slow his nervous system down long enough to harness the brain power necessary to complete an assignment.

The hyperactive child often feels separated and apart from peers, but doesn't understand why he is so different. He is bewildered by his own incapacities. Without the ability to complete normal childhood tasks in school, in the schoolyard, or in the home, the hyperactive child may suffer from stress, sadness, and low self-esteem.

A specialist in child behavior can help you distinguish between a normally active, energetic child and one who is truly hyperactive. Children, even toddlers, can run and play and create a happy commotion for hours without napping, sleeping, or looking the slightest bit tired. To ensure that a truly hyperactive child is properly treated—and to avoid inappropriate treatment of a normally active child—it is important that your child be accurately diagnosed.

During the first one or two visits to a new doctor, a hyperactive child may behave quietly and politely. Knowing what's expected, he may turn into a "model" child. Be prepared to describe, accurately and objectively, your child's behavior at home and in his social activities. If your child is having trouble at school, ask his teacher to speak with the doctor or send a written report. It may take several office visits before the hyperactive behavior becomes apparent. Don't worry. A child specialist can usually make an accurate diagnosis.

When treating a hyperactive child, your goal is to help him do the best he can, at home, at school, and with friends. Always remind yourself that your child is struggling mightily to overcome a nervous system handicap. Explain, if you must, but do not feel ashamed or guilty when your child misbehaves.

Parents of hyperactive children deserve an enormous amount of credit. It takes a lot of patience—and stamina—to love and support a hyperactive child through all the trials and frustrations that come with the condition. Parents of a hyperactive child are always concerned and watchful, always "on the alert." Consequently, it's easy to feel tired, overwhelmed, and frustrated at times. It is vitally important for parents of a hyperactive child to be good to themselves, to take appropriate breaks, to search out, and accept, help and support for themselves as well as for their child.

CONVENTIONAL TREATMENT

■ Before any treatment, a physical examination should be done to rule out other causes for your child's behavior, such as chronic middle ear infection, sinusitis, visual or hearing problems, or other neurological problems.

■ Methylphenidate (Ritalin) is the most commonly prescribed medication for hyperactivity. This is a stimulant that has the paradoxical effect of calming the nervous system and enhancing the ability of a hyperactive child to pay attention. Ritalin can be taken when needed, so that a child need not take it, for example, on weekends or during vacations, when all that extra energy can find an outlet. Be sure, however, that you check with your doctor before taking your child off this medication. Potential side effects of Ritalin include insomnia, decreased appetite, weight loss, slowed growth, increased heart rate and blood pressure, and an initial period of increased tearfulness and irritability.

■ Pemoline (Cylert) is a central nervous system stimulant that is often prescribed for hyperactivity. This medication enhances nerve impulse transmission in the brain. It can cause insomnia and so should be given at least six hours before bedtime. It is not recommended for children under six years of age.

■ Dextroamphetamine (Dexedrine) is another medication sometimes prescribed for hyperactivity. This drug is also a stimulant, but has the same paradoxical calming effect as Ritalin, as well as similar side effects.

■ Tricyclic antidepressant drugs, such as desipramine or nortriptyline (Pamelor) are less frequently prescribed. They are used mainly when an underlying depression is suspected.

■ Thiordazine (Mellaril) is a major tranquilizer that may be resorted to if a child is extremely aggressive, and then only in the most difficult situations.

■ In most circumstances, medication for hyperactivity can be stopped during the summer and resumed when school starts in the fall. This regimen may limit some of the long-term side effects of these drugs. After a summer without medication, it may be useful to permit your child to attend the first several weeks of school without medication. Consider this a trial period to determine whether your child can do without drugs. (Always talk to your doctor before discontinuing any medication for any length of time.)

DIETARY GUIDELINES

■ Before trying any other treatments, begin by eliminating refined sugar and food additives from your child's diet. Read labels carefully, and eliminate processed foods that contain artificial colors, flavors, sweeteners, and preservatives, commonly listed as benzoates, nitrates, and sulfites. Common food additives also include calcium silicate, BHT, BHA, benzoyl peroxide, emulsifiers, thickeners, stabilizers, vegetable gums, and food starch.

■ Salicylates are often implicated in hyperactivity. These are a bit trickier to eliminate from the diet; they occur naturally in addition to being used as additives. A number of popular fruits and vegetables contain salicylates, including almonds, apples, apricots, bananas, blueberries, cherries, grapes, grapefruits, lemons, melons, nectarines, oranges, peaches, plums, prunes, raisins, raspberries, cucumbers, peas, green peppers, hot peppers, pickles, and tomatoes.

■ A study cited in the journal *Pediatrics* reported that more than 50 percent of hyperactive children showed fewer behavior problems and had less trouble sleeping when put on a restricted diet. The diet that helped was free of all artificial and chemical food additives, chocolate, monosodium glutamate (MSG), preservatives, and caffeine.

■ For an in-depth look at diet and hyperactivity, investigate the findings described by Dr. Benjamin Feingold in his book *Why Your Child Is Hyperactive* (Random House, 1975). Dr. Feingold says that his study and clinical practice have convinced him that eliminating all synthetic food additives from a child's diet will resolve hyperactivity. The book offers explanations, food lists, recipes, and menus to help you design a diet for your child.

NUTRITIONAL SUPPLEMENTS

■ A liquid calcium and magnesium supplement is calming to the nervous system. After you have eliminated preservatives and sugar from your child's diet, give him this supplement. Children from five to seven years old should take 1 teaspoon, once daily. Children seven to ten years old should take 1 teaspoon, twice daily. Children ten years and older should take 1 tablespoon, once or twice daily. Follow this regimen for two months, then decrease the dose to five days a week for three months. Then stop giving the supplement altogether.

■ Choline appears to improve memory and attention span in some children. If your child is fourteen years of age or older, try giving him 500 milligrams a day for one month.

■ A liquid vitamin-B complex supplement is very important for hyperactive children. It helps to relax a stressed nervous system and improve mental functioning and concentration. Follow the dosage directions on the product label and

SOME FACTS ABOUT HYPERACTIVITY

• Although many parents of energetic children ask their doctors about hyperactivity, it is *not* a common disorder. According to an article in the *British Journal of Psychiatry*, only 3 percent of children are actually diagnosed with an attention deficit hyperactive disorder.

• Hyperactivity is ten times more common in boys than in girls.

• The exact cause or causes of hyperactivity are unknown. The medical community theorizes the disorder may result from genetic factors; chemical imbalance; injury or disease at or after birth; or a defect in the brain or central nervous system, with the result that the mechanism responsible for controlling attention capabilities and filtering out extraneous stimuli does not work properly.

• As many as half of all hyperactive children have fewer behavior problems when put on a diet free of such substances as artificial flavorings, food colorings, preservatives, monosodium glutamate, caffeine, sugar, and chocolate.

give the recommended dose for two months. Then decrease the dosage to five days a week for three months. Thereafter, stop giving the supplement altogether.

HERBAL TREATMENT

For age-appropriate dosages of herbal remedies, see page 81.

■ Chamomile tea is a noted relaxant. Give your child one dose at bedtime, as needed.

■ Minor bupleurum is a Chinese herbal formula that works to relax the nervous system and can help relieve stress. Give your child one dose daily for one month, followed by wild oat for one month (see below).
   Note: Minor bupleurum should not be given to a child who has a fever or any other sign of an acute infection.

■ Skullcap is a relaxant and calms the mind. Give your child one dose, three times a week, for three months.
   Note: This herb should not be given to a child less than six years old.

■ Wild oat calms the nervous system. Give your child one dose daily for one month.

■ Certain botanical scents may calm a hyperactive child. Mix 1 drop each of rosemary, sage, lavender, and chamomile oil in ⅛ cup of olive oil, and use this aromatic oil to rub your child's feet and spine at bedtime. Native Americans traditionally use rosemary and sage to relax the mind.

HOMEOPATHY

It is best to see a homeopathic physician to determine a constitutional remedy for a hyperactive child. The remedies that follow will help alleviate symptoms, however. Whichever remedy you choose, unless otherwise indicated, try giving your child one dose, three times a day, for five days. Do this every other month for six months.

■ For the child who is thin, excited, anxious, and always in a hurry, use *Argentum nitricum* 30x or 9c. This child craves sweets, which adversely affect his behavior. He may be susceptible to conjunctivitis and tonsillitis. This child is afraid of crowds and dislikes going to any public places, including school. He prefers being outdoors.

■ *Calcarea phosphorica* 30x or 9c benefits the devilish young child, usually a boy, who is restless, shy, and fearful, but who loves to take chances and play tricks. This child tends to have abdominal gas, has a slightly swollen abdomen, and may have enlarged tonsils.

■ If your fidgety child stops being fidgety once he has attracted attention, give him *Chamomilla* 30x or 9c. This type of child can become so hyperactive that he will get exhausted and begin to cry.
   Note: Do not give your child both homeopathic *Chamomilla* and herbal chamomile tea. They will cancel each other out. To achieve the calming effect of chamomile, choose one form or the other.

■ Give *Kali bromatum* 30x or 9c to the restless child who is constantly doing something with his hands—throwing a ball, shooting marbles, flying an airplane. If no toy is at hand, this child cracks his knuckles. *Kali bromatum*'s hands are never still.

■ Give *Lycopodium* 30x or 9c to the child who is more tired, more restless, or more irritable between 4:00 and 8:00 P.M. Tired or not, this child doesn't want to sit down at the dinner table, but prefers to run around. This child looks older than his years and is usually of above-average intelligence.

■ One dose of *Medorrhinum* 200x or 1m will help the child who is irritable, agitated, and in a hurry. This child may have a history of diaper rash as a baby, and later skin rashes and asthma.

■ *Stramonium* 30x is for the child with severe hyperactivity and possible violent agitation. His speech is loud, fast, and possibly incoherent.

ACUPRESSURE

For the locations of acupressure points on a child's body, *see* ADMINISTERING AN ACUPRESSURE TREATMENT in Part Three.

■ Four Gates helps to relax a child's stressed nervous system.

GENERAL RECOMMENDATIONS

■ Eliminate preservatives and sugar from your child's diet. This is the first and most important thing you can do for a hyperactive child. For further improvement, follow all of the recommendations under Dietary Guidelines, page 267.

■ Give your child a liquid calcium and magnesium supplement.

■ Give your child the Chinese herb minor bupleurum.

■ Select a symptom-specific homeopathic remedy. If you are not satisfied with the results, work with a homeopathic physician to find a constitutional remedy.

■ Seek counseling and try behavior modification. These disciplines help a child understand the problem he is wrestling with, how to set goals and standards, and how to recognize and evaluate his behavior. They can be immensely helpful. Such programs teach internal controls that can be used in various situations. Your child will learn to provide rewards for accomplishments, and how to learn from his mistakes. Work with your doctor or counselor in developing behavior modification programs. It is important that the program be clear, easily understood, and easily executed by all who are involved in it—the child as well as the adults. It is essential that these interventions be undertaken with care and compassion, in a calm and loving environment. The child should be a willing participant. Make certain you both understand that these programs are meant to help, not punish.

■ Develop a stable routine at home. To lessen the amount of confusion and day-to-day stimuli, set specific mealtimes and bedtimes.

■ Try assigning a small, quickly finished task, and gently insist that it be completed. Then make sure to thank and praise your child when the job is done.

■ Engage the child in projects he enjoys to help him learn to focus attention. Learning to focus will alter his response to the world, little by little. Always remember that, in addition to having a nervous system imbalance that makes sitting still a torture, a bright hyperactive child becomes bored easily. Work with your child to help him actually finish a project. Finishing a project will provide a sense of competence and increased self-esteem. Mastery and completion of a task call for praise.

■ Seek counseling for yourself and your partner. To help decrease feelings of frustration and isolation, parents of a hyperactive child need information and support. Reach out; it's available. You'll learn how to be with and support your child, and how to feel calm and connected even when the situation seems out of control. You'll also learn that it is important for parents to take some time off without feeling stress or guilt for leaving a "difficult" child with competent others.

■ It is impossible to overemphasize how necessary it is for parents to take time out from the situation. Take an afternoon or evening or weekend off. Get a babysitter. Call your parents or a friend. If you won't do it for your own sake, do it for your child. You will likely come back refreshed and more calm and loving.

PREVENTION

■ During pregnancy, keep exposure to environmental lead to a minimum and eliminate alcohol during pregnancy. Both have been correlated with hyperactivity.

■ Keep your child from being exposed to lead. The most common sources of lead exposure are lead-based paint, drinking water, and improperly glazed pottery.

Immunization-Related Problems

An immunization, or vaccination, is an injection of weakened or killed bacteria, viruses, or, in some cases, deactivated toxins that is given to protect against or reduce the effects of certain infectious diseases. When your child receives an injection of, for example, a small amount of tetanus toxoid, her immune system produces antibodies to fight this foreign substance. Should your child later be exposed to tetanus, her body's defense system will remember and rapidly form antibodies against the bacteria, thus preventing the disease from gaining a hold within the body.

The following vaccinations are among those most commonly recommended for children.

- DPT, or diphtheria/pertussis/tetanus, is designed to protect against three different diseases: diphtheria, a rare but potentially fatal disease that affects the upper respiratory tract, the heart, and kidneys; pertussis, or whooping cough, a disease that is particularly dangerous for children under one year of age and can lead to pneumonia, seizures, and other complications; and tetanus, a potentially deadly infection of the central nervous system.

- DT, or diphtheria/tetanus, is an alternative to DPT, without the pertussis vaccine. It is designed to protect against diphtheria and tetanus only.

- *Hemophilus influenzae* (H. flu.) meningitis type B vaccine, or Hib vaccine, protects against a common bacterial infection that can lead to meningitis, a potentially fatal brain disease. Complications of H. flu. meningitis include pneumonia, hearing loss, and possible learning disabilities. There is now a combination DPT and Hib vaccine available that reduces the number of injections a child must receive to be immunized against all of these diseases.

- The hepatitis B vaccine, the most recent addition to the list of routinely administered vaccines, protects against one of the more serious forms of hepatitis, hepatitis B. This is an infection of the liver that, while not highly contagious, can lead to chronic liver disease or even liver cancer. This vaccine is now being recommended for all children, starting a day or two after birth. Parents are also being encouraged to arrange for the vaccination of unimmunized older children and adolescents.

- MMR—or measles/mumps/rubella—also works to prevent three different diseases: measles, a highly contagious viral disease characterized by fever and rash, whose danger lies in the possibility of such serious complications as pneumonia, strep infections, and encephalitis; mumps, a contagious viral disease that causes fever and swollen glands around the neck and throat (and, rarely, the testicles); and rubella, or German measles, a viral disease involving fever and a mild rash that causes relatively little discomfort to the affected child, but that can cause miscarriage, stillbirth, or birth defects if a woman is exposed to the virus during pregnancy. Because there have been outbreaks of measles among previously vaccinated college students in the past few years, it is now recommended that children receive a total of two MMR injections, the first at fifteen months and the second either before entering school or at the age of eleven or twelve years.

- The polio vaccine is designed to protect against poliomyelitis, an acute viral infection that can lead to paralysis and death. Vaccination against polio involves a more complicated set of decisions than other vaccinations do. Immunization against polio may be accomplished either by an injection of inactivated, dead vaccine, or by live vaccine, which is taken by mouth. The live vaccine present in the oral form appears to give somewhat better immunity than the injectible form does, and has therefore been generally recommended in the United States. However, it also poses a higher risk of complications. An estimated six or seven children come down with polio every year as a result of receiving this vaccine. For this reason, this form of polio vaccine is specifically *not* recommended for a child with a compromised immune system. Also, it is possible for an unimmunized person to contract polio from a child who has been given the live vaccine, even if the child has no noticeable reaction to it. This poses a particular danger if a child has friends or family members who have not been vaccinated, or who have impaired immune function. In such cases, the injectible, inactivated form is recommended. A newer, more potent form of the injectible vaccine now appears to give better immunity than the original one did, while still avoiding the risk of a child (or others with whom she comes in contact) getting the disease as a result of the immunization. Some doctors who recommend the oral, live vaccine take other measures to reduce the chance of a child contracting the virus from it, such as giving the injectible version for the first dose, then switching to the oral form for the additional doses.

- Immunization against rubella may be recommended if your child is a girl between thirteen and sixteen years old who has not received the MMR vaccine (see above) or had German measles.

- The tetanus toxoid vaccine protects against tetanus, an infection of the central nervous system that can be fatal. It is usually given to children in the form of a DPT or DT immunization (see above), but it can be administered individually.

Other immunizations, or changes in the conventional immunization schedule (see the table on page 273) may be recommended for special reasons, such as illness or travel.

Any immunization can produce an adverse reaction. Some of the more common reactions include irritability, malaise, low-grade fever, and soreness or irritation at the site of the injection. These discomforts can be treated simply, at home, with the natural remedies outlined in this entry. More rare, but more serious, reactions include allergic reactions, seizures, neurological problems, and "screaming syndrome," persistent screaming that lasts for three or more hours. After your child receives a vaccination, keep a watchful eye out for any possible reaction. If your child develops a fever higher than 102°F, screams inconsolably, goes into shock, has a seizure, or becomes fretful and irritable after an immunization, call your doctor or seek emergency treatment immediately. These symptoms could indicate a dangerous reaction to a vaccine.

CONVENTIONAL TREATMENT

■ After a vaccination, the site of the injection will probably be red and slightly swollen. A warm wash or compress may help relieve the discomfort, but do not rub the area.

■ If your child experiences pain after an immunization, you can give her acetaminophen (Tylenol or the equivalent).

Note: In excessive doses, this drug can cause liver damage. Read package directions carefully so as not to exceed the proper dosage for your child's age and size.

NUTRITIONAL SUPPLEMENTS

For age-appropriate dosages of some nutritional supplements, see page 81.

■ Begin giving your child vitamin C with bioflavonoids prior to the administration of any vaccine, to help strengthen her immune system. Give a child two years or older one dose daily for one week before and one week after the vaccine. For a nursing infant, a mother can take 1,500 milligrams of vitamin C with bioflavonoids a day, starting one week before the injection.

■ *Lactobacillus bifidus* helps to reestablish healthy flora in the bowel and clear the body of the aftereffects of an immunization. Give your child the bifidus either one hour before or one hour after a meal, following the dosage directions on the product label.

HERBAL TREATMENT

■ Echinacea can be helpful for a baby who has a relatively minor reaction to an immunization, such as a localized infection, low-grade fever, or mild irritability. These herbs boost the immune system. A breastfeeding mother should take 40 drops, twice daily, for three days after her child has been vaccinated.

HOMEOPATHY

■ *Thuja* will help prevent a fever or irritability, whether your baby or older child has a noticeable negative reaction after receiving a vaccine or not. If there is a complication, *Thuja* becomes even more important. Give your child a dose of *Thuja* 200x immediately after the injection.

Conventional Immunization Schedule

Doctors generally recommend that children be immunized against different diseases at different times. Some vaccinations are repeated at intervals to achieve immunity. The schedule that follows indicates the recommended ages for childhood vaccinations and how they are administered.

Age	Vaccine	How Administered
1–2 days	Hepatitis B	By injection
1–2 months	Hepatitis B	By injection
2 months	DPT or DT Hemophilus B[1] Polio	By injection By injection By mouth or injection
4 months	DPT or DT Hemophilus B[1] Polio	By injection By injection By mouth or injection
6 months	DPT or DT Polio	By injection By mouth or injection
6 or 12 months	Hemophilus B[1]	By injection
6–18 months	Hepatitis B	By injection
15 months	MMR Hemophilus B[1]	By injection By injection
15–18 months	DPT or DT	By injection
4–6 years (before entering school)	DPT or DT Polio	By injection By mouth or injection
4–6 years or 11–13 years[2]	MMR	By injection
13–16 years	Rubella[3]	By injection
14–16 years	Tetanus	By injection

1 May be given in combination with DPT.

2 U.S. Centers for Disease Control and Prevention recommends that a second dose of this vaccine be given before a child enters school; the American Academy of Pediatrics recommends that this be done later, when a child is entering middle or junior high school.

3 For girls only, this vaccine may be recommended if a child is unimmunized (i.e., did not receive the MMR vaccine) and has not developed sufficient antibodies as a result of having the disease.

■ *Ledum* is useful for all puncture-type wounds, and can help alleviate some of the reaction at the injection site. Give your child one dose of *Ledum* 12x or 6c immediately after the vaccination, and another dose four hours later.

BACH FLOWER REMEDIES

■ Give your child Bach Flower Rescue Remedy to relieve emotional stress and fright after a vaccination. We recommend that you bring Rescue Remedy to your

The Controversy Over Immunization

Immunization is a controversial issue in pediatric medicine today. Deciding whether or not to have your child receive vaccinations is a complex and, ultimately, a personal matter. It is up to you, as a parent, to make informed, thoughtful decisions for your child.

Any vaccination has the potential to cause a reaction in some children. More than anything else, though, it was probably the serious and frightening side effects observed in some children who had been given the pertussis vaccine (the P in the DPT vaccine) that brought the question of the safety of immunizations to the public's attention. Short-term complications of the standard DPT vaccine can include fever, irritability, screaming syndrome, excessive sleepiness, seizures, and localized inflammation. A newer version of the DPT that uses a more purified pertussis vaccine developed in Japan has become available and seems to cause fewer side effects. The controversy over immunization continues, however. For one thing, critics note, Japanese children are not usually given the vaccine until they are two years old, at which time their nervous and immune systems are more mature and perhaps better able to handle the challenge. And DPT is not the only vaccine that causes concern. Other common vaccines have also been associated with serious side effects, including neurological complications, seizures, fevers, encephalitis, retinopathy, blindness, joint pain, and death.

In addition to citing the risk of side effects, opponents of immunization question the efficacy of vaccines in the first place. For example, some studies have shown that as many as 5 to 10 percent of children who have been vaccinated against pertussis go on to contract the disease anyway (although vaccination may lessen its severity). Measles outbreaks have been known to course through school populations despite the fact that 99 percent of the children had been immunized against it. Further, opponents remind us that the long-term effects of vaccinations are not known. Some propose that there may be a correlation between early immunization and later developmental problems, learning disabilities, autism, hyperactivity, and depression of the immune system.

Conventional medical opinion holds that, as a result of widespread immunization in the United States, many dangerous diseases have been eliminated or inhibited in this country. Consequently, universal immunization against a wide variety of diseases continues to be recommended by the medical establishment. Opponents argue, however, that the lower incidence of many illnesses might just as easily be related to improved sanitation, nutrition, and living conditions as to vaccination programs. They also observe that illnesses seem to follow a natural life cycle, becoming more prevalent at times, and seeming to die away at others. Indeed, there is research showing that the incidence of certain diseases, such as polio and diphtheria, were declining on their own *before* the vaccines designed to combat them were introduced.

The authors of this book believe that the decision to immunize or not to immunize involves risks that every parent should weigh carefully. There is probably no single answer that will feel right to all parents. It is your responsibility to become as informed as possible, so that you can consider both the risks and benefits, and decide whether or not you want to give your child a particular vaccine. Look into the potential side effects of different vaccines—both the short-term and any known long-term ones. Research the incidence, severity, and consequences of different illnesses. You should also call your state health department and ask for any recommendations and/or statistics they have on the subject, as well as school requirements. Once you have considered all of this information, you may choose not to have your child vaccinated, or to have your child receive only one or two of the vaccines, or you may choose to have them given when your child is one or two years old, rather than one or two months. If your child has a history of neurological disorders or seizures, you should definitely have a thorough discussion with your doctor before your child receives any vaccination.

Regardless of what decision you make, keep in mind that immunity is more than immunization. You can boost your child's resistance to disease by supporting her immune system, first by breastfeeding (a mother's immunities are temporarily transferred to her baby this way), and later by providing a nutritious diet. Creating a loving, nurturing, and (as much as possible) stress-free home environment will also help to promote overall health and well-being.

For further discussion of the immunization controversy, consult the following:

Vaccines: Are They Really Safe and Effective? by N.Z. Miller (Santa Fe, NM: New Atlantean Press, 1993).

The Immunization Decision, A Guide for Parents by R. Neustaedter (Berkeley, CA: North Atlantic Books, 1990).

Immunizations, a collection of articles from *Mothering* magazine (contact them at P.O. Box 8410, Santa Fe, NM 87504; telephone 505–984–8116).

doctor's office, and give it to your child right after she receives an injection. Mix 1 or 2 drops in a bottle or glass of water and have her sip it over the next several hours, or put one or two drops of the undiluted remedy under her tongue. (*See* BACH FLOWER REMEDIES in Part One.)

GENERAL RECOMMENDATIONS

■ Discuss with your doctor the pros and cons of any vaccine for your individual child before she receives it, to make sure it is right for her.

■ Give your child one dose of Bach Flower Rescue Remedy immediately after any vaccine is administered.

■ To minimize discomfort at the site of the injection, give your child a dose of homeopathic *Thuja*.

PREVENTION

■ The only sure way to prevent your child from having a reaction to a vaccine is to not have your child receive it. If you have your child immunized, your best defense against reactions is to watch your child closely following all vaccinations, and if symptoms of a reaction develop, contact your doctor right away.

■ A child who has had an immediate, severe reaction to a previous immunization—such as a seizure, screaming syndrome, or a fever of 105°F or higher—should not be given that vaccine again. If your child's doctor is unwilling to take this concern seriously, you may wish to consider seeking another doctor.

Impetigo

Impetigo is a highly contagious skin infection caused by either streptococcus or staphylococcus bacteria. Direct contact with fluid from the infected area or contaminated clothing can transmit the disease. Inadequate hygiene does not cause impetigo. Although good skin hygiene is important, a child who contracts impetigo is not necessarily unclean.

The infection first appears as a rough, cracked, reddened area, commonly on the face or legs. The redness gives way to itching lesions ranging from pinhead- to bean-sized. The fluid-filled blisters quickly form the telltale honey-colored crusts that are typical of the disease. When the crusts are removed, another crust quickly forms. The fluid from the blisters spreads the condition.

Impetigo occurs in a variety of forms and among all age groups, but it is most prevalent in children. In newborn infants, impetigo is a disease of great toxicity and requires prompt treatment. Ecthyma is a virulent or untreated form of impetigo, characterized by large, angry-looking boils, thick golden-yellow crusts, and sores encircled by red skin.

CONVENTIONAL TREATMENT

■ Penicillin and erythromycin are oral antibiotics that may be prescribed for a seven- to ten-day course. Penicillin is sometimes given by injection for impetigo.

• If your child is an infant and you suspect he may have impetigo, contact your doctor.

• If you are treating an older child for impetigo at home, be alert for signs of developing complications. Glomerulonephritis, or acute kidney disease, is a complication that occurs in about 5 percent of cases of streptococcus-caused impetigo not treated with antibiotics. Puffiness around the eyes or the presence of blood in the urine may be a sign that the disease has affected the kidneys. If this happens, contact your doctor. Prompt medical treatment is essential.

These drugs work by killing the bacteria that cause the infection. A possible side effect of erythromycin is the development of mouth sores; both drugs can cause stomach upset and diarrhea.

■ Neosporin and Mycitracin are over-the-counter antibiotic creams that sometimes help clear the infection and are useful for moistening and removing the crusty scabs. If these are ineffective, a prescription ointment called Bactroban may be more potent.

■ A compress made with Burow's solution, an antibacterial agent with cleaning and drying properties, can be applied to the lesions after the crusts are carefully removed.

■ Povidone-iodine (found in Betadine) and hexachlorophene (in pHisoHex, pHisoScrub) are topical antiseptics that may be recommended for cleaning the infected area. After using hexachlorophene, rinse the area thoroughly with water.
Caution: Hexachlorophene should not be used on infants.

■ If your child shows signs of the development of kidney disease, a complication that occurs in a small percentage of cases, he may need to be hospitalized for intensive care.

DIETARY GUIDELINES

■ Eliminate refined sugars and fried foods from your child's diet while he is healing.

■ Offer a diet based primarily on soups, vegetables, grains, and clean, lean protein.

NUTRITIONAL SUPPLEMENTS

For age-appropriate dosages of some nutritional supplements, see page 81.

■ Acidophilus helps restore the beneficial flora in the intestines. This is particularly important if your child is taking antibiotics. Follow the dosage directions on the product label.

■ Bioflavonoids decrease inflammation and stimulate the immune system. Give your child one-half dose, four times a day, until he is better.

■ Chlorophyll contains many vitamins and minerals, and helps to detoxify the blood. Follow dosage directions on the product label.

■ Vitamin C has anti-inflammatory and antibacterial properties. Give your child one dose of vitamin C, in mineral ascorbate form, two to three times a day, for one week to ten days.

■ Zinc helps to boost the immune system. Give your child one dose, once or twice a day, for one week to ten days.
Note: Excessive amounts of zinc can result in nausea and vomiting. Be careful not to exceed the recommended dosage.

HERBAL TREATMENT

For age-appropriate dosages of herbal remedies, see page 81.

■ Goldenseal powder applied topically as a paste is very effective in drying up and healing impetigo.

■ Calendula is a mild disinfectant and is soothing to the skin. Apply calendula tincture, oil, cream, or gel to the rash twice a day.

■ Grapefruit seed extract has antibacterial, antifungal, and antiviral properties. Choose a highly concentrated form, such as Citricidal, Nutrabiotic, or Paramicrocidin, and give your child 5 drops in a glass of juice, three times a day, for up to one week. This liquid has a very bitter flavor that some children may not be able to tolerate, however.

■ Tea tree oil has strong antibacterial and antifungal properties. Dilute 8 to 10 drops of tea tree oil in 1 quart of warm water, and apply the mixture to the infected area twice a day.

■ Garlic has antibacterial and detoxifying properties. Give your child a garlic supplement, following the dosage directions on the product label, until the impetigo heals.

■ Give your child an echinacea and goldenseal combination formula. Echinacea has antiviral properties; goldenseal has antibacterial properties and is soothing to mucous membranes. Give your child one dose, four times a day, for ten days. It can also be applied topically to the affected area, three times a day, for ten days.

Note: You should not give your child echinacea on a daily basis for more than ten days at a time, or it will lose its effectiveness.

■ Usnea moss is a very effective topical agent. Apply usnea salve to the affected area once or twice a day. One recommended product is Super Salve, which contains a combination of usnea, echinacea, chaparral, and hops, and helps to fight infection and soothe irritation.

HOMEOPATHY

Unless otherwise indicated, give your child one dose of any of the following remedies every hour, for up to six hours.

■ *Arsenicum album* 30x or 9c is for the child who has blisters with fatigue, anxiety, and coldness.

■ *Croton* 12x or 6c is for a child with blisters on the scrotum, and/or blisters that are oozing.

■ *Mezereum* 12x or 6c is for a child whose impetigo is predominantly on the scalp.

■ *Mercurius corrosivus* is for a child who has blisters with bad breath and/or body odor.

■ If none of the above remedies seems right, try *Sulphur* 30x or 9x. Give your child one dose an hour, for up to four hours.

ACUPRESSURE

For the location of acupressure points on a child's body, *see* ADMINISTERING AN ACUPRESSURE TREATMENT in Part Three.

■ Spleen 10 helps to detoxify the blood.

GENERAL RECOMMENDATIONS

■ Give your child a daily bath to prevent the infection from spreading to other parts of the body. Put oatmeal (or Aveeno, an oatmeal-based product) or calendula in the bath to moisturize the crusty lesions, ease itching, and help heal the skin.

■ Try to keep your child from scratching and picking at the lesions, a great temptation. When the crusts are removed, the liquid they exude will spread the infection.

■ A child with impetigo should not share clothing, towels, washcloths, combs, pillowcases, or other items that may become contaminated.

■ Keep your child's fingernails cut short. Put mittens on a very young child's hands. Scratching and breaking the skin can spread the infection.

■ Careful hand-washing is the most important element in preventing the infection from spreading from one child to another.

Influenza

Influenza is a viral infection of the respiratory tract. It can occur in epidemic proportions during the winter. Because the structure of the virus may change every two or three years, people will periodically be susceptible to a virus they have never been exposed to before. This creates the possibility of an epidemic outbreak of influenza, or "the flu," every two to three years. Between epidemics, smaller outbreaks may occur as people or young children not exposed in the last outbreak are infected.

Influenza is very contagious and is spread by contact with an infected person. A person is contagious from about two days before symptoms occur until about the fifth day of the illness. Symptoms of influenza include chills, fever, headache, achiness, fatigue, and lack of appetite.

Treatment is generally directed at alleviating symptoms, which can make the sufferer truly miserable. Although the illness generally runs its course in three to four days, complications such as encephalitis, pneumonia, croup, or seizures can occur. If any of these develop, your child will need immediate medical attention.

CONVENTIONAL TREATMENT

■ The cornerstones of treatment for influenza are fever control, rest, and plenty of fluids. Acetaminophen (in Tylenol, Tempra, and other medications) or ibuprofen (Advil, Nuprin, and others) can be used to reduce fever and alleviate achiness.

Note: In excessive amounts, acetaminophen can cause liver damage. Read package directions carefully so as not to exceed the proper dosage for your child's age and size. Ibuprofen can cause stomach upset in some children. To avoid this problem, try giving this medication with food.

■ *Do not* give aspirin to a child or teenager with the flu. The combination of aspirin and viral infection is associated with Reye's syndrome, a dangerous disease affecting the brain and liver (*see* REYE'S SYNDROME).

■ Because influenza is caused by a virus, antibiotics have no effectiveness and are not used. A drug containing amantadine hydrochloride (Symmetrel) is sometimes used in epidemics known to be caused by influenza type A. This drug is

WHEN TO CALL THE DOCTOR ABOUT INFLUENZA

• If your child develops a very high fever, if she has a seizure, or if you notice any changes in her level of consciousness or mental function, seek medical advice immediately. These may be signs that she is developing encephalitis.

• A child with influenza who has a high fever is at risk for having a seizure. If your child has a seizure, call your physician immediately. (*See* SEIZURE.)

• If your child shows signs of increased respiratory distress, such as an increased respiratory rate, gasping, wheezing, nasal flaring, or a pale or bluish color to the skin, call your doctor. Your child may have developed pneumonia and needs medical attention.

effective only if started in the first two days after the onset of symptoms, and it is not used in younger children.

DIETARY GUIDELINES

■ If your child doesn't feel like eating, it's best not to force food. Suggest juices, applesauce, soups, and herbal teas.

■ All fluids, including soups, help alleviate a respiratory illness. Fluids help to thin secretions, making it easier for the body to clear them. If secretions are thick and dry, they are more difficult to expel. Offer your child diluted juices, homemade lemonade (hot or cold), and lots of nourishing broth and homemade soups. Miso and chicken soup are good choices.

■ Avoid giving your child dairy products, which have a tendency to increase and thicken mucus.

■ A child with a cold and fever may get dehydrated and constipated. Flush your child's body with as much fluid as she can take. The constipation will probably resolve once your child starts feeling better and resumes eating a normal diet.

NUTRITIONAL SUPPLEMENTS

For age-appropriate dosages of nutritional supplements, see page 81.

■ Bioflavonoids have potent antiviral properties, and can be useful at any stage of an infection. Give your child one-half dose, five times a day, for five days to one week.

■ Vitamin C has anti-inflammatory properties and helps to ease the course of a respiratory illness. Choose a supplement made without sugar, and avoid chewable forms, as these can erode tooth enamel. Give your child one-half dose, five to six times a day, for five days to one week.

■ To help boost your child's immune system, give her a 5-milligram chewable zinc tablet or lozenge, twice daily, for five days to one week.

Note: Excessive amounts of zinc can result in nausea and vomiting. Be careful not to exceed the recommended dosage.

HERBAL TREATMENT

For age-appropriate dosages of herbal remedies, see page 81.

■ Give your child the Chinese botanical formula yin qiao at the first sign of the flu. This remedy is not helpful after the third day of symptoms. Give your child one dose, every two hours, while the symptoms are acute.

Note: The liquid extract is the preferred form because it contains no aspirin. The tablet form should not be given to a child under four years of age.

■ To help your child rest and relax, give her one dose of chamomile tea, twice daily.

■ The antiviral echinacea and antibacterial goldenseal both stimulate the immune system. Goldenseal also helps to soothe mucous membranes. Give your child one dose of an echinacea and goldenseal combination remedy, three times daily, for five days.

■ Garlic helps to detoxify the body. Give your child one capsule or one fresh clove of garlic, three times a day, until she is better.

■ Ginger tea is excellent if your child's stomach is affected. Give your child one dose as needed.

HOMEOPATHY

■ At the very first sign of influenza, give your child ⅓ tube of *Anas barbariae* (marketed under various brand names, including Oscillococcinum) every hour, for a total of three doses.

■ For the child who feels chilly, restless, and weak, choose *Arsenicum album*. This is for a child who feels worse in a cold room, but wants something cold to drink. She will have a red nose with runny nasal secretions that burn the nose and upper lip. When ill, she wants to sit in bed with books, magazines, and a television. This child wants to be left alone, but will demand attention and reassurance every once in a while. When comforted and cuddled, she will quiet down and go to sleep. Give this child one dose of *Arsenicum album* 30x or 9c, four times a day, for up to three days.

■ *Bryonia* is helpful for a child with a headache, cough, constipation, thirst, and irritability. Give this child *Bryonia* 30x or 9c, three to four times a day, for up to three days.

■ *Eupatorium* is helpful for the child who complains of a severe aching deep in her bones. She feels sore "everywhere." Give this child one dose of *Eupatorium* 12x or 6c, three to four times a day, for up to three days.

■ Give *Gelsemium* to a child who has heavy, droopy eyes and feels weak and tired, with aches and chills up and down her back. This child wants to be alone. Give her one dose of *Gelsemium* 12x or 6c, three to four times a day, for up to three days.

■ *Mercurius solubilis* is for a lingering flu that just doesn't seem to go away. This child may have a sore throat, bad breath, and tender, swollen glands. Give her one dose of *Mercurius solubilis* 12x or 6c, three times a day, for up to three days.

■ *Rhus toxicodendron* is for the restless child who complains of achy, stiff muscles. Give her one dose of *Rhus toxicodendron* 30x or 9c, three times a day, for up to three days.

BACH FLOWER REMEDIES

■ Impatiens helps to ease a child who is whiny, impatient, and tired of being sick. Give the remedy three times a day for three days. (See BACH FLOWER REMEDIES in Part One.)

ACUPRESSURE

For the locations of acupressure points on a child's body, *see* ADMINISTERING AN ACUPRESSURE TREATMENT in Part Three.

■ Bladder 11, 12, 13, and 14 clear and balance the respiratory system.

■ Large Intestine 4 controls the head. This acupressure point relieves congestion and headaches.

■ Lung 7 helps to clear upper respiratory tract infections.

■ Massaging your child's feet is comforting and helps to bring energy down from the head to aid healing.

GENERAL RECOMMENDATIONS

■ Begin treating your child's influenza with homeopathics and herbs as soon as symptoms appear.

■ Encourage your child to take plenty of fluids.

■ Most children naturally want to sleep and rest when suffering through the flu, sparing body energy to fight the virus. A cozy bed and an open window bringing in fresh air (when weather permits) will help. Keep your child from getting chilled.

■ *See also* COUGH; FEVER; SINUSITIS; and/or SORE THROAT if your child's flu is accompanied by these symptoms.

PREVENTION

■ Flu vaccines are offered yearly. These are sometimes recommended by family physicians for people who are most likely to be exposed to or endangered by the illness, such as health care workers, the elderly, and people with chronic heart, lung, or kidney diseases. The flu shot may cause mild flulike symptoms. Also, since flu vaccines are formulated based on viruses that have caused outbreaks in the past, they may or may not be effective in preventing flu caused by this year's virus.

■ Astragalus helps to build the immune system, and thus make your child less vulnerable to the flu. Give your child one dose, three times a week, during the flu season. You can give this herb in capsule form or added to soup.

Note: This herb should not be given if a fever or any other signs of infection are present.

■ American ginseng helps to boost the immune system and strengthen the body. Give your child one dose, in capsule form or in soup, once or twice a week, during the winter months.

■ Echinacea and goldenseal combination formula stimulates the immune system and helps keep the body clear of infections. A liquid extract is the preferred form. You can give your child one dose, twice weekly, during the flu season.

■ Give your child one dose of homeopathic *Anas barbariae* each week or every other week during the flu season.

■ Make it a rule to feed your child a low-sweet diet and no fried foods. During the flu season, prepare lots of vegetable and astragalus soup to help boost her immune system (*see* THERAPEUTIC RECIPES in Part Three).

■ A child under emotional stress may fall ill more easily. Talk out problems and be supportive of your child during times of emotional turmoil.

■ Physical stress can also create bodily imbalances that make a child's body more vulnerable to illness. Exposure to dust and chemicals, too much sugar and/or fat in the diet, even sudden and extreme temperature changes may add to your child's susceptibility to illness.

■ Vitamin C and bioflavonoids, taken daily, help to prevent colds and flu. Give your child 150 milligrams of each daily during the cold season.

Insomnia

Childhood insomnia may take the form of difficulty falling asleep when put to bed, or difficulty remaining asleep throughout the night. When assessing your child's sleep pattern, the most important factors to consider are the quality of his sleep—whether he sleeps through the night or wakes up repeatedly—and how rested and active he is during the day. A child suffering from sleeplessness may not have enough energy to get up in the morning or keep up with peers through the day. He may have dark circles under his eyes.

Normal sleep patterns include alternating cycles of rapid-eye-movement (REM) sleep and non-REM sleep. It is during REM sleep, a lighter sleep, that we dream. Newborns average about sixteen hours of sleep a day, with about half of that time spent in REM sleep, during which time they yawn, squirm, make soft noises, and awaken easily. A two-year-old needs about twelve to fourteen hours of sleep each day, including naps. As children get older, they spend less time in the lighter, REM phase of sleep, and more time time in deeper sleep. About 30 percent of a toddler's sleep time is spent in REM sleep. School-age children need about ten to eleven hours of sleep a day to replenish their active, energetic bodies. Adolescents generally want to assert their independence and determine their own sleep patterns.

As children master new tasks, experience changes in their lives, and move from one developmental stage to another, sleeplessness is a common temporary problem. A young child who is learning to sleep in a new room, a child who has just moved to a new house, or a teenager who is anxious about an upcoming event may experience a few nights of sleeplessness.

If sleeplessness persists and begins to interfere with your child's ability to keep up during the day, however, consult your doctor. Insomnia may be related to depression or anxiety, a physical problem such as a chronic ear infection or fever, or night terrors. Night terrors are characterized by screaming, thrashing, confusion, sweating, and rapid breathing. They usually occur a couple of hours after a child has fallen asleep or as he is coming out of a deep, nondreaming sleep. Another problem to consider—if your child snores heavily, is excessively sleepy through the day, and performs poorly in school—is *sleep apnea*, a temporary cessation of breathing during sleep. Brief periods of sleep apnea are common among newborns and premature infants. Obese children and children with enlarged tonsils and chronic tonsillitis may also experience sleep apnea, due to obstruction of the airway. If you suspect your child may have sleep apnea, check with your doctor.

If your newborn infant is experiencing difficulty sleeping, *see* PREGNANCY AND YOUR NEWBORN in Part One. This entry addresses temporary sleeplessness in toddlers through adolescents.

CONVENTIONAL TREATMENT

■ Diphenhydramine, an antihistamine better known as Benadryl, is one of the most benign sleep-inducing drugs. However, you should never give a child Benadryl, or any other over-the-counter drug, to help him sleep without consulting your medical practitioner.

■ Antidepressants, such as amitriptyline (Elavil) or imipramine (Tofranil) are occasionally used for sleep problems, especially if the patient is suffering from depression. These should be given only when prescribed by a child psychiatrist.

■ Tranquilizers, such as diazepam (Valium), are potent and potentially addictive prescription medicines. They are not recommended, especially for children, except in the most extreme circumstances.

DIETARY GUIDELINES

■ Avoid giving your child any stimulants, such as foods and beverages containing caffeine or refined sugars, or chocolate, which can keep him awake at night.

■ Avoid serving large meals late at night.

■ To maintain a steady blood sugar level throughout the night, give your child a light snack, such as crackers or toast, before bedtime. Avoid heavy, hard-to-digest foods.

■ Make sure your child eats foods containing the amino acid tryptophan, which helps to stabilize moods and alleviate stress. It is used by the brain to produce serotonin, a chemical that regulates the mechanisms of normal sleep. Foods high in tryptophan include bananas, cottage cheese, fish, dates, milk, peanuts, and turkey. Having complex carbohydrates such as pasta or rice for dinner is a good sleep inducer, too.

NUTRITIONAL SUPPLEMENTS

■ Brewer's yeast is high in B vitamins, as well as other vitamins and minerals that help to calm the nervous system. Give a child who is twelve years of age or older 1 teaspoon at bedtime.

■ A calcium and magnesium supplement will help calm your child's nervous system. This supplement is very helpful for the child who experiences sleeplessness accompanied by leg cramps. Give your child one dose of a supplement containing 250 milligrams of calcium and 125 milligrams of magnesium in the morning and then again at bedtime for a couple of months.

HERBAL TREATMENT

For age-appropriate dosages of some herbal remedies, see page 81.

■ To help your child unwind and relax before going to bed, give him a cup of chamomile tea, an herbal relaxant, an hour before bedtime. A combination herbal tea, such as Celestial Seasonings' Sleepytime tea, may also be used.

■ Passion flower is a mild relaxant that is safe for children over four. Give your child a cup of passion flower tea at bedtime.

■ Skullcap is an effective relaxant. Give your child one dose, in tea, tincture, or capsule form, one hour before bedtime.
   Note: This herb should not be given to a child under six years of age.

■ Valerian root can be effective for children twelve years of age or older. Give your child one dose, in capsule, tea, or tincture form, at bedtime.

■ For an older child, you can make a tea combining equal amounts of valerian, chamomile, passion flower, and skullcap, and give him a cup at bedtime.

■ Rather than giving your child the same relaxant herb consistently, it is more effective to rotate them. For example, give your child chamomile for several nights, then passion flower for several nights, and so on.

HOMEOPATHY

■ Homeopathic *Carbo vegetabilis* is for the child who awakens in the middle of the night with a stomachache. Give this child one dose of *Carbo vegetabilis* 30x or 9c when he wakes in the middle of the night.

■ *Coffea cruda*, homeopathic coffee, relieves symptoms similar to those adults feel after drinking a cup of coffee. This remedy effectively relieves mental and physical nervousness and excitement that may be interfering with sleeping. For example, the night before a big event such as a test or athletic competition, a child may lie sleepless in bed with racing thoughts. One dose of *Coffea cruda* 12x or 6c, given one hour before dinner, and another dose half an hour before bedtime, is helpful for this type of insomnia.

ACUPRESSURE

For the locations of acupressure points on a child's body, *see* ADMINISTERING AN ACUPRESSURE TREATMENT in Part Three.

■ Bladder 60 helps to take energy down and away from the head.

■ Four Gates helps relax the nervous system.

■ Pericardium 6 helps relax the mind and alleviate excitement.

■ Massaging the muscles on either side of the spine will contact a series of points that help to relax the entire system.

GENERAL RECOMMENDATIONS

■ Slow down your child's metabolic rate and allow time to unwind in the evening. A warm bath, a back rub, or a foot rub will help a child settle down comfortably.

■ Give your child a calcium and magnesium supplement.

■ Give your child a cup of herbal tea before bedtime.

■ Teach an older child relaxation techniques (*see* RELAXATION TECHNIQUES in Part Three).

■ For occasional sleeplessness, give your child homeopathic *Coffea cruda*.

PREVENTION

■ Set a sleep schedule and stick to it. Initiate a regular bedtime and wake the child at the same time every day.

■ Initiate a simple but routine bedtime ritual, such as reading a story, talking over the day, or going through a guided imagery exercise together (*see* RELAXATION TECHNIQUES in Part Three). A regular sleep cycle and familiar bedtime rituals serve to comfort, reassure, and foster healthy sleep habits. Adhere to your schedule even on weekends and during holidays. However, you should be flexible enough to adjust the schedule if it does not match your child's normal cycle. Some children are "larks," who naturally awaken early, while some are "owls," who prefer to stay up a little later.

■ With older children, discourage late afternoon or evening naps.

■ Encourage discussion of any frightening or disturbing experiences that may have occurred during the day. This is especially important for highly sensitive or impressionable children.

■ To reassure a fearful child, leave the door open and a small, comforting night light burning.

■ Encourage vigorous physical activity in the morning or afternoon.

■ Avoid frightening television shows or scary stories before bedtime.

Itching

See SKIN RASH.

Lice

Head lice are tiny insects that attach themselves to the scalp. Head lice do not jump or fly, but spread from one infested child to another by direct contact. A lice infestation (medically termed *pediculosis*) has nothing to do with hygiene, but everything to do with proximity. If two children have their heads together sharing a book, working on a project, playing a video game, wrestling, or just rumpusing around, one child can transmit lice to the other. If just one classmate has lice, the whole class can become infested. A child at summer camp is a prime candidate for infestation, if a cabinmate has head lice. Lice spread easily through shared hats, clothing, sheets, pillows, combs, and brushes.

If your child complains of an itchy head, or you notice persistent scratching, take a close look at her scalp. If you see nothing under natural light, use a flashlight. Head lice look like tiny round graying lumps on the scalp. You might see eggs, called nits, along the hair shaft. Check the lymph nodes in your child's neck and the back of her head; enlarged lymph nodes are a possibility if the scratching leads to a secondary infection.

Female lice lay four to five eggs every day, and continue to do so until stopped, so early, aggressive treatment is necessary. If your child has head lice, inform the authorities at school, camp, or any other communal area where the infestation may have been contracted (or communicated to other children). To prevent your child from becoming reinfested, a quick and thorough community cleanup is necessary.

Head lice are very irritating and cause severe itching. Your child's scalp may get raw from scratching, and an impetigolike infection is a possible complication (*see* IMPETIGO). When washing and combing your child's hair, check for signs of local infection. If you have a reason for concern, consult your health care provider.

CONVENTIONAL TREATMENT

■ Permethrin creme rinse (sold as Nix or Elimite) kills lice, ticks, mites, and fleas by attacking their nervous systems. Permethrin is relatively safe and requires only one application to get rid of a very high percentage of the mites. Follow directions on the product label.

■ Lindane shampoo (Kwell) is sometimes used for a lice infestation, but it requires two applications and can be toxic to the nervous system. One recent study has linked its use to the development of brain cancer. Because of these disadvantages, this product has largely been replaced by permethrin.

■ Crotamiton cream (Eurax) is safer than lindane, but still must be applied twice in order to be effective. It has the advantage of anti-itch properties, however.

HERBAL TREATMENT

■ Balsam of Peru has antiparasitic properties and destroys the mite *Acarus* and its eggs. It is useful against scabies, eczema, and other skin conditions as well. It can be applied to the scalp alone, or diluted with oil. After application, comb your child's hair with a fine-toothed comb to remove lice and eggs from the hair shaft.

■ In the event of a secondary infection, give your child an immune-boosting echinacea and goldenseal combination formula. Give your child one dose, three times daily, for five days.

■ Because of its antiparasitic properties, garlic will help your child's body fight a head lice infestation. Give your child one dose, three times daily, for five days.

■ Goldenseal tincture, or a strong goldenseal tea, can be used to wash the scalp.

■ Tea tree oil (*Melaleuca alternifolia*) is a strong herbal disinfectant that will help get rid of head lice. Add 25 drops of tea tree oil to 1 pint of distilled or spring water. Rub this mixture into your child's hair and scalp three times daily, and comb your child's hair with a fine-toothed comb to remove lice and eggs from the hair shaft.

HOMEOPATHY

■ Give your child one dose of *Sulphur* 30x or 9c, three times daily, for up to three days. If you are using herbal tea tree oil, give the *Sulphur* one hour before or one hour after applying the oil to your child's scalp. Otherwise, the strong odor of tea tree oil may cancel out the effectiveness of this homeopathic remedy.

GENERAL RECOMMENDATIONS

■ Rub diluted tea tree oil into your child's hair and scalp.

■ Using a fine-toothed comb, carefully and thoroughly comb your child's hair. Examine her scalp minutely. In order to see and pick out all the lice and eggs, separate the hair into fine strands. This is a tedious and unpleasant process, but it is the only way to be sure of ridding your child of a lice infestation.

■ To stimulate your child's immune system against a secondary infection, give her echinacea and goldenseal combination formula.

■ To avoid a reinfestation, wash anything and everything that comes in contact with an infested child's head in very hot water.

■ Alert neighborhood families, and call your child's school or camp to warn about the possibility of infestation. There is no reason to be embarrassed. A lice infestation does not mean that your child is uncared-for or dirty. Other children should be checked and treated, if necessary.

PREVENTION

■ To prevent an infestation of head lice from traveling through the family, don't use community towels. Until you are certain your child is free of lice, wash her clothes, bedding, and towels separately, in very hot water. An infested child should not place her head on furniture (other than her own bed), such as when reading or watching television.

■ Teach your child not to share combs and brushes, hats, or clothing with other children.

Lyme Disease

Lyme disease is a potentially serious long-term illness caused by a spirochete (a slender, spiral-shaped type of bacterium) called *Borrelia burgdorferi*. The disease is spread by infected deer ticks, which are minute ticks that commonly feed on deer and mice. It was first identified as a distinct, separate illness in the area of Lyme, Connecticut (hence the name), but it is now found in most of the United States, and there have been cases in other countries as well. In fact, in some parts of the country, infected ticks may now be found in suburban back yards. Although the incidence of the disease in any given area seems to be related to the level of the deer population, other animals, including jackrabbits, lizards, and field mice, have been found to carry the infection as well. Fortunately, the illness is not spread from one person to another.

A person becomes infected by being bitten by a tick that carries the bacteria. Because deer ticks are so tiny, however, it is quite possible to overlook their presence on the body, and the tick bites themselves are usually painless. The symptoms experienced vary from person to person, and they often mimic those of other ailments. As a result, a diagnosis of Lyme disease can easily be missed in the early stages.

The first sign noted in most people with Lyme disease is a characteristic "bull's-eye" marking at the site of the tick bite (usually, but not always, on the arm or leg). This is a round, raised reddish lesion that typically is paler, even white, in the center. In some cases, the bull's-eye rash gradually expands around the center; in others, a bumpy rash develops on the torso. These signs may come and go throughout the course of the disease. Often accompanying the development of the bull's-eye mark and/or rash are flulike symptoms, including fever, chills, headache, and overall achiness. Some people develop an enlarged spleen and lymph glands, some complain of sore throat and severe headache, and some suffer from nausea and vomiting. The symptoms can occur singly or in any combination, and they can develop anywhere from three days to three weeks (or even more, in some cases) after the initial tick bite. The course of recovery is similarly variable. Some people get better after suffering the initial illness; others go on to develop long-term, even chronic, complications, including arthritis, neurological problems, and even enlargement of the heart and irregular heartbeat. The fatigue and achiness frequently last for weeks.

The critical factor in the treatment of Lyme disease is early diagnosis. If you suspect that your child may be developing Lyme disease, it is wise to consult your doctor. There is a blood test that can confirm whether or not your child has been infected with the *Borrelia burgdorferi* bacterium. This test may have to be repeated, as it usually is not positive for several weeks after the infection is contracted.

CONVENTIONAL TREATMENT

■ Lyme disease is treated with a course of oral antibiotics that can run from ten to twenty days in length, depending on the severity and/or persistence of symptoms. Tetracycline is usually the antibiotic of choice for older children; amoxicillin or erythromycin may be recommended for younger children and infants.

■ If the disease has progressed significantly before being diagnosed, and particularly if neurological problems or arthritis have developed, a ten-day course of intravenous antibiotic, such as penicillin or ceftriaxone, may be prescribed.

■ To alleviate the symptoms of fever and achiness, your doctor may recommend giving your child acetaminophen (Tylenol, Tempra, or the equivalent) or aspirin (because Lyme disease is bacterial, not viral, in origin, it is possible to use aspirin for fever and pain with this illness). If you give your child acetaminophen, read package directions carefully so as not to exceed the proper dosage for your child's age and size. This drug can cause liver damage if given in excessive amounts. If you give your child aspirin, you may wish to give it with food to prevent possible stomach upset.

DIETARY GUIDELINES

■ As when fighting any illness, encourage your child to take plenty of fluids, and to eat plenty of well-cooked whole grains and fresh vegetables.

■ To foster a more healing internal environment, reduce the amount of fat, sugar, refined carbohydrates, and dairy products in your child's diet.

NUTRITIONAL SUPPLEMENTS

For age-appropriate dosages of some nutritional supplements, see page 81.

■ A calcium and magnesium supplement may be helpful for relieving achiness. Give your child one dose of a formula containing 250 milligrams of calcium and 125 milligrams of magnesium, twice a day, for up to two weeks.

■ Chlorophyll is full of trace minerals that are helpful in the healing process. Give your child one dose, as directed on the product label, twice a day, for two months.

■ Vitamin C is both antibacterial and anti-inflammatory; bioflavonoids stimulate the immune system and decrease inflammation, especially of the joints. Give your child one dose of vitamin C with bioflavonoids, three times a day, for two months.

■ A child with Lyme disease may have impaired digestion, resulting in stomach gas. A mild digestive enzyme can be of great help during the first month or two of treatment. Follow dosage directions on the product label.

WHEN TO CALL THE DOCTOR ABOUT LYME DISEASE

• Because early diagnosis is so important to the successful treatment of Lyme disease, if you notice a suspicious bull's-eye-type lesion (a raised reddish bump that is paler in the center) anywhere on your child's body, consult your doctor.

• If your child develops flulike symptoms within a few days after spending time outdoors, particularly in a wooded area or an area with long grass or weeds, you may wish to explain the situation to your doctor and have your child examined for the possibility of a Lyme infection.

■ Give your child a good balanced vitamin-B complex multivitamin for two months to strengthen his overall nutritional status.

■ If your child is twelve years of age or older, supplement his diet for one to two months with bromelain, a natural enzyme extracted from pineapple that acts as an anti-inflammatory. Follow dosage directions on the product label. This should be taken on an empty stomach.

■ Give your child one dose of zinc, in tablet or lozenge form, twice a day, for two weeks. Zinc promotes healing and stimulates the immune system.

Note: Excessive amounts of zinc can result in nausea and vomiting. Be careful not to exceed the recommended dosage.

HERBAL TREATMENT

For age-appropriate dosages of herbal remedies, see page 81.

■ An echinacea and goldenseal combination formula will help to clear infection and support your child's immune system. Give him one dose, three times a day, for up to two weeks.

Note: Echinacea should not be given on a daily basis for more than ten days at a time, or it may lose its effectiveness.

■ Garlic has antibacterial properties. Give your child one dose, twice a day, for two months.

GENERAL RECOMMENDATIONS

■ Pay close attention to any suspicious-looking insect bites or other marks on your child's body, especially after he has been playing outdoors. If you have any doubts, consult your physician.

■ If your child has a flulike illness with fatigue or malaise that seems to linger for an unusually long time, consult your physician to rule out the possibility of a Lyme infection. Often a diagnosis of Lyme disease is missed or delayed because the symptoms are similar to those of other common diseases, but treatment is more likely to be successful if it is begun early. If your doctor doesn't suggest the possibility, ask about it.

PREVENTION

■ If your child will be walking or spending time in an area likely to have deer ticks, make sure he wears clothing that offers some protection. Long-sleeved shirts, long pants, hats, and socks and shoes are recommended. It is a good idea to pull your child's socks up and over the bottoms of the pants legs, because ticks often climb up from the ground and will bite as soon as they find exposed skin. It may also be helpful to spray permethrin — a medication usually used for head lice — on your child's clothes. Permethrin is sold under the brand names Nix, Permanone, and Duranon. It is safe when used this way and is highly effective at repelling insects, including ticks.

■ After your child has been walking, hiking, or otherwise spending time in a wooded or high-grass area, check his body, hair, and clothing thoroughly. Keep in mind that deer ticks are *very* tiny. It may also be a good idea to have your child shower or bathe as soon as possible.

■ If you find a tick on your child, remove it by using tweezers. Grab the head of the insect, as close to your child's skin as possible, and firmly but gently pull it out of the skin. Try not to crush the tick, but save it in a small plastic bag or jar for identification. After removing the tick, wash your hands and the bite wound thoroughly with soap and water, and consult your physician.

Measles

Measles is a serious, highly contagious viral infection of childhood. Symptoms of measles include fever, malaise, cough, runny nose, and conjunctivitis. The symptoms get worse over a period of a few days, and on approximately the fourth day, a rash appears. The rash is raised, splotchy, reddish-brown or purplish-red in color, and mildly itchy. It begins on the face and neck and spreads to the trunk, extremities, and feet, lasting about five to seven days. Red spots with a bluish-white center (known as Koplik's spots) appear on the inside of the mouth about twelve hours before the red rash first appears.

Once a person is infected with the measles virus, it can incubate for nine to fourteen days before signs of illness develop. A child with the measles is considered contagious for at least seven days after the beginning of the illness. Usually, the disease is self-limiting and runs its course within ten days. The fever falls, making the sufferer feel more comfortable in general, and the rash fades to a brownish color that gradually disappears as the outer layer of skin is shed. Once this happens, the child is no longer contagious.

The seriousness of measles lies in the potential for complications following the illness itself. Ear infections are one common complication. Pneumonia and encephalitis (an inflammation of the lining of the brain) are also possible, and more serious, complications. If your child's fever climbs to a very high level, if she has a seizure, or if you notice any changes in her level of consciousness or mental function, seek medical advice immediately. These may be symptoms of encephalitis, which can be fatal.

SYMPTOMS OF MEASLES

The first signs that a child is coming down with the measles usually include some combination of the following:

- Fever.
- A stuffy and/or runny nose.
- A cough.
- Red and possibly itchy eyes that may be sensitive to light.
- Small red spots in her mouth.

Three to five days after these initial symptoms, a child with measles will develop a rash with the following general characteristics:

- It is splotchy and brownish-pink in color.
- It begins around the ears and/or on the face and neck, then spreads over the rest of the body (although in mild cases, the arms and legs may not be affected).
- It is mildly itchy.
- It lasts for four to seven days before fading away.

CONVENTIONAL TREATMENT

■ Treatment for measles is primarily aimed at alleviating symptoms while the virus runs its course. A child with the measles may run a fever as high as 104°F (in some cases higher), so fever control is a principal concern. You can give your child acetaminophen (in the form of Tylenol, Tempra, and other medications) or ibuprofen (Advil, Nuprin, and others) to bring down fever and ease overall achiness and malaise.

Note: In excessive amounts, acetaminophen can cause liver damage. Be careful not to exceed the proper dosage for your child's age and size. Ibuprofen is best given with food to prevent possible stomach upset.

■ *Never* give aspirin to a child who has—or who you suspect may be coming down with—the measles. The combination of aspirin and a viral infection has been linked to the development of Reye's syndrome, a serious disease of the liver and brain (*see* REYE'S SYNDROME).

■ Because measles is a viral illness, antibiotic therapy is ineffective and therefore not appropriate. If your doctor confirms that your child has developed a secondary, bacterial infection, such as an ear infection, antibiotics may be prescribed to fight the secondary infection.

■ Make sure your child gets plenty of rest and drinks plenty of fluids. Also, because measles often causes a heightened sensitivity to light, your child will probably be more comfortable in a dimly lit room.

DIETARY GUIDELINES

■ Lots of fluids are essential to prevent dehydration. Keep a feverish child well hydrated. Offer fruit-juice popsicles, spring water, herb teas, soups, and diluted juices. During the recovery period, immune-boosting astragalus and vegetable soup is a good choice as well (see THERAPEUTIC RECIPES in Part Three).

■ Eliminate fats as much as possible. Fats are difficult to digest under normal circumstances, and are even harder to digest when the digestive system is weakened by infection. Undigested fats contribute to a toxic internal environment.

NUTRITIONAL SUPPLEMENTS

For age-appropriate dosages of nutritional supplements, see page 81.

■ Vitamin A aids in healing mucous membranes. Give your child one dose of vitamin A, once a day, for ten days.

■ Vitamin C and bioflavonoids help to stimulate the immune system. Three to four times a day, give your child one dose of vitamin C in mineral ascorbate form, and an equal amount of bioflavonoids, for one week. The following week, give the same dosage, but two to three times a day. During the third week, give the same dosage, two to three times, every other day. Then continue to give one-half dose, once a week, for three weeks.

■ Zinc stimulates the immune system and promotes healing. Give your child one dose, twice a day, for ten days.

Note: Excessive amounts of zinc can result in nausea and vomiting. Be careful not to exceed the recommended dosage.

HERBAL TREATMENT

For age-appropriate dosages of herbal remedies, see page 81.

■ If your child is feeling very restless, give her one dose of chamomile tea, twice a day.

■ Echinacea and goldenseal combination formula helps clear an infection, supports the immune system, and soothes the skin and mucous membranes. Echinacea is a powerful antiviral. Give your child one dose, every two hours, until the fever breaks. Then give her one dose, three times a day, for one week.

Note: You should not give your child echinacea on a daily basis for more than ten days at a time, or it will lose its effectiveness.

■ An herbal fever-reducing tea will help to bring down your child's temperature, decrease chills, and increase perspiration. Combine equal parts of some or all of the following: lemon balm leaf, chamomile flower, peppermint leaf, licorice root, and elder flower. For an older child, a little honey can be added to improve flavor. Give your child one dose, four times a day, for two or three days. A nursing mother may take one adult dose, four times a day, instead of giving the tea directly to her baby; its healing properties will be passed to her baby in her breast milk. The tea should be taken as hot as possible.

Caution: Do not put honey in the tea if you are giving it to a child less than one year old. Honey has been associated with infant botulism, which can be life threatening. Also, if you are using peppermint in the tea and also giving your child a homeopathic preparation, allow one hour to elapse between the two treatments. Otherwise, the strong smell of the mint will decrease the effectiveness of the homeopathic remedy.

■ Ginger tea can be effective against a fever. It is most helpful for the child who tends to feel cold, especially in the hands and feet. To decrease chills and increase perspiration, snuggle your child under light covers after giving her the tea. Give your child one dose, four times daily, for one day. If your child finds the taste too pungent, mix the tea with fruit juice.

■ Shiitake mushrooms have immune-stimulating properties. They may be eaten fresh, or taken in capsule form. Give a child twelve years old or older one capsule, three times a day, as long as signs of infection are present.

■ Give your child cool oatmeal baths to lessen the itching. Wrap a handful of oatmeal in a washcloth and let it soak in your child's bath water. For extra relief, gently rub the oatmeal-filled washcloth over your child's skin.

HOMEOPATHY

Choose the most appropriate symptom-specific remedy from the suggestions that follow and give your child one dose, every two hours, up to a total of four doses a day, for up to two days.

■ *Apis mellifica* 30x or 9c is recommended for a child who has a swollen throat and difficulty breathing, and has a cough that causes pain in the chest. This child does not feel thirsty and is less comfortable in a warm room.

■ Choose *Arsenicum album* 30x or 9c if your child is restless but weak, feels worse after midnight, and wants frequent small drinks. This child's skin may be itchy, and she may have diarrhea as well.

■ *Belladonna* 30x or 9c is the remedy for a child who has a high fever, red eyes, and a flushed face, and complains of a throbbing head and difficulty swallowing.

■ *Gelsemium* 30x or 9c is for the feverish child with droopy eyes and a croupy cough, who complains of feeling chilly and having a runny nose. This child's rash is likely to be very red and itchy, and she may have a headache.

■ *Pulsatilla* 30x or 9c is helpful for a child who is tearful, with eyes that are sticky, discharging, and very sensitive to light. This child's rash is dark red and spotty. She has thick yellow nasal mucus and a cough that is dry at night but looser during the day. She may have an upset stomach as well.

ACUPRESSURE

For the locations of acupressure points on a child's body, *see* ADMINISTERING AN ACUPRESSURE TREATMENT in Part Three.

■ Four Gates helps to relax a feverish child.

GENERAL RECOMMENDATIONS

■ To prevent dehydration, encourage a feverish child to drink plenty of fluids. The increased metabolic rate that results from a fever causes the body to lose fluids rapidly.

■ Make sure your child gets plenty of rest. Keep the lights in your child's room dim.

■ Give your child an echinacea and goldenseal combination formula.

■ Select and administer a symptom-specific homeopathic remedy.

■ To promote perspiration and bring down a moderate to high temperature, give your child fever-reducing herbal tea.

■ If your child is uncomfortable and restless, give her soothing and calming chamomile tea.

■ Give your child vitamin C with bioflavonoids, zinc, and vitamin A.

■ If your child has the measles, be alert for signs that a secondary infection may be developing. If symptoms seem to get worse, or if new symptoms develop, seek medical advice.

PREVENTION

■ A vaccine that protects against measles is available. It is usually given in the form of the MMR vaccine, which also contains vaccines against mumps and rubella (German measles), when a child is approximately fifteen months old. An additional dose is recommended either before a child enters school or when she is between the ages of eleven and thirteen. (*See* IMMUNIZATION-RELATED PROBLEMS.)

■ A child who has recently been exposed to measles and may be incubating the disease should not be given the measles vaccine at that time. It may suppress the rash at the time, but it could leave her vulnerable to developing a more serious case of the illness in adolescence.

■ As much as possible, try to keep your child from contact with contagious children, particularly if she is not (or is not yet) immunized against the disease.

Meningitis

Meningitis is an infection and inflammation of the three *meninges*, which are thin membranes that cover the brain and spinal cord. The infection can be caused by either a virus or bacteria. *Hemophilus influenzae*, or "H. flu.," is the most common among the bacterial organisms that cause meningitis in children. An infection in the blood (bacteremia), ears, jaw, or sinuses can also lead to an infection of the meninges.

A newborn with meningitis may have poor muscle tone, difficulty feeding, a weak suck and cry, vomiting, irritability, sleepiness, and/or jitteriness. In infants, symptoms of meningitis include a high-pitched cry, irritability, loss of appetite,

SYMPTOMS OF MENINGITIS

The symptoms of meningitis usually come on quickly, especially in children, and involve some combination of the following:

- Fever;
- Headache, often severe;
- Malaise;
- Vomiting;
- Stiff neck and back;
- Changes in consciousness, from irritability through confusion to drowsiness, stupor, and coma.

In an infant, symptoms may be somewhat different, including:

- A high-pitched cry;
- A bulging or tight fontanel (soft spot);
- Seizure and/or loss of consciousness.

If your child displays any of these symptoms, particularly after or while recovering from a respiratory illness or sore throat, call your doctor right away.

vomiting, lethargy, and possibly a fever or convulsions. An older child is likely to have a fever, chills, vomiting, irritability, headache, and/or a stiff neck. Seizures and changes in consciousness, such as stupor or coma, are possible as the infection progresses.

Meningitis is a serious infection that is potentially life threatening and can cause such long-term consequences as hearing or vision problems. It requires immediate medical attention. If treated early and appropriately, there is a low likelihood of complications or lasting harm to your child.

CONVENTIONAL TREATMENT

■ Meningitis is diagnosed by looking for signs of infection and the presence of an infectious organism in the spinal fluid. To perform a "spinal tap," a needle is inserted into a space between two vertebrae and a small amount of fluid is withdrawn for inspection. The process can be difficult, as it requires the child to curl up and lie still. The doctor will use a numbing medicine on the skin before putting the needle in to lessen the pain, but it still feels like pressure in the back. The doctor will probably also take a sample of your child's blood to look for other signs of infection.

■ If meningitis is suspected, antibiotic therapy will be started immediately after the spinal fluid samples are taken. A doctor will not wait to get the results back to find out whether the meningitis is bacterial or viral, because the risks of not treating a possible bacterial infection immediately are too great. The antibiotic will be given intravenously, usually for a minimum of seven days. Ampicillin, penicillin, and chloramphenicol are commonly used antibiotics for bacterial meningitis.

■ If the meningitis is determined to be viral in origin, antibiotics are ineffective and will be discontinued. Rest, fluids, and nutrition, as well as measures to control fever and relieve pain, will be recommended to ease the discomfort and aid in recovery.

■ If there is *even a suspicion* of viral meningitis, aspirin should not be given as a painkiller, because the combination of aspirin and viral infection has been linked to the development of Reye's syndrome, a dangerous disease affecting the brain and the liver (*see* REYE'S SYNDROME).

NUTRITIONAL SUPPLEMENTS

The nutritional supplements listed below are aimed at supporting your child's recovery from meningitis. They should not be considered a substitute for appropriate antibiotic therapy. For age-appropriate dosages of some nutritional supplements, see page 81.

■ Floradix is an herbal iron supplement that will give your child vitamins and minerals necessary to rebuild his strength. Follow the dosage directions on the product label, and give it to your child for two weeks.

■ Green Magma is a product that supplies trace minerals and beta-carotene and helps to restore strength. Give your child the dose specified on the label for two weeks.

■ *Lactobacillus acidophilus* and/or *bifidus* is very good for restoring bowel health after a regime of potent antibiotics. Follow the dosage directions on the product label, and give your child one dose a day for one month.

■ The B vitamins help to restore strength. Give your child a vitamin-B complex supplement for two weeks, following the dosage directions on the product label.

■ Vitamin C and bioflavonoids help stimulate the immune system. Give your child one dose, four times daily, for two weeks.

HERBAL TREATMENT

Herbal treatment for meningitis is aimed at supporting your child's recovery from the illness. It should not be considered a substitute for appropriate antibiotic therapy. For age-appropriate dosages of herbal remedies, see page 81.

■ The antibacterial properties of garlic will help resolve infection. Give your child one capsule or one fresh clove, three times a day, until the infection clears.

■ American ginseng is an excellent source of trace minerals and micronutrients. It will also support and strengthen your child's immune system. Give your child one dose, three times a day, for two weeks.

Note: This herb should be used during recovery only. It should not be given if fever or any other signs of infection are present.

■ Astragalus (*Astragalus membranaceous*), with its rich concentration of trace minerals and micronutrients, will help strengthen your child's immune system. Give your child one dose, three times a day, for two weeks.

Note: This herb should be used during the recovery phase only, not while fever or any other signs of acute infection are present.

HOMEOPATHY

Homeopathic treatment for meningitis is aimed at supporting your child's recovery from the illness once the acute phase of the infection has passed. It should not be considered a substitute for appropriate antibiotic therapy. Choose a symptom-specific remedy and give your child one dose, four times a day, for up to two days.

■ *Belladonna* 30x or 9c is helpful for a child who has a fever, with dilated pupils and perhaps delirious behavior.

■ *Bryonia* 30x or 9c is good for a child who experiences eye pain and constipation. This child will complain that his entire body is in great pain.

GENERAL RECOMMENDATIONS

■ During the acute phase of meningitis, a quiet, dimly lit room will help ease the headache pain. Stories, a soothing massage, and holding will help reassure your child and ease his discomfort.

■ If your child contracts bacterial meningitis, be aware of the possibility of a subtle injury to the brain. Don't hesitate to talk to your doctor if you are worried about persistent hearing loss, problems with balance or coordination, difficulties with schoolwork, or similar difficulties.

PREVENTION

■ Most medical doctors now recommend that children be routinely given the Hib vaccine, which offers immunity against *Hemophilus influenzae* bacteria (the most common cause of bacterial meningitis), starting when they are two months of age. This can be given either by itself or in combination with the DPT vaccine.

Menstrual Cramps

The menstrual cycle is a normal and predictable cycle that involves the shedding of the uterine lining once a month. The cycle repeats itself throughout a woman's reproductive years. Medically, menstrual cramps are known as *dysmenorrhea*, which literally means painful menstruation.

If your daughter suffers from cramps, we suggest that you both read this entry. To understand how to nurture and care for her body during what can be a difficult time of the month, she should first understand what happens during the menstrual cycle.

A complete menstrual cycle can be anywhere from twenty-one to thirty-five days long, with a twenty-eight-day cycle being average. The menstrual period, which marks the beginning of the cycle, lasts from three to seven days. During the rest of the cycle, intricate physical and hormonal changes occur that prepare the body for the possibility of pregnancy. During the first half of the cycle, the ovary prepares to release an egg. During this time, the body increases production of the hormone estrogen. This causes the lining of the uterus, the endometrium, to grow and await a fertilized egg. Meanwhile, the pituitary gland has released a follicle-stimulating hormone, causing an egg-bearing follicle in the ovary to develop. About halfway into the menstrual cycle, ovulation occurs and an egg is released from the follicle. This is followed by a rise in the hormone progesterone, which prepares the uterus for implantation of a fertilized egg. Progesterone influences the lining of the uterus to become rich in blood vessels and glandular tissue—a nourishing soft, spongy "nest." If the egg is not fertilized, however, the nest the body has prepared is not needed and, approximately two weeks after ovulation, the levels of both estrogen and progesterone drop. This triggers menstruation, and the enriched spongy lining of the uterus leaves the body as menstrual blood. About one-quarter cup of blood is lost with each menstrual period.

When menstrual cramps occur, it is usually just before the cycle starts or with the onset of menstruation. They can last anywhere from a few hours to a few days. Menstrual cramps feel like muscle contractions or sharp spasms in the lower abdomen. They may radiate to the back or down the thighs, and range from mildly achy to wrenchingly painful. In the severely afflicted, cramping may be accompanied by nausea, vomiting, headache, nervousness, fatigue, diarrhea, fainting, bloating, breast tenderness, mood swings, backache, and/or dizziness.

Women who suffer from cramps seem to produce greater amounts of prostaglandins, which are hormones secreted by the uterine lining, than other women do. These hormones affect the smooth muscle of the uterus, causing an increase in uterine contractions. The contractions interfere with blood flow, reducing the amount of oxygen reaching the uterus and resulting in pain. A large increase in prostaglandins can also cause strong gastrointestinal contractions, which may be responsible for the diarrhea, nausea, and vomiting associated with severe menstrual cramps.

When a teenager experiences menstrual cramps, she may not feel up to socializing, going to gym class, or participating in her usual daily activities. Because most teenagers thrive on social contact, suffering through a day or two of menstrual cramps can be difficult.

A teenager who suffers severe pain during her menstrual period should see her health care provider for advice. Severe abdominal pain may be a sign of an ectopic pregnancy, pelvic inflammatory disease, endometriosis, ovarian cysts, pelvic adhesions, fibroid cysts, or endometrial cancer. A medical diagnosis is essential.

A young woman who experiences persistently irregular menstrual cycles, a change in the normal pattern of her cycle, or an unusual amount of blood loss should call her doctor. Irregular or changing cycles may indicate an endocrine problem. Prolonged or excessive bleeding can lead to anemia.

If your daughter is fitted with an intrauterine device (IUD) or is taking birth control pills and develops cramping, see your doctor to be sure that her symptoms are properly diagnosed.

CONVENTIONAL TREATMENT

■ The drugs most often suggested for menstrual cramps are nonsteroidal anti-inflammatory drugs (NSAIDs), including ibuprofen (Advil, Motrin, Nuprin, and others), naproxen (Anaprox, Naprosyn), and mefenamic acid (Ponstel). Some are available over the counter; others require a prescription. These medications work by blocking the production of prostaglandins, thereby decreasing the intensity of uterine contractions. Because they typically take up to two hours to work, they should be taken when cramping first starts. Prostaglandin inhibitors are generally well tolerated, although they can cause gastrointestinal upset and bleeding in the stomach in some cases. Taking them with food can help to lessen stomach upset.

Note: These drugs are not recommended for women or girls with ulcers, asthma, or liver or kidney disease, or for those with a sensitivity to aspirin or any other of these drugs.

■ Oral contraceptives are sometimes recommended for the relief of menstrual cramps. They work by interfering with the hormonal process that leads to ovulation. As a result, the body does not build up or shed the lining of the uterus, so fewer cramp-inducing prostaglandins are released. A doctor may recommend oral contraceptives for a young woman with menstrual cramps who cannot tolerate NSAIDs, or for a woman who wants birth control coupled with pain relief. Oral contraceptives are associated with many different side effects, some of them potentially serious. They should not be taken for menstrual cramps without serious consideration.

DIETARY GUIDELINES

■ Dietary treatment is directed toward making the lower abdomen a friendly and relaxed place prior to the onset of the menstrual period. Cramps are often exaggerated by a poor diet. Many young women experience tremendous relief from cramps when their diet improves. A good diet is so beneficial that it alone may completely resolve menstrual cramps. (*See* Choosing Food and Water for Your Child in DIET AND NUTRITION in Part One.)

■ Avoid foods that cause gas. These include sugar, fats, and any other foods that make the lower abdomen uncomfortable, such as cucumbers, peppers, and the like. These foods, especially if indulged in during the week before menstruation, will often exacerbate cramps. Fats in particular are difficult to digest and contribute to a toxic environment. Excess amounts of saturated fats can also lead to production of "bad" prostaglandins, which contribute to uterine contractions.

WHEN TO CALL THE DOCTOR ABOUT MENSTRUAL PROBLEMS

• Severe abdominal pain—as opposed to cramping or an achy feeling—can be a sign of a more serious problem, such as an internal infection, ectopic pregnancy, or a gynecological syndrome like endometriosis or cysts in the genitourinary tract. If a young woman experiences extreme pain with her period, she should be examined by a doctor as soon as possible.

• Menstrual cycles that fail to develop a regular pattern, or a significant change in a young woman's menstrual cycles, should be reported to her health care provider. Changes in menstrual cycles can include periods that become noticeably more or less frequent, as well as significant changes in the length and amount of bleeding.

SOME FACTS ABOUT MENSTRUAL CRAMPS

• Menstrual cramps are one of the most common gynecological complaints. About 50 percent of women experience menstrual cramps at some point in their lives.

• More than 10 percent of those who suffer from menstrual cramps have pain severe enough that they cannot carry on with their usual daily routines.

• A young girl just entering puberty will not usually experience cramps. Cramps usually only begin with the onset of ovulatory cycles, which typically happens six months to two years after the first menstrual cycle.

• Physically active, athletic girls and women are less likely to suffer from menstrual cramps, as are women who have had children.

• Anemia, fatigue, and diabetes may predispose a young woman to menstrual cramps. Obesity may also be a factor. In some cases, the tendency to have menstrual cramps seems to run in families.

■ Menstrual cramps can be related to or made worse by constipation. Eat a diet high in fiber to promote regularity.

■ Eat plenty of cooked green vegetables, which are rich sources of vitamins and minerals.

■ Avoid alcohol and caffeine. Both promote inflammation and can increase cramping.

NUTRITIONAL SUPPLEMENTS

■ Magnesium relaxes the uterine muscles and is the most helpful nutrient for menstrual cramps. Beginning one week before the expected onset of menstruation, take 100 milligrams of magnesium, two to three times daily. The day before menstruation begins, take 100 milligrams, three times daily, and on the first day of menstruation, take 100 milligrams, four to five times daily. If the magnesium causes loose stool, reduce the dosage. Try it again, at a lower dose and in combination with calcium, during the next cycle: One week before menstruation, take 100 milligrams of calcium and 50 milligrams of magnesium, twice daily; the day before menstruation, take the same dosage, three times daily; and on the first day of menstruation, take the same dosage four to five times daily.

■ If you are unable to tolerate taking magnesium orally, try taking an Epsom salts bath each day on the two days before the expected onset of menstruation and on the first day of your period.

■ Niacin makes blood vessels dilate and can improve blood flow to a contracting uterus. Take 50 to 100 milligrams, but not more, every four to six hours. Higher doses may result in intense flushing. Keep your dosage slightly below the amount that causes a flush.

Note: Niacin should not be taken by itself for more than five days in a row. In general, when taking any B vitamin (such as niacin or B_6) individually, you should also take a B-complex supplement at a different time of the day.

■ Vitamin B_6 is often used as a supplement in the treatment of menstrual cramps and other menstrual symptoms. Beginning five days before the anticipated onset of menstruation, take 50 milligrams, twice daily, between meals.

■ Take mineral ascorbate vitamin C with bioflavonoids. Vitamin C is a mild anti-inflammatory; bioflavonoids enhance the action of vitamin C. Five days before the expected onset of menstruation, start taking 250 milligrams, three times a day, and continue until the cramping subsides.

■ Vitamin E, the B vitamins, and zinc can also be helpful against menstrual cramping, especially for those who can't resist the temptation to eat junk foods. Take 100 international units of vitamin E, twice a day (once in the morning and again at bedtime); a vitamin-B complex that contains 25 milligrams of each B vitamin, twice daily; and 5 to 10 milligrams of zinc, also twice daily, starting ten days before the anticipated onset of menstruation and continuing for as long as cramping lasts.

Note: Excessive amounts of zinc can result in nausea and vomiting. Be careful not to exceed the recommended dosage.

■ Gamma-linolenic acid (GLA), an extract of evening primrose oil or borage oil, helps to balance out the inflammatory prostaglandins by acting as a source of anti-inflammatory prostaglandins. Take 250 milligrams of GLA daily for three months.

HERBAL TREATMENT

■ Chamomile is an herbal relaxant. Drink a cup of chamomile tea as needed.

■ The Chinese herb dong quai helps to regulate the menstrual cycle by balancing female hormones. When taken for a few months, it will help alleviate cramping, particularly when taken in combination with red raspberry leaf. Begin by taking 40 drops of dong quai tincture, or dong quai and red raspberry leaf combination formula, twice daily, from Day 6 through Day 20 of the menstrual cycle (calculated from the first day of menstrual bleeding). Continue taking 40 drops, twice daily, for three weeks. If the cycle is irregular, take the herbs for two to three weeks out of every month, and repeat this program for at least three menstrual cycles. Do not take this remedy during the menstrual period itself, however.

■ A hot ginger-tea compress placed on the lower abdomen helps to relax muscle cramping. Boil 6 ounces of fresh ginger root in 1 quart of water for fifteen to twenty minutes, and dip a washcloth or hand towel in the tea. You can either place the saturated cloth directly on the abdomen, or wrap it first with a dry cloth. Ginger is warming and increases circulation in the lower abdomen. This compress will feel like a deep heating rub.

■ True cramp bark, a little-known botanical, is effective in treating menstrual cramps. Take 1 cup of true cramp bark tea, twice daily, for three days before the expected onset of the menstrual period, and 1 cup, three times daily, during the menstrual period if cramping occurs.

■ Prepare a soothing herbal bath. Mix 1 quart of strong chamomile tea and 1 quart of ginger tea with warm to hot bath water, and enjoy a leisurely soak.

HOMEOPATHY

For long-term relief of menstrual cramps, it may be most helpful to consult a homeopathic physician for a constitutional remedy. Otherwise, try the most appropriate of the symptom-specific remedies below.

■ *Colocynthis* is especially effective against cramps that cause a sharp, stabbing pain and for those that feel better with mild pressure on the abdomen. Take one dose of *Colocynthis* 6x, 12x, or 6c, every fifteen minutes, for one hour. Then take one dose, three times daily, until the cramping subsides.

■ *Magnesia phosphorica* relieves menstrual cramps that feel better with heat on the lower abdomen. Start by taking one dose of *Magnesia phosphorica* 6x or 6c, every fifteen minutes, for one hour. Thereafter, take one dose, three times daily, until the cramping subsides.

■ *Colocynthis* and *Magnesia phosphorica* can be alternated to relieve menstrual cramps. First take one dose of *Colocynthis*; fifteen minutes later, take one dose of *Magnesia phosphorica*. Repeat the cycle, alternating the remedies every fifteen minutes, for one hour, or until the cramping is relieved. Resume the regimen if the cramps return.

■ *Pulsatilla* is for the young woman with late and/or irregular periods and menstrual cramps. This young woman has blue eyes and fair hair, and is timid and perhaps somewhat frightened of men. She may cry easily, especially during the premenstrual period. Take one dose of *Pulsatilla* 30x or 9c, three times daily, the day before the expected onset of menstruation and as cramping occurs.

■ *Sepia* will benefit the brown-eyed, brunette young woman. This woman is thin, enjoys exercising, and often experiences low back pain with menstrual cramping. Take one dose of *Sepia* 30x or 9c, three times daily, the day before the anticipated onset of menstruation and as cramps occur.

■ *Viburnum* 30x or 9c is recommended for a young woman whose period comes late, with diminished blood flow and pain in the abdomen that extends into her legs. Take one dose, three times daily, for up to three days.

ACUPRESSURE

For the locations of acupressure points, *see* ADMINISTERING AN ACUPRESSURE TREATMENT in Part Three.

■ Bladder 20 to 28 relaxes the nerves of the uterus.

■ Gallbladder 34 helps to relax muscles.

■ Large Intestine 4 removes energy blocks in the large intestine, thus promoting a healthier lower abdomen. Massaging this point also relaxes the nervous system.

■ Liver 3 is a general acupressure point for relieving muscle cramps and spasms.

■ Spleen 6 relaxes uterine cramps.

■ Stomach 36 helps to regulate digestion.

GENERAL RECOMMENDATIONS

■ Eat a diet low in fat and high in grains, fresh fruits, and vegetables, to create a healthy environment in the abdomen.

■ Get plenty of exercise. Swimming, biking, and walking are all very helpful.

■ Take magnesium and vitamin B6.

■ Take homeopathic *Magnesia phosphorica* or *Colocynthis*, as needed.

■ Use acupressure, especially Spleen 6, and massage the abdomen and lower back. Massage can be particularly helpful for relieving lower back pain.

■ Acupuncture has been shown to relieve menstrual cramps. Licensed acupuncturists have established practices in most larger cities. You might ask your health care provider to recommend one.

■ Simple stretching will often relieve the abdominal cramps and lower back pain that can accompany menstruation. One helpful exercise is to put your hands on your hips and rotate your hips in a circle—15 times in one direction and then 15 times in the other direction. You can do up to a total of 120 circles. Start doing this exercise one week before menstruation begins and continue throughout your period. The idea is to keep energy moving in the pelvis and abdomen.

■ Yoga can be very helpful. *A Gem for Women* by Geeta S. Iyengar (Timeless Books, 1990) is a good resource book.

■ Investigate biofeedback, visualization, and other relaxation techniques. All can be very effective.

■ Try using sanitary pads instead of tampons, at least during the first two days of menstruation. The presence of a tampon may cause cramping by itself. Tampons can also cause a low-grade infection that will exaggerate cramping. It may be helpful to try going without them for a couple of months to see if there is any change in symptoms.

■ Learn to welcome the menstrual cycle as a natural and important part of the body's functions. Tension and negative feelings can make cramping worse. This is a good time to learn about and get in touch with your body. *Understanding Your Body* by Felicia H. Stewart (Bantam, 1987) is a good, readable reference that thoroughly covers topics such as anatomy, physiology, the menstrual cycle, birth control, premenstrual syndrome, and menstrual discomfort.

PREVENTION

■ Follow a healthy diet, starting with the dietary guidelines above.

■ Get plenty of vigorous exercise. Women who are physically active are less likely to suffer from menstrual cramps.

■ Take dong quai and red raspberry leaf herbal combination as suggested above.

Mononucleosis

Infectious mononucleosis is an acute infection of the throat and lymph nodes caused by the Epstein-Barr virus (EBV). Youngsters are often affected with "mono," which is commonly mistaken for influenza. In childhood, the disease is mild and can pass unnoticed. However, when a teenager contracts mononucleosis, the symptoms are usually more severe.

Because the virus is transmitted through infected saliva, mononucleosis is sometimes called the "kissing disease." Some teenagers are initially amused when they come down with mono—until they discover that their activities must be severely restricted to ensure a full recovery. The virus may also be spread through coughing or sneezing.

The condition gets its name from a characteristic increase in the number of mononuclear white blood cells. Symptoms can include fever, sore throat, swollen lymph glands and spleen, abnormal liver function, and a bumpy red rash. A child with mononucleosis usually feels weak and very tired.

The infection generally lasts from two to four weeks, although the older a person is when it strikes, the more severe the symptoms and the longer the recovery time. It is not uncommon for a child to feel more tired than usual for several months. Potential complications of the disease include obstruction of the upper airway, difficulty swallowing, depression of the immune system, and liver disease. In exceptionally severe cases, the spleen may become very enlarged and then rupture (usually after a fall or similar trauma), making emergency surgery necessary.

CONVENTIONAL TREATMENT

■ Mononucleosis must be diagnosed by a blood test that detects an elevated concentration of antibodies to the Epstein-Barr virus, an elevated lymphocyte (white blood cell) count, or other characteristic abnormalities. When the diagnosis is confirmed, liver functions are usually measured as well. A physical examination

SYMPTOMS OF MONONUCLEOSIS

The symptoms of mononucleosis often resemble those of other infectious illnesses, but tend to be more persistent. They include:

• A vague feeling of achiness and discomfort.

• A pronounced feeling of fatigue or weakness.

• Headache.

• A tendency to feel chilled.

• Moderate to high fever.

• Sore throat.

• Lymph nodes that become enlarged and remain that way for a week or more.

If you suspect that your child may have mononucleosis, consult your physician for a professional diagnosis.

is done to check for an enlarged spleen or liver, and to look for pus and inflammation in the back of the throat.

■ There is no cure for mononucleosis. Treatment is aimed at relieving the symptoms and monitoring the patient for the development of complications while the virus runs its course.

■ To prevent serious damage to the liver and spleen, bed rest will be recommended, usually for one to four weeks. As long as the spleen is enlarged, strenuous exercise should be avoided, especially contact sports.

■ If your child is uncomfortable or has a fever, ibuprofen or acetaminophen may be helpful to relieve pain and reduce fever. If the liver is inflamed, however, acetaminophen should be used with caution. Consult your doctor. Ibuprofen is best given with food.

■ *Do not* give aspirin to a child with mononucleosis. The combination of aspirin and a viral illness is associated with Reye's syndrome, a serious liver complication (*see* REYE'S SYNDROME).

■ Steroids, such as dexamethasone (Decadron) are sometimes used, but only for patients with such severe complications as an airway obstruction.

■ A strep throat often accompanies mononucleosis. If a throat culture reveals a strep infection, an oral antibiotic will be prescribed. Although penicillin is often the drug of choice for strep, it can cause an allergic rash in children with mononucleosis and should be used cautiously. Erythromycin is a better choice.

DIETARY GUIDELINES

■ Encourage your child to drink plenty of pure spring water to flush toxins from the body. If swallowing is difficult, as it often is for people with mononucleosis, encourage frequent small sips of fluids to prevent dehydration.

■ Fresh-squeezed lemonade helps to dilute mucus and soothes the throat. Fruit-juice popsicles can also be soothing to an inflamed throat. Offer your child pure fruit juices and fresh, whole fruits as well.

■ To support the healing process, prepare healthy, nutrient-rich, whole foods for your child. Base his diet primarily on grains, fruits, vegetables, and lean proteins. Hot soups are a good source of nutrients, and are easier to take than whole foods.

■ Eliminate fats. This virus affects the spleen and the liver. The liver has to work very hard to metabolize fats. Give the liver time to rest and heal by taking fats off the menu.

■ Eliminate sugary foods, commercially prepared and additive-laden convenience foods, soft drinks, and all processed foods. All of these contribute to a toxic internal environment.

NUTRITIONAL SUPPLEMENTS

For age-appropriate dosages of some nutritional supplements, see page 81.

■ Calcium and magnesium help to relax the nervous system. Give your child one dose of a liquid formula containing 250 milligrams of calcium and 125 milligrams of magnesium at bedtime.

■ Chlorophyll has many vitamins and trace minerals that speed healing. Follow dosage directions on the product label.

■ B vitamins increase energy. Once the fever has subsided and the acute phase of the infection resolved, give your child a liquid vitamin-B complex twice a day.

■ Vitamin C and bioflavonoids have antiviral and anti-inflammatory properties. Give your child one dose of mineral ascorbate vitamin C with an equal amount of bioflavonoids, three to four times a day during the acute phase, and once a day thereafter, until the illness is completely resolved.

■ Vitamin E boosts the immune response and helps to protect the liver from inflammation. Give your child a double dose of vitamin E every day for one month.

■ Zinc helps to stimulate the immune system. Give your child one dose, twice a day (at the beginning of a meal), for one month.

Note: Excessive amounts of zinc can result in nausea and vomiting. Give zinc supplements with food, and be careful not to exceed the recommended dosage.

HERBAL TREATMENT

For age-appropriate dosages of herbal remedies, see page 81.

■ Yin qiao is a Chinese formula that is the first herb to give in the initial stages of mononucleosis. It is helpful for relieving the initial feeling of achiness associated with mono. Give your child one dose, three times daily, for the first three days.

Note: The liquid extract is the preferred form, because it contains no aspirin. The tablet form should not be given to a child under four years of age.

■ Echinacea and goldenseal combination formula has antiviral and antibacterial properties. It helps to boost the immune system and fight infection. Give your child one dose, three times daily, for the first week. The second week, discontinue it, and then resume it for the third week.

■ Garlic has antiviral properties helpful in the treatment of mononucleosis. Give your child one capsule, twice a day, for two to three weeks.

■ Marshmallow root and licorice root are soothing for a sore throat. Make a combination herbal tea and give your child 2 to 3 cups a day, for two days, to relieve throat pain.

Note: A child with high blood pressure should not be given licorice.

■ Milk thistle helps to detoxify, restore, and protect the liver. Give your child one dose, once or twice a day, for one month.

■ Shiitake mushrooms help the immune system fight off viruses. After the fever has subsided, you may give a child over twelve years old one capsule, three times daily, for two weeks. Then give him the same dosage, twice daily, for one month.

■ Astragalus is a Chinese botanical that helps to strengthen the immune system and increase energy and is helpful in the recovery stage. This herb should not be given if a fever or any other signs of infection are present. After the fever subsides, you may give your child one dose, three times daily, for one month.

HOMEOPATHY

■ If a sore throat persists, give your child one dose of *Mercurius corrosivus* 12x or 6c, four times daily, for up to three days.

■ For swollen lymph glands in the neck, give your child one dose of *Phytolacca* 12x or 6c, four times daily, for up to four days.

■ If your child has heavy, droopy eyes, feels weak and tired, and has aches and chills running up and down his back, give him one dose of *Gelsemium* 9x or 30c, three to four times a day, for two days.

■ Consult a homeopath for a constitutional remedy for your child.

ACUPRESSURE

For the locations of acupressure points on a child's body, *see* ADMINISTERING AN ACUPRESSURE TREATMENT in Part Three.

■ Gallbladder 20 and 21 help to bring down energy from the head and keep it circulating throughout the body to promote healing.

■ Liver 3 helps to ease headache pain.

■ Liver 4 helps to bring down a fever.

■ Stomach 36 energizes the digestive and immune systems, and helps to bring down fever.

■ Massaging down both sides of the spine helps to relax the nervous system.

GENERAL RECOMMENDATIONS

■ For a full recovery, unlimited rest is absolutely essential. Limit physical activity in accordance with your doctor's orders. In the acute stage, your patient will probably be glad to rest. When he begins to feel restless, be ready with "effort-free" distractions, such as a favorite movie, books, magazines, puzzles, or board games.

■ Adequate nutrition and hydration are important to recovery. Follow the dietary guidelines above.

■ Remember that recovery is a gradual process. Returning to full activity too soon can prolong the time it takes for full healing.

■ Make sure your child avoids strenuous exercise, especially contact sports, until your doctor certifies that recovery is complete. The spleen can become enlarged with mononucleosis, and an enlarged spleen can rupture easily, necessitating surgery.

■ Once your child is able to be up and about, a modest twenty-minute walk every day will help to increase circulation and build strength.

■ *See also* FEVER; HEADACHE; and/or SORE THROAT if your child's mononucleosis is accompanied by any of these symptoms. A mild form of hepatitis is also a possible complication (*see* HEPATITIS).

PREVENTION

■ Because mononucleosis is often mistaken for a case of the flu, it is sometimes impossible to avoid contact with a contagious person. There are no overt danger signals. If you know that a person is infected, however, keep your child out of the range of coughs and sneezes, which carry the virus.

Motion Sickness

Whether you are traveling by car, boat, or plane, motion sickness can spoil a good time. Motion sickness is caused by excessive stimulation of the vestibular apparatus, located in the inner ear, which is responsible for maintaining a sense of balance and equilibrium.

Abnormal or irregular body motions or postures, as well as repeated acceleration and deceleration, such as occur in a moving car, on the deck of a boat, or in an airplane, disturb the delicate balance mechanisms in the inner ear. Because the eyes transmit messages to this seat of balance, visual cues also play a part. When the body is passively being transported while the landscape rushes by, the contradictory stimuli can confuse and disrupt the vestibular apparatus, resulting in symptoms of motion sickness.

Symptoms vary from child to child. Motion sickness usually starts with a general sense of discomfort and uneasiness. Your child may look noticeably pale, even a little green. She may feel dizzy and complain of a sick headache. Motion sickness can escalate into vomiting and unremitting nausea.

Expecting instant relief at journey's end, your child may ask repeatedly, "Are we there yet?" Unfortunately, it can take several hours for the body to recover completely from motion sickness, even once out of a vehicle.

Motion sickness is easier to prevent than it is to cure. If your child tends to get carsick, keep in mind that whatever treatment you choose, it is best initiated *before* you get in the car.

CONVENTIONAL TREATMENT

■ Dimenhydrinate (better known as Dramamine) is an over-the-counter drug that is often effective in preventing motion sickness. It must be taken before motion sickness arises, however; it is not as effective once symptoms have started. Common side effects include drowsiness and dry mouth. It is not safe for children less than two years old.

■ Meclizine (in Bonine and Antivert) and scopolamine (in Transderm Scōp, a medicated skin patch) are prescription medications that are not recommended for children under twelve, but can be effective for older children, especially when the problem is persistent.

■ There are many over-the-counter drugs that promise relief from motion sickness. Consult your doctor before giving any drug to your child.

DIETARY GUIDELINES

■ Use your judgment. Determine whether your child travels best on a full stomach or an empty stomach, and act accordingly.

■ Avoid giving your child fried or fatty foods before traveling. Greasy foods are more likely to cause an upset stomach.

HERBAL TREATMENT

For age-appropriate dosages of herbal remedies, see page 81.

■ Ginger is an effective treatment for nausea and motion sickness. Prepare and carry a thermos of warm or room-temperature ginger tea to give your child as needed. Ginger is also available in tincture and capsule form. Give your child one dose, every one to two hours, until the symptoms of motion sickness are eased.

HOMEOPATHY

Choose the most appropriate of the following symptom-specific homeopathic remedies and give your child one dose, one hour before traveling, another upon entering the vehicle, and another one hour into the trip.

■ *Cocculus* 12x or 6c will help the child who feels nauseous and refuses to eat anything. The smell of food makes this child feel sick, and she insists on cuddling under warm blankets.

■ If your child feels less nauseous after eating, when resting quietly with her eyes closed, and when she knows the trip will end soon, give her *Petroleum* 12x or 6c.

■ If your motion-sick child is pale, in a cold sweat, feels faint, and is nauseous and vomiting, give her *Tabacum* 6x, 12x, or 5c.

ACUPRESSURE

For the locations of acupressure points on a child's body, *see* ADMINISTERING AN ACUPRESSURE TREATMENT in Part Three.

■ Four Gates will help relax your child during a trip.

■ Pericardium 6 helps relieve nausea.

GENERAL RECOMMENDATIONS

■ Plan ahead. When it comes to motion sickness, prevention is easier—and more likely to be successful—than treatment.

■ When traveling, carry a thermos of ginger tea or a bottle of ginger tincture to give to your child as needed.

■ Based on the particular symptoms your child displays, choose a suitable homeopathic remedy.

■ A child who is motion sick may be restless and think that moving around will ease the discomfort. But not only does movement actually exacerbate motion sickness, it is unsafe to release your child from a safety seat or seat belt in a moving vehicle to satisfy a desire to move around. *Never* take your child out of a safety seat or permit her to take off the seat belt. It really is better to be sick than sorry.

PREVENTION

■ Teach your child to hold her head very still. A strategically placed pillow will help.

■ To avoid the confusion arising in the balance mechanism when the body is being passively transported and the eyes are viewing the landscape rushing by, teach your child to focus on a fixed point on the far-distant horizon. The horizon is a constant and will appear to remain still.

■ Air blowing across the face is very helpful in preventing and/or lessening motion sickness. Open a car window. Sit on the open deck of a boat. Direct the air valve above your child's airplane seat toward her face.

■ Practice distraction. Try to keep your child entertained and her mind off the trip. Avoid anything involving reading, as attempting to read in a moving vehicle can often bring on an attack of motion sickness. Instead, sing with your child, or permit her to select the radio station. Tell stories. Most children love to listen to stories about when they were babies or toddlers.

Mumps

Mumps is a viral infection of childhood that affects the salivary glands, most commonly the parotid glands, located near the ear (hence its medical name, *parotitis*). The illness begins with a fever, headache, loss of appetite, malaise, and muscle aches. Pain in the ear and under the jaw begins about twenty-four hours later. Over the next one to three days, the salivary glands swell and become very tender. The swelling typically lessens over a course of three to seven days.

The illness is spread by contact with infected saliva. It is somewhat less contagious than either measles or chickenpox. Once a child is infected with the virus, it can incubate for two to three-and-a-half weeks before signs of infection appear. A child is contagious from about six days before the onset of illness to nine days after the glands have become swollen.

Mumps is most common in children from age five through fifteen. It is usually self-limiting and runs its course without complications. One possible long-term complication that does exist occurs in boys, when the virus attacks the testicles. This may result only in pain and swelling initially, but in some cases it can cause infertility in the long run, especially if a boy contracts the disease as a teenager or young adult.

CONVENTIONAL TREATMENT

■ Treatment of mumps is aimed at helping your child feel comfortable through the illness. Acetaminophen (in the form of Tylenol, Tempra, and other medications) or ibuprofen (Advil, Nuprin, and others) will bring down fever and ease the headache, muscle aches, and malaise that accompany the disease.

Note: In excessive doses, acetaminophen can cause liver damage. If you give your child acetaminophen, follow age-appropriate dosage instructions carefully. Giving ibuprofen with food is advised to prevent possible stomach upset.

■ *Do not* give a child aspirin if you think he may have the mumps. The combination of aspirin and a viral infection has been linked to the development of Reye's syndrome, a dangerous liver disease (*see* REYE'S SYNDROME).

■ Because mumps is a viral illness, antibiotic therapy is ineffective and therefore not appropriate.

■ Warm or cool compresses applied to the site of the swollen glands may help relieve the pain and tenderness.

■ If your son has a case of mumps that causes testicular pain, bed rest is particularly important. It may help lessen the pain if you support the scrotum by

SYMPTOMS OF MUMPS

The first signs that a child is coming down with mumps usually include some combination of the following:

• An all-over achy and chilled feeling.
• Headache.
• Low to moderate fever.

Twelve to twenty-four hours after these initial symptoms, a child with mumps will have the characteristic signs of swollen salivary glands:

• Pain upon swallowing, especially swallowing acidic foods.
• Pain and swelling in the jaw and under the ear or ears. The affected areas will be quite sensitive when touched.
• Possible loss of appetite.

using cotton held in place by an adhesive-tape "bridge" between the thighs, and/or if you apply ice packs. In rare cases, where pain and swelling are extremely severe, a corticosteroid may be prescribed to combat these symptoms.

DIETARY GUIDELINES

■ Because mumps causes pain when chewing or swallowing, a diet of soft foods may minimize discomfort.

■ Avoid giving your child citrus fruits or other acidic foods, which can be painful to swallow.

■ To keep your child well hydrated, encourage him to take plenty of fluids. Offer fruit-juice popsicles, spring water, herbal teas, soups, and diluted fruit juices. Once the acute phase of the infection has subsided, immune-boosting astragalus and vegetable soup is very good for supporting recovery (*see* THERAPEUTIC RECIPES in Part Three).

■ Eliminate fats as much as possible. Fats are difficult to digest under normal circumstances, and are even harder to digest when the digestive system is weakened by infection. Undigested fats contribute to a toxic internal environment.

NUTRITIONAL SUPPLEMENTS

For age-appropriate dosages of nutritional supplements, see page 81.

■ Beta-carotene is the precursor to vitamin A, which helps heal mucous membranes. Give your child a double dose of beta-carotene, twice daily, for ten days.

■ Vitamin C and bioflavonoids help to stimulate the immune system. Three to four times a day, give your child one dose of mineral ascorbate vitamin C with an equal amount of bioflavonoids, for one week. (If your child develops loose stool as a result of taking this supplement, cut back on the dosage.) The following week, give him the same dosage, but two to three times a day. During the third week, give the same dosage, once or twice a day. Then continue to give one-half dose daily for the fourth week, and three times a week for the next two weeks.

■ Zinc stimulates the immune system and promotes healing. Give your child one dose of zinc, twice a day, for one week to ten days.

Note: Excessive amounts of zinc can result in nausea and vomiting. Be careful not to exceed the recommended dosage.

HERBAL TREATMENT

For age-appropriate dosages of herbal remedies, see page 81.

■ A tincture of arnica or peppermint oil, used as a rub, can help to relieve headache. Rub arnica tincture into the temple or forehead area; rub peppermint oil into the temple area. Be very careful to keep tinctures away from your child's eyes and do not use them on broken skin.

Note: If you are using peppermint oil as well as a homeopathic preparation, allow one hour between the two. Otherwise, the strong smell of the mint may interfere with the action of the homeopathic remedy.

■ If your child is feeling very restless, give him a cup of chamomile tea, twice a day, as needed.

■ Echinacea and goldenseal combination formula helps to fight viruses and boost the immune system. It also soothes mucous membranes. Give your child one dose, three times a day, for up to one week, until the fever is resolved and his salivary glands have returned to their normal size.

■ Shiitake mushrooms have immune-stimulating properties. They may be taken in capsule form. Give a child over twelve years old one capsule, three times a day, for up to ten days.

■ Castor oil packs can be soothing to swollen glands. Heat castor oil to a soothing (but not too hot) temperature, soak clean cotton cloths in it, and apply these compresses as often as needed.

HOMEOPATHY

Choose a symptom-specific remedy from the suggestions that follow, and give your child one dose of a 30x or 9c potency, four times a day, until the symptoms improve. If the remedy produces no improvement within forty-eight hours, try another remedy.

■ *Belladonna* 30x or 9c is for a child whose right gland is much more swollen than the left. This child has a high fever, a flushed face, and is easily chilled.

■ *Bryonia* 30x or 9c is also for a child whose right gland is more swollen than the left, and who is probably also constipated. This child's symptoms are worse with movement.

■ *Mercurius solubilis* 12x or 6c is for a child with swollen glands and a sore throat. A boy may have testicular swelling as well.

■ *Phytolacca* 12x or 6c is for a child whose glands are swollen and hard, and who has pain that goes into his ears. This child will not want anything hot to drink.

■ *Rhus toxicodendron* 30x or 9c is for a child whose left gland is much more swollen than the right, and who may feel stiff and achy in the morning.

ACUPRESSURE

For the locations of acupressure points on a child's body, *see* ADMINISTERING AN ACUPRESSURE TREATMENT in Part Three.

■ Four Gates helps to relax an uncomfortable child.

■ Large Intestine 4 controls the head. This acupressure point can be helpful for relieving the headache that may accompany mumps.

GENERAL RECOMMENDATIONS

■ A child with the mumps should be isolated until the swelling of the glands has gone down, to decrease the possibility of spreading the disease.

■ Make sure your child gets plenty of rest and drinks plenty of fluids. The increased metabolic rate that results from a fever causes the body to lose fluids rapidly.

■ Give your child an echinacea and goldenseal combination formula.

■ Select and administer a symptom-specific homeopathic remedy.

■ Apply warm or cool compresses to ease the discomfort of the swollen glands.

■ Use an herbal arnica or peppermint oil rub to help relieve headache.

■ If your child is uncomfortable and restless, give him soothing and calming chamomile tea.

■ Give your child vitamin C with bioflavonoids, zinc (once your child is eating meals), and beta-carotene.

■ If your child has the mumps, be alert for signs that a secondary infection may be developing. If symptoms seem to get worse, or if new symptoms develop, seek medical treatment.

PREVENTION

■ As much as possible, try to keep your child from contact with contagious children.

■ A vaccine that protects against mumps is available, usually given in the form of a combination vaccine that also protects against measles and rubella (the MMR vaccine). Doctors recommend that this vaccine, which is given by injection, be administered when a child is approximately fifteen months old, and that an additional dose be given later, when a child is either four to six years old (before entering school) or between eleven and thirteen years old (in middle school or junior high school). (*See* IMMUNIZATION-RELATED PROBLEMS.)

Nail Injuries, Finger and Toe

EMERGENCY TREATMENT FOR NAIL INJURIES

✚ If there is intense pain and pressure after a nail injury, it is possible that a "blood blister" is forming underneath the nail that may need to be drained. See your health care provider or take your child to a hospital emergency room for evaluation and care. If necessary, a doctor can relieve the pressure by making a small hole in the nail so that the blood can drain. This may also be an opportunity to update your child's tetanus vaccination, if necessary.

Injuries to the fingernails and toenails are common in childhood. Children are curious, and their hands seem to get into everything. Little fingers and car doors sometimes come together with disastrous results. Splinters find their way underneath fingernails. A badly caught ball can jam a finger and injure a nail. Rocks can get dropped, and bare toes often get stubbed.

Depending on the extent and type of injury, a bruise may form immediately. The area may appear red and swollen, or white and scraped. More seriously, a nail can be completely torn off.

Any injury to tissue makes infection a possibility. If a nail injury does not improve within twenty-four hours, or if the area begins to show increasing redness, warmth, swelling, or other signs of infection, call your physician.

CONVENTIONAL TREATMENT

■ Cleanse the area by holding the injured nail under running water. If there is bleeding, use cold water. Unless you can readily see a foreign object protruding from under or around the nail, do not try to remove anything that might be under the skin. Poking and probing can result in infection later on.

■ Unless the nail is completely torn at the base, do not remove it. Even a badly broken nail can and should be taped in place to provide protection for the very tender nail bed underneath until the tissue has healed. The nail will eventually fall off by itself, or else grow out again.

Nail Problems and Your Child's Health

Many different health problems can affect the condition of fingernails. If your child develops any of the problems that follow, you may wish to bring it to your doctor's attention:

- **Pitted nails.** This condition may be associated with psoriasis.

- **Very pale colored nail beds.** This may be a sign of anemia.

- **Vertical ridges.** This may point to poor absorption of nutrients.

- **Horizontal ridges.** This can be an indicator of injury, infection, or illness.

- **White spots.** These may signify a zinc deficiency.

- **Spoon-shaped nails.** This condition is associated with iron deficiency.

- **Easily broken nails.** These can be a sign of a deficiency of calcium, silica, and/or certain trace minerals.

- **Crumbly, whitish nails, with surrounding skin that is dry and peeling.** This can be caused by a fungal infection.

- **Blackish, splinterlike bits in the nails.** This may be a sign of bacterial endocarditis, a serious infection of the heart.

■ If the wound involves a puncture or is dirty, cleanse it with hydrogen peroxide, gently pat dry, and apply an antibiotic ointment such as bacitracin or Betadine before covering it.

HERBAL TREATMENT

For age-appropriate dosages of herbal remedies, see page 81.

■ If a nail injury becomes infected, apply a green clay and goldenseal poultice to help draw out the infection. Apply the poultice for fifteen minutes, twice a day, until the infection is resolved.

■ If your child develops an infection at the site of the injury, give her one dose of an echinacea and goldenseal combination formula, three times daily, for three days.

HOMEOPATHY

■ If your child suffers a nail injury, give her one dose of *Arnica* 200x or 30c as soon as possible to help alleviate the initial pain.

■ To help alleviate bruising, give your child one dose of *Ledum* 12x or 6c, three times daily, for two to three days.

■ *Hypericum* helps to lessen the pain in an injured finger or toe. Give your child one dose of *Hypericum* 12x or 6c, three times a day, for two to three days.

■ *Hepar sulphuris* helps to resolve a minor infection following a nail injury. Give your child one dose of *Hepar sulphuris* 12x or 6c, three times daily, for up to three days.

BACH FLOWER REMEDIES

■ After any injury, give your child Bach Flower Rescue Remedy to relieve fear and apprehension, and to restore her equilibrium. (*See* BACH FLOWER REMEDIES in Part One.)

GENERAL RECOMMENDATIONS

■ Cleanse the area with cold water.

■ If the nail has been partially torn from the finger or toe, bandage it lightly with the remaining nail held loosely in place. Keep the area protected against further injury with a small splint or finger cup.

■ If part of the nail bed is exposed, or if there is an open wound, apply an antibiotic ointment before bandaging. Keep the area bandaged until the injury heals.

■ Give your child Bach Flower Rescue Remedy.

■ Select and administer a suitable homeopathic remedy.

PREVENTION

■ The only *sure* method of preventing injury is to wrap your child in tissue paper and not allow her to move! But there are a number of things you can do to reduce the possibility of an accident that could cause a nail injury. For suggestions, *see* HOME SAFETY in Part One.

Nausea and Vomiting

Symptoms of stomach upset may begin with loss of appetite, proceed to queasiness or nausea, then actual pain—either constant or crampy—in the upper stomach, followed by vomiting and, occasionally, diarrhea. A child may complain of a "headache in my stomach," or his abdomen may feel "full" or crampy. The pain may be in one spot, all over the abdomen, or travel around. The abdomen may be tender to the touch. Vomiting may occur, perhaps with waves of nausea right before an episode and temporary relief afterwards.

Childhood stomachaches have a wide variety of physical and emotional causes. In an infant, a stomachache and vomiting can be associated with serious problems, including meningitis, urinary tract infection, feeding difficulties, and anatomical defects. In older children, a stomachache and vomiting can be the result of food poisoning, overeating, motion sickness, infection, hepatitis, appendicitis, constipation, muscle strain, tiredness, food allergies, or the accidental ingestion of drugs and poisons. Emotional upsets, such as homesickness, sorrow, nervousness, anger, or anticipation of an upcoming event, can translate into stomach upsets. A child wrestling with feelings surrounding divorce, a new sibling, holidays, a final exam, or school phobia can develop a stomachache.

A single episode of nausea or vomiting is likely to be a reaction to some food your child has eaten, or a sign of emotional upset. When nausea is severe or persists for more than a few hours, the most likely cause is either food poisoning or an infection. Bacterial infections can be caused by a wide variety of organisms, including *Campylobacter*, *Escherichia coli* (E. coli), *Salmonella*, *Shigella*, or *Staphylococcus*. Most often vomiting related to a bacterial infection of the intestine will be accompanied by diarrhea and fever, whereas food poisoning caused by a bacterial toxin is less likely to cause a fever. Viral infections can also cause diarrhea. By listening to your child's history and symptoms, and by performing tests and a physical examination, your doctor can help diagnose the underlying cause of your child's stomachache and/or vomiting so that you can treat the illness properly.

If an underlying illness has been ruled out and your child is still complaining of a stomachache, you might want to consider emotional causes for his distress. Talking to your child and to your child's doctor, teachers, school counselors, or even a child therapist can be a good place to start. Keep in mind that even if your child's symptoms are emotional in origin, the discomfort they cause is real and they deserve treatment and attention, just as they would if they were physically based.

CONVENTIONAL TREATMENT

■ Your child's doctor will perform an examination to determine whether the nausea and vomiting are caused by an infection or toxin, emotional distress, or an internal obstruction. He or she will look for signs of dehydration, fever, abdominal tenderness, or blood in the stools. If diarrhea is present, a stool culture may help to determine if the vomiting is related to a bacterial infection. Your doctor will recommend treatment based on the likely cause of your child's distress.

■ Antiemetics are drugs that are sometimes prescribed to ease nausea and stop vomiting. Trimethobenzamide (Tigan), prochlorperazine (Compazine), and promethazine (Phenergan) are among the ones most commonly used. They can be given in tablet or suppository form, or by injection. Because these drugs can have serious side effects, they should be used with caution in children. Never administer more than the prescribed dose.

■ Over-the-counter antacids, such as Maalox, Mylanta, and Rolaids, may be helpful for an occasional stomachache caused by acid indigestion or heartburn. Antacids neutralize acidic secretions in the stomach. However, because some antacids can actually end up increasing the production of acids in the stomach, or cause constipation or diarrhea, they are not routinely recommended for children.

■ Emetrol is a safe, over-the-counter syrup that settles the stomach. It is useful for relief of nausea caused by infections, overeating, or emotional upset, and produces no side effects. Give your child one teaspoon every few hours, as directed on the product label.

■ Bismuth subsalicylate, more commonly known as Pepto-Bismol, absorbs toxins and provides a protective coating along the gastrointestinal tract. It is helpful for relief of nausea as well as of diarrhea.

■ Unless specifically prescribed by your doctor, *do not* give a child with a stomachache a pain reliever, such as acetaminophen, aspirin, or ibuprofen. In relieving stomach pain whose cause has not been diagnosed, you may mask an underlying condition that could become worse without treatment.

DIETARY GUIDELINES

■ Guard against dehydration. The small body of a child loses fluids at an alarming rate when coping with episodes of vomiting or diarrhea. Refer to the guidelines for fluid intake in DIET AND NUTRITION in Part One to learn how much fluid intake your child needs. Do not ask or expect him to drink a whole glass of liquid at one time, however. Instead, offer frequent small sips throughout the day. Give fluids that are relatively high in glucose and salts, such as soups and fruit juices. Avoid carbonated beverages, which stretch the stomach and may aggravate vomiting.

WHEN TO CALL THE DOCTOR ABOUT NAUSEA AND VOMITING

• If your child has projectile vomiting—a particularly violent episode in which the vomit is ejected in a forceful stream and lands at a distance from his mouth—call your doctor right away. This can be an indication of a serious problem.

• If your child experiences nausea and vomiting with progressive pain and tenderness in the lower right abdomen, seek medical help immediately. It may signify the development of appendicitis. Typically, appendicitis pain starts around the umbilicus and gradually travels to and localizes around the lower right-hand quadrant of the abdomen. Appendicitis is often associated with a fever. (*See* APPENDICITIS.)

• If your child experiences any of the following, consult your physician: persistent vomiting; blood in the vomit; abdominal pain so severe that it keeps your child from eating, playing, or other normal activities; persistent abdominal pain that lasts more than a few hours.

■ When your child is vomiting, give him only clear liquids to give the gastrointestinal tract time to heal and rest. Once the vomiting is under control, slowly progress to solid foods to give the digestive tract time to readjust itself.

■ When a child refuses food, follow his lead. A child often instinctively knows what's best for his body. When his appetite improves, offer a bland, simple diet. Thin, weak cooked oatmeal, dry toast, applesauce, and yogurt are good foods to begin with. Once your child begins to feel better, he will feel hungry and will most likely ask for specific foods.

■ To lessen stomach acidity, a mixture of baking soda and water is effective. However, this old standby should be used only once. Dissolve ¼ teaspoon of baking soda in ½ cup of spring water.

NUTRITIONAL SUPPLEMENTS

■ *Lactobacillus acidophilus* or *bifidus* can help ease a stomachache by restoring healthy flora to the intestines. Give your child one dose, as directed on the product label, three times daily, for at least two to three weeks following an infection.

HERBAL TREATMENT

For age-appropriate dosages of herbal remedies, see page 81.

■ Aloe vera juice helps to clear and resolve a stomachache that a child may describe as "burning." Make sure to get a food-grade product. Give your child 1 tablespoon diluted in 6 ounces of water, up to three times daily. Use it sparingly; it can be a strong cathartic.

■ To help calm a sick and restless child, make chamomile tea and give him one dose with or between meals twice daily.

■ Ginger tea is helpful for nausea, vomiting, and stomachache. Give your child one dose, as needed. If the tea tastes too strong for your child, mix it with apple juice or make it with equal amounts of ginger and licorice root to sweeten the taste.

■ Green clay helps to neutralize an acid stomach. Mix 1 teaspoon of clay in 1 cup of spring water. The mixture can be taken immediately, but most children won't like the taste. It's usually better to permit the mixture to stand overnight to allow the clay to settle out and have your child drink it in the morning.

■ Either raw honey or barley malt extract can be used to settle an irritated stomach. Give your child ½ to 1 teaspoon every hour.
Caution: Never give honey to a child under one year old. It is associated with infant botulism, a potentially life-threatening form of food poisoning.

■ Licorice root is very settling to the stomach. Give your child one cup of licorice root tea, three times a day.
Note: This herb should not be given to a child with high blood pressure.

■ Peppermint tea is an effective and safe digestive aid. It is especially helpful for stomachache or vomiting that occurs after a heavy meal. Give your child one dose of tea, with or between meals, twice daily.

■ For a stomachache that is accompanied by gas, brew a beneficial stomach tea by blending one part each anise seed, fennel, peppermint, and thyme. Give your child one dose, as needed.

■ Umeboshi plum paste is very settling to an upset or acidic stomach. Give your child ⅛ teaspoon every thirty to sixty minutes. It can be combined with ginger and/or kuzu root. (*See* THERAPEUTIC RECIPES in Part Three.)

■ A 2,000-year-old Chinese herbal formula, available today as a product called Curing Pills, is effective for any stomach upset. Follow the age-appropriate dosage directions on the product label.

HOMEOPATHY

The following symptom-specific homeopathic remedies are useful for combating nausea. Please note that if you are also giving your child a tea containing peppermint, you should allow one hour between the tea and any homeopathic preparation. Otherwise, the strong smell of the mint may interfere with the action of the homeopathic remedy.

■ Give *Arsenicum album* to the child who has vomiting with diarrhea. Give him one dose of *Arsenicum album* 30x or 9c, every hour, up to a total of six doses.

■ *Carbo vegetabilis* is good for a child who has a specific pain in the center of his stomach. He will have gas with burping, possibly heartburn, and his abdomen will be distended. Give this child one dose of *Carbo vegetabilis* 30x or 9c, three times a day, up to a total of eight doses. There are also homeopathic combination remedies containing both *Nux vomica* and *Carbo vegetabilis*. Your health food store should have them.

■ *Ignatia* 30x or 9c is effective for emotionally based nausea. Your child will probably complain of a "lump" in his throat. Give him one dose, three times a day, for up to three days.

■ If your child experiences incessant vomiting and heaving, homeopathic *Ipecac* can bring relief. It also helps to relieve unrelenting nausea. Give your child one dose of *Ipecac* 12x or 6c every hour, up to a total of three or four doses.

Caution: Do not confuse homeopathic *Ipecac* with conventional syrup of ipecac. That is an entirely different product, and it should never be used except at the direction of a doctor or Poison Control Center.

■ *Nux vomica* benefits the child who develops a stomachache after overeating, after eating too many sweets, or after eating too much fried or fast food. This child feels nauseous, may have a headache, and is generally irritable. Give him one dose of *Nux Vomica* 30x or 9c, three times a day, up to a total of six doses.

ACUPRESSURE

For the locations of acupressure points on a child's body, *see* ADMINISTERING AN ACUPRESSURE TREATMENT in Part Three.

■ Pericardium 6 helps to lessen nausea and vomiting.

■ Stomach 36 harmonizes and tones the digestive system.

GENERAL RECOMMENDATIONS

■ Guard against dehydration. Be sure your child gets enough fluids.

■ Select a symptom-specific homeopathic remedy.

■ Give your child ginger or peppermint tea, or umeboshi paste.

■ Give your child a kuzu and salt plum paste mixture, especially if diarrhea is present.

■ To comfort and soothe stomach and/or abdominal muscles that are sore from vomiting, put a hot water bottle on your child's stomach. Don't fill the bottle so full that it becomes hard. Instead, fill it only about halfway, so that the bottle remains light enough to mold to your child's body.

■ Give your child Emetrol syrup, barley malt, or rice syrup. In children over two years of age, a teaspoon of honey every hour or two can help settle the stomach.

■ Remember that emotionally based nausea is still nausea, and therefore uncomfortable. A child who is emotionally upset is not feeling well, and needs your loving care and attention.

■ *See also* CONSTIPATION or DIARRHEA if your child's nausea is accompanied by either of these symptoms.

■ *See also* APPENDICITIS; CELIAC DISEASE; EMOTIONAL UPSET; FOOD ALLERGIES; FOOD POISONING; HEPATITIS; MOTION SICKNESS; or POISONING if you suspect that your child's nausea or vomiting may be related to any of these problems.

PREVENTION

■ To reduce the possibility of bacterial or viral infection, or a parasitic infestation, teach children to keep dirty fingers out of their mouths and to wash their hands regularly and thoroughly, especially before eating.

■ Caution against overeating. Serve appropriate amounts of food for your child's body. Prepare a healthy, moderate diet, and limit sugar and fats.

■ Encourage children to eat slowly and to chew their food thoroughly. Make mealtimes a pleasant, relaxed family gathering.

■ Be aware of your child's preferences and sensitivities. Eliminate foods that seem to bring on an upset stomach.

■ Avoid taking long car trips immediately after eating.

■ Anticipate the emotional stresses that come with difficult or exciting life events. Encourage your child to talk openly about his feelings.

Nose, Chronic Runny

See ALLERGIES.

Nosebleed

There are a great many tiny blood vessels in the delicate lining of the nose. These small capillaries are easily broken. Any number of things can rupture some of these small vessels and cause a nosebleed.

A fall from a jungle gym or bicycle, or a swat from an angry playmate or sibling, may cause a child's nose to bleed. If your child suffers a bloody nose from one of these causes, expect some hollering. A blow to the nose can be very painful.

If your child puts something in her nose, a nosebleed can occur from the trauma. Even just blowing the nose can start one. Inflammation from a cold, an allergy, even dry winter air, can cause the vessels to swell and rupture. Your child may even awaken with blood on her sheets or staining her nightclothes. When a nosebleed from one of these causes occurs, it seldom hurts.

Blood can be swallowed during a nosebleed, especially one that occurs during the night. If enough blood is involved, your child may vomit it up, or pass a dark, tarry-looking stool after the nosebleed has stopped.

The amount of blood coming from the nose during a nosebleed can be a continuous stream, or just a small trickle. It may look as if your child is losing a lot of blood, but not much blood is actually lost during the typical nosebleed. Although a bloody nose can be frightening to a child, it can usually be managed easily at home. Like most wounds, ruptured capillaries inside the nose will heal completely in about ten days.

If your child has a medical condition that makes her prone to nosebleeds, such as high blood pressure, leukemia, or hemophilia, ask your doctor for advice. If your child's nosebleeds recur more than once a month or so, have her examined by a doctor to rule out a possible underlying cause.

EMERGENCY TREATMENT FOR NOSEBLEED

See How to Stop a Nosebleed on page 318.

CONVENTIONAL TREATMENT

■ In the event of a severe nosebleed, your doctor may pack your child's nose with gauze, and instruct you to leave the packing in place for one or two days.

■ For an exceptionally serious nosebleed, your physician may recommend cauterizing the broken blood vessels within the nose. This involves applying an electrical current or silver nitrate stick directly to the broken vessel to solidify blood at the site. In very rare cases of severe, recurrent nosebleeds, a surgical tie-off of one of the larger blood vessels that supplies the tiny capillaries in the lining of the nose is recommended. Fortunately, this procedure is rarely necessary.

NUTRITIONAL SUPPLEMENTS

For age-appropriate dosages of some nutritional supplements, see page 81.

■ Vitamin C with bioflavonoids helps prevent capillary fragility. Give your child one to two doses, four times daily, for two days after a nosebleed. Then give her one-half dose, twice a day, for at least one month.

■ Give your child a multiple vitamin, once a day, for one month.

■ Vitamin K helps the blood to clot more efficiently. If your child suffers from recurring nosebleeds, give her 15 micrograms, once or twice daily, for one month.

How to Stop a Nosebleed

➕ To stop the bleeding, apply pressure to the bridge of your child's nose, as follows.

1. Sit your child upright.

2. Tilt her head forward (*not* backward).

3. Place your thumb and forefinger on either side of the bridge of the nose and apply pressure firmly enough to slow bleeding, but not so strongly as to cause discomfort. Pressure decreases the blood flow through the affected area, slowing bleeding. To give a clot time to form, maintain the pressure for about ten minutes.

4. After ten minutes, check to see if the bleeding has stopped. If not, apply pressure for another ten-minute period.

5. If your child's nose is still bleeding steadily after twenty minutes of pressure, call your doctor.

➕ Another way to stop a nosebleed is to put an ice pack across the bridge of your child's nose. This will constrict the blood vessels and help stop the bleeding. Hold the ice pack firmly in place. After ten minutes, check to see if bleeding has stopped. If not, reapply the ice pack for another ten-minute period. If your child's nose is still bleeding steadily after twenty minutes, call your doctor.

➕ Try wetting a bit of cotton or plain sterile gauze with white vinegar and placing it in your child's nose. Leave it in place for at least ten minutes. The acid of the vinegar will gently cauterize the inside of the nose and stop the bleeding.

HOMEOPATHY

■ *Ferrum phosphoricum* will help resolve a nosebleed and speed local healing of the injured tissue. Give your child one dose of *Ferrum phosphoricum* 6x, 12x, or 6c, every ten minutes, for a total of three to four doses.

PREVENTION

■ Teach your child not to pick her nose, or to put any object into her nose.

■ Do not smoke in your child's environment. Protect your child from exposure to secondhand smoke.

■ If your child is prone to recurring small nosebleeds, give her nettle leaf tea, several times a week, as a preventive. Nettle contains vitamins A and C, which strengthen the mucous membranes, as well as many trace minerals, including an easily absorbed form of iron.

Note: Some children experience stomach upset as a result of taking nettle. If this happens, stop giving it. This herb should not be given to a child under four.

■ Give your child bioflavonoids as recommended above.

■ To keep the lining of the nose moist and lessen the chance of small capillaries swelling and rupturing, humidify the air in your home, especially during the dry winter months. Use a humidifier in your child's room, making sure to fill it with purified distilled water only. Clean your humidifier once a week to keep bacteria from building up and to make certain that allergens are not being spread.

■ Moisten the lining of your child's nose with a salt-water spray. Follow the procedure for a SALINE NASAL FLUSH in Part Three to flush the nasal membranes twice daily (*do not* suction out mucus afterward). Over-the-counter saline (salt water) nasal sprays, such as Ocean, Ayr, and Salinex, serve the same purpose. A small amount of ointment such as Aquaphor, calendula, or aloe vera applied after a saline spray can help nasal membranes heal.

■ Avoid the use of decongestant nasal sprays. They constrict blood vessels and can lead to bleeding.

■ For some suggestions of things you can do to reduce the possibility that your child will suffer a bump to the nose that leads to a nosebleed, *see* HOME SAFETY in Part One.

Obesity

Many parents, especially parents of small children, complain that their children "won't eat." Yet despite this, the number of children, even young children, who are overweight has been increasing significantly in recent years.

A child is considered obese if he weighs 20 percent more than an average child of the same sex and similar age, height, and body build. In the simplest terms, obesity results from an imbalance in energy exchange: Too much energy is taken in (food) without an equal amount of energy output (activity). The body takes these excess calories, turns them into fat, and stores them, which can lead to a weight problem. A child who establishes a pattern of too much eating, too little activity, and obesity early on is at risk for continued weight problems throughout life, as well as for the health risks that accompany obesity. Heart disease, certain cancers, and adult-onset diabetes, among other things, are potential concerns. An obese child can also suffer greatly from unkind remarks made by his peers.

A particular problem for young people these days is a dependence on convenience and junk foods, which supply lots of calories but very little nutrition. Heavy consumption of these foods creates an obese child who—despite the excess weight—may also be malnourished, because he is missing the essential nutrients he should be getting from fresh, whole foods.

Although in the simplest terms, obesity is a result of imbalance between the consumption and expenditure of calories, people have been trying for years to determine the underlying causes—that is, why certain people become obese and others do not. The fat-cell theory, proposed in 1967 by Dr. Jules Hirsch of Rockefeller University in New York, postulates that in a growing child who has been programmed to overeat, or one who consumes a high-fat and/or high-sugar diet, particularly during growth spurts, the body is stimulated to manufacture an excessive number of new fat cells. The body also manufactures new fat cells when the existing fat cells become full, a process that occurs with alarming frequency in overweight children as well as in adults. According to the fat-cell theory, every fat cell the body manufactures stays with the body for life, and short of surgery, there is no way to rid the body of even one fat cell once the body has manufactured it.

Another theory concerns the possibility that some people are simply destined to be obese because overweight runs in families. Indeed, studies have shown that just 7 percent of children born to normal-weight parents will grow up to be overweight. However, if one parent has a weight problem, there is a 40-percent chance that a child will also have a weight problem. If both parents are overweight, a child faces an 80-percent probability of being overweight. Is this heredity at work? Are overweight parents passing on a genetic tendency to put on pounds?

Both theories probably contain elements of the truth, but there is reason to doubt that either one is entirely correct. Research data do show that 75 percent of children who are overweight between the ages of nine and twelve will grow into overweight adults. The odds are even more disturbing for overweight teenagers. Ninety percent of overweight adolescents will be overweight for life. But recent research shows that it may be possible to reduce the number of fat cells in the body, *if* there is a major weight loss. Other laboratory studies have been done showing that while overweight rats give birth to offspring that quickly match their parents in body size, and slender parents give birth to babies who grow into slender adults, even obese rats slim down to healthy proportions when their rations are adjusted and they are forced to exercise. In other words, an inherited tendency to pack on the pounds does *not* mean that a person has no choice but to become (or stay) overweight, just as the number of fat cells in the body is probably not a life sentence. In the final analysis, the experts say, environmental factors are the greatest determinants of which children end up overweight. Eating patterns learned at the family dining table during childhood are responsible for most of the chubby babies, chunky toddlers, overweight schoolchildren, and teens who suffer because of weight problems—as well as adults who continually battle the bulge.

The best approach to obesity is to prevent it by fostering a healthy lifestyle from the very beginning. But it is never too late to begin. In DIET AND NUTRITION in Part One, we discuss the ways in which parents unintentionally, and perhaps unknowingly, "program" their children to become overweight, the pitfalls to avoid, and suggestions for feeding your child a clean and lean diet that builds a healthy body. We also talk about the scientific and medical findings that point to ways responsible parents can help their offspring sidestep potential childhood weight problems—problems that can lead to a lifetime of struggling with obesity.

There's no one solution to weight loss. Self-discipline helps. A supportive family approach helps. A nutrient-rich, appetite-satisfying diet of whole foods helps. Exercise helps. And medical science and natural medicine can help. The key to success is a healthy, consistent approach to eating and activity—crash dieting and fad diets are *not* the answer.

An essential part of your approach to your child's weight concerns is a realistic, nonjudgmental perspective. Too much anxiety or control, or a too narrow view of the "right" body weight, can lead to anxiety, body image disturbances, or even eating disorders for your child (*see* Eating Disorders: Anorexia and Bulimia, on page 321). This is a sensitive and complicated arena. It deserves your thoughtful communication, consistency, and loving support. Doctors, nurses, nutritionists, naturopathic physicians, counselors, and physical therapists are among the people who can offer you support and guidance.

Be particularly sensitive if your child is a teenager. A teenager with a weight problem is usually very unhappy. Not only does excess weight expose your teenager to potential health problems, it can also create potentially significant emotional problems. Body image, self-esteem, and issues of physical attractiveness are paramount during adolescence.

Because many teens equate food with emotional comfort, overeating during adolescence is common. Your teen may eat to cope with feelings of depression, rejection by peers, or low self-esteem. Another common reason for overeating is eating out of habit, such as munching when doing homework or sitting in front of the television.

Family eating habits can play a large role with overweight adolescents. When family eating habits include large meals, incessant snacking, and sweet treats, these come to be regarded as the norm, and teenagers can overeat without think-

Eating Disorders: Anorexia and Bulimia

Anorexia and bulimia are complicated and serious eating disorders related to distorted self-image and self-control issues. Both of these conditions occur much more frequently among girls than boys, although the number of boys suffering from eating disorders has been growing in recent years.

Anorexia is characterized by a strong fear of gaining weight, a refusal to maintain appropriate body weight, self-imposed starvation, and a distorted view of one's sexuality. In girls, menstruation often ceases. A child with anorexia will have a very distorted view of her body size, insisting that she is not too thin. A child with anorexia may also display unusual eating habits, such as cutting food into tiny pieces or eating only one or two foods. She may become obsessed with food—obsessed with not eating and obsessed with preparing food for others. She may also exercise excessively. In addition, a child with anorexia is not likely to admit her problem or be willing to receive treatment.

As anorexia and malnutrition continue, serious physical consequences can result. Weakness, fatigue, dizziness, constipation, low blood pressure, a slowed heart rate, a low body temperature, abdominal swelling, thinning hair, decreased muscle tone, and slowed physical development may ensue. Hospitalization is required for some children whose physical status is so compromised that they are at risk for heart complications.

Like anorexia, bulimia is characterized by a strong fear of gaining weight and a distorted body image. However, it is distinguished by episodes of secretive binge eating followed by guilt, shame, self-hatred, and sometimes the use of laxatives or vomiting. A child with bulimia often fears that she doesn't have the self-control to stop eating. Depression and low self-esteem are likely also to be part of the picture. Tooth erosion, irritation of the throat and esophagus, chest pain, salivary gland swelling, and dehydration may result from the persistent vomiting. A child with long-term bulimia is also at risk for heart problems, even a sudden heart attack, due to the imbalance of electrolytes caused by vomiting.

Underlying both of these behaviors are very low self-esteem and poor coping abilities. A child who develops anorexia or bulimia fears losing her autonomy. To friends, teachers, and parents, she may appear to be the perfect "good girl," while underneath she may be struggling with feelings of helplessness, anger, or a fear that her life is not in her control.

Treating either of these illnesses involves addressing the underlying psychological issues that are contributing to the problem and restoring and maintaining a child's nutritional needs. Individual and family therapy, behavior modification, and nutritional counseling are important components of a successful treatment plan. Cultural, familial, psychological, and physiological issues need to be addressed when treating a young person with either of these eating disorders.

Anorexia and bulimia are multifaceted and serious illnesses. A thorough discussion of the causes and treatments of these eating disorders is beyond the scope of this book. The information provided here is only a brief introduction. If you feel concerned that your child may have an eating disorder, talk with your health care provider regarding diagnosis and approaches that can help restore your child's health. These are problems that can rarely be treated successfully without the help of a skilled professional, and it is often a long-term commitment. There are also toll-free hot lines you may call for assistance:

Anorexia Helpline
800–888–4673

Bulimia Abuse Helpline
800–888–4680

ing. A teen who has been programmed from his early years to regard food as a comfort or a reward can end up comforting and rewarding himself far too often.

Healthy exercise is as important as a healthy diet in maintaining a clean and lean body. Physical activity actually reduces appetite and increases the metabolic rate so that more calories are burned more efficiently.

Basal metabolism, the rate at which the body burns calories while at rest, varies from child to child. There is no standard or norm. On the whole, though, naturally active children—the ones who never seem to sit still—use up more calories, and burn calories faster and more efficiently, than a dreamy child who is content with quiet play. An active child will typically burn 10 percent more calories per hour than a sedentary child. Exercise helps in weight control because it stimulates and increases a child's metabolic rate. Remarkably, this higher rate of caloric burn continues even after the physical activity ceases.

Exercise also inhibits appetite. The appetite-control center of the body is the *hypothalamus*, or "appestat." This gland, located in the brain, tells the body when it's hungry and when the stomach is full. The appestat is triggered by certain chemicals (glucose, serotonin, noradrenaline, adrenaline, dopamine), which continually circulate through the body in varying amounts. Physical activity reduces the levels of the hunger-stimulating chemicals that cause the appestat to start the stomach growling for food, and increases the levels of the chemicals that signal to the appestat that the body is humming along at peak efficiency and doesn't require food.

All these complex exercise-driven chemical changes vary from child to child. They are very difficult to measure precisely. However, research indicates that exercise can inhibit hunger for as long as six hours after a high level of physical activity. If your child comes home after several hours of physical activity, he may very well say, "I'm not hungry." When this happens, believe it. The appestat, the master control, is simply responding to all the complex chemical changes that exercise initiates.

If you have a sedentary child whose favorite activity is eating, you can help him by insisting on a period of physical activity each day. Help your child discover a pastime that is both physically active and fun. When exercise time is a good time, you won't have to nag a reluctant child into getting up and getting going.

If you have a teenager with a weight problem, you might want to have him take a look at a calorie-burning chart (*see* How Many Calories Are You Burning? on page 324). There may be some surprises in store. For example, low-intensity aerobic dancing and mowing the lawn burn approximately the same number of calories per hour. Given a choice between cutting the grass and dancing, most teens will opt for dancing. If your teenager prefers privacy to an aerobic exercise class, you might want to look into getting a video workout tape.

It is also revealing to translate numbers of calories into actual foods, and see how long it takes to burn off, say, a handful of potato chips by engaging in different activities. For example, it takes 190 minutes (over three hours) to use up the calories in ten potato chips if you're watching television, but dancing will burn up the calories in those chips in just twenty minutes.

In maintaining a lean, healthy body, exercise and diet go hand in hand. It's difficult to say which is more important. One of the most loving things you can do for your child is to foster a lifelong love of physical activity.

Research indicates that there are some people who will probably be overweight no matter what they do. There are also a number of metabolic and endocrine imbalances, including hypothyroidism and hypopituitarism, that cause abnormal weight gain. These conditions are rare, but they do occur, so if you have a real reason to suspect that your child's excess weight is a result of something other than eating habits, consult your physician. In most cases, however, a healthy lifestyle—combining exercise and a diet based on grains, vegetables, fruits, complex carbohydrates, and lean proteins (and without refined sugar and fatty foods)—is the best way to prevent, or combat, obesity.

CONVENTIONAL TREATMENT

■ In rare cases, an obese child may have an underlying medical condition that is causing the problem. A doctor's examination and blood testing may be worthwhile to rule out endocrine or metabolic problems, such as hypothyroidism, adrenal disease (Cushing's syndrome), pituitary disorders, or genetic diseases.

■ If your child has no signs of underlying disease, your doctor will probably recommend dietary changes and regular exercise. Many will design a special diet and, in severe cases, supervised fasting. Some will mandate specific periods of exercise.

■ Behavior modification is a commonly used tool for weight problems (*see* BEHAVIOR MODIFICATION FOR WEIGHT CONTROL in Part Three).

■ Medications to suppress appetite, whether prescription or over-the-counter drugs, are to be avoided. They do nothing to address the behavior patterns that led to obesity in the first place, and can produce serious side effects.

DIETARY GUIDELINES

■ To help flush toxins from the system and fill a hungry stomach, encourage your child to drink at least eight glasses of spring water every day.

■ Crash diets don't work. Skipping meals doesn't work. When the body is provided with too few calories (or no calories at all), it automatically slows down the rate at which it is burning calories so as to conserve and use every nutrient. A steady intake of a reasonable number of calories is the quickest and most efficient way to lose weight. Also, most teenagers can't function on less than 1,600 calories per day.

■ Foster healthy eating habits. A diet of whole nutrient-rich foods satisfies the appetite. Junk foods do not. Your child will discover that dieting is a lot easier when he is on a healthy diet. When whole foods are on the menu, blood sugar levels are maintained and cravings are first minimized, then disappear. Meanwhile, energy levels remain high.

■ Encourage your child to avoid foods with additives, preservatives, or sugar, as well as sodas, soft drinks, caffeine, chocolate, and all sweets. Sugar and caffeine cause a tremendous surge in blood sugar levels—followed by a great downward crash. When blood sugar levels are low, dieters tend to eat undesirable foods.

■ Give your child a breakfast including a cereal made from finely ground whole grains (millet, wheat, rice, oats, etc.) every morning to sustain blood sugar and give a full feeling in the stomach.

■ When buying and preparing food for a dieting child, keep in mind that simple, whole foods have fewer calories than manufactured food products. Most commercially prepared foods are loaded with excess calories. If you must use prepared foods, check the labels carefully for calories per serving, as well as fat (especially the percentage of calories that come from fat), sugar, and sodium content.

■ Encourage your child to eat a diet consisting primarily of vegetables, fruits, lean protein, and whole grains. Fiber-rich foods provide low-calorie, stomach-filling bulk, making it easier to eat less. Vegetables should be eaten either steamed or raw. Lean proteins include fish and the white meat of chicken and turkey. (Red meat should be limited to one serving a week, or better yet, eliminated altogether.)

How Many Calories Are You Burning?

Everything a person does burns calories. However, some activities burn more calories than others. The number of calories burned also depends, to some extent, on a person's body size and metabolic rate. The following table gives approximations of how many calories a teenager is likely to burn up in the course of many everyday activities. If you have a teenager with a weight problem, he can use this table to estimate how many calories he currently uses in the course of a day, and then to set a goal for increasing his expenditure of calories while engaging in activities he enjoys.

Activity	Calories Burned per Hour, by Body Weight (in Pounds)					
	105–115	116–126	127–137	138–148	149–159	160–170
Aerobics						
low-speed	215	230	245	260	275	290
high-speed	515	550	585	620	655	690
Baking	130	140	150	155	165	175
Busing tables	235	250	270	285	300	315
Cooking	105	110	120	125	135	140
Dancing						
slow	195	210	225	240	250	265
vigorous	235	250	270	285	300	315
Doing yoga	180	195	205	220	230	245
Driving a car						
standard transmission	105	110	120	125	135	140
automatic transmission	75	80	85	90	95	100
Eating	70	75	80	85	90	95
Gardening	305	325	245	365	390	410
Mountain climbing	470	500	535	565	600	630
Mowing the lawn (with a hand-operated power mower)	210	225	240	255	270	285
Playing basketball	435	465	495	525	555	585
Playing chess	70	75	80	85	90	95
Playing football						
touch	470	500	535	565	600	630
tackle	660	705	750	795	835	885
Playing handball	470	500	535	565	600	630
Playing the piano	95	100	110	115	120	130
Playing table tennis						
recreational	235	250	270	285	300	315
competitive	355	375	380	405	425	450
Playing tennis	335	355	380	405	425	450
Reading	70	75	80	85	90	95
Riding a bicycle						
at 5 miles per hour	175	185	195	210	225	235
at 10 miles per hour	325	370	395	415	440	460
at 13 miles per hour	515	550	585	620	655	690
Riding a motorcycle	160	170	180	295	205	215
Running						
11-minute miles	515	550	585	620	655	690
8-minute miles	550	585	625	660	700	735
7-minute miles	705	755	805	850	900	950
5-minute miles	955	1025	1090	1155	1220	1285

Activity	Calories Burned per Hour, by Body Weight (in Pounds)					
	105–115	116–126	127–137	138–148	149–159	160–170
Shopping	130	140	150	155	165	175
Shoveling snow	825	885	940	995	1055	1110
Skiing						
cross-country	470	500	535	565	600	630
downhill	465	500	530	560	595	625
Sleeping	50	55	60	60	65	70
Studying	65	70	75	80	85	90
Typing	80	90	95	100	105	110
Watching television	60	65	70	75	80	80
Waiting on tables	190	205	215	230	245	255
Walking						
at 2 miles per hour	145	155	165	175	185	195
at 3 miles per hour	235	250	270	285	300	315
at 4 miles per hour	270	290	310	330	345	365
at 5 miles per hour	435	465	495	525	555	585
Writing	70	75	80	85	90	95

Another way to look at your calorie consumption is to consider how long it takes to burn off different foods. The following table shows how many minutes of different kinds of activities are required to burn the calories in specific foods.

Food, Portion Size	Number of Minutes Required to Burn Calories, by Activity							
	Sitting	Standing	Walking	Bicycling	Dancing	Doing Dishes	Running	Swimming
Apple, 1 medium	133	107	27	21	14	53	8	7
Banana, 1 medium	168	135	34	27	18	67	10	8
Butter, 1 pat	60	48	12	10	6	24	3	3
Candy bar, 1 ounce	245	196	49	39	26	98	14	12
Carrot, 1 small	35	28	7	6	4	14	2	2
Green beans, ½ cup	27	21	5	4	3	11	1	1
Greens, ½ cup	28	23	6	5	3	11	2	2
Hamburger, 3 ounces	310	248	62	50	33	124	18	16
Ice cream, ½ cup	230	184	46	37	24	92	13	12
Milkshake, 1½ cups	652	521	130	104	69	261	37	33
Orange juice, ½ cup	93	75	19	15	10	37	5	5
Pastry, 1 plain	457	365	91	73	48	183	26	23
Pizza, ¼ of 14" pie	590	472	118	94	62	236	34	30
Popcorn, 1 cup plain	38	31	8	6	4	15	2	2
Pork chop, 3 ounces	513	411	103	82	54	205	29	26
Potato								
baked, 1 large	220	176	44	35	23	88	12	11
French fries, 20	388	311	78	62	41	155	22	19
Potato chips, 10	190	152	38	30	20	76	11	10
Skim milk, 1 cup	133	107	27	21	14	53	8	7
Soft drink, 1 cup	160	128	32	26	51	64	9	8
Tossed salad, 1 cup	22	17	4	3	3	9	1	1
White bread, 1 slice	102	81	20	16	11	41	6	5

Filling and nutritious grains include oatmeal, rye, sweet brown rice, millet, buck-wheat, and quinoa.

■ Prepare a diet low in fat. Avoid creamed dishes, foods with creamed fillings, and rich gravies. Do not add extra butter, oil, mayonnaise, cream, or salad dressings to foods. Do not deep-fry or pan-fry foods. Bake, broil, poach, or steam them instead. Dieters should not eat fried foods of any kind. They are both high in calories and difficult to digest. The only exception to this rule is stir-frying, where only a tablespoon or two of oil (preferably olive oil) is needed to cook an entire meal quickly. Using no-stick cookware helps reduce the amount of oil you need for cooking as well.

NUTRITIONAL SUPPLEMENTS

■ Chromium picolinate, or glucose tolerance factor, helps to control blood sugar levels and diminishes cravings for sugar. Remember, low blood sugar sends hunger signals to the brain, causing your child to want to eat something—any-thing—quickly. An overweight teenager can take 50 micrograms of chromium picolinate, once or twice daily, for up to one month.

■ Lipotropics (choline, inositol, methionine) help to control blood sugar levels, improve liver function, and enhance fat and carbohydrate metabolism. Lipotropics help the body use nutrients more efficiently, making it easier to eat less. Give a child over twelve years of age a lipotropic combination supplement twice daily with meals, following dosage directions on the product label.

■ It is best to satisfy the body's vitamin and mineral needs with a healthy diet. However, if your dieting child experiences a notable drop in energy level, select a good multiple vitamin and mineral supplement that includes all the basic vitamins and minerals in at least the recommended daily allowances (100 percent of RDA). Follow the dosage directions on the product label.

■ Anorexia has been linked to a vitamin-B complex and zinc deficiency. If your child has an eating disorder, or if you suspect he may be developing one, ask your physician about introducing these nutrients into his nutritional program.

HERBAL TREATMENT

For age-specific dosages of herbal remedies, see page 81.

■ Dong quai is a Chinese herb that is helpful for dieters, especially females, who become tired and have little energy. It is particularly good for a young woman who finds it difficult to stay on a diet around her menstrual period. A girl who is thirteen years or older may take one dose, once daily, two weeks out of every month, for up to three months.

■ Licorice root, in tea or tincture, is a natural herb that reduces cravings for sweets by strengthening the adrenal glands, thereby helping sustain a regulated blood sugar level. Licorice tastes sweet. It can be added to other teas, such as those below, to sweeten them. Give your child one dose, once daily, one week out of every month, for up to three months.

Note: This herb should not be given to a child with high blood pressure.

■ Cleansing and chlorophyll-rich parsley tea is a mild diuretic. Give your child one dose, once daily, for one week when beginning a new dietary routine.

■ Red clover aids in detoxifying a body burdened with excess pounds. Give your child one dose of red clover tea, once daily, for one week out of every month, for up to three months.

■ Red raspberry leaf tea reduces the appetite, balances the hormonal system, and increases energy—and it tastes good. Give your child one dose, twice a day, one week out of each month, for up to three months. Do not give this tea before bed, though; it may be too energizing.

■ Siberian ginseng helps to stabilize blood sugar and reduce cravings for sweets. It is also a natural energizer. Give your child one dose daily, one week out of every month, for up to three months.

HOMEOPATHY

■ *Argentum nitricum* reduces cravings for sweets. Give your child one dose of *Argentum nitricum* 30x or 9c, twice daily, for up to one week.

■ If a teenager has difficulty controlling his appetite and eats to calm his nerves, give him one dose of *Calcarea carbonica* 12x or 6c, three times daily, for up to one week when beginning a diet.

■ If an excitable and nervous teenager eats primarily to calm down, *Coffea cruda* will help. After he has tried *Calcarea carbonica* for three days, try one dose of *Coffea cruda* 12x or 6c, three times daily, for up to three days.

ACUPRESSURE

For the locations of acupressure points on a child's body, *see* ADMINISTERING AN ACUPRESSURE TREATMENT in Part Three.

■ Four Gates relaxes the nervous system.

■ Neck and Shoulder Release will help to relax and calm a child on a diet.

GENERAL RECOMMENDATIONS

■ The parents of an overweight child should approach this topic with care and compassion. You are the most important adults in your child's life. Whether he shows love or not, your growing child needs your love and support to learn to respect the uniqueness of his body. The issue of weight needs to be dealt with gently and compassionately.

■ An overweight child, especially a teenager, may "hate" himself and everything and everyone around him. Help him to understand that he is unique. Emphasize that losing weight is about being healthy, not about having the "right" body—in fact, there is no "right" shape or size. Every one of us has a different body, with different strengths and capabilities. An adolescent should be helped to realize that each individual must care about all aspects of himself—body, heart, soul, and mind. Only when your child has been gently encouraged to love and care for himself is it time to begin a weight-loss regimen.

■ Follow the dietary guidelines above.

■ To lessen appetite, give your child red raspberry tea.

■ It's easy to start a weight-loss program, but hard to follow one. Biofeedback, meditation, and visualization will all help. Encourage your child to visualize having a slimmer, fitter body, and feeling stronger and healthier.

■ Encourage your child to avoid chewing gum. The calories in gum are few, but chewing increases the appetite by fooling the stomach into "thinking" that food is on the way. The stomach begins to prepare. It floods the area with digestive juices and churns and growls. Appetite increases. Because hunger signals have been activated, your child may end up eating.

■ Encourage exercise. Although the initial response may seem slow, results come faster. When the first few pounds are lost, it will be much easier for your child to stay enthusiastic. To rev up the system, burn fat, tone muscles, and lose weight, exercise is essential. Once your child understands this, it should be easier for him to get up and get going. Encourage a teenager to engage in the exercise of his choice, at least four days a week, for at least thirty minutes per session. Fun exercises for teens include dancing, hiking, walking, yoga, swimming, bicycling, roller skating, and team sports.

■ If an overweight teenager is self-conscious and prefers to exercise alone, be supportive. Investigate a local club or spa. Don't choose one frequented by 105-pound girls in leotards or 165-pound guys in muscle shirts. The sight of all those toned bodies could send your teen home to raid the refrigerator for consolation. Find a spa where your child will feel comfortable and encouraged, not self-conscious and discouraged.

■ A vigorous massage is a wonderful way for a teenager to care for himself, whether dieting or not. Provide a natural vegetable fiber (loofah) mitt or brush. A dry-brush massage before showering enhances circulation, stimulates a sluggish nervous system, and hastens detoxification of the system, as well as getting rid of dead skin cells and making the skin shine.

■ Encourage your child to express himself. Sharing thoughts, accomplishments, and frustrations—if not with you, with a friend—will help keep him on track. If an extra boost is needed, investigate a support group or engage a counselor.

■ Realize that the miraculous claims for many food products and/or services are designed to sell the product or service, not to transform an overweight individual into a slim one. Help your child sort out fiction from fact when evaluating a product or service that promises painless weight loss. A simple rule of thumb is: If it sounds too good to be true, it probably is.

■ A teenager may find it helpful to join a support group. Having a place to listen to others, share experiences, and receive encouragement can be an invaluable part of the process.

PREVENTION

■ Encourage an active lifestyle, starting at a very young age.

■ To prevent weight gain or to maintain weight loss, make sure your child eats a healthy diet of nutrient-rich, appetite-satisfying whole foods. Avoid refined sugar and caffeine. Limit fats.

Pain Relief

Pain is nature's alarm system, a signal that something is hurt and needs to be attended to. Pain in the form of a headache can signal muscle tension. Other types of pain can alert you to a strained muscle, a broken bone, an infection, or an inflamed appendix. Pain is a response that helps protect the body from harm. For example, it is the lightning-fast transmission of a pain signal that causes a child to snatch her hand away from a fire or hot stove. Even before the brain signals "danger," or the hurt fully registers consciously, the body knows what action to take.

Pain is experienced as a wide variety of sensations, including throbbing, stabbing, and aching. Pain may be localized at the site of an injury, or "referred" to another part of the body. It may be acute and resolve after a short time, or chronic, lasting for six months or more, and it can be anywhere from mild to severe in intensity.

Pain can also be a signal that something has gone wrong internally. Listen carefully when a child complains of pain. Ask questions, such as where it hurts, how much it hurts, what makes it hurt, and what makes it feel better. If the answers you get don't give you some idea of what's happening, it may be helpful to seek medical advice. Pain is a basic symptom of inflammation, and an important clue to many disorders. If your child experiences pain that gets progressively worse, does not improve with ordinary pain-control measures, interferes with the child's normal activity level, or starts in a small area and involves an increasingly larger area, or if the pain is severe and unremitting, consult with your doctor.

The suggestions offered here are ways to treat the type of mild pain that may be related to a headache, sore muscles or bruises, or recovery from surgery, an injury, or a broken bone.

Children are often unable to describe their pain accurately. Because of their inability to express themselves, children may not receive the pain control they need. Infants and children do feel pain, and they need to be listened to and cared for when they show signs of being in pain. If your child says she hurts or seems uncomfortable, start with the basic assumption that the pain is real, and ask questions that will help your child describe what she is feeling.

Both the physical and emotional aspects of pain need to be addressed and respected. The physical component of pain is relatively straightforward; it is the result of information being transmitted from the site of injury or illness to the brain. At the same time, however, another impulse runs through the central nervous system to another part of the brain, the limbic system. This system transmits the perception of pain and generates an emotional reaction to it. For example, when you stub a toe, the immediate pain of the injury is felt. But an emotional reaction also occurs that may cause you to feel angry, afraid, sick to your stomach, or even sad. Because both physical and emotional aspects are involved when your child is feeling pain, comforting her and acknowledging her emotional response may be as important as anything else you can do.

CONVENTIONAL TREATMENT

■ Acetaminophen (found in Tylenol, Panadol, Anacin-3, Tempra, and other medications) is generally thought to be the safest over-the-counter analgesic. Side effects are rare, but they can include liver toxicity, primarily in cases of overdose. Always read labels carefully and be sure not to exceed the recommended dosage for your child.

■ Ibuprofen (Advil, Medipren, Motrin, Nuprin, Pediaprofen, and others) is an anti-inflammatory that some doctors consider to be the most effective pain reliever. The liquid form allows for more flexible dosage adjustments.

■ Codeine is a prescription narcotic that is effective for moderate to severe pain that is not relieved by less potent medications. Narcotics like codeine work by binding with opiate receptors in the central nervous system to alter the *perception* of pain. In other words, the pain still exists, but the narcotic tricks the body into not recognizing it. Possible side effects of codeine include sedation, slowed breathing, low blood pressure, stomach upset, and constipation. If your doctor prescribes codeine, encourage your child to consume more fluids and a high-fiber diet to help keep her from becoming constipated (*see* CONSTIPATION).

■ An acetaminophen and codeine combination can be very effective and is sometimes prescribed for pain control in children. Acetaminophen works at the site of the illness or injury, lessening pain and inflammation, while codeine works in the central nervous system and blocks the perception of pain.

■ Because of the connection between aspirin and Reye's syndrome, aspirin is *not* recommended for a child or teenager without a doctor's approval. However, it is useful for some types of pain, such as for the relief of pain from an injury or childhood arthritis.

HERBAL TREATMENT

For age-appropriate dosages of herbal remedies, see page 81.

■ Brew a pain-relief tea as follows: Simmer 1 tablespoon of white willow bark in 1 quart of water for fifteen minutes. Add 1 tablespoon of valerian root, 1 tablespoon skullcap, 1 tablespoon chamomile, and ½ tablespoon licorice root. Simmer for another ten minutes; then strain and cool. Give your child one dose, every hour, for four consecutive hours, to help relieve generalized pain. White willow bark is an anti-inflammatory similar to aspirin; valerian and skullcap have sedative and antispasmodic properties; chamomile is an effective relaxant; licorice is an anti-inflammatory and enhances the action of the other herbs, in addition to sweetening the tea.

Note: Skullcap should not be given to a child under six years of age. Licorice should not be given to a child with high blood pressure.

HOMEOPATHY

■ *Arnica* is very helpful for pain related to overexertion, injury, or bruising. Give your child one dose of *Arnica* 30x or 9c every hour, for three to four hours, until the pain subsides.

■ *Hypericum* benefits an injury to fingers or toes, pain after surgery, or injury to a nerve. Give your child one dose of *Hypericum* 12x or 6c, three times daily, for up to two days.

■ *Ledum* is good for a puncture wound that results in bruising. Give your child one dose of *Ledum* 12x or 6c, three times daily, for two days.

ACUPRESSURE

For the locations of acupressure points on a child's body, *see* ADMINISTERING AN ACUPRESSURE TREATMENT in Part Three.

■ Four Gates helps to calm and soothe.

■ Neck and Shoulder Release helps to release pain centered in the head, neck, and shoulder area, and will help relax your child.

GENERAL RECOMMENDATIONS

■ When a child is in pain, start by comforting, listening, and verbally acknowledging the hurt. This helps to lessen fear and anxiety.

■ Help your child relax. A quiet room, soothing music, a warm bath, or a gentle massage can be helpful. Help your child practice slow, deep breathing.

■ Relaxation exercises and visualization techniques are very helpful, and also teach children tools they can use on their own, should the need arise. Maureen Murdock's book *Spinning Inward: Using Guided Imagery with Children for Learning, Creativity, and Relaxation* (Shambhala, 1987) is a good source for techniques you may wish to teach your child.

■ When appropriate, practice distraction. Playing a game, reading a story, talking to friends, watching a movie, or any other form of pleasant distraction will help take attention away from the discomfort.

PREVENTION

■ Many types of pain a child may suffer cannot be prevented. But there are steps you can take to childproof your home and also to minimize hazards your child will encounter outside. *See* HOME SAFETY in Part One.

Pertussis

See WHOOPING COUGH.

Pinkeye

See CONJUNCTIVITIS.

Pinworms

Pinworms (*Enterobius vermicularis*) are small, thin white worms a little less than half an inch long. One of the most common parasitic infections, pinworms can affect people of any age, culture, or socioeconomic status.

The infestation occurs when eggs are ingested. The eggs are usually transferred by fingernails, clothing, bedding, house dust, and food. If the house is infested, pinworms will very likely spread to all members of the family. When pinworm eggs are swallowed, they hatch, then migrate to the large intestine. In this hospitable environment, the worms live and grow into adult form. At night, adult females travel through the intestine to the area around the anus, where they deposit their eggs.

This egg deposit is itchy and irritating, which leads to scratching around the anal area. Scratching usually results in some of the eggs getting under the fingernails. Then, if the fingernails aren't well scrubbed, it's very likely the eggs will get into the mouth, either through eating or touching the lips, and the cycle starts all over again. Because of the persistent itching, the sufferer may experience difficulty sleeping.

There are many types of parasitic worms. Some of them can cause serious problems, such as diarrhea and malnutrition, so it is important that a correct diagnosis is made. This can be done by putting cellophane tape on the perianal area early in the morning. When the tape is removed, it can be examined for eggs that may have been deposited during the night. Sometimes live worms will be seen as well, either by direct examination of the anus or on the cellophane tape.

If pinworms or other parasitic infestations are not completely eradicated, the worms can cause an intestinal blockage, primarily of the appendix. In a child, they can slow normal growth and development. Urinary tract infections can be associated with pinworms. In girls, scratching from pinworms can lead to a vaginal infection.

To prevent spreading pinworms, or to prevent reinfestation, your doctor may suggest that all family members be examined and treated, especially in persistent cases.

CONVENTIONAL TREATMENT

■ Mebendazole (available under the brand name Vermox) is the drug most frequently prescribed for pinworms. It is also effective against many other worms. This drug prevents the worms from getting the sugar and nutrients they need to live. Usually a single dose is given, but another dose may be given after three weeks if there are any signs of recurrence. This drug is usually well tolerated, with minimal side effects.

DIETARY GUIDELINES

■ Eliminate refined carbohydrates and sugar from your child's diet. These are the primary foods for pinworms. A high-fiber diet of grains and raw vegetables, especially greens, is not only useful for prevention but also aids in treatment. Less sugar means fewer pinworms.

NUTRITIONAL SUPPLEMENTS

■ An acidophilus or bifidus supplement will help to restore the healthy flora in intestines that have been disrupted by the presence of worms. Give your child one capsule, twice daily, for one month, then one capsule daily for two months.

HERBAL TREATMENT

For age-appropriate dosages of herbal remedies, see page 81.

■ Black walnut tincture can be helpful in clearing a pinworm infestation. This is a strong botanical, however, and not suitable for infants or small children. For a child age twelve or older, give three drops, three times daily, for no more than seven days.

■ Garlic is a natural antiparasitic. Give your child one to two capsules, twice daily, for two weeks. If your child is over one year old, you can give him one fresh clove mashed in honey instead, two to three times a day, for two to three weeks.

■ Wormwood (artemesia) has antiparasitic properties that will help to clear a case of worms. Give your child one dose, twice daily, for up to one week.

■ Grapefruit seed extract is a strong antiparasitic. A highly concentrated form, such as Citricidal, Nutrabiotic, or Paramicrocidin, is preferred. For three to seven days, two or three times a day, dilute 5 to 10 drops in a glass of water or juice and have your child drink it. The flavor is very bitter, and your child may need a lot of encouragement to take it.

HOMEOPATHY

■ *Cina* is often very effective for children with pinworms. Give your child *Cina* 12x or 6c, three times daily, for up to four days.

■ If homeopathic *Cina* is not effective, the guidance of a homeopathic physician may be helpful in finding a constitutional remedy. It is often necessary to address the entire body when fighting a pinworm infestation.

GENERAL RECOMMENDATIONS

■ To prevent a recurrence, the entire family should practice meticulous hygiene during a pinworm infestation.

■ Give your child homepathic *Cina*.

■ Give your child an acidophilus or bifidus supplement.

■ Discourage scratching. Calendula ointment may help to relieve irritation. Cotton swabs dipped in witch hazel are also useful for relieving minor irritation. If the itching is intolerable, a low-potency over-the-counter cortisone cream, such as Lanacort or Cort-Aid, may help.

■ Cut your child's fingernails very short and make sure he washes his hands and scrubs under the fingernails with a nail brush, especially after going to the bathroom and before eating.

■ Change your child's underpants every day.

■ Change and wash bed linens every day.

PREVENTION

◼ Teach your child to wash his hands carefully, particularly before eating and after going to the bathroom.

◼ Try to discourage any hand-to-mouth habits, such as thumb-sucking and fingernail-biting.

Pneumonia

Pneumonia is an acute inflammation and infection of the lung tissue that can result in the tiny air sacs becoming filled with fluid, mucus, and pus. It can be caused by a number of different infectious agents, including viruses, bacteria, mycoplasma, and fungi.

Viral pneumonia often begins as an upper respiratory infection, such as the flu. The illness may progress suddenly or gradually, and may be accompanied by either a low-grade fever, cough, and mild fatigue, or by a high fever, severe cough, and lethargy. The cough is usually not productive until the later stages of the illness. A stomachache may also be present. It is important to treat viral pneumonia, because if left untreated, it creates fertile ground for the development of a secondary bacterial infection in the lungs.

Bacterial pneumonia usually comes on suddenly, often as a complication of other illnesses. Pneumococci, staphylococci, and chlamydia are the bacteria most often responsible. A child with bacterial pneumonia will feel and appear very sick, with a high fever, lethargy, difficulty breathing, a cough, and possibly pain in the chest, particularly upon breathing. She is likely to be pale and sweating; in severe cases, her fingernails may turn bluish in color. Bacterial pneumonia is a dangerous illness, more dangerous than either viral or mycoplasmal pneumonia. Fortunately, it is much less likely than viral or mycoplasmal pneumonia to be transmitted from one person to another.

A full recovery from pneumonia, no matter what the cause, may take several weeks, and a cough may sometimes last up to two months, even after the infection is gone.

SYMPTOMS OF PNEUMONIA

Pneumonia often occurs as a complication of other infectious illnesses, including the common cold. The symptoms of pneumonia usually include a combination of one or more of the following:

• A persistent, possibly severe cough;

• Fever, whether low-grade or high;

• Lethargy and malaise;

• Difficulty breathing and/or pain in the chest.

If you suspect that your child may be developing pneumonia, call your physician promptly, especially if the symptoms come on suddenly. The most ominous signs include rapid breathing, straining the chest muscles in order to breathe, high fever, and extreme weakness. If your child experiences serious difficulty breathing, call for emergency medical assistance or take him immediately to the emergency room of the nearest hospital for treatment.

CONVENTIONAL TREATMENT

◼ If pneumonia is suspected, it is likely that your physician will first want to look at a chest x-ray (to determine which part of the lungs is involved), as well as a blood test and/or a sputum sample (to determine what type of infectious agent is responsible). This determination is essential for proper treatment.

◼ If the child is having difficulty breathing, an ear or finger oximetry test is a quick and easy way to find out how much oxygen is in the blood.

◼ If it is determined that your child has viral pneumonia, treatment will be aimed at promoting comfort and preventing bacterial pneumonia from developing. To lower fever and ease your child's discomfort, your doctor may recommend acetaminophen (Tylenol, Tempra, or the equivalent), as well as plenty of bed rest. Chest physiotherapy to promote the drainage of mucus from the lungs may also be indicated.

Note: In excessive amounts, acetaminophen can cause liver damage. Read package directions carefully so as not to exceed the proper dosage for your child's age and size.

■ For mycoplasmal pneumonia, an antibiotic (usually tetracycline or erythromycin) may or may not be recommended. This treatment may somewhat reduce the length of time your child has such symptoms as fever, cough, and general discomfort. However, it does not actually kill the mycoplasma responsible for the infection, and although the recovery period may be a little longer, it is possible that your child might recover just as well without the antibiotics.

■ If bacterial pneumonia is diagnosed, your child has a serious infection that requires aggressive treatment with either intravenous or oral antibiotics. Oxygen therapy may be called for, as well as chest physiotherapy to promote the drainage of mucus from the lungs.

■ Cough suppressants should be used with great care in a child with pneumonia. It is important for her to be able to cough out the mucus that is in her lungs in order to recover, and any medication that interferes with this may slow recovery. However, if a persistent hacking cough keeps a child from resting, a mild suppressant, such as benzonatate (Tessalon perles) may be a reasonable compromise.

DIETARY GUIDELINES

■ Make sure your child gets plenty of fluids. This will help prevent dehydration and will thin secretions so that they are easier to cough out. Try offering a drink of lemon water sweetened with a bit of maple syrup. Offer lots of soups and juices.

■ Avoid giving your child dairy products. These can increase the production of mucus. Also avoid foods that contain fats, refined sugar, refined carbohydrates, and caffeine.

■ Offer your child small, frequent meals featuring nutrient-dense foods such as grains, fruits, vegetables, and lean proteins. Hot soups are a good choice, because they are soothing and may be easier than solid foods for a sick child to take.

NUTRITIONAL SUPPLEMENTS

For age-appropriate dosages of nutritional supplements, see page 81.

■ Beta-carotene helps to protect, soothe, and repair mucous membrane tissue. It is also a precursor of vitamin A, which is essential for the health of the respiratory passage linings. Give your child one dose, twice a day, for two weeks or until symptoms have resolved.

■ Vitamin C is an anti-inflammatory and helps to stimulate the immune system. Choose a mineral ascorbate form of vitamin C with bioflavonoids and give your child one dose, three to four times a day, for two weeks.

■ During the recovery phase, give your child a vitamin-B complex supplement for two weeks.

■ Also during the recovery phase, give your child one dose of zinc, twice a day, for two weeks.

Note: Excessive amounts of zinc can result in nausea and vomiting. Be careful not to exceed the recommended dosage.

HERBAL TREATMENT

For age-appropriate dosages of herbal remedies, see page 81.

■ Depending on the type and severity of your child's pneumonia, you can use a variety of herbs either along with conventional treatment or during the recuperation phase, once the conventional treatment regimen is completed. You can use these herbs on an alternating basis, giving one herb for the first two weeks, another for the second two weeks, and so on. Or you can make a tea that combines several or all of them. Give your child one dose, three times a day, for two weeks, of one, several, or all of the following, as appropriate:

- Ginger tea will help to break up mucus and enhance circulation. Applying warm ginger compresses to the chest several times a day may also help to ease breathing.

- Isatis is a Chinese herb with antiviral properties. It can be useful if your child's pneumonia is viral or mycoplasmal. However, it may be difficult for your child to tolerate if she has a sensitive stomach.

- Licorice root helps to increase energy and soothe the lungs, and eases coughing.
    Note: This herb should not be given for extended periods of time, as prolonged use can cause high blood pressure. For a lengthy disease like pneumonia, it is best to use licorice for two to three days, then switch to another herb for one week, then repeat the licorice for another two to three days.

- Marshmallow root is a demulcent and is soothing to the lungs.

- Mullein activates the lymph circulation in the neck and chest.

- Nettle is full of trace minerals and chlorophyll and also helps to break up mucus.
    Note: Some children experience stomach upset as a result of taking this herb. If this happens, stop giving it. This herb should not be given to a child under four years old.

- Oat straw is a mild calmative.

- Osha root helps to strengthen the lungs and decrease inflammation.

■ A combination herbal tea can be made by simmering 1 teaspoon each of licorice, osha root, slippery elm, and marshmallow root, plus ¼ teaspoon of wild cherry bark, in a quart of water. Simmer the mixture for fifteen minutes. For a child over one, the tea can be sweetened with honey.
Caution: Wild cherry bark should not be taken by children under four, nor by pregnant women. If your child is under four, omit the wild cherry bark. Also, licorice should not be given to a child with high blood pressure.

■ Mix a couple of drops of thyme, peppermint, or eucalyptus oil in ¼ cup of almond or sesame oil and rub this on your child's back and chest to relax her and increase circulation to the chest area.
Note: If you are giving your child a homeopathic preparation in addition to this treatment, allow one hour between the two. Otherwise, the strong smell of the herbs may interfere with the action of the homeopathic remedy.

HOMEOPATHY

If your child has viral or mycoplasmal pneumonia, choose the most suitable symptom-specific remedy from the list below, and give her one dose, four times a day, for up to two days. If your child has bacterial pneumonia, you may do the same once your child is past the acute stage and is recovering from the illness. Be aware, however, that for acute bacterial pneumonia, homeopathic remedies should not be considered a substitute for appropriate antibiotic therapy.

■ Give *Arsenicum album* 30x or 9c to the child who is coughing with a wheeze. This child is also anxious and restless.

■ *Bryonia* 30x or 9c is recommended for the child whose chest hurts every time she moves, who feels pain when she inhales, and who is constipated.

■ If your child developed pneumonia following exposure to cold wind or an episode involving great fear and is running a temperature, try *Belladonna* 30x or 9c.

■ *Hepar sulphuris* 12x or 6c is for the child who has a hacking cough and wants hot drinks.

■ If your child has a cough with ropy or stringy phlegm, give her *Kali bichromicum* 12x or 6c.

■ *Nux vomica* 30x or 9c is for the child who has a dry cough, is irritable, and has a stomachache and, possibly, vomiting.

■ For a child with a tickle in her throat, some vomiting, and a craving for cold drinks, try *Phosphorus* 30x or 9c.

■ *Pulsatilla* 30x or 9c is for the child who is fearful and weepy and wants company. She may be coughing up yellow and/or green phlegm.

■ *Spongia* 30x or 9c is for the child with a barking cough that feels better after drinking warm liquids.

ACUPRESSURE

For the locations of acupressure points on a child's body, *see* ADMINISTERING AN ACUPRESSURE TREATMENT in Part Three.

■ Lung 7 helps to clear upper respiratory infections.

■ Pericardium 6 helps to relax the chest.

■ Stomach 36 supports and improves circulation and digestion.

■ Hold Four Gates to help relax and calm a sick and fussy child.

GENERAL RECOMMENDATIONS

■ Make sure your child gets plenty of fluids and plenty of rest. Rest is essential for the recovery process.

■ A cool mist humidifier will help to soothe your child's respiratory tract and thin secretions so that they are easier to cough out. A drop of thyme, eucalyptus, pine, or orange oil added to the water in the humidifier may also help to ease breathing. Be certain to clean the humidifier every few days to avoid the buildup or bacteria and fungi.

■ For further suggestions on relieving the symptoms of pneumonia, *see* COUGH and FEVER.

PREVENTION

■ Whenever your child comes down with a viral illness, especially an upper respiratory infection, be sure to treat it promptly and keep your child from overexertion until she is completely recovered. Be alert for any signs that pneumonia may be developing.

■ As much as possible, keep a child with pneumonia isolated, and keep healthy children from coming into contact with those who have, who are recovering from, or who have recently been exposed to viral or mycoplasmal pneumonia. The microorganisms that cause the illness may remain in an infected person for several weeks.

Poison Ivy, Poison Oak, and Poison Sumac

The rash associated with a case of poison ivy, oak, or sumac is an allergic reaction to a resin contained in the leaves, stems, and roots of these poisonous plants. Because these plants are most abundant during springtime, most cases occur at that time of the year.

The rash and treatment of these three conditions are similar. This entry focuses mainly on poison ivy, the most common of the three, but what is true for poison ivy is true also for poison oak and poison sumac.

A child can get poison ivy from the plant itself or by touching anything that has come in contact with the plant and has some of the resinous oil on it. For example, if a child picks up a rake that has been resting in a bed of poison ivy, the characteristic rash may develop. If clothing or the part of the body that touched the plant is not carefully washed, the oil can be spread to other parts of the body, or even be transmitted to another person. Another, and potentially quite serious, form of exposure can occur through the inhalation of smoke from burning leaves if there are parts of the poison ivy plant among them.

A poison ivy rash can appear anywhere from a few hours to a few days after contact with the resin. The rash can last from one to four weeks, and is usually at its worst four to seven days after exposure. The severity of the condition depends on the amount of contact with the resinous oil, as well as how sensitive the child is to the plant. Not everyone is allergic to poison ivy. The resin may not bother some children at all, while others develop a serious and extensive rash.

The rash first appears as red, very itchy pimples that may develop into small fluid-filled blisters. If the contact occurred with the edge of a leaf, the eruption may form in a straight line. As with all skin rashes and wounds, it is possible for the area to become infected. If you notice signs of local infection, such as increased redness, swelling, or warmth or tenderness at the site, seek medical advice.

If your child experiences pain or swelling on the face or genitals and is uncomfortable because of this, or if the rash is very extensive, medical care may be warranted. Otherwise, most cases of poison can be treated successfully at home.

CONVENTIONAL TREATMENT

■ Calamine lotion is an old standby that temporarily eases the itching of poison ivy. However, if used for more than one week, calamine lotion can harden and dry the skin, causing more problems.

■ Rhulicream and Rhuligel are over-the-counter preparations that may be more effective than calamine at relieving the itching of poison ivy. Follow the application directions on the product label.

■ Benadryl and Chlor-Trimeton are two over-the-counter oral antihistamines that can help with the itching and swelling of poison ivy.

■ In severe cases, an oral or topical steroid, such as prednisone, may be prescribed to lessen itching and especially to decrease inflammation. Steroids are strong and work quickly, but because of potential side effects, they are not suitable for long-term use and are generally reserved for very serious cases. Also, if steroids are stopped too soon or too abruptly, the rash may get worse as a result of a "rebound" effect.

■ Cold compresses applied for twenty minutes every few hours are useful for soothing and decreasing the swelling.

■ If the rash is inflamed, red, and oozing, Burow's solution may help. This over-the-counter product is both astringent and antiseptic, but it is mild on the skin. It may be diluted even further than the label directions indicate if it seems to irritate your child's skin.

HERBAL TREATMENT

■ Apply soothing aloe vera gel to the rash three or four times a day.

■ To relieve itching and help the skin heal more quickly, apply calendula tincture to your child's rash several times a day, as needed.

■ To relieve both itching and inflammation, apply jewelweed juice. Use the fresh plant. Simply slit the stem and put the juice on the rash. Jewelweed will also help keep the rash from spreading. Jewelweed is a native perennial wildflower that is sometimes also referred to as impatiens. However, it should not be confused with the cultivated annual called impatiens that is commonly sold in nurseries and garden centers, which is an entirely different plant that has no usefulness in treating poison ivy. Jewelweed should be available at herb shops and through qualified herbalists.

HOMEOPATHY

■ *Rhus toxicodendron*, homeopathic poison ivy, will help relieve itching quickly. Give your child one dose of *Rhus toxicodendron* 12x or 6c, three to four times daily, until symptoms lessen.

ACUPRESSURE

For the locations of acupressure points on a child's body, *see* ADMINISTERING AN ACUPRESSURE TREATMENT in Part Three.

■ Four Gates will help relax your child.

WHEN TO CALL THE DOCTOR ABOUT POISON IVY

• If there is any sign that your child is developing difficulty breathing as a result of an allergic reaction to poison ivy, oak, or sumac, seek emergency medical treatment.

• If your child experiences pain or swelling on the face or genitals, or if the rash is very extensive and/or causing extreme discomfort, call your doctor.

• As with any skin disorder, it is possible for an area affected by poison ivy to become infected. If you notice signs of a developing local infection, such as increased redness, swelling, warmth, or tenderness at the site, consult your physician.

Recognizing Poison Ivy, Oak, and Sumac

The best way to prevent a bout with poison ivy, poison oak, or poison sumac is to know how to recognize these plants and avoid them.

Poison ivy (*Rhus radicans*), by far the most common of the three, is usually thought of as a vine, but it can also grow straight up, like a shrub, to a height of anywhere between two and seven feet. It grows equally happily in woods, partly wooded areas and thickets, and suburban back yards, and can be found virtually anywhere in the United States and southern Canada. Its leaves are often shiny bright green, but not always; the edges can be smooth or jagged. In the fall, the leaves can turn a brilliant bronze-red, and drooping clusters of white berries appear. The distinctive feature of poison ivy, and the thing to look for, is that its leaves always occur in groups of three, with the end leaflet pointed and on a slightly longer stalk than the side pair (see illustration). If you see any plant whose leaves match this description, avoid it and warn your child to stay well away from it. Touching any part of the poison ivy plant is dangerous.

Poison oak (*Rhus toxicodendron*) is similar to poison ivy in most respects. The only important differences to note are that this plant always grows in shrub form, and that the leaves, while still occurring in trios, are shaped more like oak leaves (see illustration).

Poison sumac (*Rhus vernix*) is less common than poison ivy or poison oak, which is a good thing, because it is much more toxic. Touching any part of the plant can result in a severe rash and allergic reaction. The poison sumac plant, which is found primarily in swampy, partly wooded areas in the eastern half of the United States and Canada, takes the form of a shrub or small tree with leaves consisting of seven to thirteen (but always an odd number) pointed leaflets. The edges of the leaflets are smooth, not jagged. From late summer to early spring, the plant puts out berries that are whitish in color and occur in clusters.

If your child does come into contact with any of these plants, you should take measures immediately to wash off the resin with either soap and water or jewelweed juice (*see* General Recommendations, this entry).

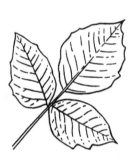
Poison Ivy

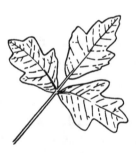
Poison Oak

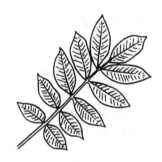
Poison Sumac

■ Spleen 10 helps detoxify the blood.

GENERAL RECOMMENDATIONS

■ After known exposure to poison ivy, thoroughly wash the area of contact with soap and water as soon as possible. Because unexposed areas of skin may come in contact with the oil as clothing is stripped off, a thorough shower is probably the best way to make sure all of the resin is washed off. If no washing facilities are available, do what you can to cleanse the area that made contact with the plant. Change clothes as soon as possible, taking care to avoid contact with contaminated areas. Washing or rinsing with jewelweed juice may also be helpful. The resinous oil of poison ivy penetrates the skin in about ten minutes. After ten minutes, it cannot be washed off.

■ Use alternate applications of jewelweed juice and herbal or homeopathic calendula tincture, three times daily, until the itching and discomfort are relieved.

■ Give your child homeopathic *Rhus toxicodendron*.

■ Prepare an old folk remedy by making a paste of 2 tablespoons of sea salt and 1 cup of buttermilk. Apply it to the affected area to reduce itching and promote healing.

■ Soak a clean cotton cloth in a blend of 1 tablespoon sea salt dissolved in one pint of spring water. To relieve itching, apply the compress to the affected area for fifteen to thirty minutes several times daily.

■ Cold cucumber slices applied to the affected area can help dry out an oozing rash.

■ Clothing that has come in contact with the oil should be washed in a strong detergent with chlorine bleach added.

PREVENTION

■ When your child will be in an area where poison ivy may be flourishing, dress him in shoes, socks, long pants, and a long-sleeved shirt to reduce the possibility of contact with the oil.

■ Teach your child how to identify poison ivy, oak, and sumac (*see* Recognizing Poison Ivy, Oak, and Sumac on page 340)—and to avoid these plants. Poison ivy and poison oak grow as bushy plants or vines. They are easily identified by the three leaflets on each major leaf. Poison sumac carries a row of double leaflets.

Poisoning

Eighty percent of all poisonings occur in children under five years old. Small children use their mouths to learn about the world. Anyone who has watched an infant knows that everything—clothes, toes, fingers, toys—goes into a baby's mouth.

Accidental poisonings in childhood most often occur as a result of ingesting harmful substances found around the home. In the 1980s, the Environmental Protection Agency reported that there were over 58,000 chemical substances available in the United States. Since new products are being created all the time, we can safely assume that there are now considerably more than that. Medicines, cleaning products, paints, varnishes, pesticides, hobby supplies, and cosmetics all contain harmful chemicals. Worse, these products are often packaged in bright and attractive colors that catch the eye of an exploring child. The chemicals they contain can cause serious injury or even death if a curious child ingests them.

Another type of childhood poisoning occurs as a result of a child receiving too much medication, or an incorrect medication. This can happen if a child is given a prescription originally written for another person. To share medications is to risk the possibility that your child may receive a toxic dose of a drug.

Some common houseplants and outdoor plants are poisonous. A number of children are poisoned every year by ingesting a toxic leaf, flower, or berry from a plant.

EMERGENCY TREATMENT FOR POISONING

See the inset on page 342.

Emergency Treatment for Poisoning

A child who has ingested a poisonous substance needs emergency treatment. However, proper treatment depends on the nature of the poison involved. If you know that your child has ingested a poisonous substance, follow the appropriate steps outlined below. If you are not certain about the nature of the poison, call your local Poison Control Center and ask for advice. For a list of Poison Control Centers in the United States and Canada, see page 344.

✚ **If your child has ingested a noncaustic, nonpetroleum-based product, such as medication or a poisonous plant:**

1. Immediately remove any toxic substances visible in your child's mouth.

2. Call the local Poison Control Center at once for information on what steps to take. Try to remain calm, and be as specific as possible in describing your child's age and weight, the possible source of the poisoning, the amount of poison ingested, and the time elapsed. Poison Control may tell you to administer syrup of ipecac to induce vomiting, and then to call an ambulance or take your child to the emergency room of the nearest hospital.

3. Administer ipecac according to the directions given by the Poison Control Center (see Administering Syrup of Ipecac on page 343).
   Caution: Do not give syrup of ipecac to a child less than one year old or to a child who is unconscious, who has a history of heart disease, or whose gag reflex may not be working properly.

4. After your child has vomited, take her at once to the emergency room. Take the bottle or package of suspect material with you. It may save valuable time in determining what treatment is necessary.

✚ **If your child has ingested a caustic acid or alkali product, such as lye, drain cleaner, oven cleaner, toilet bowl cleaner, electric dishwasher detergent, or swimming pool cleaner:**

1. Immediately remove any toxic substances visible in your child's mouth.

2. If a caustic substance is in her eyes or on her skin, immediately flush the area with large amounts of clean running water to prevent damage to the area and absorption into the body.

3. *Do not induce vomiting.* Causing a child to vomit after ingestion of caustic substances can cause additional damage to the esophagus and mouth as the substance comes back up.

4. To dilute the substance in your child's stomach, give her two glasses of water or milk immediately. Either one will dilute the substance and help to minimize damage.

5. Call the local Poison Control Center at once for information on what steps to take. Try to remain calm, and be as specific as possible in describing your child and identifying the possible source of the poisoning. Poison Control may tell you to dilute the substance in your child's stomach, and then to call an ambulance or take your child to the emergency room of the nearest hospital.

6. When taking your child to the emergency room, take the bottle or package of suspect material with you. It may save valuable time in determining what treatment is necessary.

✚ **If your child has ingested a petroleum-based product, such as gasoline, oil, turpentine, benzene, kerosene, lighter fluid, furniture polish, mothballs, or lubricating fluid:**

1. Immediately remove any toxic substances visible in your child's mouth.

2. If a caustic substance is in her eyes or on her skin, immediately flush the area with large amounts of clean running water to prevent damage to the area and absorption into the body.

3. *Do not induce vomiting.* Causing a child to vomit after ingestion of a petroleum-based substance can cause additional damage to the esophagus and mouth as the substance comes back up.

4. Call an ambulance or take your child to the emergency room of the nearest hospital at once. Take the bottle or package of suspect material with you. It may save valuable time in determining what treatment is necessary.

Although most children who ingest poisons are very young, the incidence of poisonings among adolescents is rising in the United States. The adolescent who ingests a toxic or poisonous substance may be making a suicide gesture, which must be taken seriously. An adolescent who intentionally takes an overdose of a toxic substance may be seeking attention or adventure, or may seriously wish to end her life. Once the immediate crisis has been handled, professional counseling is crucial for both child and parents to determine and deal with the deeper issues involved.

Administering Syrup of Ipecac

Syrup of ipecac is an over-the-counter drug that usually causes a person to vomit quickly when it is swallowed. In certain cases of poisoning, the best treatment is to get the toxic substance out of the victim's stomach as quickly as possible. Syrup of ipecac is excellent for this.

Sometimes, however, inducing vomiting will do more harm than good. This largely depends on the nature of the poisonous substance ingested. Ipecac should *not* be used if your child has swallowed any of the following:

- Alkalis, such as lye, dishwasher detergent, drain cleaner, oven cleaner, etc.

- Petroleum distillates, such as furniture polish, kerosene, gasoline, oil-based paint, lighter fluid, etc.

If your child has ingested a poisonous substance and your local Poison Control Center advises you to use syrup of ipecac to induce vomiting before taking your child to the emergency room, follow the instructions they give you on how to administer the drug. *Do not* use ipecac unless you are instructed to do so by the Poison Control Center. The amount you will be told to use will depend on your child's size. Generally, if your child weighs 25 pounds or less, the dosage should be 1 tablespoon; if your child weighs over 25 pounds, the dosage should be 2 tablespoons. After your child has swallowed the ipecac, have her drink at least 12 ounces of water to ensure vomiting. Try to keep her walking around. If she has not vomited in twenty minutes, you may be instructed to administer another dose of ipecac, followed by another 12 ounces of water. *Do not give any child more than two doses of ipecac.* The vomiting caused by ipecac can be very violent. If the second dose is unsuccessful, abandon the attempt and take your child at once to the emergency room of the nearest hospital.

When your child vomits, have her lie on her side with her mouth lower than her chest, so that the vomited material will not reenter the airway and cause more trouble. If she leans over a toilet to vomit, make sure her chest is lower than her stomach.

There are a number of situations in which syrup of ipecac should *never* be used:

- Never give ipecac to a child less than twelve months old.

- Never attempt to give ipecac to a child who is unconscious.

- Never give ipecac to a child with a history of heart disease.

- Never give ipecac to a child whose gag reflex may not be working properly, such as a child who has ingested sedatives or tranquilizers, a child who is drowsy, or one who may be drunk.

CONVENTIONAL TREATMENT

■ In the emergency care unit, charcoal may be instilled into your child's stomach in order to bind with the toxic substance and prevent it from being absorbed by the body.

■ Emergency personnel may perform *gastric lavage*, better known as stomach pumping. This procedure involves passing a tube through the nose and into the stomach to pull the toxic substance out of the stomach.

■ Depending on the severity of the injury, your child may be admitted to a pediatric intensive care unit or a general pediatric unit for further treatment and/or observation.

NUTRITIONAL SUPPLEMENTS

■ Charcoal capsules help to absorb poisons. Give your child one capsule, twice a day, for five days after she returns home.

■ After a poisoning episode, *Lactobacillus acidophilus* or *bifidus* will help reestablish

Emergency Poison Control Center Telephone Numbers

The following are telephone numbers for local Poison Control Centers in the United States and Canada. In an emergency, call your regional center. Because area codes and phone numbers are subject to change, it is a wise precaution to know the current phone number of your local center and post it near every telephone in your home. If you can program your telephone for automatic dialing, add the number to your phone's programming as well.

ALABAMA

205–939–9201
205–933–4050
800–292–6678 (AL only)

ALASKA

907–261–3193

ARIZONA

Statewide
800–362–0101 (AZ only)

Phoenix Region
602–253–3334

Tucson Region
602–626–6016

ARKANSAS

501–686–6161

CALIFORNIA

Davis Region
916–734–3692
800–342–9293 (N. CA only)

Fresno Region
209–445–1222
800–346–5922 (CA only)

Orange County Region
714–634–5988
800–544–4404 (S. CA only)

San Diego Region
619–543–6000
800–876–4766 (619 area only)

San Francisco/Bay Area
415–476–6600

San Jose/Santa Clara Valley
408–299–5112
800–662–9886 (CA only)

COLORADO

303–629–1123

CONNECTICUT

203–679–1000
800–343–2722 (CT only)

DELAWARE

302–655–3389

DISTRICT OF COLUMBIA

202–625–3333
202–784–4660 (TTY*)

FLORIDA

813–253–4444
800–282–3171 (FL only)

GEORGIA

404–589–4400
800–282–5846 (GA only)

HAWAII

808–941–4411

IDAHO

208–378–2707
800–632–8000 (ID only)

ILLINOIS

217–753–3330
800–543–2022 (IL only)
800–942–5969

INDIANA

317–929–2323
800–382–9097 (IN only)

IOWA

800–272–6477 (IA only)
800–362–2327 (IA only)

KANSAS

Topeka/Northern Kansas
913–354–6100

Wichita/Southern Kansas
316–263–9999

KENTUCKY

502–629–7275
800–722–5725 (KY only)

LOUISIANA

800–256–9822 (LA only)

MAINE

800–442–6305 (ME only)

MARYLAND

Statewide
410–528–7701
800–492–2414 (MD only)

* teletype, for the hearing-impaired

D.C. Suburbs
202–625–3333
202–784–4660 (TTY*)

MASSACHUSETTS

617–232–2120
800–682–9211

MICHIGAN

Statewide
800–632–2727 (MI only)
800–356–3232 (TTY*)

Detroit Region
313–745–5711

MINNESOTA

Statewide
800–222–1222

Duluth/Northern Minnesota
218–726–5466

Minneapolis/St. Paul Region
612–347–3141
612–337–7474 (TDD**)
612–221–2113

MISSISSIPPI

601–354–7660

MISSOURI

314–772–5200
800–366–8888

MONTANA

303–629–1123

NEBRASKA

Statewide
800–955–9119 (NE only)

Omaha Region
402–390–5555

NEVADA

702–732–4989

NEW HAMPSHIRE

603–650–5000
800–562–8236 (NH only)

NEW JERSEY

800–962–1253

NEW MEXICO

505–843–2551
800–432–6866 (NM only)

NEW YORK

Albany Region
800–336–6997

Binghamton/Southern Tier
800–252–5655

Buffalo/Western New York
716–878–7654
800–888–7655

Long Island
516–542–2323
516–542–2324
516–542–2325
516–542–3813

New York City
212–340–4494
212–POISONS
212–689–9014 (TDD**)

Nyack/Hudson Valley
914–353–1000

Syracuse/Central New York
315–476–4766

NORTH CAROLINA

Statewide
800–672–1697

Charlotte Region
704–355–4000

NORTH DAKOTA

800–732–2200 (ND only)

OHIO

Statewide
800–682–7625

Columbus/Central Ohio
614–228–1323
614–461–2012
614–228–2272 (TTY*)

Cincinnati Region
513–558–5111
800–872–5111 (OH only)

OKLAHOMA

800–522–4611 (OK only)

OREGON

503–494–8968
800–452–7165 (OR only)

PENNSYLVANIA

Hershey/Central Pennsylvania
800–521–6110

Philadelphia/E. Pennsylvania
215–386–2100

Pittsburgh/W. Pennsylvania
412–681–6669

PUERTO RICO

809–754–8535

RHODE ISLAND

401–277–5727

SOUTH CAROLINA

803–777–1117

**telecommunication device for the deaf

SOUTH DAKOTA

800–952–0123 (SD only)

TENNESSEE

Memphis/Western Tennessee
901–528–6048

Nashville/Eastern Tennessee
615–322–6435

TEXAS

214–590–5000
800–441–0040 (TX WATS)

UTAH

801–581–2151
800–456–7707 (UT only)

VERMONT

800–562–8236 (VT only)

VIRGINIA

Statewide
800–451–1428

Charlottesville/Blue Ridge
804–925–5543

D.C. Suburbs
202–625–3333
202–784–4660 (TTY*)

WASHINGTON

800–732–6985 (WA only)

WEST VIRGINIA

304–348–4211
800–642–3625 (WV only)

WISCONSIN

Madison/S.W. and N. Wisconsin
608–262–3702

Milwaukee/S.E. Wisconsin
414–266–2222

WYOMING

800–955–9119 (WY only)

CANADA

ALBERTA

403–670–1414

BRITISH COLUMBIA

604–682–5050

MANITOBA

204–787–2591

NEW BRUNSWICK

Fredericton
506–452–5400

Saint John
506–648–6222

NEWFOUNDLAND

709–722–1110

NOVA SCOTIA

902–428–8161

ONTARIO

613–737–1100 (E. Ontario)
800–267–1373 (Ontario only)

PRINCE EDWARD ISLAND

902–428–8161

QUEBEC

800–463–5060 (Quebec only)

SASKATCHEWAN

306–359–4545

healthy flora in the bowel. Give your child the dosage recommended on the product label for at least one month after the episode.

■ Beta-carotene, vitamin C, vitamin E, and selenium help the body to detoxify itself. Choose a combination formula and give it to your child, following the dosage directions on the product label, for two weeks after the crisis is over and your child is at home.

HERBAL TREATMENT

Herbal treatment for poisoning is directed at helping your child recover once the acute phase of the crisis is over. If you suspect poisoning, seek emergency treatment for your child immediately. For age-appropriate dosages of herbal remedies, see page 81.

■ Once your child is well enough to come home from the hospital, give her echinacea to help detoxify the blood and ginger tea to stimulate a return to proper functioning of the digestive system. Give her one dose of each, twice daily, for five days.

■ Ginger tea helps to "clean" the digestive tract. Give your child one to two doses of ginger tea daily for three to five days after a poisoning episode.

HOMEOPATHY

Homeopathic treatment for poisoning is directed at helping your child recover once the acute phase of the crisis is over. If you suspect poisoning, seek emergency treatment for your child immediately.

■ *Nux vomica* helps to neutralize poisons and reestablish proper functioning of the stomach. Give your child one dose of *Nux vomica* 12x or 6c, twice a day, for three days after she returns home.

■ *Arsenicum album* 200x or 30c is useful if diarrhea persists after a poisoning episode (*see* DIARRHEA).

BACH FLOWER REMEDIES

■ After medical personnel have your child resting comfortably and it is safe to give her something by mouth, give her Bach Flower Rescue Remedy to calm fears and anxiety. Place one or two drops under her tongue and repeat every half hour or so if needed. (*See* BACH FLOWER REMEDIES in Part One.)

PREVENTION

■ The best way to prevent accidental poisoning is not to have poisonous products in your home at all. There are nontoxic alternatives to many poisonous commercial cleaning products. For example, mix equal parts of vinegar and water in a spray bottle to use as a glass cleaner. A handful of baking soda mixed with ½ cup of white vinegar can be used to help unclog a slow drain, replacing highly toxic drain cleaners. Baking soda makes as good a scouring powder as the commercial powders, which are loaded with bleach, detergents, and artificial dyes. *Nontoxic, Natural & Earthwise*, by Debra Lynn Dadd (J.P. Tarcher Inc., 1990) is a great reference to natural and homemade household products.

■ You can use the "Mr. Yuk" stickers distributed by some Poison Control Centers or design your own way of labeling any dangerous products you do have, to teach and caution children about poisonous substances. However, you should be aware that there is some disagreement about the use of these systems (see margin inset).

■ Dispose of toxic products responsibly—away from children and in a way that doesn't damage the earth. Call your state or local environmental administration, the Environmental Protection Agency, or your local health or sanitation department to find out how to dispose of hazardous materials. Ammonia cleaners, chlorine bleach, drain openers, furniture polish, and batteries (especially the "button batteries" used in watches and calculators) are examples of hazardous

THE "MR. YUK" CONTROVERSY

Some Poison Control Centers and children's advocates recommend using "Mr. Yuk" stickers to label any dangerous substances present in the home, and teaching children that they must never touch anything bearing the Mr. Yuk label. Even toddlers, they say, can be taught to recognize this symbol and avoid danger. But other experts contend that the stickers may actually make potentially harmful items more attractive to a curious child. There is also some concern that the stickers may give parents a false sense of security, causing them to be less vigilant about dangerous products.

You may wish to discuss this issue with your local Poison Control Center. And whether you choose to use Mr. Yuk stickers or not, always keep in mind that the most important thing you can do to protect your child against accidental poisoning is to keep any potentially harmful substances in your home securely locked up and out of your child's reach at all times.

materials that should not be thrown away with your daily household garbage. And don't let the "empty" containers pile up in your basement or garage. Even tiny quantities of these toxins can do damage.

■ For suggestions on ways to childproof your home and guard against accidental poisonings, *see* HOME SAFETY in Part One.

Poliomyelitis

EMERGENCY TREATMENT FOR POLIOMYELITIS

✚ A child with polio can develop respiratory problems so severe that they can be life threatening. If your child seems to be having serious and/or increasing difficulty breathing, seek medical attention immediately. He may need to be hospitalized to receive mechanical respiratory support.

Polio is a viral infection that can cause either a mild illness with a fever, or a severe illness resulting in paralysis or death. There are three distinct, but related, types of the polio virus, and the severity of the disease is linked to which of the three is the cause.

The virus is highly contagious and is spread by fecal contact. Once in the intestines, the virus reproduces. The incubation period varies widely, but the average is five to seven days. The virus is found in the throat and blood for three to five days after exposure. Once symptoms start, it is found in large amounts in the stool for six to eight weeks. This is why contaminated water is a principal source of infection, especially in developing countries, and why public swimming pools can be dangerous for unimmunized children.

The symptoms and prognosis of a polio infection can take several courses. For some, an infection with the virus will cause absolutely no discernible illness. Some people develop a fever, sore throat, headache, nausea, and vomiting, as well as abdominal pain that lasts from one to three days, and then recover fully. Others have symptoms similar to these, but accompanied by pain and stiffness in the neck, back, and legs. The most serious form of the disease can lead to muscle weakness, paralysis, and respiratory difficulty. Some recover from these symptoms; some do not, and may suffer lasting paralysis. If strength has not returned in two years' time, it is likely that weakness or paralysis will be permanent.

CONVENTIONAL TREATMENT

■ If your child develops a serious case of polio, he may have to be hospitalized for treatment.

■ Treatment for less severe cases of polio is aimed at relieving discomfort. You can give your child acetaminophen (found in Tylenol, Tempra, and other medications) or ibuprofen (Advil, Nuprin, and others) to bring down fever and ease pain and achiness.

Note: In excessive amounts, acetaminophen can cause liver damage. Before giving your child this drug, read package directions carefully so as not to exceed the proper dosage for your child's age and size. Ibuprofen is best taken with food to prevent possible stomach upset.

■ *Never* give aspirin to a child with polio. The combination of aspirin and a viral infection has been linked to the development of Reye's syndrome, a potentially fatal disease of the liver and brain (*see* REYE'S SYNDROME).

■ Because polio is a viral illness, antibiotic therapy is ineffective and therefore not appropriate.

■ Bed rest is important. Keep your child in bed as much as possible.

■ Apply hot, moist compresses to help decrease muscle spasms and pain.

GENERAL RECOMMENDATIONS

■ Always be alert for changes in your child's condition, especially his breathing. If symptoms continue to get worse, or new symptoms develop, consult your physician.

■ Because polio is spread by fecal contact, teach your child to wash his hands thoroughly, scrubbing well under the fingernails, after using the bathroom. Because large amounts of virus are found in the stool of infected individuals for six to eight weeks after the onset of symptoms, if one of your children develops polio, use a separate bathroom for the sick child or clean and disinfect the toilet and bathtub after each use during this period. Also, don't allow children to share a bed or clothing.

PREVENTION

■ Two different vaccines are available that prevent polio: an oral form and an injection. Whichever form is used, it is usually given four different times: at two, four, and eighteen months of age, and again between four and six years. The injected form, consisting of inactivated, dead vaccine, appears to be somewhat safer and less likely to produce a bad reaction. The oral form, which contains live vaccine, is believed by some to give better immunity and is therefore generally recommended, even though an estimated six or seven cases of disease a year result from its use. The oral form should not be given to children with compromised immune systems, or to a child with family members who have not been vaccinated, since unvaccinated people can contract the disease from a child who has been given the live vaccine. Before having your child immunized against polio, discuss your situation and the available options with your doctor.

■ If your child is not (or is not yet) immunized against polio, keep him from coming into contact with any child who has received the oral polio vaccine within the last month. A recently immunized child can transmit the virus to the unimmunized child. For this reason, facilities such as daycare centers and public swimming pools can be hazardous to an unimmunized child.

■ Avoid contact with water that may be contaminated, especially when traveling.

Prickly Heat

Prickly heat—medically termed *miliaria* and also known as heat rash or summer rash—is a rash that affects infants and small children. It is caused by profuse sweating with blocked and inflamed sweat glands. Because of the blockage and inflammation, the sweat does not reach the surface of the skin, but is trapped within it, causing irritation and, frequently, itching. Prickly heat is common after a sunburn, on a hot and humid day, with a fever, or as a result of excessive warmth from too many clothes or an overheated environment.

The rash is characterized by red areas, with small, blisterlike bumps at the center. This rash can appear on the face, neck, shoulders, stomach, or chest. It may be somewhat itchy and stinging.

CONVENTIONAL TREATMENT

■ Treatment for prickly heat is aimed at relieving the discomfort, principally by cooling and drying the affected area. Baths, cool clothes, and avoidance of conditions likely to cause sweating are the primary recommendations for a child with prickly heat. An air-conditioned environment is often helpful.

■ Applying a topical steroid cream such as Cort-Aid or Lanacort to the affected area may offer some relief, but this is not as effective at resolving the problem as changing your child's clothing and/or her environment.

DIETARY GUIDELINES

■ While your child has this rash, eliminate sweets and greasy foods. These can increase internal heat and aggravate the rash.

NUTRITIONAL SUPPLEMENTS

■ A vitamin-C spray, applied topically, can hasten healing of the rash. Mix 2 tablespoons of powdered vitamin C with ½ cup of aloe vera gel in a spray bottle and spray the mixture on the rash two or three times a day until the rash heals.

HERBAL TREATMENT

■ Topical aloe vera gel is soothing and cooling. Apply aloe gel to the rash to take the heat and stinging out of the skin. Repeat as often as necessary.

■ Apply calendula gel or lotion to the skin to help ease the discomfort and promote healing.

HOMEOPATHY

■ *Apis mellifica* 30x or 9c is helpful if the rash is red and very swollen looking. Give your child one dose, three times a day, for two days.

■ *Sulphur* is good for a child who is sweaty, feels warm, and has red, dry, hot-looking patches of skin. This child tends to throw off the covers, wants her skin to be exposed, and dislikes being washed. Give this child one dose of *Sulphur* 30x or 9c, twice a day, for three days.

GENERAL RECOMMENDATIONS

■ Give your child tepid oatmeal baths to help cool the skin and relieve itching. Dry the skin by patting gently, not by vigorous rubbing.

■ Do not apply cornstarch or any perfumed lotions or ointments to the skin. These can aggravate the condition.

■ Dress your child in cool natural-fiber clothing that breathes.

PREVENTION

■ Avoid overdressing your child, especially in hot weather.

■ If your child is prone to prickly heat, try to keep her as cool as possible, particularly in the summer. As much as possible, have her avoid activities that cause sweating.

Rash

See SKIN RASH.

Reye's Syndrome

Reye's syndrome is a serious, potentially life-threatening illness that involves several vital organs—primarily the brain and the liver, but also the pancreas, heart, kidney, spleen, and lymph nodes. It most commonly occurs in children up to the age of eighteen, and most cases occur in late fall and winter. As of this writing, the precise cause is not known, although a connection has been established between the taking of salicylates (aspirin) in the presence of a viral illness and the development of the disease. This is why it is no longer recommended that children be given aspirin for most infectious illnesses.

The onset of the disease usually comes several days to a few weeks after a child suffers a viral illness such as chickenpox or influenza. Often, just as a child seems to be recovering from one illness, she will get sick again, with flulike symptoms such as fatigue, fever, headache, nausea, and vomiting. She may also seem unusually irritable, confused, apathetic, or aggressive. The disease progresses rapidly, causing changes in consciousness including hallucinations, decreased awareness, and seizures. The child may also hyperventilate and become very weak.

Any child who exhibits these symptoms needs immediate medical attention. Early intervention is critical to success in treating this disease. A child with Reye's syndrome may need to be hospitalized. If the diagnosis is made soon enough, and treatment begun early, most children will recover from the disease without complications, but some will require rehabilitation and continued care after they leave the hospital, especially when there is severe brain involvement.

CONVENTIONAL TREATMENT

■ Diagnosis is based on the history of the illness, a physical examination, and the results of certain blood tests. A doctor may also recommend that a liver biopsy be done to confirm the diagnosis and/or determine damage to the liver, as well as an electroencephalogram (EEG) to assess brain function.

EMERGENCY TREATMENT FOR REYE'S SYNDROME

✚ If your child develops any of the following symptoms, call your doctor immediately or take your child to the emergency room of the nearest hospital and explain the situation:

● Prolonged and heavy vomiting followed by drowsiness that occurs as a child is starting to recover from a viral infection such as the flu or chickenpox.

● Agitation and disorientation.

● Fatigue, lethargy, and lapses in memory.

Your child may be developing Reye's syndrome and may need to be hospitalized for treatment.

■ A child who has been diagnosed as having Reye's syndrome is usually admitted to the hospital's intensive care unit. Because the disease causes rapid and dangerous changes in metabolic functioning, your child's breathing, heartbeat, fluid levels, neurological status, and electrolyte status must be monitored continuously, and measures must be taken to cope with whatever difficulties arise. Your child may require assistance with breathing or intravenous infusions of glucose, insulin, vitamin K, plasma, and/or anticonvulsant medication, depending on her particular situation. These processes may involve tubes and other equipment that can be upsetting to see, but that may be necessary to help your child through the acute phase of this illness.

HERBAL TREATMENT, HOMEOPATHY, AND ACUPRESSURE

Natural medicine can be used to help ease the discomforts associated with this illness and to help your child recover her strength once she is out of the hospital. Because this illness is so severe and its symptoms and effects vary from child to child, the authors recommend that you work closely with a qualified practitioner, preferably one who is willing to work with a medical doctor (and vice versa). Each of these professionals will need to know what the other is doing, so that the treatments they recommend can work together for the health of your child.

GENERAL RECOMMENDATIONS

■ Having a child in an intensive care unit can be stressful and draining, both emotionally and physically. Ask friends and family for their emotional support. If people ask what they can do to help, don't be too proud or shy to ask for assistance with day-to-day responsibilities such as preparing meals, doing the grocery shopping, or caring for other children. Make a conscious effort not to let yourself get run down and, consequently, more vulnerable to illness. As much as possible, eat regular, nutritious meals; try to get sufficient rest, sleep, and exercise. If you become ill or exhausted, you will not be able to be the comforting and nurturing presence your child needs.

PREVENTION

■ *Never* give aspirin, or any product containing aspirin, to a child who has a viral illness. Viral illnesses include many of the infections most common in childhood, such as colds, flu, bronchitis, chickenpox, ear infections, measles, mumps, rubella (German measles), croup, roseola, and sinus infections. In addition, any time your child has a cough, sore throat, fever, headache, conjunctivitis, diarrhea, nausea, or vomiting, it may be caused by a virus. A good rule of thumb is not to give your child aspirin or an aspirin-based product unless your doctor *specifically* recommends it.

Rheumatic Fever

Rheumatic fever is an illness that occurs as a complication of a streptococcus infection, such as strep throat or scarlet fever. It most commonly occurs in children between the ages of four and eighteen. Although the strep infections that precede this illness are contagious, the rheumatic fever itself is not. Rather, its occurrence seems to be a matter of individual susceptibility, which may run in families.

Symptoms of rheumatic fever include fever; arthritic joint pain in two or more joints (most commonly the ankles, knees, elbows, or wrists), with redness, heat, and swelling; emotional instability; a flat, painless rash on the trunk and extremities that may come and go; uncontrollable twitching of the arms or legs; and bumps or nodules in the joints, scalp, or spine. The primary danger of rheumatic fever is the possibility of carditis, an inflammation of the heart tissue, which can result in permanent damage to the heart valves. Carditis may produce symptoms including coughing, shortness of breath, or an uncomfortable feeling in the chest. However, in many cases it is detectable only by a doctor's examination and medical tests. In fact, many people do not find out that they have had the condition until years later, when damage to the heart valves is discovered.

The symptoms of rheumatic fever can appear singly or in any combination, so the illness follows many different patterns and variations. It usually develops between seven and twenty-eight days after a strep throat, and can take anywhere from two weeks to three months to resolve. The length of time required for recovery usually depends on the degree to which the heart is affected. Once a child has been diagnosed with rheumatic fever, it is important that any subsequent strep infections be treated promptly and aggressively to prevent further complications.

CONVENTIONAL TREATMENT

■ The diagnosis of rheumatic fever is based on a description of major and minor symptoms, according to a formula known as the "modified Jones criteria." Special blood tests may be performed and an ultrasound examination of the heart may be done to look for carditis.

■ If there is heart involvement, your child may be given a steroid, such as prednisone, to reduce the inflammation. In serious cases, treatment in an intensive care unit may be required.

■ Because rheumatic fever is a complication of a bacterial rather than a viral infection, aspirin may be given for pain relief and to reduce inflammation.

■ If a child still has an active strep infection, he will be given a course of antibiotics for at least ten days. Penicillin is the most often prescribed antibiotic for strep; erythromycin is an alternative for children who are sensitive to penicillin.

DIETARY GUIDELINES

■ Encourage your child to take plenty of fluids. Warm miso soup and chicken soup are excellent.

■ Barley water is good as well; barley is soothing to the entire digestive tract. Simmer 1 cup of barley in 2 quarts of water for one-and-a-half hours. Strain and serve the resulting broth.

■ Reduce the amount of sugar, refined carbohydrates, and dairy products in your child's diet.

■ Encourage your child to eat lots of fruits, simple whole grains (make sure they are well cooked), and fresh raw vegetables.

NUTRITIONAL SUPPLEMENTS

For age-appropriate dosages of some nutritional supplements, see page 81.

■ A calcium and magnesium supplement may be helpful for joint pain. Give your child one dose of a liquid combination formula containing 250 milligrams of calcium and 125 milligrams of magnesium, twice a day, for up to two weeks.

■ Vitamin C and bioflavonoids have anti-inflammatory properties and will help ease the course of the illness. Choose a supplement made without refined sugar, and avoid the chewable forms, as they can erode tooth enamel. Give your child one dose, three times a day, for three to six months.

HERBAL TREATMENT

For age-appropriate dosages of herbal remedies, see page 81.

■ The Chinese herbal formula yin qiao may be given at the first sign of fever. Give your child one dose, three times a day, for up to three days, starting as soon as symptoms begin.
    Note: The liquid extract is the preferred form because it contains no aspirin. The tablet form should not be given to a child under four years of age.

■ Garlic has antibacterial properties that help to clear the body of infection. Give your child one capsule or clove of garlic, three times a day, until he recovers.

HOMEOPATHY

■ At the onset of illness, when your child is first diagnosed and may be frightened, give him one dose of *Aconite* 200x or 30c.

■ If your child is thirsty, irritable, and describes pain with every movement, give him one dose of *Bryonia* 30x or 9c, three to four times a day, for up to three days.

■ If your child is weak and has a low-grade fever that does not seem to be resolving, give him one dose of *Ferrum phosphoricum* 12x or 6c, three to four times a day, for up to three days.

■ *Pulsatilla* is helpful for pain that moves from one joint to another, and for a child who is very tearful. Give your child one dose of *Pulsatilla* 30x or 9c, three to four times a day, for up to three days.

■ *Rhus toxicodendron* helps to resolve the red, blotchy rash that can accompany rheumatic fever. Give your child one dose of *Rhus toxicodendron* 30x or 9c, three to four times a day, for up to three days.

■ To help your child regain strength and vitality after the rheumatic fever is resolved, a constitutional remedy prescribed by a homeopath may be helpful.

ACUPRESSURE

For the locations of acupressure points on a child's body, *see* ADMINISTERING AN ACUPRESSURE TREATMENT in Part Three.

■ Applying pressure to Liver 3 and Large Intestine 4 simultaneously will help to calm and relax your child.

GENERAL RECOMMENDATIONS

■ If you suspect your child may have rheumatic fever, consult your doctor. It is important to begin treatment promptly to reduce the risk of permanent heart damage.

■ Follow your doctor's recommendations exactly regarding treatment with antibiotics, steroids, and/or aspirin.

■ Encourage rest. A rested body generally heals more quickly than an active one.

■ Select and administer an appropriate homeopathic remedy.

■ Give your child calcium and magnesium, vitamin C, and bioflavonoids.

PREVENTION

■ It may not be possible to prevent your child from developing rheumatic fever. Your best defense is to be aware of the disease's various symptoms so that you can seek treatment for the condition as soon as possible. When your child has or is recovering from a strep throat (or other streptococcus infection), be on the alert for any changes in his symptoms that might point to the development of rheumatic fever.

■ If your child has had rheumatic fever, consult your health care provider for advice regarding any subsequent suspected strep infections, to prevent the development of further complications.

■ As much as possible, protect children from contact with sick playmates or infected others.

Ringworm

Ringworm is not actually a worm, but a fungal infection that thrives on the outer layers of the scalp, skin, and nails. This is the same fungus (tinea) that causes "jock itch" and athlete's foot. Ringworm is highly contagious. Like athlete's foot, it spreads from one child to another via contaminated gymnasium floors and shower stalls in schools and other communal facilities. A child away at camp can contract ringworm from contaminated showers and shared bedding. Contact with an affected animal will also spread the infection.

Ringworm typically appears as a slightly scaly lesion on the skin that starts as a small, round, itchy red spot. The infection heals from the inside of the lesion to the outer rim of the circle, giving rise to the typical ringlike look. It often spreads from one area of the body to another.

Ringworm is not a serious infection, but it can be persistent. To confirm a diagnosis, your doctor may gently scratch off some scaly particles from a lesion and examine them under a microscope. The fungus also tends to have a characteristic glow under ultraviolet light. With prompt treatment, ringworm generally clears up in a few weeks. If the fungus is not correctly treated, however, it can lead to a chronic rash or hair loss.

A related problem, tinea versicolor, shows up as a blotchy white discoloration of the skin. The darker the skin tone of the infected person, the more obvious the discoloration is. In a very light-skinned person, it may not be visible at all unless she gets a suntan (the affected areas will remain white) or unless it is looked at under ultraviolet light. Other than the characteristic skin discoloration, tinea versicolor produces few, if any, symptoms, but it is extremely persistent and difficult to get rid of completely. Normal color cannot return to the affected area unless the fungus is completely eradicated and the skin is exposed to the sun. Treatment is similar to that for ringworm. In addition, the overnight application of a selenium sulfide shampoo, such as Selsun Blue, for three or four days, is often recommended.

CONVENTIONAL TREATMENT

■ Topical antifungals, available in cream and lotion form, usually bring about an improvement in ringworm within seven days. To decrease the chance of a recurrence, however, it is best to continue applying the medication for a full course of treatment of up to three weeks. Over-the-counter antifungals include miconazole (in Micatin and Monistat), clotrimazole (Lotrimin, Mycelex), and undecylenic acid (Desenex).

■ If thorough treatment with a topical antifungal medication does not resolve the problem, it may be necessary to use an oral medication such as griseofulvin (Fulvicin, Grifulvin, Grisactin). This drug can have significant side effects, however, including allergic reactions, gastrointestinal upset, and liver toxicity, so it should be reserved for severe, resistant cases. Only in very rare cases is it necessary to resort to this medication for the treatment of ringworm.

■ If your child's ringworm is on her scalp, use a shampoo that contains selenium sulfide (such as Selsun Blue) for at least one week.

DIETARY GUIDELINES

■ Give your child a diet containing plenty of vegetables. Vegetables are high in important vitamins and trace minerals. Green and yellow vegetables are especially recommended. The beta-carotene they contain is an important nutrient for all conditions involving the skin.

HERBAL TREATMENT

For age-appropriate dosages of herbal remedies, see page 81.

■ Balsam of Peru is useful for many skin conditions. It can be applied to the affected area either full strength or diluted with olive, almond, or sesame oil, two or three times a day, for two to three weeks.

■ Echinacea, goldenseal, and burdock root all boost the immune system and can help resolve ringworm. Give your child one dose of an echinacea, goldenseal, and burdock combination formula, three times daily, for ten days.

Note: You should not give your child echinacea on a daily basis for more than ten days at a time, or it will lose its effectiveness.

■ Tea tree oil is one of the strongest known botanical antifungals, and is very effective against ringworm. Mix 8 to 10 drops of tea tree oil in 1 pint of spring or distilled water and apply the mixture to the affected area three times daily, until the rash goes away. Tea tree oil has a strong, turpentinelike odor.

WHEN TO CALL THE DOCTOR ABOUT RINGWORM

It is possible for a secondary infection to develop alongside a case of ringworm. If you are treating a child for ringworm, be alert for signs of a worsening rash. If the area gets increasingly red, warm, tender, or swollen, or if your child develops a fever or swollen glands, consult your doctor for advice about further treatment.

356

HOMEOPATHY

■ Give your child one dose of *Sulphur* 30x or 9c, three times a day, for three days. *Sulphur* should be taken at least one hour before or after an application of tea tree oil. The pungent odor of tea tree oil may cancel the effectiveness of this homeopathic.

GENERAL RECOMMENDATIONS

■ Give your child homeopathic *Sulphur*.

■ Apply tea tree oil to affected areas, either one hour before or one hour after giving her the homeopathic *Sulphur*.

■ Give your child an echinacea, goldenseal, and burdock combination formula.

■ Keep your child's skin clean, cool, and dry. Fungus thrives in warm, moist environments. Loose cotton clothing is best, as it allows air to circulate next to the skin.

■ To decrease the possibility of reinfection and to prevent the spread of ringworm to other family members, wash your child's clothing after each wearing. Do not allow your child to share clothing, combs, hats, socks, pillows, or sheets.

PREVENTION

■ Teach your child good hygiene practices, especially careful hand-washing.

■ Avoid contact with affected animals. The signs and symptoms of ringworm in animals are the same as in humans. If you notice the telltale ring or patches of hair loss on the family pet, take the animal to a veterinarian for treatment. Do not let your child touch or play with a pet or with any other animal that is actively infected.

Roseola

Roseola is an illness that occurs in young children and is characterized by a high fever (as high as 104° to 106°F) and a mild pink, itchy rash that appears as the fever goes down. The fever can last from one to five days; the rash may resolve quickly or it may last about two to four days, beginning first on the chest and back and then spreading to the face and extremities. The lymph glands in the neck will likely be swollen and the spleen may be enlarged. Loss of appetite, irritability, sore throat, and runny nose may also be present. Once the rash disappears, these other symptoms will disappear as well.

Roseola—known to doctors as *roseola infantum*—is thought to be caused by a virus that is probably a member of the herpes family (human herpes virus type 6). This illness is most common in children between the ages of six months and three years. Roseola is contagious and appears to be spread through respiratory contact, with an incubation period of about ten to fifteen days. A child remains infectious for about five days after the fever goes down.

The principal danger associated with roseola is the possibility of a seizure due to the high fever. In fact, because the fever can come on so suddenly, a seizure is sometimes the first sign that a child has roseola.

CONVENTIONAL TREATMENT

■ Treatment for roseola is aimed at reducing fever and keeping your child comfortable. Acetaminophen (found in Tylenol, Tempra, and other medications) lowers fever and is also an analgesic, so it eases the discomfort and body aches that can accompany a fever. It is available in liquid or pill form, as well as in suppositories for infants.

Note: In excessive amounts, acetaminophen can cause liver damage. Read package directions carefully so as not to exceed the proper dosage for your child's age and size.

■ Ibuprofen (available as Advil, Nuprin, and others) is another drug that can be used to reduce fever and relieve mild to moderate achiness and pain. It is available in liquid or pill form. If you give your child ibuprofen, be sure to give it to him with food to prevent an upset stomach. Follow the dosage directions on the product label.

■ *Do not* give aspirin to a child with roseola. The combination of aspirin and a viral infection has been linked to the development of Reye's syndrome, a serious disease affecting the liver and brain (*see* REYE'S SYNDROME).

DIETARY GUIDELINES

■ A child with a fever can become dehydrated easily, so make sure your child gets plenty of fluids. If you are breastfeeding, feed your child as frequently as he can be persuaded to nurse. Offer an older child lots of spring water, herbal teas, soups, and diluted fruit juices.

NUTRITIONAL SUPPLEMENTS

For age-appropriate dosages of nutritional supplements, see page 81.

■ Vitamin C has anti-inflammatory properties and can help to resolve a fever that is due to infection. Give your child one dose, three to four times a day, until the illness resolves.

■ Bioflavonoids are antiviral and anti-inflammatory. Give your child one dose, four times a day, until he is better.

■ Zinc boosts the immune system and aids in healing. Give your child one dose daily.

Note: Excessive amounts of zinc can result in nausea and vomiting. Be careful not to exceed the recommended dosage.

HERBAL TREATMENT

■ A combination herbal tea can help to lower fever, decrease chills, and increase perspiration. Use lemon balm leaf, chamomile flower, peppermint leaf, licorice root, and elder flower, either singly or in any combination (use ½ teaspoon of licorice root and 1 teaspoon each of the others). Give a child two years of age or older ½ cup of tea, four times daily, for one day. A child under two can take up

EMERGENCY TREATMENT FOR A FEBRILE SEIZURE

✚ A child with roseola may have a seizure, called a febrile seizure, as a result of the high fever that accompanies this illness. If your child has a febrile seizure, he needs medical attention *immediately*. Call for emergency assistance.

✚ While you wait for help to arrive, stay with your child. Clear the area around your child to prevent injury. Keep him upright and make sure he is breathing well. *Do not* try to restrain him, hold him down, or force anything into his mouth, but stay with him and talk reassuringly to him.

✚ Watch your child closely for any changes in breathing and/or color. Be sure his airway stays open. If your child vomits, turn his head (if possible, his whole body) to the side so that there is no risk of choking on inhaled vomit.

to ¼ cup of tea or, if you are breastfeeding, you can take 1 cup yourself. The tea should be taken as warm as possible.

Note: If you are using peppermint in the tea and also giving your child a homeopathic preparation, allow at least one hour between the two. Otherwise, the strong smell of the mint may interfere with the effectiveness of the homeopathic remedy.

■ Give your child an immune-boosting echinacea and goldenseal combination formula. These herbs have antibacterial and antiviral properties, and soothe mucous membranes. Give your child one dose, every two hours, until the fever breaks. Then give him one dose, three times a day, for two or three days.

■ If your child's rash is itchy, try giving him soothing lukewarm oatmeal baths.

HOMEOPATHY

■ Try *Belladonna* 200x or 15c for a child with high fever and enlarged pupils. This child's eyes have a glazed look. Start giving this remedy at the first sign of a fever. Give one dose, three times a day, for one day.

■ *Phytolacca* will help to ease tender, swollen glands. Give your child one dose of *Phytolacca* 12x or 6c, four times a day, for up to two days.

■ *Pulsatilla* 30x or 9c is for a child who cries easily and does not want to be left alone. Give this child one dose, three times a day, for up to three days.

■ If your child's illness is lingering and he has a sore throat and bad breath, give him one dose of *Mercurius solubilis* 12x or 6c, four times a day, for up to two days.

GENERAL RECOMMENDATIONS

■ Roseola is usually a self-limiting condition. Treatment is aimed primarily at controlling fever and keeping your child as comfortable as possible.

■ Make sure your child gets plenty of rest and lots of fluids.

PREVENTION

■ Roseola is a common infection of childhood and may not be preventable. It goes without saying, however, that you should keep a healthy child from coming into contact with a child with a known case of the disease.

Rubella

See GERMAN MEASLES.

Runny Nose

See ALLERGIES; COMMON COLD.

Scabies

Scabies is a skin rash caused by a tiny crablike mite. The mites burrow into and lay eggs in soft areas of the skin, such as the buttocks, genitals, wrists, armpits, and between the toes and fingers.

The rash is characterized by small red lumps that may become dry and scaly. It can be very itchy, especially at night. You may also notice tiny, thin light-gray or pink lines on your child's skin. These are the burrowing tunnels.

Scabies is highly contagious and spreads through skin-to-skin contact or through contact with infested clothing, sheets, or towels. It can also be caught from infested animals. If your child develops scabies, all the members of the household should be checked for this infestation.

Scabies can usually be treated successfully at home. If the inflammation persists after one week of treatment, if it becomes worse, or if new bumps develop, call your doctor.

CONVENTIONAL TREATMENT

■ The diagnosis of scabies is made by examination of the distribution and characteristic appearance of the rash. Sometimes the mites can be scraped off and seen under a microscope.

■ Permethrin lotion (sold as Nix or Elimite) kills the mites by attacking their nervous systems. It is safer and more effective than the better known lindane, or gamma benzene hexachloride (found in Kwell), which is chemically related to DDT and can cause headaches and nervous system damage. Another alternative is crotamiton cream (Eurax), which is safer than gamma benzene hexachloride and also has anti-itch properties.

■ An over-the-counter spray called RID is useful for treating infested clothes and bedding.

■ A topical steroid, such as cortisone, or an oral antihistamine, such as Benadryl or Atarax, may be suggested to help lessen the itching while the medication is taking effect. You should be aware that an antihistamine will also likely have the effect of making your child sleepy.

■ An antibiotic is not necessary unless a secondary bacterial infection results from scratching and breaking the skin.

DIETARY GUIDELINES

■ To decrease your child's vulnerability to infestation and boost her immune system, make sure she eats foods that contain plenty of zinc. Foods that are high in zinc include egg yolks, fish, milk, blackstrap molasses, sesame seeds, soybeans, sunflower seeds, turkey, wheat bran, wheat germ, whole-grain products, and yeast.

HERBAL TREATMENT

■ Tea tree oil (*Melaleuca alternifolia*) is a strong herbal disinfectant. Paint the affected area with undiluted tea tree oil twice a day.

■ Balsam of Peru has antiparasitic properties and is useful against scabies. It can be applied either full strength or diluted with olive, almond, or sesame oil.

■ Comfrey root also makes an excellent topical salve. Apply this three times a day.

■ Calendula and goldenseal ointments are commercially available. The calendula is healing and soothing to the skin; the goldenseal helps to heal infection. Apply the mixture to the affected area three times a day.

HOMEOPATHY

■ *Antimonium crudum* is good for a dry skin rash with pimples or vesicles, when the itching is often worse at night. Give your child one dose of *Antimonium crudum* 12x or 6c, three times a day, for up to three days.

■ *Arsenicum album* is for a dry, rough, scaly rash. The itching may be accompanied by a burning sensation and restlessness. The rash feels worse when your child is exposed to cold. Give your child one dose of *Arsenicum album* 12x or 6c, three times a day, for up to three days.

■ *Sulphur* will benefit the child, usually a boy, who is sweaty, feels warm, and has red, dry, hot-looking skin patches. This child typically throws off the covers and wants the skin exposed. Give this child one dose of *Sulphur* 30x or 9c, twice a day (at 11:00 A.M. and 3:00 P.M.), for up to three days.

GENERAL RECOMMENDATIONS

■ Thoroughly wash all bedding, towels, and clothing in very hot water. Spray them with RID according to the directions on the product package.

■ Give your child cool oatmeal baths to help lessen the itching.

PREVENTION

■ Discourage the sharing of clothes, bedding, and towels. Do not allow your child to share these items with a child who has a known case of scabies.

■ Do not allow your child to handle wild animals.

Scarlet Fever

See SORE THROAT.

Seizure

A seizure, or convulsion, is a sudden, uncontrollable contraction of a group of muscles. It may be mild or violent. When a child experiences a convulsion, all or

EMERGENCY TREATMENT FOR A SEIZURE

✚ Stay with your child. Talk reassuringly to him.

✚ Watch closely for changes in breathing and color. Be sure your child's airway stays open.

✚ Clear the area around your child to prevent injury, such as might occur if he knocks into a table or chair. Do not try to hold your child down. Restraining a thrashing child can cause additional injury.

✚ If vomiting occurs, turn your child's head to the side to prevent him from choking on inhaled vomit. If possible, keep his whole body turned on the side.

✚ Do not try to force anything into your child's mouth to hold down his tongue. You might cause choking, or suffer a bite.

✚ Try to place a soft pillow or blanket under your child's head and loosen clothing to prevent injury and ease discomfort.

✚ If the seizure lasts for less than ten minutes, allow your child to sleep afterwards, but keep watch and call your doctor.

✚ If the seizure lasts longer than ten minutes, or if your child is having difficulty breathing, is turning blue, or is hurting himself, call for emergency help.

✚ If your child has a seizure in combination with fever, vomiting, headache, irritability, lethargy, a stiff neck, or (in infants) a bulging fontanel (soft spot), call your doctor immediately. These can be signs of meningitis, a dangerous infection of the brain or spinal cord.

✚ After a seizure, take your child to the doctor for an examination.

part of his body may stiffen and jerk either with tiny, almost imperceptible movements, or with large, obvious movements.

Although a seizure usually lasts only a few minutes, seeing a child undergo this is a frightening experience for a parent. The child loses consciousness. His body may twitch or shake. His eyes may roll back and his teeth may clench. Breathing may be labored and heavy. The child may froth at the mouth, and may wet himself.

Seizures can have a variety of causes, including high fever, a head injury, poisoning, shock, epilepsy, brain infection, or an allergic reaction. It may be an isolated occurrence or the result of a chronic disorder.

After a seizure has run its course, the child will sleep. Upon awakening, he will feel fatigued, disoriented, and dazed.

CONVENTIONAL TREATMENT

■ A child who has a seizure should be examined by a doctor. An initial evaluation may include a neurological examination, blood and urine tests, a spinal tap, and/or a brain scan. The recommended course of treatment, if any, will depend on the cause of your child's seizure.

■ If your doctor determines that your child has suffered an epileptic seizure, *see* EPILEPSY for more information.

NUTRITIONAL SUPPLEMENTS

Nutritional treatment for seizures is directed at supporting recovery once the seizure has run its course and emergency medical care, if appropriate, has been administered.

■ A combination calcium and magnesium supplement helps to relax the nervous system. Give your child one dose of a liquid formula containing 250 milligrams of calcium and 125 milligrams of magnesium, twice a day, for one month; then give him one dose daily for six months.

■ The B vitamins help to strengthen the nerves. Give your child a vitamin-B complex supplement, three times a week, for six months.

HERBAL TREATMENT

Herbal treatments for seizures are directed at supporting recovery once the seizure has run its course and emergency medical care, if appropriate, has been administered. For age-appropriate dosages of herbal remedies, see page 81.

■ Chamomile, licorice, passion flower, skullcap, and valerian root are all herbs that help to relax the nervous system. Give your child one dose of any of these herbs, either individually or in any combination, twice a day, for one week following a seizure.

Note: Licorice should not be given to a child with high blood pressure. Skullcap should not be given to a child less than six years old.

■ The following twelve-week regimen is helpful for supporting recovery from a seizure.

Weeks 1–4: Minor bupleurum is a Chinese herb that helps to regulate the nervous system. Give your child one dose, twice a day, for the first week after a seizure. Then give your child one dose daily for three weeks.

Note: Minor bupleurum should not be given to a child with a fever or any other sign of an acute infection.

Weeks 5–8: Milk thistle detoxifies and protects the liver. Give your child one dose, once a day, for the second month after a seizure.

Weeks 9–12: Skullcap and oat straw are calmative herbs. Give your child one dose of either, once a day, for the third month after a seizure.

Note: Skullcap should not be given to a child under six years old; oat straw should not be given to a child under four.

HOMEOPATHY

Homeopathic treatment for seizures is directed at supporting recovery once the seizure has run its course and emergency medical care, if appropriate, has been administered.

■ Give your child one dose of *Aconite* 200x following a seizure to ease his fright and shock.

■ Working with a homeopath to find a constitutional remedy for your child can be very beneficial in strengthening your child's overall health.

PREVENTION

■ Because the most common cause of seizures in infants and young children is high fever, it is useful to take measures to control a child's fever and keep him well hydrated (*see* FEVER).

■ If your child has a febrile (fever-induced) seizure, your physician may recommend that he take phenobarbital or a similar drug to prevent a recurrence. You should be aware that this form of treatment is controversial, and appears to be falling out of favor among many doctors. If your doctor recommends this type of treatment, make sure you first have a thorough discussion about its pros and cons in relation to your child's individual case before agreeing to it. (*See* FEVER.)

■ Be alert for symptoms of meningitis, which can lead to a seizure. These include fever, vomiting, headache, irritability, lethargy, a stiff neck, a bulging fontanel (soft spot), or decreased level of consciousness. Bacterial meningitis is a serious, rapidly progressing illness that must be treated promptly and aggressively with antibiotics. If you have any reason to suspect your child may be developing meningitis, seek emergency treatment.

Shock

Although many people use the word to describe an emotional reaction, in medical terms, shock is a physical state in which circulation is so severely compromised that blood cannot reach the body's tissues and organs. Without the essential nutrients and oxygen carried by the blood, the body becomes less and less able to perform its vital functions. This creates an emergency situation that requires immediate medical attention. If untreated, shock leads to complete circulatory collapse and death.

Shock can be caused by a variety of problems, including a severe allergic reaction, major blood loss, drug overdose, severe dehydration, serious infection, major emotional trauma (such as after a serious accident), or, in a person with diabetes, a sudden and dangerous rise in the amount of insulin in the body.

Signs and symptoms of shock include nausea, vomiting, weakness, cold and clammy skin, pale white or grayish skin color, dizziness, a cold sweat, increased breathing and heart rate, and restless or frightened behavior.

EMERGENCY TREATMENT FOR SHOCK

✚ If an injured child appears to be in shock, call for emergency medical help immediately.

✚ While waiting for an ambulance to arrive, wrap the child in a warm blanket or extra clothes. Put a blanket between the child and the ground to help keep her body protected from the cool earth. If no blanket or extra clothing is available, use leaves, newspaper, or anything else on hand that can act as insulation.

✚ Keep the child on her back and raise her feet about a foot off the ground, so that they are at a level higher than her heart. If she has an injured arm or leg, raise it above the level of the heart as well. These measures decrease the workload of a heart that is already under stress.

✚ If the child is not breathing, turn to CARDIOPULMONARY RESUSCITATION (CPR) on page 426. Start CPR at once.

✚ If the child is bleeding, turn to BLEEDING, SEVERE on page 122. Take action immediately to stop the bleeding.

✚ If the child is unknown to you, look for a Medic Alert necklace or bracelet that might explain the child's condition. For example, a child with diabetes may have a bracelet relating this information, which would guide medical personnel in their treatment.

✚ If the child vomits or begins bleeding from the mouth, turn her onto her side so that the fluid can drain from her mouth.

CONVENTIONAL TREATMENT

■ If shock is related to a large blood loss, your child will be given intravenous fluids to increase blood volume. Cardiopulmonary resuscitation (CPR), blood transfusion, and/or a ventilator for breathing assistance may be required in severe situations.

■ If shock is caused by an allergic reaction, your child will be given epinephrine by injection to counteract the body's severe reaction to the allergen. Most often children respond to this treatment quickly and recover with little or no long-term treatment (*see* ANAPHYLACTIC SHOCK).

HERBAL TREATMENT

Herbal treatment for shock is directed at supporting recovery once the acute phase of the crisis is over and your child is home from the hospital. If you suspect shock, seek emergency treatment for your child. For age-appropriate dosages of herbal remedies, see page 81.

■ Gotu kola is a general tonic that is also very useful for wound healing. Give your child two to three doses daily for one week.

Note: This herb should not be given to a child under four years of age.

■ Nettle and yellow dock help build healthy blood cells. After the crisis is over, give your child one dose of either or both herbs, twice daily, for one week.

Note: Some children experience stomach upset as a result of taking nettle. If this happens, stop giving it. This herb should not be given to a child under four.

■ American ginseng helps to restore energy. Try giving your child one dose, twice daily, for two days after the nettle and/or yellow dock.

Note: This herb should not be given if fever or any other signs of infection are present.

HOMEOPATHY

Homeopathic treatment for shock is directed at supporting recovery once the acute phase of the crisis is over and your child is home from the hospital. If you suspect shock, seek emergency treatment for your child.

■ *Ferrum phosphoricum* 6x assists in recovery from a major blood loss. Give your child one dose, three times daily, for five days.

BACH FLOWER REMEDIES

■ If your child is conscious (or once she becomes conscious), give her Bach Flower Rescue Remedy. Following any injury or crisis, this remedy helps to calm and stabilize. Mix a few drops of Rescue Remedy in a glass of water, and have your child take sips of the mixture. Or place one or two drops under her tongue directly from the bottle. (*See* BACH FLOWER REMEDIES in Part One.)

PREVENTION

◼ It may not always be possible to prevent a child from going into shock. The authors strongly recommend that all parents and other child-care providers take a first aid course that includes instruction in infant and child CPR. Hopefully, you will never be called upon to use these skills, but CPR is a technique that should be learned *before* the need arises.

◼ Keep smelling salts on hand. These can be used to distinguish an episode of fainting from true shock. If an emergency arises when smelling salts are unavailable, try using a bottle of perfume instead. Open the bottle and wave it under your child's nose. (*See* FAINTING.)

◼ If your child is prone to severe allergic reactions, ask your doctor to prescribe a home emergency kit containing epinephrine, such as the Ana-Kit or EpiPen, and be sure you learn how to administer it correctly. Having a supply of epinephrine on hand may someday save your child's life.

◼ There are many things you can do to decrease the possibility that your child will suffer an accident that might lead to shock. See HOME SAFETY in Part One of this book.

Shock, Electric

See ELECTRIC SHOCK.

Sinusitis

Sinusitis is an inflammation or infection that occurs in the sinuses. The sinuses are four sets of open spaces within the bones of the skull. They come in matched pairs. The *sphenoid sinuses* are centered in the skull, nestled just behind the bridge of the nose. The *ethmoid sinuses* are way back in the upper nose. The *frontal sinuses* are located in the forehead, just above the eyebrow. The *maxillary sinuses* are located under each eye, on either side of the nose. Sinusitis most often occurs in the frontal and/or maxillary sinuses.

The sinuses are lined with mucous membranes similar to the lining of the nasal passages. Their apparent function is to warm, moisten, and filter incoming air on its way to the trachea and lungs. The trouble starts when the membranes lining the nasal passages swell and block the ducts that lead to the sinuses, preventing them from draining freely. Congestion results. The swelling, blockage, and congestion then predispose the sinuses to bacterial infection.

When the sinuses are blocked, congested, irritated, and inflamed, secondary

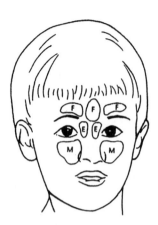

A. Front View

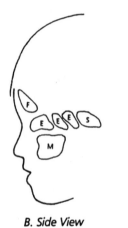

B. Side View

Location of the Sinuses

There are four sets of sinuses: the sphenoid (indicated by the letter S), located behind the bridge of the nose; the ethmoid (E), in the upper nose; the frontal (F), above the eyebrows; and the maxillary (M), below the eyes and on either side of the nose.

symptoms may include headache, earache, toothache, and/or facial pain and pressure, with marked tenderness over the forehead and cheekbones. There may be a high fever, loss of the ability to smell, and bad breath. Swelling and puffiness around the eyes, as well as drainage from the eyes, can be danger signals that a more serious condition is developing. If left untreated, sinusitis can lead to meningitis or pneumonia. Chronic sinusitis, even when mild, can also be an underlying factor in asthma. If it is, often the asthma will not improve until the sinusitis is treated.

Many cases of sinusitis occur after the onset of a cold. Hay fever and food allergies, especially a sensitivity to milk and dairy products, are common sources of allergic sinusitis. Exposure to environmental pollutants, including cigarette smoke, can also predispose a person to allergic sinusitis, as can nasal polyps.

The only truly accurate way to diagnose sinusitis is by a magnetic resonance imaging (MRI) scan or ultrasound. X-rays are sometimes useful, but can be misleading. A physical examination and diagnostic tests may reveal other indicators of sinus infection, including teeth that are tender when tapped, tenderness in the maxillary area, puffy lower eyelids, thick green-yellow nasal discharge, an elevated white blood cell count, and a culture of the nasal discharge that reveals the presence of an infection.

CONVENTIONAL TREATMENT

■ For bacterial infections, antibiotics are prescribed. Most commonly prescribed are amoxicillin and trimethoprim (Bactrim). For an acute infection, the medication is usually prescribed for ten to fourteen days. A host of newer antibiotics have become available in recent years that are much more expensive—but not necessarily more effective—than the old standbys. Their primary usefulness is in treating patients who are allergic to penicillin or sulfa drugs.

■ Decongestants may be suggested to help drain the sinuses. Topical decongestants like Afrin and Neo-Synephrine are probably more effective than the oral variety, but nasal sprays or drops should not be used for longer than three days in a row. Their initial effect is an opening of nasal passages, but after several days the body can become dependent on them and then, when use is discontinued, the nasal ducts may swell up and fail to respond as they normally would.

■ Acetaminophen (in Anacin-3, Panadol, Tempra, Tylenol, and other medications) can be used to ease discomfort and to bring down a fever.

Note: In excessive amounts, this drug can cause liver damage. Read package directions carefully so as not to exceed the proper dosage for your child's age and size.

■ A severe case of sinusitis that does not respond to antibiotics may have to be treated by a surgical procedure to open the sinuses and allow them to drain adequately.

DIETARY RECOMMENDATIONS

■ To thin mucus, promote drainage, and relieve congestion, encourage your child to drink a lot of clean water and hot herbal teas.

■ Offer your child chicken or vegetable soup. A recent medical study showed that hot chicken soup promotes sinus drainage.

■ In any case of sinusitis—no matter what the cause—eliminate milk and dairy products from your child's diet. Dairy products can increase the production of mucus and cause it to thicken, making drainage even more difficult.

■ To identify food sensitivities or allergies that may be fostering a chronic sinus condition, try a rotation or elimination diet (*see* ELIMINATION DIET or ROTATION DIET in Part Three). Start by targeting dairy products and wheat, two of the most common offenders.

■ Make a drink of hot lemonade to help cut mucus and improve blood flow. Mix the juice of two freshly squeezed lemons with an equal amount of water. Sweeten the drink with maple syrup, and give it to your child three times a day. If your child will tolerate it, you can try adding 1/8 teaspoon of cayenne pepper to the lemonade as well.

NUTRITIONAL SUPPLEMENTS

For age-appropriate dosages of nutritional supplements, see page 81.

■ Beta-carotene helps to heal mucous membranes. Give your child one dose, twice a day, for four or five days.

■ Vitamin C and bioflavonoids help reduce inflammation and fight infection. Give your child one dose of each, three to four times a day, for four or five days.

■ Zinc helps tissue to heal. Lozenges are a particularly good form. Give your child one dose, twice a day, for up to one week.

Note: Excessive amounts of zinc can result in nausea and vomiting. Be careful not to exceed the recommended dosage.

HERBAL TREATMENT

For age-appropriate dosages of herbal remedies, see page 81.

■ Make an herbal tea combining 1 tablespoon of fenugreek, 1 tablespoon of thyme, 1 tablespoon of rose hips, and 1/2 tablespoon of licorice. Fenugreek and thyme help to relieve nasal and sinus congestion; rose hips contain vitamin C; and licorice will sweeten the tea. Give your child one dose, twice a day, during the acute phase of the infection.

Note: Licorice should not be given to a child with high blood pressure.

■ Give your child an herbal vapor inhalation treatment by adding 4 or 5 drops of rosemary oil or eucalyptus oil to a sinkful or large pot of water (*see* PREPARING HERBAL TREATMENTS in Part Three).

■ Echinacea and goldenseal stimulate the immune system and help in clearing infections. These herbs are antibacterial and soothe mucous membranes. Give your child one dose of an echinacea and goldenseal combination formula, every two hours, while symptoms (including fever and sinus pain) are acute, up to a total of six doses. After the acute phase is resolved, give him one dose, three times a day, for up to ten days.

Note: You should not give your child echinacea on a daily basis for more than ten days at a time, or it will lose its effectiveness.

■ Garlic has antibacterial properties and helps to clear infection. Select an odorless capsule variety and give it to your child, according to the dosage directions on the product label, for up to ten days.

■ Menthol lozenges help to clear respiratory passages. Menthol is a purified and refined form of peppermint oil. Lozenges made without sugar are preferable. Give your child one lozenge per hour, up to a total of three or four lozenges a day, as needed.

Note: If you are giving your child menthol lozenges as well as a homeopathic preparation, allow one hour between the two. Otherwise, the strong smell of the lozenges may interfere with the action of the homeopathic remedy.

■ Shiitake mushrooms have an immune-stimulating effect. Give a child over twelve years of age one capsule, three times daily, for one week after the acute infection is over.

■ Alkalol is a commercially available "mucus solvent" made from salt water and a combination of aromatic oils. It is very soothing to the sinus membranes and helps clear out infection. Dilute it with an equal amount of water and gently flush your child's sinuses with the mixture three or four times daily.

HOMEOPATHY

■ *Hepar sulphuris* is helpful for sinus infections when the nasal discharge is yellow or yellow-green. Give your child *Hepar sulphuris* 12x or 6c, four times a day, for up to two days.

■ For a sinus infection with white, ropy mucus, give your child one dose of *Kali bichromicum* 12x or 6c, four times a day, for up to two days.

■ Give *Mercurius solubilis* 12x or 6c to a child with a stuffed nose that isn't getting better. This child is likely to have bad breath as well. Give him one dose of this remedy, four times a day, for up to two days.

■ Homeopathic combination sinus formulas are available that may offer relief for your child. Follow the dosage directions on the package.

ACUPRESSURE

For the locations of acupressure points on a child's body, see ADMINISTERING AN ACUPRESSURE TREATMENT in Part Three.

■ Large Intestine 4 clears the head and sinuses.

■ Large Intestine 20 clears the sinuses.

GENERAL RECOMMENDATIONS

■ Use nasal saline flushes to cleanse the sinuses and thin mucus (*see* NASAL SALINE FLUSH in Part Three). You can do this four to six times a day, as needed.

■ In a case of chronic sinusitis, eliminate all dairy products for two weeks and monitor your child's overall level of congestion throughout this period. If there is a significant improvement, this is a good indication of a sensitivity or allergy to dairy products.

■ Teach your child the proper technique for blowing his nose. He should *not* hold one nostril closed, and he should *not* blow hard. Holding one nostril closed and blowing with force can send mucus back up into the sinus cavities. A gentle blow with both nostrils open is more effective.

■ The use of a cool mist vaporizer may be helpful. To prevent the buildup of bacteria, keep the equipment scrupulously clean. During an acute infection, a humidifier can help to thin and drain secretions.

■ A warm, moist compress of water and ginger root placed over the sinuses helps to drain the area and relieve congestion. Grate a large ginger root into a pot containing 1 pint of water and simmer for fifteen minutes. Use the resulting tea to make a hot compress.

■ A rosemary steam inhalation is very soothing to the nasal passages and helps the sinuses to drain. Follow the stovetop instructions for an herbal vapor inhalation treatment (*see* PREPARING HERBAL TREATMENTS in Part Three), using 1 tablespoon of rosemary for each quart of water.

PREVENTION

■ Eliminate all known and suspected allergens from your child's environment.

■ Avoid exposing your child to cigarette smoke and wood smoke. Studies have shown that children who live with parents who smoke, or who live in extremely well insulated homes with wood stoves, have upper respiratory infections more often than other children do.

Skin Rash

"Rash" is a general term that describes an eruption of the skin. A rash may be the result of a bacterial infection such as impetigo, a viral infection such as chickenpox or herpes, a fungal infection such as ringworm or yeast, or an allergy to food, a plant, or medicine.

When your child develops a rash, there are many possibilities for how it will look and feel. A rash may be flat, raised, or blistered. It may be pink, red, purple, or brown. The rash may be made of discrete circular lesions, patches, or a diffuse reddened area. It may be moist and "weepy" or dry and scaly. The rash may start on one part of the body and spread to other parts, or it may appear in one area only. There may be no sensation with it, or it may be itchy or burning.

The more you know about the rash, the better able you will be to treat it. Look at it closely and observe what it looks like. Take note of where it appears on the body, whether it spreads or not, and any other symptoms your child has, even if they seem unrelated. Also take into account where your child was or what he may have been doing in the day or days before the rash appeared, as well as environmental factors such as the temperature or exposure to possible allergens. All of these clues can be important for the correct diagnosis of a rash.

If you feel unsure about your child's rash, consult your health care provider for advice. If your child develops a rash accompanied by a high fever, weakness, and lethargy, seek medical attention immediately.

GENERAL RECOMMENDATIONS

■ Appropriate treatment, if any, depends on the cause of the rash. For example,

Common Childhood Rashes

In order to know how to treat a rash, it is best to know the cause. The following chart lists some of the illnesses that most commonly cause childhood rashes, together with a description of characteristic features. It is not meant to be a list of all possible causes of skin rash, however. Consult your health care provider for a definitive diagnosis of your child's rash.

Cause of Rash	Description
Athlete's foot	Clusters of tiny blisters and scaly sores that appear on the feet, especially between the toes. Itchy and burning. Goes away with treatment, but can be persistent; a complete cure can take up to a month in some cases.
Chickenpox	Appears first as a flat, reddish rash, then turns into batches of tiny pimples and blistered lesions that crust over as they heal. Usually preceded by a day or two of typical viral symptoms—fever, headache, fatigue, and general malaise. In most cases the rash begins on the trunk and spreads to the extremities. Usually there are comparatively few lesions on the neck and head. Very itchy.
Cradle cap	Thick, yellowish crusty patches, usually on the scalp but also possibly on the face and ears or in the groin area. Most common in children between two and twelve weeks of age. It is not itchy, and it usually goes away on its own as the child gets older.
Diaper rash	Ordinary diaper rash causes red patches on the groin, buttocks, and inguinal creases. The skin may be swollen and/or dry and scaling. Fungal diaper rash is smooth, shiny, raised, and very red, and the skin appears raw and painful. Usually heals within one week with treatment.
Food or drug allergy (hives)	Pink or red flat and raised lesions. The skin may appear swollen, and it may be itchy. Usually resolves once the offending food or drug is identified and avoided, but in rare cases a drug allergy can lead to a prolonged skin disease called Stevens-Johnson syndrome.
Eczema	A raised red rash that may be dry and scaly or comprised of weepy, fluid-filled lesions. Itching can be severe. Usually an allergic reaction that improves once the allergen is identified and avoided.
Erythema toxicum	Red areas that are flat or raised, with small white dots that are tiny pus-filled lesions. May appear anywhere on a child's body. Most often occurs during the first two weeks of life and fades away in two to three days.
German measles (rubella)	A pink or red rash with tiny lesions that have well-defined edges, usually accompanied by mild symptoms of a viral infection, including swollen lymph glands and general malaise. The rash most often begins on the head and neck and spreads to the trunk and extremities. Lasts about three days, then fades as the virus runs its course.
Herpes virus	Small blisters and ulcers, either around the mouth or in the genital area, that may be preceded by an itching or burning sensation. Itchy and painful. An outbreak usually lasts four to ten days, but outbreaks can be a recurring problem.
Impetigo	Appears first as irregularly shaped discolored spots, then turns into weepy honey-colored lesions that crust and scab. Most often occurs on the hands, face, and perineum. Heals with treatment.
Lyme disease	A round, raised reddish lesion that is usually paler or whitish in the center occurs at the site of the tick bite that transmits this disease. May or may not be accompanied by flulike symptoms, including headache, fever, and general malaise. The rash may come and go throughout the illness.

Cause of Rash	Description
Measles	A splotchy purplish-red rash of irregularly shaped raised and flat lesions. Begins as small spots that coalesce into larger patches. Usually preceded by several days of viral symptoms, including fever, cough, and general malaise, as well as conjunctivitis. In most cases the rash begins on the face and spreads to the trunk and extremities. Lasts four to seven days, then fades as the virus runs its course.
Poison ivy	Small fluid-filled lesions, with redness and swelling, weeping and crusting. Can appear several hours or several days after contact with the plant. Itching and burning can be severe. Lasts from two to four weeks, then gradually heals.
Prickly heat	Small, raised red lesions with tiny blisters at the center. Appears suddenly, usually in hot weather, and resolves quickly. May be itchy and stinging.
Ringworm	Small, flat lesions that grow to be approximately $\frac{1}{4}$-inch circular lesions. The skin may appear scaly; there may be fluid-filled blisters. Itchy. Usually appears on the face, arms, and/or trunk. Goes away with treatment.
Roseola	Widespread flat, pink rash. Usually preceded by a fever, often a high fever; the rash appears as the fever subsides. Most common in young children. The rash may last a few hours to a few days.
Scabies	Small red lumps that may become dry and scaly. You may also see thin light-gray or pinkish lines under the skin. Often very itchy. Most commonly occurs on the buttocks, genitals, wrists, armpits, and between the fingers and toes. Resolves with treatment.
Scarlet fever	Widespread light pink or red rash that feels like sandpaper to the touch. Usually preceded by a day or so of fever, sore throat, and headache. The rash appears first in the warm areas of the body, such as under the arms, behind the knees, and in the groin area, and then spreads to the trunk and extremities.

a rash resulting from a viral infection usually doesn't need any specific treatment except for comfort measures, while a rash caused by a bacterial infection may need to be treated with antibiotic cream and herbs with immune-stimulating properties. *See* Common Childhood Rashes on page 370 to help you determine what may be causing your child's rash, and then refer to the relevant entry in this book. *See* ACNE; ALLERGIES; ATHLETE'S FOOT; BITES AND STINGS, INSECT; CHICKENPOX; CRADLE CAP; DIAPER RASH; ECZEMA; FOOD ALLERGIES; GERMAN MEASLES; HERPES VIRUS; IMPETIGO; LYME DISEASE; MEASLES; POISON IVY; PRICKLY HEAT; RINGWORM; ROSEOLA; SCABIES; or SORE THROAT for further information.

■ Regardless of the cause, if your child's rash is itchy and/or inflamed, cool compresses can provide quick relief. Soak a clean cloth in cool water, wring it out, and apply it to the affected area for ten minutes. Repeat as often as necessary.

Sleep Problems

See FATIGUE; INSOMNIA.

Sore Throat

The medical terms for sore throat are *pharyngitis* (inflammation of the throat), *laryngitis* (inflammation of the larynx, or voice box), and *tonsillitis* (inflammation of the tonsils).

The throat, or pharynx, is a tubelike passageway that separates into the breathing and digestive tracts. It is made of smooth muscle and lined with a mucous membrane. The throat facilitates speech by changing shape to allow the formation of vowel sounds. It also contains openings for the hearing (eustachian) tubes, nasal space (posterior nares), larynx, gullet (esophagus), and the tonsils.

Most sore throats are caused by viruses or bacteria. Other causes may be a local irritation, such as exposure to cigarette smoke, environmental pollutants, dust, or dry winter air. A long episode of screaming may give rise to a sore throat. A sore throat can also be caused by an abscess in the back of the throat or on the tonsils.

Childhood sore throats occur most often in late winter and early spring. A sore throat may be accompanied by a head cold, runny nose, or ear infection. The majority of sore throats are minor viral illnesses that can be treated easily at home. However, about one-third of childhood sore throats are diagnosed as "strep" throat, an infection caused by the bacteria *Streptococcus*. The strep bacteria is highly contagious and persistent. Strep throat can run through a family like wildfire. The distinguishing signs and symptoms of strep infection, as opposed to a viral infection, are not always consistent. Definitive diagnosis of a strep infection must therefore be based on a throat culture. But there are some general features that can help you make an initial evaluation of your child's sore throat (*see* Strep Infection Versus Viral Infection on page 374).

If your child's symptoms are characteristic of a strep infection, call your physician. Your doctor can then diagnose your child's condition by performing a throat culture and prescribe appropriate treatment. Because the streptococcus bacteria is so highly contagious, it may be wise to check other family members for strep symptoms, too. If left untreated, a strep infection can lead to a number of complications. The most serious of these is rheumatic fever, an inflammatory disease that can cause heart damage (*see* RHEUMATIC FEVER). If you have a child who has already had a case of rheumatic fever, call your physician immediately if she develops a sore throat of any kind.

A strep infection may also be accompanied by scarlet fever. This illness begins with a fever, sore throat, headache, and possibly vomiting. Twelve hours to two days after symptoms begin, the child will develop a characteristic red rash that feels like fine sandpaper to the touch. The rash usually appears first on the neck, under the arms, behind the knees, and in the groin area, and then it spreads to the extremities. It lasts for about seven days, after which the skin begins to peel or flake off. Another common sign of scarlet fever is a red, swollen "strawberry tongue." If you suspect your child's sore throat may be related to a case of scarlet fever, call your physician.

CONVENTIONAL TREATMENT

■ A throat culture provides the only conclusive diagnosis of streptococcus infection. Using a swab, the physician gently removes mucus from the back of the throat for examination. In a modern laboratory, a culture can be done very quickly, and the results can be in your doctor's hands within twenty-four hours. A chemically based test, known as "quick-strep," can give a tentative answer in fifteen to twenty minutes. This test is only 85- to 90-percent accurate, however, and will miss a few cases. A quick-strep test should therefore always be backed up with a regular throat culture, especially when the initial results are negative. A newer test, called Strep OIA, also gives a result in fifteen minutes, but is more sensitive. According to the manufacturer, BioStar Medical Products, it yields accurate results and no backup throat culture is required.

■ If the diagnosis is strep, an antibiotic will be prescribed. Penicillin is usually the antibiotic of choice. Your physician may prescribe a course of penicillin in pill form, to be taken over a ten-day period, or he or she may opt for a one-dose injection of penicillin. If your child is allergic to penicillin, erythromycin is the preferred alternative. If pills are prescribed, it is important that the entire ten-day course be taken to ensure complete eradication of the bacteria.

■ Your doctor may recommend a three-day wait before treating your child with antibiotics. There are both potential risks and benefits involved in initiating immediate antibiotic treatment for acute strep throat, as opposed to waiting three days before beginning treatment. A 1987 article in *The Journal of Pediatric Infectious Diseases* reported that discomfort and fever were reduced more quickly in children who were given antibiotics immediately, but these children suffered a higher incidence of reinfection. Children whose treatment was delayed for three days took longer to get better, but showed higher resistance to developing another case of the disease. Some doctors now believe that this is because immediate treatment with antibiotics inhibits the immune system by slowing the production of antibodies needed to fight off the existing infection. It appears that if the body is permitted to initiate healing on its own, it may be more able to mobilize the defenses required to heal itself in the long run. You may wish to discuss with your doctor the possibility of using natural treatments for the first few days instead of starting with antibiotics immediately.

■ If a strep throat is ruled out, your child's sore throat is most likely caused by a viral infection. If this is the case, antibiotics are ineffective and therefore not appropriate. Medical science has not yet discovered medications that fight most viral infections effectively. Fortunately, most viruses are self-limiting, even though viral infections can be quite uncomfortable. Treatment for a viral infection is aimed at helping the child stay as comfortable as possible.

■ A pain reliever, such as acetaminophen (found in Tylenol, Tempra, and other medications), helps to control fever and ease the pain of a sore throat, as well as any other accompanying aches and pains.

Note: In excessive doses, this drug can cause liver damage. Follow the age-appropriate dosage directions on the package carefully.

■ *Do not* give aspirin to a child or teenager with a sore throat unless your doctor specifically recommends it. Most sore throats are caused by viruses, and the combination of a viral infection and aspirin has been associated with Reye's syndrome, a dangerous liver disease (*see* REYE'S SYNDROME).

■ Chloraseptic, available in lozenge or spray form, is an oral anesthetic and antiseptic that can help relieve the pain of a sore throat. Follow the directions on the product label.

WHEN TO CALL THE DOCTOR ABOUT A SORE THROAT

● If your child has a fever over 102°F or other symptoms of a strep infection, see your doctor (see STREP INFECTION VERSUS VIRAL INFECTION, page 374). Only a doctor can accurately diagnose a strep throat.

● If your child has, or has recently recovered from, a strep throat and develops renewed fever, joint pain or swelling, muscle spasms or twitching, a flat, painless rash, and/or bumps on her joints, scalp, or spine, contact your doctor right away. These are signs that she may be developing rheumatic fever.

● If your child's sore throat is accomanied by a red, slightly rough rash on her neck, arms, legs, and/or groin area, or a red, swollen tongue, call your doctor promptly. These are symptoms of scarlet fever.

● If your child has ever had rheumatic fever or scarlet fever in the past, you should consult your doctor whenever she gets a sore throat, no matter what the suspected cause, to protect against further complications. If anyone else in your household has had either of these diseases in the past, he or she should also consult with a health care practitioner concerning measures to protect against further illness or complications.

Strep Infection Versus Viral Infection

Although not all viral or strep infections cause identical symptoms, there are some general tendencies to look for when your child has a sore throat. Review the following symptoms to see which match your child's condition. If you suspect a strep infection, contact your child's doctor. Only a throat culture can accurately confirm a diagnosis of strep.

Sign	Strep Infection	Viral Infection
Age	Most common in children over three years of age.	Possible at any age.
Onset	Comes on suddenly. One minute, the child seems fine—the next, tired, listless, and complaining.	Comes on gradually, escalating from a mild scratchiness to a full-fledged sore throat.
Symptoms	A very painful sore throat, often accompanied by headache, stomach pain, vomiting, and/or tender or very firm lymph nodes. There can be much difficulty swallowing. The child will look and feel very sick.	A sore, thick, or scratchy-feeling throat that may be accompanied by cough, headache, runny nose, hoarseness, enlarged lymph nodes, some difficulty swallowing, and/or conjunctivitis.
Fever	A temperature that escalates to as much as 104°F is possible.	Mild to moderate fever.
Tonsils	Most likely red and swollen with white splotches.	May or may not be swollen; may or may not have a white coating.

DIETARY GUIDELINES

■ An ice-cold fruit-juice popsicle can be an effective temporary anesthetic for a sore throat.

■ Encourage your child to take plenty of fluids. Warm miso soup and chicken soup are excellent.

■ Reduce the amount of sugar, refined carbohydrates, and dairy products in your child's diet.

■ Encourage your child to eat lots of simple whole grains, fresh vegetables, and fruits.

NUTRITIONAL SUPPLEMENTS

For age-appropriate dosages of some nutritional supplements, see page 81.

■ Vitamin C is both antibacterial and anti-inflammatory. Dissolve 1 teaspoon (1,000 milligrams) of buffered vitamin-C powder in 8 ounces of water. Have your child sip this throughout the day, for the first forty-eight hours of a sore throat.

■ Herbal-based, sugar-free lozenges fortified with vitamin C or zinc, a mineral that speeds healing, are very helpful. Give your child one lozenge every hour, as needed, up to a total equivalent to two doses of zinc daily, for up to one week.

Note: Excessive amounts of zinc can result in nausea and vomiting. Be careful not to exceed the recommended dosage.

■ Bioflavonoids help to ease inflammation in the throat and fight infection. Give your child one dose, three or four times a day, for the first three to four days.

■ Give your child one dose of beta-carotene, twice a day, for the first forty-eight hours.

HERBAL TREATMENT

For age-appropriate dosages of herbal remedies, see page 81.

■ Echinacea and goldenseal combination formula is important for helping to clear any kind of infection. Both of these herbs stimulate the immune system. Give your child one dose, every two hours, during the acute phase. Then reduce the dosage to one dose, three times a day, for up to one week.

Note: You should not give your child echinacea on a daily basis for more than ten days at a time, or it can lose its effectiveness.

■ Garlic is antibacterial and supports the immune system. Choose an odorless form, which will be better tolerated by children. You can give it to your child in whole capsule form, or dissolve the liquid in hot water or soup. Follow the dosage directions on the product label and give it to your child until she is better.

■ Brew a sore throat tea. In 1 quart of water, boil some or (preferably) all of the following: 1 tablespoon of licorice root, 1 tablespoon of hyssop, 2 tablespoons of slippery elm bark, and 1 teaspoon of sage. Licorice and slippery elm soothe irritated mucous membranes and ease a sore throat. Hyssop and sage detoxify the blood. Give your child one dose of tea, three times daily, for a couple of days or until she feels better. She can also gargle with this tea when it has cooled.

Note: Licorice should not be given to a child with high blood pressure.

■ At the first sign that your child may be developing scarlet fever, give her one dose of the Chinese botanical formula yin qiao, twice a day, for two days. This remedy is not helpful after the third day of symptoms.

Note: The liquid extract is the preferred form because it contains no aspirin. The tablet form should not be given to a child under four years of age.

■ Yarrow may be helpful because it promotes sweating and helps to lower fever. Give your child one dose, two to three times a day, as needed, for the first one or two days.

■ Grapefruit seed extract can be taken internally or used as a gargle. A highly concentrated form, such as Citricidal, Nutrabiotic, or Paramicrocidin, is preferred. Place 5 to 10 drops in a glass of water for a gargle. Or have your child drink 3 to 5 drops of extract in 6 ounces of water, three or four times daily, for up to three days.

HOMEOPATHY

■ If your child has a mild to moderate fever along with a sore throat, give her *Ferrum phosphoricum* 6x, three times daily, until the fever is resolved, along with one of the other symptom-specific remedies recommended in this entry.

■ *Apis mellifica* is good for the child with swollen, red tonsils and a sore throat that comes on suddenly. This child has little thirst, although the mucous membranes are dry, and there is no coating on the throat. Her tongue may be red. Give this child one dose of *Apis mellifica* 30x or 9c every hour, up to a total of four doses, as long as symptoms last.

■ Give your child *Belladonna* if her tonsils, throat, and uvula are extremely red, and the sore throat came on suddenly. This child will have a fever and possibly dilated pupils. Give her one dose of *Belladonna* 30x or 9c every hour, up to a total of three doses, as long as symptoms last.

■ *Hepar sulphuris* is for the child whose sore throat is accompanied by a cough that brings up thick white or yellow plugs of mucus, and whose throat is coated with mucus. This child feels better with a hot washcloth on her throat. Give her *Hepar sulphuris* 30x or 9c, three times a day, for two days.

■ *Lachesis* will benefit the child with a sore throat that is localized on the left, or one that moves from left to right. The throat and tonsils will be dark red. This child is understandably in a very bad mood; she is in a lot of pain and doesn't want to be touched. Give this child *Lachesis* 30x or 9c, three times a day, for up to two days.

■ *Lycopodium* will help the child with a sore throat that is localized on the right side. The pain may move from the right to left side. This child feels worse during afternoon and early evening, between the hours of 4:00 and 8:00 P.M. Give this child *Lycopodium* 30x or 9c, three times a day, for up to two days.

■ If your child's sore throat is accompanied by hoarseness and worsens in the evening, give her one dose of *Phosphorus* 30x or 9c, three times a day, for up to two days.

■ *Phytolacca* is for the child with a very dark, red throat and much pain with swallowing. This child will have swollen glands, with pain that radiates to the ears. Give her *Phytolacca* 12x or 6c, four times a day, for up to two days.

ACUPRESSURE

For the locations of acupressure points on a child's body, *see* ADMINISTERING AN ACUPRESSURE TREATMENT in Part Three.

■ Large Intestine 4 helps to clear infection.

■ Lung 7 moistens a dry and irritated throat.

GENERAL RECOMMENDATIONS

■ If you suspect that your child's sore throat may be caused by a strep infection, contact your physician. The only way to ensure proper diagnosis and treatment is with a throat culture.

■ Encourage rest. A rested body generally heals more quickly than an active one.

■ Give your child an echinacea and goldenseal combination formula.

■ Select and administer an appropriate homeopathic remedy.

■ Give your child vitamin C and bioflavonoids.

■ Prepare an herbal tea and gargle as described above. Or make a gargle by dissolving ¼ teaspoon of salt in 4 ounces of water and adding a small pinch each of cayenne pepper, lemon juice, and honey.

■ Give your child sugar-free lozenges enriched with vitamin C and zinc. Lozenges increase saliva production and help soothe a dry, irritated throat. Avoid lozenges made with unnecessary chemicals and sugar.

■ Use a cool mist vaporizer to humidify the air. Humidified air soothes irritated respiratory membranes and helps relieve a cough or hoarseness.

■ To decrease the risk of spreading infection, minimize a sick child's contact with others.

■ *See also* COMMON COLD; COUGH; or FEVER if your child's sore throat is accompanied by these symptoms.

■ Be alert for symptoms of scarlet fever (described in the introduction to this entry) or rheumatic fever (*see* RHEUMATIC FEVER). These are serious complications that can accompany a streptococcus infection.

PREVENTION

■ Protect your child from environmental pollutants and respiratory irritants, such as cigarette smoke and wood smoke. It goes without saying that every child should be strongly discouraged from taking up smoking.

■ As much as possible, protect children from contact with sick playmates or infected others.

■ If recurrent strep infections are a problem, consider checking out the family pet. Cats have been known to harbor streptococcus bacteria.

■ If your child has had a strep infection, be sure to throw out her toothbrush and replace it with a new one.

Stomachache

See NAUSEA AND VOMITING.

Streptococcus Infection

See BAD BREATH; IMPETIGO; RHEUMATIC FEVER; SORE THROAT.

Stye

A stye is an infection on the edge of the eyelid that occurs in an oil-secreting gland located near the root of an eyelash. Often, more than one gland is affected. Styes are usually bacterial in origin, primarily caused by *Staphylococcus* bacteria. A more chronic but less inflamed bump in the same area is called a chalazion.

An emerging stye appears as a red, swollen, tender area on the rim of an eyelid. As pus forms, the red area may develop into a fluid-filled blister with a small but visible yellowish spot in the center, and the eye may water. Eventually, the blister opens and drains, and healing can begin.

Because it's irritating to have a bump within one's line of sight, a child may find it irresistible to scratch or rub at the stye, but it is important not to squeeze or try to puncture the lesion. This only worsens the infection. A stye should begin to improve within two or three days. A chalazion can last for several weeks without getting either better or worse.

CONVENTIONAL TREATMENT

WHEN TO CALL THE DOCTOR ABOUT A STYE

If you are treating your child's stye and the stye shows no signs of improvement after two or three days, or if it begins to spread, with increased swelling, consult your health care provider.

■ Warm-water compresses are the treatment of choice, since they help to bring the lesion to a head so that it can drain. Conventional medical treatment includes cleansing the area with sterile water and applying warm compresses, for ten minutes, four to six times daily. Cleanse the eyes with warm water after applying the compresses, and wash your hands both before and after administering the treatment. Use a clean compress each time. The compresses should not be scalding hot, but they should be as warm as your child can tolerate.

■ If the stye is persistent or the infection seems to be growing worse, an ophthalmic-formula antibiotic, such as erythromycin (Ilotycin), tobramycin (Tobrex), Sodium Sulamyd, or Polysporin, may be prescribed.

■ In rare cases, a stye may have to be opened with a needle to facilitate drainage. This procedure must be performed by a physician.

NUTRITIONAL SUPPLEMENTS

For age-appropriate dosages of nutritional supplements, see page 81.

■ Vitamin A is a specific for the eyes, and helps to soothe and heal mucous membranes. Give your child one dose of vitamin A daily. Beta-carotene can also be taken, along with vitamin A. Give your child one dose of beta-carotene a day, or one-half dose of each, twice daily, until the stye clears.

■ Vitamin C and bioflavonoids have anti-inflammatory and antibacterial properties. Give your child one-half dose of each, three to four times a day, for up to one week.

■ Zinc boosts the immune system, thus helping the body to fight infection. Give your child one dose of zinc, two to three times a day, for up to one week.

Note: Excessive amounts of zinc can result in nausea and vomiting. Be careful not to exceed the recommended dosage.

HERBAL TREATMENT

For age-appropriate dosages of herbal remedies, see page 81.

■ Use warm herbal compresses. Simmer 1 teaspoon of herb in 1 pint of water for ten minutes. Cool the resulting tea to a comfortably warm temperature and soak a clean cloth in it. Apply this warm, wet compress to the stye for ten minutes, four to six times a day. Any of the following herbs is recommended:

- Eyebright helps relieve redness and swelling of the eye, and will help clear an eye infection.
- Oregon grape root is a source of berberine, a potent natural antibiotic.
- Goldenseal is antibacterial and is also a good source of berberine.

■ To support your child's immune system and help clear infection, give him an echinacea and goldenseal combination formula orally. Echinacea is antiviral and antibacterial; goldenseal is antibacterial and helps to soothe mucous membranes. Give your child one dose, three times daily, for one week.

HOMEOPATHY

■ Give your child one dose of *Aconite* 30x or 9c when you first notice a stye developing. After this initial dose of *Aconite*, choose one of the other remedies recommended in this entry, based on your child's symptoms.

■ If your child's eyelid is red and swollen, give him one dose of *Apis mellifica* 30x or 9c, three times a day, for up to two days.

■ If the stye looks as if it is going to burst, give your child one dose of *Hepar sulphuris* 12x or 6c, three times a day, for up to two days. This remedy will help the stye to drain.

■ *Myristica* 12x or 6c is useful if the stye is taking a very long time to open. Give your child one dose, three times a day, for up to two days.

■ To help alleviate pain, give your child one dose of *Staphysagria* 12x or 6c, four times a day.

GENERAL RECOMMENDATIONS

■ Flush your child's eye with sterile water.

■ Apply warm Oregon grape root, eyebright, or goldenseal compresses.

■ Follow the appropriate homeopathic protocol.

■ Explain to your child that touching, rubbing, or scratching the eyelid will make the infection worse. Offer distractions to keep his fingers busy.

PREVENTION

■ Teach your child to keep his hands clean and to avoid rubbing his eyes.

■ If your child has a tendency to develop recurrent styes, the aptly named herb eyebright may be helpful. Give your child one dose in tea form, several times a week, for a few months.

■ Encourage your child to eat plenty of green and yellow vegetables. These vegetables are rich in beta-carotene, the precursor of vitamin A, the "eye vitamin." Vitamin A benefits the eyes in general and supports healthy membranes in particular.

Sunburn

Sunburn is caused by exposure to radiation from the sun. It is usually a first-degree burn. In other words, it involves the epidermis, the outer (superficial) layer of the skin. If your child is sunburned, the exposed skin will be hot, red, and painful. If the skin blisters and swelling develops, a second-degree burn has occurred, and the dermis, the underlying layer of skin, has been affected (*see* BURNS).

The radiation that causes sunburn comes down to the earth in the form of ultraviolet (UV) rays. There are two types of UV radiation: ultraviolet-A (UVA), which is present year round, and ultraviolet-B (UVB), which is present primarily in the summer months. While it was once believed that only UVB radiation presented the danger of damage from the sun, it is now known that UVA radiation is harmful also. As a result, experts recommend taking precautions against sun exposure no matter what the season.

A child's skin is tender and fragile. Without the protection of sunscreen, a hat, or clothing, it burns quickly. The sun's rays are further intensified when they are reflected by water or sand, and by suntan oils and lotions that do not contain sunscreen. Even if a child is wearing a T-shirt and sitting under a beach umbrella, reflected radiation can burn through the shirt.

A child's delicate skin should be sheltered from the sun. The long-term hazards of sun exposure have long been well known. More recent evidence suggests that skin cancer may be even more closely related to sunburn—even a single bad case, and especially a burn that occurs in childhood—than to total long-term sun exposure.

Just because your child doesn't seem to be getting burned as she plays outside, you cannot assume that she is unaffected by the sun's rays. A sunburn can develop and deepen even after your child is home and in bed. The pain of sunburn is most intense six to forty-eight hours after exposure to the sun. Skin that is lightly pinked when your child goes to bed may turn red, burning, and painful by the next morning. A severe sunburn can cause nausea, chills, and fever, as well as intense stinging.

CONVENTIONAL TREATMENT

WHEN TO CALL THE DOCTOR ABOUT SUNBURN

Most cases of sunburn can be cared for at home, with natural remedies. Under certain circumstances, however, you should seek your doctor's advice:

• If your child's sunburned skin becomes blistered or swollen, call your health care provider. When blisters open, as with any open wound, there is an increased risk of infection.

• If a sunburned child develops secondary symptoms, such as chills, fever, or nausea, consult your physician. These may be signs of sun poisoning.

■ Painkillers such as aspirin, ibuprofen, and acetaminophen can be used to decrease the severity of sunburn pain if given soon after exposure, but before a full-blown burn develops. Do not give your child aspirin if there is any possibility that she may have a viral illness, however. If you give your child acetaminophen, read the dosage instructions on the package carefully, as excessive amounts of this drug can cause liver damage. Ibuprofen is often best given with food to avoid possible stomach upset.

■ Cool showers, baths, or compresses are very soothing, and may prevent worsening of the burn, especially if used soon after sun exposure.

■ If your child suffers itching as a sunburn heals, an antihistamine such as Atarax, Benadryl, or Chlor-Trimeton may be recommended to counter the itching and swelling.

■ Anesthetic sprays that contain benzocaine are of value in some cases, especially if pain is severe. They can cause an allergic skin reaction and eczema in some children, however, and should not be used routinely on a child's sensitive skin.

■ For extremely severe sunburns, cortisone-like drugs such as prednisone may be prescribed, to be taken orally or used in a topical spray. Although this can be dramatically effective when given early on, there are potentially serious side effects.

NUTRITIONAL SUPPLEMENTS

For age-appropriate dosages of nutritional supplements, see page 81.

■ Give your child one dose of beta-carotene, twice a day, for two weeks after a sunburn. This nutrient also helps protect against burns.

■ Give your child one dose each of mineral ascorbate vitamin C and bioflavonoids, twice a day, for two weeks following a sunburn.

■ Zinc boosts the immune system and aids in healing. Give your child one dose of zinc, once or twice a day, for up to two weeks after she suffers a sunburn.

Note: Excessive amounts of zinc can result in nausea and vomiting. Be careful not to exceed the recommended dosage.

HERBAL TREATMENT

■ Aloe vera has been used for centuries to soothe and cool burns. To take the heat and stinging out of your child's sunburned skin, gently rub 100-percent aloe vera gel on the hurt area. Apply it as often as needed.

■ To take the heat out of the skin and help promote healing, soak a clean white cloth in cool comfrey-root tea and apply the compress to the affected area. Comfrey is high in allantoin, a compound that helps to promote healing.

■ Infection-fighting gotu kola is effective against sunburn. Give a child over four years of age 1 to 2 cups of gotu kola tea or two capsules of gotu kola daily.

■ To relieve stinging and burning, you may apply nettle lotion, tincture, or ointment directly to the burned area.

HOMEOPATHY

■ *Urtica urens*, homeopathic stinging nettle, will quickly reduce the stinging and burning pain of sunburn. Give your child one dose of *Urtica urens* 12x or 6c, every fifteen minutes, for a total of four doses. Thereafter, give your child one dose every hour, up to a total of three more doses.

■ If your child develops a slight fever after the pain has been relieved, *Ferrum phosphoricum* will help. Give your child one dose of *Ferrum phosphoricum* 12x or 6c every hour, up to a total of four doses.

GENERAL RECOMMENDATIONS

■ If you suspect your child may be developing a sunburn, take her out of the sun right away.

■ To soothe and cool a sunburn quickly, apply aloe vera gel to the affected area.

■ Give your child homeopathic *Urtica urens*.

■ After your child has been overexposed to the sun, have her soak in a cool bath. This will help to take the heat out of the burn, lessen the pain, and moisturize parched skin. Reapply aloe vera after the bath.

■ For an extra-soothing soak, treat your child's bath water with ½ cup of oatmeal (or Aveeno, a commercial product that is an oatmeal derivative). Wrap the oatmeal in a washcloth and let it soak in the tub. You can also *gently* rub the oatmeal-filled washcloth on your child's skin.

■ To soothe the worst areas of the burn, apply cool compresses where needed.

■ Dehydration often accompanies excessive exposure to the sun. Make sure your child gets sufficient fluids after spending time in the sun.

PREVENTION

■ *Always* apply a sunscreen to your child's skin when she will be in the sun. Make sure you select a formula that screens out both UVA and UVB rays, that has an SPF of 10 or higher, and that is specifically designed for a child's delicate skin. Apply generously before your child goes out in the sun, and reapply the sunscreen every three or four hours throughout the day for as long as your child is outside.

■ Make sure your child wears sunglasses and, if possible, a hat when she is in the sun. Like sunscreen, sunglasses should screen out both UVA and UVB rays to provide effective protection.

■ Limit your child's outdoor play in bright sunlight during the middle of the day (between 10:00 A.M. and 2:00 P.M.), when the sun is at its highest and strongest point.

■ Divide outdoor playing time between sunlight and shade. Do not permit your child to be in the sun for more than a total of three or four hours on any day.

■ In the summer, start your child off with short exposures to sunshine. As her skin becomes accustomed to the sun, she can gradually work up to longer periods of exposure by the end of the season.

■ Don't be fooled by cloudy or hazy days. Approximately 80 percent of the sun's rays pass through clouds. Take the same precautions on hazy days as you would on bright, sunny days.

■ When exposure to sunshine is inevitable, protect your child with a hat and cover exposed skin with loose, light-colored clothing. Because the sun can burn through clothing, monitor your child's exposure continuously.

■ Explain the dangers of sunbathing, and especially tanning salons, particularly if your child is a teenager. Tanning salons sometimes advertise that their machines are "safe" because they emit only UVA rays. This is simply not true. Exposure to UVA radiation can cause skin cancer just as well as UVB radiation can. Both should be avoided. As one dermatologist put it, a suntan is really just a sign of skin damage.

Surgery, Recovering From

There may be a time in your child's life when surgery is a necessary intervention. After any surgery, no matter how minor, a certain amount of time is required for the body to heal itself. Generally speaking, a child's tissues heal quickly. By the time you take your child home from the hospital, the healing process will probably be well underway. You can support and speed that process by implementing a healthy regimen for your child both before and after the surgery, and by following your doctor's suggestions.

CONVENTIONAL TREATMENT

■ After consultation with the surgeon, your private physician may give you specific instructions for your child's diet, activity level, or special exercises, as well as any precautions you should take to guard against complications. Take these recommendations seriously, especially those regarding activity level.

■ After a surgical procedure, even a minor one, a child may suffer pain. The pain may be mild and easily managed with an analgesic such as acetaminophen (Tylenol, Tempra, or the equivalent) or ibuprofen (Advil, Nuprin, and others). Follow package directions for proper dosage and administration. If your child's surgery was extensive, however, the pain associated with the healing process may be severe and require stronger, perhaps prescription, medication. Try to make certain that your child receives adequate pain relief. Children, especially young children, may not be articulate when it comes to describing pain. This does not mean they don't feel pain, however. Nonverbal signs that a child may be in pain include irritability, restlessness, lack of interest in usually engaging activities, unusual quietness or withdrawal, a tendency to "protect" a part of the body, lack of appetite, and an inability to sleep. If not relieved, pain is a source of stress, and stress can slow down the healing process. If your child requires powerful medication for pain, keep in mind that it is rare for anyone, including a child, to become addicted to pain medications if they are used to treat a short-term problem. For more information about pain management, *see* PAIN RELIEF.

DIETARY GUIDELINES

■ Depending on the type of surgery your child had, your physician will prescribe a regulated diet for a time for medical reasons. Follow your doctor's instructions.

■ Even after your doctor gives full permission for your child to eat, he may have little or no appetite. Once your child feels like eating, begin by offering clear liquids, such as broth, fruit juices, and herbal teas. Applesauce and toast also make good "starter" foods.

■ To allow your child's gastrointestinal tract to readjust to food, gradually work up to a full diet. Prepare whole foods full of the many vitamins and minerals your child's body needs to heal and regain energy. Begin with foods that are easier to digest and work up to a normal diet gradually. As your child recovers, a healthy whole-foods diet will help him feel better than he did before the operation.

NUTRITIONAL SUPPLEMENTS

For age-appropriate dosages of some nutritional supplements, see page 81.

■ If your child needs surgery, you can help his body prepare for and recover from it with a simple program of nutritional supplements and natural remedies. Begin the following program anytime up to two weeks before the day of surgery, and maintain it for one month afterwards.

- Beta-carotene, a precursor of vitamin A, soothes injured mucous membranes and helps heal tissue. Give your child one dose daily.

- Vitamin C with bioflavonoids helps with tissue repair and in decreasing inflammation. Give your child one dose, two to three times a day.

- Zinc hastens wound and tissue healing. Give your child one dose, two to three times a day.
    Note: Excessive amounts of zinc can result in nausea and vomiting. Be careful not to exceed the recommended dosage.

■ If your child has gastrointestinal surgery, give him a *Lactobacillus acidophilus* or *bifidus* supplement for one month following the operation. Follow dosage directions on the product label.

■ Vitamin E is an antioxidant nutrient and is a mild but effective anti-inflammatory. Give your child one dose, twice a day, for up to one month following surgery.

HERBAL TREATMENT

For age-appropriate dosages of herbal remedies, see page 81.

■ Echinacea and goldenseal combination formula helps to detoxify the blood after anesthesia, and can help prevent infection of the surgical wound. These herbs also support the immune system. Give your child one dose, twice daily, on the first, second, and third days following surgery.

■ With its rich concentration of trace minerals and micronutrients, astragalus (*Astragalus membranaceous*) will help strengthen your child's immune system and support healing. Give your child one dose, three times daily, on the fifth, sixth, and seventh days after surgery.

Note: This herb should not be given until fever or other signs of infection are no longer present.

■ American ginseng is an excellent source of trace minerals and micronutrients. It will support and strengthen your child's internal defenses. Give your child one dose, three times daily, on the eighth through fifteenth days after surgery.

Note: This herb should not be given if a fever or any other sign of infection is present.

■ Gotu kola is a general tonic that also speeds wound healing. Give a child four years of age or older one to two doses of tea or two capsules daily, for three to four weeks after surgery.

HOMEOPATHY

■ To begin detoxifying the blood after general anesthesia, give your child one dose of *Nux vomica* 30x or 200x when he awakens from anesthetic sleep. This homeopathic will also help to reduce the nausea associated with anesthetics. Wait three hours and if your child is still nauseous, give one more dose.

■ If your child received general anesthesia, *Phosphorus* will help detoxify his overloaded liver. The liver is the organ responsible for clearing anesthetic chemicals from the body. One to two hours after giving the second dose of *Nux vomica* as described above, give your child one dose of *Phosphorus* 30x or 200x.

■ The following regimen will support and hasten the healing process.

Days 1–2: Give your child one dose of *Arnica* 30x or 9c, three to four times daily, to help decrease inflammation following surgery and speed the healing process.

Day 3: To further hasten healing of tissues injured by surgery, give your child one dose of *Ledum* 12x or 6c, three to four times during the day.

Days 4–5: For nerve pain following surgery, give your child one dose of *Hypericum* 12x or 6c, three to four times daily.

■ If your child's abdomen is bloated and he is looking weak, give him one dose of *China* 30x or 9c, three times a day, for up to two days.

BACH FLOWER REMEDIES

■ On the day of surgery, immediately following the procedure (as soon as your physician gives you the okay), give your child one dose of Bach Flower Rescue Remedy. You may wish to take a dose of Rescue Remedy yourself as well. One hour later, give your child a dose of homeopathic *Arnica* 30x, 200x, 9c, or 15c.

GENERAL RECOMMENDATIONS

■ To ensure a full and strong recovery after surgery, or any serious illness, adequate rest is essential. Limit visitors. Minimize distractions. Create a calm and familiar environment. A cozy, dimly lighted room, thick blankets, and soft music are conducive to rest and relaxation. For a restless, uncomfortable child, try reading and/or playing audiocassette tapes of stories.

■ Keep your child well hydrated. Offer plenty of water, nourishing broths, apple juice, and herbal teas. Even a child who isn't thirsty will often sip water or juice through a straw.

■ As healing progresses and appetite returns, provide a healthy whole-foods diet for your child.

■ Select and administer appropriate homeopathic remedies.

■ Give your child mineral ascorbate vitamin C and bioflavonoids, beta-carotene, and zinc.

■ A surgical wound, like any wound, can become infected. Watch for signs and symptoms of a local infection. If the area becomes red, warm, swollen, or tender, or if a fever develops, call your surgeon or physician.

■ Once your physician has told you that the surgical wound is *completely closed*, rub castor oil or vitamin-E or evening primrose oil into it to speed healing and minimize scarring.

Tantrums

See EMOTIONAL UPSET.

Teething

Teething is the process by which an infant's first deciduous (baby) teeth erupt through the gums. Teething normally begins between the sixth and eighth months of life. Once your baby's first tooth arrives, another new one will appear about every month. Although the rate and order of emerging teeth is different for different children, the two middle teeth on the bottom tend to erupt first, followed by the lower teeth that surround them, and then the upper two middle teeth. The molars are the last to appear. Eruption continues until the child's complete set of twenty baby teeth has appeared, usually by the age of thirty months.

A child's permanent teeth begin to come in at the age of six or seven years. As a permanent tooth emerges, the baby tooth it is replacing is nudged out. Fortunately, emerging permanent teeth do not create the same irritation and discomfort that babies experience when teething (with the exception of the last set of molars, also known as wisdom teeth, which usually erupt sometime in the late teen or early adult years).

Signs of teething include sore, inflamed gums, a low-grade temperature, drooling, a fondness for biting on hard objects, irritability, difficulty sleeping, and, often, loss of appetite. Teething is also sometimes accompanied by a tendency toward increased nasal congestion, which can lead to colds or ear infections. The pain, discomfort, and inflamed gums a teething child experiences result from the pressure that is exerted against the gum tissue as the crown of a tooth breaks through the membranes. A baby's cheeks may become red and chapped as a result of much drooling. Your infant may chew or suck her fingers, or seek an object to bite and chew on. A teething baby is easily irritated and more restless than usual, sometimes awakening as often as once an hour through the night.

CONVENTIONAL TREATMENT

WHEN TO CALL THE DOCTOR ABOUT SYMPTOMS ACCOMPANYING TEETHING

Because the teething process itself causes stress to the body, a teething infant is more susceptible to illness. Fever and diarrhea may occur during teething. These symptoms indicate illness. The teething process alone does not cause a high fever or diarrhea, so if these symptoms occur, or if your child seems acutely uncomfortable, seek medical advice.

■ To numb the area and provide temporary relief from teething pain, your physician may recommend lidocaine or benzocaine ointment. These local anesthetics can be rubbed (sparingly) onto your baby's gums. Anbesol is a good choice.

■ A mild pain reliever, such as acetaminophen (in Tylenol, Tempra, and other medications) or ibuprofen (Advil, Nuprin, and others) can help reduce the pain an emerging tooth causes. Follow age-appropriate dosage directions on the product label.

HERBAL TREATMENT

■ Clove oil acts as a natural anesthetic. It has a pleasant taste and quickly eases sore gums. However, it should be used in moderation, as excessive amounts can cause blistering. So that it is not too strong for your baby, blend 1 drop of clove oil with 1 to 2 tablespoons of safflower oil. With your fingertip or a cotton swab, massage the mixture onto your child's sore gums.

■ Licorice root powder can be made into a paste that is very soothing to inflamed gums. Mix a small amount (about ⅛ teaspoon) with enough water to make a paste and gently pat the mixture onto your baby's gums.

HOMEOPATHY

■ *Calcarea carbonica* is good for a baby who has delayed teething with difficult tooth emergence. She has a round, shiny "Gerber baby" face. Give this child one dose of *Calcarea carbonica* 30x or 9c, twice a day during teething, up to a total of six doses.

■ *Chamomilla* is commonly used for teething. It is especially useful for the infant whose gums bleed easily and are red, swollen, and sensitive to the touch. This baby is very irritable, feels worse at night, worse with warmth, and is comforted when carried around. Give this child *Chamomilla* 12x or 6c, every hour, as needed, up to a total of six doses.

■ A combination teething remedy may prove helpful to your child if neither of the above remedies seems right. Follow dosage directions on the product label.

ACUPRESSURE

For the locations of acupressure points on a child's body, *see* ADMINISTERING AN ACUPRESSURE TREATMENT in Part Three.

■ Large Intestine 4 relieves face and tooth pain and calms a stressed nervous system.

■ Liver 3 relaxes the nervous system.

GENERAL RECOMMENDATIONS

■ Massage your infant's sore and irritated gums with your fingertip to help ease the pain and tension. Use a drop of clove oil diluted in safflower oil as described above.

■ Choose an appropriate homeopathic remedy.

■ Give a teething infant something hard to bite on, such as a hard rubber teething ring or toy, or a hard biscuit. Biting helps to balance the pressure exerted by an emerging tooth. When choosing items for your teething child to chew and bite down on, be sure to select unbreakable items and toys without small parts that can come loose and cause choking. Hard rubber items are safest.

■ Cold soothes and numbs sore gums. Keep several clean and sterile hard rubber items in the refrigerator or freezer for your infant to chew on. If your baby welcomes the cold, as one item warms, substitute a cold one. Or try refrigerating an apple and giving your baby a slice of it to bite on (make sure to cut a fairly thick slice, not a small chunk, which might pose a choking hazard). Some babies like mashing their gums on this better than gnawing on an iced teething ring.

PREVENTION

■ Teething is a natural process, and so cannot be prevented. Pain from teething can be minimized, however, by following the suggestions above.

Tetanus

Tetanus, also known as lockjaw, is a consequence of infection by *Clostridium tetani*, an organism found in the soil, manure, and everyday dirt. It enters the body through an open wound, particularly a puncture wound or the umbilicus of a newborn, and releases a toxin that travels to the central nervous system, causing severe muscle stiffness and spasms. Once the organism enters the body, the incubation period can be one to twelve days, or even longer. Tetanus is not transmitted from one person to another.

The wound through which the organism enters the body often heals before other symptoms appear. The illness begins with muscle stiffness in the neck and jaw and progresses over the next twenty-four hours into painful muscle rigidity and spasms. Normal muscle function can be so impaired that breathing may stop during the first three to four days. This can be a life-threatening situation that requires hospitalization and close medical attention.

If your child suffers a puncture wound, call your doctor promptly. Your child may need to have his tetanus immunization updated and the wound properly cleaned and debrided to avoid the risk of developing the disease. If your child displays symptoms of tetanus, even if he doesn't remember any injury that could have exposed him to the risk of the disease, call your doctor right away.

CONVENTIONAL TREATMENT

■ If your child develops tetanus, he will probably have to be hospitalized for treatment. This is a complex process that involves the administration of medications including antitoxin, antibiotics, painkillers, and drugs that relax muscles and decrease spasms; measures aimed at supporting nutrition and elimination and preventing the development of secondary infections, such as pneumonia; continuous monitoring of bodily functions; as well as other additional interventions as the need arises.

■ Having the disease once does not give a person lifelong immunity to it. Once your child recovers, your physician will recommend that he receive a full course of immunizations.

DIETARY GUIDELINES

■ A child who is healing from any illness or injury should not consume any refined sugars. Sugar makes the body more acidic, which slows healing. When your child's body is working to repair itself, avoiding sugar helps create a more balanced, alkaline internal environment.

NUTRITIONAL SUPPLEMENTS

The nutritional supplements listed below are aimed at supporting your child's recovery from a puncture wound. They are not intended as substitutes for appropriate tetanus immunization or professional wound treatment. For age-appropriate dosages of nutritional supplements, see page 81.

■ Mineral ascorbate vitamin C and bioflavonoids help heal skin tissue and prevent infection after an injury. Give your child approximately one-half dose of each, three times a day, for one week following a puncture wound. Then give the same dosage twice a day for two weeks. Generally, the larger the child and the dirtier the wound, the higher the appropriate dose.

■ Vitamin E and beta-carotene help to promote healing and support the immune system. Give your child one dose of vitamin E, twice a day, and one dose of beta-carotene daily, until the wound heals.

■ Zinc helps to boost the immune system. Give your child one dose, twice a day, for up to ten days following a puncture wound.

Note: Excessive amounts of zinc can result in nausea and vomiting. Be careful not to exceed the recommended dosage.

HERBAL TREATMENT

The herbal treatments outlined below are aimed at supporting your child's recovery from a puncture wound. They are not intended to substitute for appropriate tetanus immunization or professional wound treatment. For age-appropriate dosages of herbal remedies, see page 81.

■ Echinacea and goldenseal combination formula will help boost your child's immune system. Give your child one dose, three to four times a day, for three days.

■ Garlic has antibacterial properties. Choose an odorless form, and follow the dosage directions on the product label. Or you can give a child older than one year one to three cloves of fresh garlic mashed in honey each day.

■ Make an herbal poultice. Add 1 tablespoon of any or all of the following to 1 cup of water: plantain, marshmallow root, goldenseal, and Oregon grape root. Bring to a boil and simmer for twenty minutes. Soak a washcloth in the mixture and apply it to the affected area for twenty to thirty minutes. Do this three times a day for two to three days.

■ Super salve, an ointment made from chaparral, echinacea, hops, and usnea moss, fights infection and is soothing to injured skin. Apply to the wound three or four times a day.

HOMEOPATHY

The following homeopathic remedy is aimed at supporting your child's recovery from a puncture wound. It is not intended as a substitute for appropriate tetanus immunization or professional wound treatment.

■ *Ledum* is a homeopathic remedy specifically for puncture wounds. Give your child one dose of *Ledum* 12x or 6c, every thirty minutes, up to a total of three doses. Then give one dose, four times a day, for up to two days.

BACH FLOWER REMEDIES

■ If your child suffers a puncture wound, give him a dose of Bach Flower Rescue Remedy as soon as possible. This wonderful natural remedy helps to calm and stabilize the anxiety, shock, or fright a child may experience after an injury.

GENERAL RECOMMENDATIONS

■ If your child suffers a puncture wound, consult your doctor promptly for proper cleansing and possibly a tetanus vaccine update.

■ Give your child homeopathic *Ledum*, echinacea and goldenseal, garlic, and/or nutritional supplements as outlined above while he is recovering from a puncture wound.

■ If your child displays the symptoms of tetanus, even if he has no memory of an injury, call your physician immediately. A child with tetanus needs professional medical treatment.

PREVENTION

■ The tetanus toxoid vaccine, which prevents tetanus, is usually given in combination with vaccination against diphtheria (the DT vaccine) or diphtheria and pertussis (DPT), but it can be administered individually. It is normally given by injection when a child is approximately two months, four months, six months, eighteen months, four to six years, and fourteen to sixteen years of age. Thereafter, a booster may be given every ten years, or after an injury is suffered.

■ All wounds, especially punctures, should immediately be washed with plenty of water to which a small amount of hydrogen peroxide or povidone iodine solution (Betadine) has been added.

■ For suggestions of things you can do to reduce the possibility that your child will have an accident that could place him at risk of exposure to tetanus, *see* HOME SAFETY in Part One.

Throat, Sore

See SORE THROAT.

Thrush

Thrush, or *moniliasis*, is a fungal infection of the mouth. It is caused by the yeastlike fungus *Candida albicans*, which can also cause diaper rash and vaginal yeast infections. Thrush is usually seen in children under six months of age. In older children, it is much less common and its occurrence may indicate a serious illness, such as an immune deficiency.

Thrush appears as white, flaky, cheesy-looking patches covering all or part of the tongue and gums, the inside of the cheeks, and, sometimes, the lips. These patches do not scrape off easily. When they are picked or scraped off, they leave a red, inflamed area that may bleed. Milk curds look like thrush, but curds scrape off very easily without leaving a sore area. The pain of thrush may interfere with feeding. It can cause your infant to lose her appetite.

Thrush is usually self-limiting, but it should be treated to avoid a long, chronic course of infection. If pain from the infection prevents your baby from taking sufficient fluids, aggressive treatment is necessary. Insufficient feeding can compromise hydration and nutrient needs. If you are nursing your baby, it is possible for her to spread the thrush to one or both of your nipples. Nipples with a thrush infection will be red, swollen, and tender, and may be cracked. There may also be itching, flaking, and burning.

If thrush is accompanied by fever, cough, or stomach upset, call your doctor. These could be signs of a compromised immune system.

CONVENTIONAL TREATMENT

■ The most commonly prescribed medication for thrush is a liquid antifungal, such as nystatin (in the medications Mycostatin and Nilstat), given four times daily, until the infection clears. You may either swab your baby's mouth with this medicine or gently squirt the liquid into her mouth with a medicine dropper or syringe. Infants can suck the medicine directly from a syringe. Because of nystatin's high sugar content, caution should be exercised when treating a child who has teeth with this formula. Prolonged use can promote cavities.

■ A breastfeeding mother whose infant has thrush should also be treated with nystatin. To avoid a "ping-pong" effect—where infection passes from baby to mother and back again—nystatin ointment can be applied to a nursing mother's nipples. It's all right for your baby to take in a bit of nystatin from the nipples.

■ To ease the pain of infection and help your baby feed more comfortably, a pain reliever such as acetaminophen (Tylenol, Tempra, and others) may be useful. Follow the instructions on the product package, being careful not to exceed the proper dosage for your child's age and size.

■ Gentian violet in a 1-percent solution can help clear a thrush infection. This is a purple dye that is swabbed on the inside of your baby's mouth and, if necessary, over your nipples. Be careful when applying it—it does stain.

DIETARY GUIDELINES

■ The mother of a breastfed infant who has thrush should drastically reduce the amount of sugar in her diet or, better yet, eliminate it entirely. Fungus thrives on sugar and proliferates in its presence.

■ Reducing or eliminating fats can also be helpful, with one notable exception: A diet that includes cold-pressed, uncooked olive oil may inhibit the growth of yeast.

NUTRITIONAL SUPPLEMENTS

■ The antioxidant nutrients beta-carotene, vitamin C, vitamin E, zinc, and selenium can help to control yeast in a nursing mother. Follow dosage directions on the product labels.

   Note: Excessive amounts of zinc can result in nausea and vomiting. Be careful not to exceed the recommended dosage.

■ Caprylic acid, a short-chain fatty acid, helps to kill yeast. A nursing mother may take one capsule, two to three times a day.

■ *Lactobacillus acidophilus* and *bifidus* are friendly bacteria that help clear the body of fungus. Follow the dosage directions on the product label for mother and/or baby.

HERBAL TREATMENT

■ Grapefruit seed extract is very helpful for reducing the yeast in a breastfeeding mother's intestinal tract. A nursing mother may take 250 milligrams daily or 10 drops in 1 cup of water, two or three times a day, for two to three weeks.

■ Aloe vera gel has been shown to have antifungal properties. Try dipping your finger in aloe vera gel and applying it topically to the thrush, two or three times a day, until the infection clears. Use a food-grade product for this purpose.

■ Garlic has yeast-fighting properties, although it can sometimes cause colic. A nursing mother can take one odorless garlic capsule, twice daily, for two to three weeks.

■ Ginger tea has antibacterial and antifungal properties. A nursing mother can take one cup with meals.

HOMEOPATHY

■ For thrush accompanied by restlessness and/or fatigue, try one dose of *Arsenicum album* 30x or 9c, three times a day, for up to three days.

■ If your baby has thrush and is generally overheated, try giving her one dose of *Sulphur* 30x or 9c, three times a day, for up to two days.

■ If your child developed thrush after receiving a vaccination, try one dose of *Thuja* 200x or 30c.

GENERAL RECOMMENDATIONS

■ *Do not* try to scrape or pick off patches of thrush from inside your infant's mouth. You will hurt your child and leave behind an inflamed, possibly raw and bleeding area.

■ A lactobacillus mouthwash may be helpful. Mix ⅛ teaspoon of a lactobacillus supplement in ½ cup of water. Using an eyedropper, squirt the solution on your baby's gums, tongue, and the insides of the cheeks.

PREVENTION

■ Nursing mothers should keep their refined-sugar intake to a moderate or low level. Taking ginger tea with meals may also be helpful.

■ Antibiotics alter the normal flora of the mouth and body, predisposing an infant to thrush by allowing an overgrowth of candida. To maintain the friendly bacteria that help control candida within the body, a nursing mother should eat yogurt regularly or supplement her diet with *Lactobacillus bifidus* when taking antibiotics. If a bottlefed infant is taking antibiotics, add *Lactobacillus bifidus* to her formula.

■ Never underestimate the importance of simple, practical cleanliness. A nursing mother should avoid having her breasts stay moist for too long by keeping them dry between feedings and allowing them some "air time." If it is necessary to clean them, use water with a tiny bit of hydrogen peroxide added. Bottlefed babies sometimes contract oral thrush as a result of sucking on inadequately cleaned pacifiers or bottle nipples (often the result of dropping them and then putting them back into the mouth), in combination with a fruit-juice-rich diet or following antibiotic treatment for an ear infection. To avoid this, always have an ample supply of clean rubber nipples, pacifiers, and/or teething items on hand, or clean any such item that pops out of your baby's mouth with hydrogen peroxide and rinse it in water before giving it back to your baby.

Thumb-Sucking

Thumb-sucking is very common in infants. Thanks to ultrasound, a device that can show the image of a fetus in utero, we now know that some babies suck their thumbs in the womb as early as eighteen weeks of gestation.

In newborns, suckling is an instinctive response. Almost all babies suck their thumbs at one time or another. When the breast or the bottle isn't ready, it's natural for an infant to soothe himself by suckling on something, whether it's an ever-available thumb or finger, a pacifier, a toy, or the edge of a blanket. Thumb-sucking usually peaks between eighteen and twenty months of age. As a child grows and becomes older, the thumb becomes less and less important.

If your baby is a thumb-sucker, look on the habit as fulfilling a natural and instinctive need to suckle. If a young child continues sucking his thumb, experts agree that there is little need to worry about harm to emerging baby teeth. Your little one may resort to thumb-sucking when he is hungry, overtired, distressed and in need of comfort, or just plain bored. By the age of two or three, your child will likely have more exciting things to do and think about, and will be too busy to bother with his thumb.

A sensitive and shy child who has given up the thumb may return to thumb-sucking during the first few weeks in a new school or new home, or after the birth of a new sibling. This comfort-seeking behavior will normally be merely a passing phase, and will disappear with liberal love and reassurance from you. Should the habit be kept up for longer than a few weeks and appear to be becoming persistent, however, you may need to intervene.

If a child continues sucking his thumb past the age of five or six, or after the loss of his baby teeth, a visit to the dentist (or a counselor) is indicated. Prolonged and persistent thumb-sucking can lead to a malocclusion, a condition in which the upper and lower teeth do not meet properly. If your child positions his thumb pushing against the root edge of the teeth—which is common—prolonged and persistent thumb-sucking can lead to a malformation of the upper arch of the jawbone, causing the upper teeth to protrude. Long-term thumb-sucking can also cause an abnormality of the bony tissue of the favored thumb.

CONVENTIONAL TREATMENT

■ If thumb-sucking threatens the alignment of a child's permanent teeth, a good pediatric dentist should be consulted. In extreme cases, a device may be inserted behind the upper teeth that will make thumb-sucking uncomfortable or impossible. Because this will cause trauma to a child, such a device should be your very last resort.

GENERAL RECOMMENDATIONS

■ For a child under two years of age, no treatment is necessary. For a child between the ages of three and five, first try minimizing stress, giving warm and caring attention, and providing adequate stimulation. Once a child is past infancy, thumb-sucking becomes comfort-seeking behavior, rather than fulfilling a need to suckle. Heaping helpings of love may be more effective than anything else.

■ For a child over six, gently but consistently remove his thumb from his mouth every time sucking occurs. Among older children, thumb-sucking often occurs when they are tired or bored. Follow this with the positive reinforcement of a hug, and then initiate a distracting activity.

■ Never punish a child for thumb-sucking.

■ Whatever intervention may become necessary, be sure to enlist your child's support and participation. Without your child's understanding and cooperation, intervention may be perceived as punishment.

PREVENTION

■ Make sure your infant has ample time at the breast or bottle to satisfy the need to suckle. This is a good time to supply abundant cuddling as well.

■ Experts say that it is all but impossible to prevent thumb-sucking in some children. If all interventions fail, you may have to resign yourself to finding an excellent orthodontist after your child's permanent teeth are in place.

Tooth, Broken or Knocked Out

EMERGENCY TREATMENT FOR A BROKEN OR KNOCKED-OUT TOOTH

See the inset on page 395.

We often look at the structures of the mouth in a rather mechanical way—there are cavities, baby teeth, permanent teeth, perhaps braces. But if you think about the course of a child's development, you realize that for a newborn, his mouth is his primary means of communicating (through crying, cooing, and smiling) and of interacting with and learning about the world. His mouth brings relief of hunger as well as tranquil pleasure through suckling. Later, this versatile organ becomes a sensory probe for exploring our curious world—as we all know, babies and toddlers put *everything* in their mouths.

Fully one-third of the motor and sensory areas of the human brain are devoted to the mouth and oral structures. Disturbances here can therefore have far-reaching implications. Consequently, dental problems deserve serious attention. Among the most common tooth-related problems that affect children are injuries.

Toddlers and older children may suffer mouth injuries that result in a tooth being fractured or knocked out. A toddler may sink his baby teeth into the corner of the coffee table or the linoleum floor during an attempt at takeoff or landing. An older child can suffer a similar injury if he falls off his bicycle or is struck in the mouth by a softball. According to some estimates, injuries to the teeth account for as many as 50 percent of all childhood injuries.

Any child who suffers a tooth injury should be seen by a dentist, even if he seems to be fine afterwards. Complications such as an infection or abscess under the gum can develop and must be treated promptly. In addition, any tooth that has suffered trauma will have to be watched closely afterwards by your child's dentist. If your child has a baby tooth that was once pushed further into its socket, the permanent tooth that replaces it may emerge crooked or with some discoloration. Orthodontia and/or cosmetic dentistry may be necessary to treat the situation.

If your child suffers an injury that results in a fractured or knocked-out tooth, act quickly.

CONVENTIONAL TREATMENT

■ Take emergency measures to save the tooth (see page 395). Rely on your dentist to treat the injury and advise you on how to care for your child as he recovers.

394

Emergency Treatment for a Broken or Knocked-Out Tooth

➕ If your child has suffered a blow or injury to the mouth, wipe away any blood with a cool, clean, wet cloth and look at his teeth. If they are all present and properly aligned, check the *frenum* (the tissue that connects the lip to the gums) for lacerations.

➕ If a baby tooth is knocked out, don't worry about the tooth. However, if your child has a permanent tooth knocked out, and you find it within minutes, you should rinse it briefly to remove debris, but *do not* scrub it. Use one of the following (listed in order of preference) to rinse the tooth:

- A product called Save•A•Tooth, which is a nutrient-based solution designed specifically for this purpose (see the suggestions under Prevention on page 396).
- Physiologic saline solution (commercial eyewash).
- A cup (8 ounces) of water with ½ teaspoon of table salt dissolved in it.
- The child's own saliva.

➕ *Immediately* after rinsing the tooth, replace it in the tooth socket, checking its position with respect to adjacent teeth. Then call your dentist to explain the situation and arrange an emergency visit. If at all possible, it is better *not* to take the tooth to the dentist for reimplantation, but to replace it yourself and then seek your dentist's treatment. This will save precious time and prevent clotting from taking place in the socket. Also, immediately after an injury, the shock will cause your child's face to feel somewhat numb. If the tooth is reimplanted after this numbness (as well as the distraction of the event) has passed, this process will be needlessly difficult for your child.

➕ If all of your child's teeth are present but one appears to have been displaced deeper into the socket, clasp the bone and palate above the tooth firmly between your thumb and finger. Firmly but gently squeeze/massage with a downward motion to encourage the tooth to return to a normal position. Call your dentist to explain the situation and arrange an emergency visit.

➕ If your child has fractured a tooth, call your dentist. Tooth fractures vary in severity, depending on the amount of the inner tooth that has been exposed, and the severity is what determines the appropriate treatment. A chip or a very shallow fracture, for example, may require only cosmetic treatment—the fracture smoothed out to eliminate rough or sharp edges. In such a case the newly exposed area of tooth in time will calcify and become less sensitive as long as it is kept clean, brushed with a mineralizing toothpaste, and kept from contact with decalcifying foods such as carbonated sodas and apples (see TOOTH DECAY). If the fracture is somewhat deeper, your dentist may recommend restoring it by means of bonding techniques.

➕ A deeply fractured tooth requires immediate treatment to prevent infection and other complications. If your child suffers a deep tooth fracture, if possible, rinse the broken part quickly and hold it in place until it can be treated. Or place clean plastic wrap over the bleeding area and have your child secure it by biting steadily on a piece of folded gauze. This will seal off and protect the injured area until you can get to your dentist's office. If possible, save the broken piece of the tooth; it may be possible for your dentist to reattach it. Call your dentist to arrange an emergency visit.

➕ If a fracture is particularly severe, root canal therapy may be advised. A root canal is a procedure in which the nerve is removed and replaced with a sterile material such as a heavy wax or paste. Root canals are a source of controversy in dentistry, as they expose the immune system to mixtures of different metals and other foreign substances, some of which may have toxic or immune-compromising effects. Unfortunately, if a tooth is injured or decayed badly enough, there are, as yet, few alternatives except extraction. There is some research that suggests root canals may be better tolerated if they are performed before a tooth becomes seriously degenerated. Before agreeing to have root canal therapy performed on your child's tooth, it is a good idea to discuss with your dentist all of the available treatment options and the pros and cons of each for your individual child's situation.

DIETARY RECOMMENDATIONS

■ A child recovering from a tooth injury should eat a diet that contains plenty of lean protein, plus healthy concentrations of calcium, phosphorus, and vitamin D. Calcium-rich foods include all the familiar dairy products, plus green leafy vegetables, broccoli, cabbage, and Brussels sprouts. Figs, kelp, oats, prunes, sesame seeds, and tofu contain calcium as well. Phosphorus can be obtained from bananas, whole-grain breads and cereals, nuts, eggs, fish, and poultry. Vitamin D is present in fortified dairy products, eggs, and saltwater fish. The body also produces this vitamin as a result of exposure to the sun.

■ Eliminate carbonated soft drinks and sugary foods from your child's menu. The acid and phosphorus most sodas contain can cause the depletion of calcium from tooth enamel, making them weaker and slowing recovery; the dangers of sugar are well known.

HOMEOPATHY

■ One dose of *Aconite* 200x can be given immediately after an accident to alleviate some of the initial shock.

BACH FLOWER REMEDIES

■ After any injury, Bach Flower Rescue Remedy will help to ease your child's fright and anxiety. Add a few drops to a glass of water and have your child sip it, or place one or two drops of the undiluted remedy under his tongue. (*See* BACH FLOWER REMEDIES in Part One.)

GENERAL RECOMMENDATIONS

■ If your child suffers a mouth injury, take action at once. The speed of response is important. If at all possible, don't wait to have your dentist replace a knocked-out tooth or persuade a tooth that has been knocked up into its socket to come back down. Call your dentist after you have taken these measures yourself. In the case of a knocked-out tooth, if you are not able to reimplant it yourself, your next best choice is to keep the tooth in Save•A•Tooth solution and take it and your child to your dentist as quickly as you can.

PREVENTION

■ There are some injuries a parent cannot prevent. You can, however, reduce the possibility that your child will suffer a mouth injury by taking measures to childproof your house. *See* HOME SAFETY in Part One.

■ Be prepared. Keep Save•A•Tooth solution on hand in case your child knocks out or fractures a tooth. It is available in many drugstores or it can be ordered from the manufacturer, Biological Rescue Products, by calling 800–882–0505. It is a good idea to order two—one for home and one for the car. This nutrient-based product is simple to use, and research has shown that it can keep a tooth alive for hours if it cannot be reimplanted immediately (without protection, a knocked-out tooth will often die in about fifteen minutes). This reduces the possibility that a tooth will be permanently lost, causing your child stress and embarrassment and creating the need for years of expensive dental procedures and exposure to metal bridgework.

■ Teach your child to be appropriately cautious and thoughtful in all of his activities. Insist on proper headgear for activities like bicycling, skiing, and contact sports such as football or hockey. When riding in a car, always wear your seat belt and make sure your child does the same. A baby should always ride in an approved child restraint seat.

■ Proper oral hygiene and regular visits to the dentist are important. A decaying tooth is much more likely to chip or fracture than a healthy tooth. A good program of oral care should begin as soon as your baby is born—even before any teeth erupt (*see* TOOTH DECAY).

Tooth Decay

Tooth decay—known to dentists as *dental caries*—is a process by which the tooth enamel (the outer covering of the tooth) and the dentin (the body of the tooth) gradually disintegrate (see margin illustration, page 398). Tooth decay does not happen all at once. It takes months for the bacterial plaque on the surface of the teeth to dissolve its way through the outer enamel and into the dentin. After that happens, the bacteria can travel through structures called dentinal tubules toward the pulp, where it can lead to deep infection, the formation of abscesses, and possible tooth loss.

Tooth decay is a two-faceted disease. It requires, first, that a concentration of certain bacteria (which for unknown reasons seem to be more prevalent in some people's mouths than others) be left for long periods of time on the surface of the teeth. Second, it requires that an individual's teeth be susceptible to decay. This can be caused by a number of factors, including poor-quality tooth enamel, mineral imbalances in the blood, and/or acidic, mineral-deficient saliva. Certain foods are implicated in the decay process as well. At the top of the list of culprits are fermentable carbohydrates—refined starches and sugars, including fruits—and fats. Also, while a certain level of phosphorus is necessary for healthy teeth, an excessive amount of this mineral can be a problem because it may cause the depletion of calcium from tooth enamel. A child who consumes large quantities of meat, milk, and above all sodas, is probably getting more phosphorus than is good for her teeth. Finally, acidic foods, including soda pop, certain types of fruit, and chewable vitamin C tablets, also cause the loss of calcium from tooth enamel. (You'll notice that sweetened carbonated beverages—a favorite of many children, unfortunately—are actually a triple threat to healthy teeth.)

On the other hand, there are foods that can help fight and prevent tooth decay. Mineral-rich vegetables, nuts, and whole grains enhance the buffering (neutralizing) action of the saliva, and promote recalcification of the teeth. They also preserve teeth from the inside by helping to maintain proper balances of calcium, magnesium, and phosphorus. And tannin, which is found in black teas, grapes, and certain herbs, fights the bacteria that are involved in the decay process.

In the early stages of decay, there are likely to be no symptoms. Your child will probably not be aware of a developing cavity until it is pretty far advanced. Then the tooth may become sensitive to heat and cold, and your child may feel discomfort after eating sugary foods. In order to prevent your child's teeth from developing a serious decay problem, therefore, you should make sure she receives periodic dental examinations. A dentist can detect early signs of decay either visually or by probing (the spot on the surface of tooth where decay is beginning will feel softer than it should). At this stage the problem is simpler and relatively painless to treat. Your dentist should then also be able to help you identify and change the decay-promoting elements in your child's oral environment, so that you can reduce the chances of other cavities developing in the future.

CONVENTIONAL TREATMENT

■ When decay is found, treatment involves cleaning by the dentist to remove the decay and restoring the cleaned spot with a filling to seal out further decay and reconstruct the surface of the tooth.

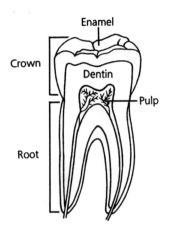

Enamel

Crown

Dentin

Pulp

Root

Structure of the Tooth

Many different materials can be used to fill teeth. Most commonly used in the United States are *amalgams*, which are silver-colored mixtures of metals that contain copper, tin, and zinc, among others, plus approximately 50 percent mercury. Because of the potential toxicity of these metals, especially mercury, there is growing concern about the safety of amalgam as a dental material. Some European countries, in fact, have set goals for the transition to mercury-free dental fillings. As a result, a number of effective nonmetallic and less potentially toxic filling materials (called *composites*) have been developed. Unfortunately, in order to use them, a dentist must spend a certain amount of time learning to handle them properly, something not all dentists are willing or able to do. If your child needs a filling, ask your dentist about the materials he or she uses. If you are concerned about metal fillings, you may wish to seek a dentist who shares your concern.

■ In cases where the decay has reached the pulp of a primary (baby) tooth, the tooth may be removed or a procedure called *pulpotomy* may be recommended. In a pulpotomy, enough of the infected pulp is removed to avoid inflammation and the formation of an abscess, thus saving the tooth, which is then restored with a crown. Most of the crowns used for this purpose are made of stainless steel or nickel-chromium. Both of these metals contain nickel, which can cause a variety of sensitivity or allergic reactions either in the mouth or, more commonly, on the skin elsewhere on the body. If avoiding these materials is important to you, discuss this with your dentist.

■ It is possible for a permanent tooth, particularly a molar, to develop deep decay that is not detectable by regular visual examination or even probing, but can be seen with the use of an x-ray or special transilluminating lights or lasers. In young children, these can often be treated by careful removal of the decay followed by the placement of a sedative dressing. As long as the pulp is still vital, this procedure will usually preserve it and allow the tooth to heal. If the decay is very deep into the pulp, a dentist may try a pulpotomy (see above), or may recommend root-canal treatment or extraction of the tooth.

■ Your dentist may recommend that a local anesthetic be injected into your child's gums to numb her mouth during a dental procedure. The injection of anesthetic itself is a source of anxiety to many children. Most small cavities should be able to be treated with minimal discomfort using modern cleaning and filling techniques, so it is probably better to bypass anesthesia in favor of less invasive measures, including distraction and the use of guided imagery. Certain procedures, however, such as pulpotomy or root canal, or the filling of deep and/or extensive decayed areas, may simply be too painful for your child if performed without anesthesia. In some cases, general anesthesia may be recommended. This is a subject you should discuss in advance with your child's dentist. What you decide will depend on the type of treatment your child needs as well as your child's feelings and past experiences with dental treatment.

DIETARY GUIDELINES

■ If your child is prone to tooth decay, eliminate sodas and sugary foods from the menu. Keep your child's consumption of fats and refined carbohydrates to a minimum. These foods promote tooth decay. Be especially wary of sticky foods that linger in the mouth. They are much more likely to cause problems than nonsticky foods.

■ Make sure your child gets plenty of vegetables and whole grains.

HOMEOPATHY

■ After your child undergoes a dental procedure, give her one dose of *Arnica* 30x, 200x, 15c, or 30c to help lessen residual pain and heal any traumatized tissue.

BACH FLOWER REMEDIES

■ If your child is fearful or apprehensive about dental treatment, give her Bach Flower Rescue Remedy immediately before and after a visit to the dentist.

ACUPRESSURE

For the locations of acupressure points on a child's body, *see* ADMINISTERING AN ACUPRESSURE TREATMENT in Part Three.

■ If your child is suffering from pain as a result of a cavity, massage Large Intestine 4. This acupressure point relieves face and tooth pain and calms a stressed nervous system.

■ Four Gates will help to relax an anxious or uncomfortable child.

GENERAL RECOMMENDATIONS

■ Choose a dentist who is skilled at working with children. A good pediatric dentist is the obvious choice, if you can find one in your area. If not, before taking your child to a dentist, visit him or her yourself for dental work to get a sense of his or her "touch" and feelings about children.

■ Dental visits need not be scary for children. Talk about visiting the dentist in an upbeat way and try to build up positive associations for your child. For example, you might talk about how good your clean teeth feel or how healthy and sparkling they look, and how nice the dentist is for helping them to get that way. Do this in short, simple comments spaced a few days apart; bring the subject up regularly but matter-of-factly, casually, and briefly. Avoid having big, serious discussions a few days before your child's dentist visit, or your child will sense that something is "up," and may either begin conjuring up scary images of the unknown or ask a more "reliable" source—a friend or sibling, who might get a kick out of scaring her—about what is going on.

■ When you take your child to the dentist's office, bring a tape or CD player with your child's favorite story or song and play it, slightly louder than usual, during the dental procedure (but not when receiving instructions from the dentist). It is also good to bring along a pair of sunglasses to help protect your child's eyes from the bright lights in the dental operatory and reduce the visual input. Your child may enjoy having her feet rubbed as a way to help her relax. This will also distract her from all the activity going on around her head.

■ Discuss your dentist's treatment plan thoroughly in advance, especially if your child needs more than one procedure performed. Many dentists routinely treat the worst cavity first, for example, but there is no reason that this has to be done, and it is often easier on a young patient if the procedure done first is the one that is least likely to be unpleasant. That way, you can avoid having your child get a

Caring for Your Child's Teeth

When it comes to your child's teeth, an ounce of prevention can be worth many pounds of cure. Proper oral hygiene begins at birth. Twice a day, use a bit of moistened gauze or a terry-cloth towel to gently clean your baby's gums and, as they erupt, her teeth, until a toothbrush can be tolerated. Don't wait until she has a mouthful of teeth to begin. One problem—unfortunately, not an uncommon one—among toddlers is "baby-bottle caries." This is tooth decay that occurs in a distinct, recognizable pattern as a result of a baby falling asleep with a bottle loosely in place in her mouth, her lips parted, and a puddle of formula or juice resting on her teeth. (Although less likely, this can even happen to a breastfeeding baby, if both mother and child doze off together frequently—breast milk is rich in sugars and fermentable carbohydrates.) If you must put your infant to bed with a bottle, fill it with clear water. Do not make it too easy for your baby to nurse from a bottle by enlarging the hole. Be especially careful with fruit juice! And be sure to cleanse your baby's teeth and tongue regularly.

As your baby gets a little older, place her near you as you brush your teeth and tongue and floss your teeth. Make your tooth-brushing a pleasant and relaxed time. It's best not to brush your teeth while leaning over the bathroom sink, because fatigue sets in quickly, reducing your effectiveness. Instead, sit down and listen to music or look at a magazine while brushing and flossing. You will find that you do a much more thorough job and feel fully refreshed. And one complete brushing job a day is better for your mouth than two "quickies," which are likely to get certain areas and miss others again and again. Begin to introduce an infant toothbrush or scrubber in a pleasurable, stimulating way, while commenting on how pretty your baby's teeth are. Toothpaste isn't necessary at this point. Regularly inspect your baby's teeth, gums, and tongue carefully.

As your child asserts more independence, you should not fully relinquish your role as cobrusher and inspector, but continue to monitor and train your child. Once your child has most of her baby teeth, flossing can begin. Your dental hygienist or dentist will usually note the effectiveness of your program and make appropriate suggestions. Continue to find opportunities to happily cleanse your own mouth in the presence of your child.

Exercise care in your choice of toothpaste for your child. Be sure to get a formula that can be swallowed without harm, because children *will* swallow. Avoid formulas with strong flavors, which can numb the tongue and create a deceptive feeling of cleanliness. Your child needs to be fully aware of the fuzzy spots she missed *while* she is brushing, not after the effect wears off and she is away from the brush. Also, strong flavorings, especially mint, can be irritating. Some of the most popular toothpaste brands have been associated with tissue reactions in children.

One recommended product is Merfluan. This is a baking soda-based powder with myrrh, natural oils, sea salt, calcium, and magnesium. It comes in a variety of flavors, including a pleasant lemon-lime formula. Your child doesn't have to use very much for it to be effective, and research has shown that it is better than fluoride at remineralizing (strengthening) tooth enamel. Another good product is Desert Essence Tea Tree toothpaste. This is reasonably mild when used sparingly, is all-vegetable and safe, and is a natural antiseptic. Homeopathic-type toothpastes, which are of necessity mild, are also available. When choosing toothpastes, read labels and ask your dentist for recommendations. Some "natural" toothpastes are overly abrasive. Fluoride toothpastes have been shown to be effective, but there are alternatives. Be sure to choose a product made without sugar.

Flossing is a must for a healthy mouth. When your child is little, you will have to do the flossing for her, but once she is old enough to do it herself, be sure to show her the correct technique and watch from time to time to make sure she is doing it properly. Most children find waxed dental floss easier to use than the unwaxed variety, and as an added incentive, it often comes in fun flavors. Also, make sure your child brushes her tongue as well as her teeth (as an alternative, the tongue can be gently scraped with a craft stick).

Finally, be sure to select soft-bristle toothbrushes and replace them frequently, at least every three months. This goes for adults as well as for children. Also, you should *always* replace your child's toothbrush after an infectious illness. It is not uncommon for a child to reinfect herself after recovering from a strep throat or other infection as a result of continuing to use the same toothbrush. Finally, toothbrushes should not be kept near the toilet, and they should be soaked or cleansed regularly using hydrogen peroxide, diluted citrus extract, salt water, or any other nontoxic solution that kills bacteria.

negative first impression of what a visit to the dentist is like, and you can build on this success in subsequent visits. If your child has more than one cavity, discuss this approach with your dentist.

PREVENTION

■ Prevention of tooth decay begins in utero and extends throughout life. Because the protective enamel on teeth is fully formed when they erupt, a good diet while the teeth are developing under the gums is the best insurance for strength and durability.

■ Other things can affect the teeth in the development stage as well. Certain drugs, especially the antibiotic tetracycline, can cause discoloration of developing teeth. The discoloration is not apparent until the teeth erupt, but by then it is too late—it cannot be reversed. This is why tetracycline should not be taken by a pregnant woman or by a child under the age of eight (or even older, if the child hasn't gotten in all of her adult teeth yet).

■ Make sure your child practices good oral hygiene. An oral hygiene program should begin even before teeth appear in your baby's mouth (*see* Caring for Your Child's Teeth on page 400). Use Merfluan or baking soda-based tooth powder regularly.

■ Discourage frequent snacking and the consumption of refined sugars and carbohydrates and sticky foods.

■ If you give your child vitamin-C supplements, avoid the chewable types. These can erode tooth enamel and promote decay.

■ Some dentists recommend fluoride treatments for the prevention of cavities. Fluoride is a mineral found in nature that, in small concentrations, stabilizes the structure of the tooth material and helps teeth to resist decay. In fact, because of this connection, many municipal water authorities now routinely add fluoride to their water supplies. In too-large concentrations, however, fluoride can cause the teeth to develop abnormal color and form, and the enamel to become softer, though it is still decay-resistant. You and your child's dentist are a team that must weigh the benefits and risks of fluoride treatment, as well as looking at other alternatives.

■ Another technique recommended by some dentists to protect against tooth decay involves the use of sealants. These are resins or other similar materials that are applied to form a hard, invisible covering over the teeth, especially the grooves and pits that occur naturally on the tops of the molars. These pits and grooves are the areas in which decay is most likely to begin, because they are easily missed during brushing and therefore tend to collect cavity-causing bacteria. Sealants prevent bacteria from getting to the teeth and causing cavities. If applied properly, sealants should be undetectable and should last for at least two years.

Toxoplasmosis

See Pets and Your Child in HOME SAFETY in Part One.

Tuberculosis

Tuberculosis is a chronic bacterial infection of the lungs caused by *Mycobacterium tuberculosis*. Although the incidence of tuberculosis in this country has decreased significantly, outbreaks still occur, primarily in such large metropolitan areas as New York, Boston, and Los Angeles. The AIDS epidemic is also implicated in recent outbreaks, because people with impaired immune systems are more likely to contract (and therefore to spread) the disease.

Tuberculosis is transmitted when an infected person coughs or sneezes and microscopic droplets containing the infecting organism dry in the air and are inhaled by others. Crowded living conditions therefore are conducive to the spread of the disease.

Tuberculosis generally affects the lungs, but it can spread to the joints and to other parts of the body, creating serious illness. Symptoms include fatigue, a chronic cough, bloody sputum, lack of appetite, weight loss, headache, and fever. A tuberculin skin test, chest x-ray, and a culture of sputum are used to confirm the diagnosis.

CONVENTIONAL TREATMENT

■ A child with an active case of tuberculosis will need to be isolated and will need to receive antibiotics. Rifampin (brand names Rifadin and Rimactane) and isoniazid are the primary antitubercular medicines. Both of these drugs are given in a single daily dose. Although a child will usually begin to feel better within a week of starting treatment, these drugs must be given for a prolonged period of time to effect a complete cure. If the full course of medication is not completed, it is possible for the bacteria to become resistant to the usual antitubercular drugs and for the child to suffer a relapse. Treatment of drug-resistant strains of tuberculosis is very complex and difficult. A full course of isoniazid usually lasts from eighteen months to two years for a child diagnosed with active tuberculosis. It can cause liver toxicity and needs to be monitored for this. Rifampin can cause drowsiness and may turn bodily fluids such as urine and sweat a red-orange color.

■ Once a child's sputum and gastric secretions are clear of the bacteria, he is no longer contagious.

■ A child with a newly positive tuberculin skin test but without symptoms will likely be given isoniazid for twelve to eighteen months to prevent the illness from developing. It is generally recommended that all the members of a household with a person diagnosed with tuberculosis take isoniazid for twelve months.

■ Vaccination with BCG (a weakened form of the tuberculosis bacteria) is sometimes suggested to increase the resistance of a child who is living with an adult who has the disease. This vaccine is used routinely in some parts of the world where the incidence of tuberculosis is high, but is rarely used in the United States. A person who is given a BCG vaccine can later have a false positive result to a TB skin test.

DIETARY GUIDELINES

■ Encourage your child to drink large amounts of fluids. Herbal teas, chicken soup, and vegetable soups will help support your child's body during recovery.

■ Avoid giving your child concentrated animal fats and greasy or fried foods.

NUTRITIONAL SUPPLEMENTS

The nutritional supplements listed below are intended to support your child's recovery from tuberculosis. They should not be considered a substitute for appropriate antibiotic therapy. For age-appropriate dosages of some nutritional supplements, see page 81.

■ Mineral ascorbate vitamin C with bioflavonoids may be given to help decrease inflammation and build the immune system. During the first month, give one dose, three to four times a day. During the second month, give the same amount, but twice a day. During the third and fourth months, give one dose daily.

■ Zinc will help build up your child's immune system. Give your child one dose, twice a day, for three months.

Note: Excessive amounts of zinc can result in nausea and vomiting. Be careful not to exceed the recommended dosage.

■ Vitamin B6 can be used to help prevent liver toxicity from isoniazid. Give your child 10 milligrams daily (one hour away from food) throughout the course of treatment with this medication.

■ Beta-carotene helps to heal mucous membranes. Give your child one dose a day while the disease is active.

HERBAL TREATMENT

Herbal treatment for tuberculosis is aimed at supporting your child's recovery from the illness. It should not be considered a substitute for appropriate antibiotic therapy. For best results, do not use a single herb continuously, but set up a rotating schedule using the herbs listed here, so that your child takes one herb a week for six months. For age-appropriate dosages of herbal remedies, see page 81.

■ American ginseng is an excellent source of trace minerals and micronutrients, and also helps strengthen the immune system. Give your child one dose, three times a day.

Note: This herb should not be given until fever and other signs of acute infection are no longer present.

■ Astragalus (*Astragalus membranaceous*) has a rich concentration of trace minerals and micronutrients, and helps to strengthen the immune system. Give your child one dose, three times daily.

Note: This herb should not be given until fever and other signs of acute infection are no longer present.

■ Licorice tea or tincture soothes the throat and respiratory tract, has antibacterial properties, and tastes sweet. For a cough, licorice works best when taken warm. Give your child one dose, three times a day.

Note: This herb should not be given to a child with high blood pressure or to any child for prolonged periods of time. Use it by itself for one week out of every month for three to four months, or use *small* amounts mixed with other herbs.

■ Marshmallow root lessens lung inflammation and coats and soothes an irritated throat. Make a tea and give your child one dose, twice a day. You can mix the marshmallow root with licorice as a tea.

■ Make a cough syrup containing slippery elm, licorice, osha root, and marshmallow root. Simmer 40 drops or 1 tablespoon of each in 1 quart of water for fifteen to twenty minutes. Sweeten with honey and give your child a teaspoon at a time, every four hours, for two days. Each of these herbs is soothing to the throat and respiratory tract.

HOMEOPATHY

■ When dealing with tuberculosis, it is most valuable to visit a homeopath who can prescribe a constitutional remedy for your child. A constitutional remedy can help strengthen your child's overall vitality as he recovers from the illness. Homeopathic treatment for tuberculosis should not be considered a substitute for appropriate antibiotic therapy.

GENERAL RECOMMENDATIONS

■ Rest is an important part of treatment and healing from tuberculosis. Encourage your child to get as much rest as possible.

■ It is important to prevent the spread of this highly contagious disease from one person to another. A child with tuberculosis should sleep and play away from other children. Dishes used by the infected child should be disposed of or sterilized. Used tissues should be disposed of carefully, preferably by burning.

■ Routine screenings are an important tool used by public health departments to track, and thereby limit, cases of tuberculosis. Have your child tested regularly, every year if possible.

■ The American Lung Association provides information on tuberculosis. Write to them at 1740 Broadway, New York, NY 10019, or phone 212–315–8700.

■ *See also* COUGH and FEVER.

PREVENTION

■ The only way to prevent tuberculosis is to avoid it. Keep children away from any adult or other child who has active tuberculosis. Be aware of the disease's tendency to spread in overcrowded and unsanitary conditions, and among people with compromised immune systems.

Unconsciousness

EMERGENCY TREATMENT FOR UNCONSCIOUSNESS

See the inset on page 405.

A child who has lost consciousness may be in serious difficulty. An unconscious state signals a lack of adequate oxygen supply to the brain. Causes may include shock and breathing problems, such as choking and near-suffocation. A loss of consciousness can also be caused by the ingestion of drugs or poisons. Other possible causes are brain injury, seizures, stroke, brain tumor, and infection.

Fainting is a term used to describe a less serious episode in which consciousness is lost. This is caused by a temporary disruption of blood flow to the brain, which may be brought on by hunger or pain, or even overwhelming emotional circumstances. Fainting is usually momentary, and a child who has fainted will revive readily, without disorientation upon awakening, although she may feel fatigued. (*See* FAINTING.)

Emergency Treatment for Unconsciousness

✛ Call the child's name. Try to provoke a response by sharply patting your child's face. Shake her gently. If she does not respond immediately, use smelling salts, if you have them readily available, to see if this revives her.

✛ If your child is limp and does not respond, call for emergency help immediately. It is best to have someone else call, so that your child is not left alone. If you must make the call yourself, do not leave your child unattended for more than thirty seconds.

✛ Quickly assess the situation. If you suspect that your child may have suffered a neck or back injury, such as might occur in a fall, *do not* move or jostle her. Rely on emergency medical personnel to know how to stabilize your child so that transport to the hospital will be safe.

✛ If you do not suspect a neck or back injury, turn your child onto her back. Roll her whole body as a unit to prevent further injury.

✛ Check for breathing. Put your cheek close to your child's mouth to feel for a breath. Watch her chest to see if it is rising and falling in normal breathing.

✛ *If there is no breath, turn to* CARDIOPULMONARY RESUSCITATION (CPR) *on page 426.* Begin artificial respiration in the manner appropriate for your child's age.

✛ Once your child's pulse and breathing have been restored and the immediate crisis is over, check and treat your child for bleeding, broken bones, concussion, or any other injury or problem she might have (*see* BLEEDING, SEVERE; BONES, BROKEN; CONCUSSION).

✛ After any episode where your child loses consciousness, it is wise to call your physician or take your child to the emergency room of the nearest hospital. Even if your child seems to be fine after such an ordeal, she should be seen by a doctor. It is important to seek the advice of a qualified medical professional.

If unconsciousness lasts for more than a few minutes, however, there may be other problems, such as internal or external bleeding, which can lead to shock. If your child loses consciousness, try to remain calm and act quickly.

CONVENTIONAL TREATMENT

■ Appropriate treatment for a child who has lost consciousness will depend on the cause of the episode. Follow your doctor's advice, and consult other entries in this book that address the cause of your child's problem, if appropriate.

HERBAL TREATMENT

For age-appropriate dosages of herbal remedies, see page 81.

■ An herbal tea made from licorice, American ginseng, and/or ginger will help to restore energy following an episode in which your child loses consciousness. Once your child has received appropriate emergency treatment and is well enough to recuperate at home, give her one dose, twice a day, for one or two days.

Note: American ginseng should not be given if fever or any other signs of infection are present.

PREVENTION

■ There are many things that can cause a child to lose consciousness. Some of these are unpreventable, but many are common dangers that you can take steps to eliminate. For suggestions on how to childproof your home and minimize the hazards your child will encounter outside, see HOME SAFETY in Part One.

Underweight

Some children fail to gain weight normally, experience unwanted weight loss, or just consistently weigh less than most other children of the same age and height. The chief concern in caring for such a child should be to try to find the underlying cause of the situation. A child who is underweight may simply not eat enough to supply his body with the calories and nutrients it needs. Or he may have a food allergy or a problem with nutrient metabolism or absorption that makes his body unable to get the nutrition it needs, even though his diet is healthy and sufficient. Underweight can also be one sign of intestinal parasites; certain chronic illnesses, such as cystic fibrosis, celiac disease, heart disease, and problems with thyroid function; or emotional issues, such as stress, depression, anxiety, or an eating disorder. Finally, it may also be that an underweight child is actually quite healthy, but is simply smaller and/or thinner than other children. A child may be lower than the fifth percentile on height and weight charts, but still be following a normal growth curve. It is a far greater cause for concern if a child's height and weight start out in the average range only to reach a plateau or "fall off" the growth curve later.

A child who is undernourished—whether as a result of insufficient intake or inadequate absorption of nutrients—may feel more tired or weak than his friends. He may feel dizzy and have a difficult time concentrating. A child with a chronically deficient nutritional status may have his growth and development affected, so that puberty is reached later than normal or sterility results. Usually, however, it is possible to track down the underlying cause of the problem and treat it so that an underweight child can gain weight and catch up with his peers.

CONVENTIONAL TREATMENT

■ The first step in treating the underweight child is to discover whether there is an underlying illness that is treatable. Your doctor will probably discuss your child's dietary routine with you and may order blood tests to determine his nutritional status and check thyroid function, glucose levels, and other key markers to either rule out or identify any metabolic disorders. A stool analysis is sometimes used to check for absorption problems or parasites. A doctor will also likely take a complete medical history, including any unusual aspects of pregnancy and birth. The height and weight of both parents will also be taken into consideration. The recommended treatment, if any, will depend on the results of the doctor's examination and diagnostic tests.

■ A child with severe weight loss or an eating disorder may need to be hospitalized in order to receive nutrition and close medical care and attention.

DIETARY GUIDELINES

■ If your infant is underweight, be patient with feeding times. It may be that your child is just not getting as much time as he needs to eat.

■ Do not give an underweight child sweets or fatty foods in an attempt to "fatten him up." Your child should eat a well-balanced, healthy diet consisting of three meals a day and at least two healthy snacks—more if the child requests it and they don't interfere with his appetite at mealtimes. *See* DIET AND NUTRITION in Part One.

■ Try serving smaller initial portions at meals. Being confronted with large amounts of food can actually cause a child, especially a small child, to lose his appetite. You can always give your child more if he's hungry after he finishes the first serving.

■ Eliminate any foods or sodas that contain caffeine from your child's diet.

■ A nutritionist may be a valuable resource in helping you plan meals for your child. He or she may also be able to counsel or advise you concerning emotional and practical issues that may be affecting your child's ability to gain weight.

NUTRITIONAL SUPPLEMENTS

■ Try giving your child *Lactobacillus acidophilus* or *bifidus* supplement. This will often improve nutritional absorption. Follow dosage directions on the product label.

■ Give an underweight child a good multiple vitamin and mineral supplement to correct for possible nutritional deficiencies.

■ Floradix, a plant-based iron supplement, sometimes helps to increase the appetite. Follow dosage directions on the product label.

ACUPRESSURE

For the locations of acupressure points on a child's body, *see* ADMINISTERING AN ACUPRESSURE TREATMENT in Part Three.

■ Massaging the bladder meridian (adjacent to the spine) and then Stomach 36 will gradually improve your child's absorption of nutrients.

GENERAL RECOMMENDATIONS

■ If you think that your infant or child may be underweight, your first concern should be to determine whether his nutritional status is truly deficient. If it is, you should try to determine the cause. A physician can help you to identify and understand the underlying issues so that the problem can be treated properly.

■ If your child's underweight is related to emotional issues, it may be helpful to find some kind of support, such as a group or therapist, that can help your child understand and manage his feelings. This is particularly important if your child is suffering from an eating disorder such as anorexia or bulimia. These are problems that can rarely be resolved without the input of a professional (*see* Eating Disorders: Anorexia and Bulimia, page 321).

■ Try to make mealtimes as relaxed and happy as possible. Do not threaten or force your child to eat if he resists. This will only set up a pointless contest between you and your child and make him dislike eating all the more. And after all, one missed (or refused) meal won't lead to malnutrition, but a negative feeling about eating, built up over years of conflict at the dinner table, might. Instead, simply invite your child to eat and to participate in mealtime conversation. Chances are, if a child sees others eating and enjoying themselves, sooner or later he will see that this is pleasurable and want to join in.

Urinary Tract Infection

A urinary tract infection is a bacterial infection of the urethra, ureters, kidneys, or bladder. An infection of the bladder, called cystitis, is the most common type of urinary tract infection.

A child with a urinary tract infection (UTI) may complain of a burning pain upon urination. There may be foul-smelling, dark, or bloody urine. The child may feel the urge to urinate frequently, but void only a small amount each time. Additional symptoms can include wetting the bed at night, stomachache, backache, or fever. An infant with a urinary tract infection may have a fever, vomiting, diarrhea, lethargy, and irritability.

Because of the structure of the female urinary tract, UTIs are more common in girls than in boys. The urethra is the small tube that drains urine from the bladder and out of the body. In females, the urethra lies close to the rectum. Bacteria from the lower intestine or vagina can easily migrate to and travel up the urethra into the bladder. In more serious situations, bacteria continue to migrate through the ureters and into the kidneys, causing an inflammation or infection of kidney tissue. Bacteria often migrate into the bladder, especially in females, but they usually don't cause an infection. This is because urination washes the bacteria out of the body, the lining of the bladder resists the invasion of bacteria, and urine itself is bacteriostatic, meaning that it inhibits bacterial growth.

Other causes of a UTI include constipation, malnutrition, and sexual intercourse, especially when a diaphragm is used for birth control. Even the chemicals in bubble baths and the scents and dyes in some toilet tissue can cause local irritation that leads to an infection.

Urinary tract infections frequently recur in girls. However, after two or three episodes, a young girl should be evaluated closely for a possible anatomical abnormality. Recurrent UTIs can be a sign of a structural problem in the urinary tract system that causes reflux to occur. That is, the urine moves back up through the urethra to the bladder, and sometimes into the kidneys, instead of moving out of the body. Continuous reflux creates a perfect environment for bacterial growth.

Urinary tract infections are much less common in boys. In boys, the symptoms of local irritation caused by scratching, masturbating, or an injury to the area can often mimic those of a UTI. If the symptoms result from a true UTI, it is important to have a complete medical investigation, including ultrasound and x-rays, because anatomical abnormalities are very commonly involved.

It is important to treat UTIs thoroughly, so that they do not spread to the kidneys.

CONVENTIONAL TREATMENT

■ To determine whether or not an infection is present, and which specific bacteria are involved, both a urinalysis and urine culture are necessary. Your child may be tested again three or four days after treatment is initiated, until the urine is free of signs of infection, to be certain that treatment is successful.

■ UTIs are usually treated with antibiotics. Nitrifurantoin (Furandantin), sulfamethoxazole (Gantrisin), trimethoprim (Bactrim, Septra), and amoxicillin are commonly prescribed. Most antibiotics are excreted through the urinary tract, so they make their way to the site of the infection and wash over it on their way out of the body, killing the organism responsible for the infection. Antibiotics are usually prescribed for a ten-day period. They can have a variety of side effects, including allergic reactions, diarrhea, upset stomach, and intestinal or vaginal yeast infections.

■ Phenazopyridine (Pyridium), a urinary tract analgesic, is sometimes prescribed to anesthetize the urethra. This eases the uncomfortable feeling of urgency that can accompany a urinary tract infection, and makes it less painful to urinate. It also turns the urine a reddish-orange color. It may be prescribed to alleviate discomfort during the two- or three-day period before antibiotic therapy has an effect on symptoms.

■ Ultrasound and x-rays of the kidney area may be ordered. These tests allow a doctor to see the anatomy of the renal system and help in the identification of anatomical abnormalities. Intravenous pyelography (or IVP, a procedure in which dye is injected intravenously, then observed via x-ray as it passes through the system), voiding cystourethrography (VCUG), renal ultrasound, and renal scanning are further x-ray studies used to evaluate the structure and functioning of the urinary system. An IVP is usually indicated for a girl under three years old or a boy of any age with a UTI. It is often recommended for girls between three and ten as well. In older girls, x-rays are usually considered necessary after three infections.

DIETARY GUIDELINES

■ To help flush out the system, encourage your child to drink as much water as possible. Diluted urine is easier on the urinary tract, and less painful as it leaves the body.

■ Avoid citrus fruits and acidic foods, which can be irritating to the urinary tract.

NUTRITIONAL SUPPLEMENTS

■ *Lactobacillus acidophilus* or *bifidus* helps to maintain or restore beneficial flora in the digestive and urinary tracts. This treatment is more preventive than curative in its effect on UTIs, but it is particularly important if your child is taking antibiotics. Follow the dosage directions on the product label.

HERBAL TREATMENT

For age-appropriate dosages of herbal remedies, see page 81.

■ Make an herbal tea from corn silk and parsley. The stringy, silky, browning material that peels away from a ripe ear of corn is a wonderful diuretic and is very soothing to a distressed urinary tract. It is available either fresh or as a tincture. Fresh parsley, also a diuretic, is rich in chlorophyll. Give your child one dose, three times daily, for three days.

■ Cranberries contain an ingredient that keeps bacteria from sticking to the bladder wall. Give your child three glasses of pure cranberry juice, or three capsules of cranberry extract (available as a product called Cran-Actin), daily.

WHEN TO CALL THE DOCTOR ABOUT A URINARY TRACT INFECTION

● An infant with a urinary tract infection (UTI) may be irritable and have a fever, vomiting, and diarrhea. If you suspect your baby may have a UTI, call your doctor right away. In an infant, a UTI may indicate a more serious underlying condition.

● If your child has a UTI and she develops fever, chills, vomiting, or severe back or side pain, or if there is blood in her urine, contact your doctor. These are signs that the infection may have spread to the kidneys.

■ Garlic is a natural antibiotic that will help to destroy intestinal bacteria that cause a UTI. Choose an odorless capsule form and give your child one to three capsules a day. Or give your child one whole clove of fresh garlic daily.

■ Uva ursi has been used for decades by Native Americans for urinary disorders. It has antiseptic and astringent properties that can be very effective for mild UTIs or for preventing recurrences. Give your child one dose, three to four times a day, for three to four days. Because uva ursi can be irritating to the urinary tract, it is best to combine it with a soothing herb, such as corn silk.

Note: Uva ursi should not be given to a child under six years of age.

■ Although harder to find, pipsissewa is less potentially irritating than uva ursi, and is just as effective. Give your child one dose, three to four times a day.

■ An echinacea and goldenseal combination formula is antibacterial and soothes mucous membranes. Give your child one dose, three times a day, for up to five days.

HOMEOPATHY

■ *Cantharis* is the premier homeopathic for urinary tract infection. It helps to relieve the burning pain experienced before, during, and after urination. Give your child one dose of *Cantharis* 12x or 6c, three to four times a day, for two to three days.

ACUPRESSURE

For the locations of acupressure points on a child's body, *see* ADMINISTERING AN ACUPRESSURE TREATMENT in Part Three.

■ Bladder 28 is the master point for the bladder.

■ Kidney 3 helps to strengthen the kidneys and bladder.

■ Stomach 36 is useful if a UTI is related to a disturbance in the digestive tract.

GENERAL RECOMMENDATIONS

■ If your child has recurrent UTIs, consult with your doctor to be sure proper tests are done confirming that your child has no anatomical abnormality that is causing them.

■ Encourage your child to drink plenty of water. This is one of the most comforting ways to treat a urinary tract infection. Diluted urine is not only easier on the urinary tract, but it causes much less pain and burning on urination.

■ If it is too painful for your child to urinate, sitting in a tub of warm water can help to relax the muscles and dilute the urine so that it is easier and less uncomfortable for her to urinate.

■ Give your child homeopathic *Cantharis*.

■ Give your child an echinacea and goldenseal combination formula.

■ Give your child uva ursi, corn silk and parsley tea, or cranberry juice or capsules.

PREVENTION

■ Encourage your child to take in lots of fluids.

■ To prevent bacteria from migrating through the urethra, teach little girls to wipe from front to back. Buy and use only unscented white toilet tissue.

■ Avoid giving your child bubble baths. Use mild soap.

■ A child who seems prone to urinary tract infections will benefit from the inclusion of acidophilus-rich foods, such as sweet acidophilus milk and yogurt, in the diet. Be sure to select brands containing active cultures.

■ Give your child a *Lactobacillus acidophilus* or *bifidus* supplement to help prevent recurrences.

Vaginitis, Yeast

Almost every female has vaginitis due to a yeast infection at some point in her life. Essentially, this is an infection that causes inflammation of the vaginal lining. Although there are other types of vaginitis, the condition most commonly occurs when a microorganism invades the vaginal environment and irritates or inflames the sensitive vaginal walls.

Itching, tenderness, burning, pain with urination, and pain with sexual intercourse are the most common complaints of those with a yeast infection. There may also be a white discharge that resembles cottage cheese. Because there are several kinds of vaginitis, it is important to get a precise diagnosis. A physician or nurse practitioner will take a sample of discharge from the vagina or cervix and look at it under a microscope to determine what is causing the symptoms.

Many of the organisms that can cause vaginitis are present in the vagina normally, but the vagina is able to maintain the delicate healthy balance required to prevent infection. Vaginal secretions are basically acidic, which inhibits the growth of most organisms. But this balance can become disrupted, allowing an overgrowth of the normal flora or allowing an organism from outside the body to invade and start an infection.

Some types of vaginitis are sexually transmitted, and vaginitis can be a symptom of a more serious underlying illness such as chlamydia or gonorrhea. An untreated infection can also travel up the genital tract to cause pelvic inflammatory disease or an infection of the fallopian tubes.

The infectious agents that cause more cases of vaginitis than any other are monilia (yeast), gardnerella (bacteria), and trichomonas (protozoa). The most common yeast organism, *Candida albicans*, lives in the vaginas of up to 20 percent of all women without creating symptoms. Changes in the normal flora of the vagina can create an environment that allows the monilia that are usually present to overgrow. Antibiotics are one of the greatest culprits when it comes to changes in the vaginal environment. Other things that change the flora and increase the likelihood of infection include stress, birth control pills, steroids, diabetes, pregnancy, tight clothing, pantyhose, warm weather, or a decrease in overall immune function. Although sexual intercourse is not a usual means of transmission, sexual partners should be checked for candida in persistent cases.

CONVENTIONAL TREATMENT

■ Antifungal creams or vaginal suppositories (Femstat, Monistat, and Gyne-Lo-trimin, among others) are available by prescription and over the counter. Both the creams and suppositories can be inserted with an applicator. A suppository is warmed and melted by the body so that it can be dispersed throughout the vagina. Antifungal creams also are dispersed throughout the vagina. Both can be messy and leaky; wearing a minipad may be helpful. If your daughter is menstruating, it is probably best for her not to wear a tampon while using these medications, as the tampon may absorb the medication.

■ A Betadine douche is good for washing out the vagina. Mix the solution according to the directions on the product label and administer (*see* ADMINISTERING A DOUCHE in Part Three). This preparation should not be used for a retention douche and should not be used during pregnancy.

■ If your child suffers from recurring yeast infections, it is important to consult a physician. Recurring infections can be a sign of a compromised immune system or another serious health problem that requires treatment. She should have a blood sugar test done to check for diabetes, which can predispose an individual to developing yeast infections. It may be advisable as well to have an HIV test done to check for the presence of antibodies to the virus that causes AIDS.

DIETARY GUIDELINES

■ Prepare a nutrient-dense diet of grains, vegetables, and lean proteins.

■ Eliminate all refined foods, alcohol, sugars, dairy products, and simple carbohy-drates from your child's diet. Yeast thrives on sugar, especially lactose (milk sugar).

■ If your teenager experiences recurrent yeast infections, use an elimination or rotation diet to identify foods to which she may be allergic or sensitive (*see* ELIMINATION DIET or ROTATION DIET in Part Three).

NUTRITIONAL SUPPLEMENTS

■ Make a retention douche by mixing 1 teaspoon of acidophilus powder with 1 ounce of water or milk. Insert the douche and lie down with your legs elevated for ten minutes (some women do a shoulder stand instead). Afterwards, wear a sanitary pad for the next several hours, as there will be some leakage (*see* ADMIN-ISTERING A DOUCHE in Part Three).

■ Taking *Lactobacillus acidophilus* or *bifidus* by mouth helps to add friendly flora to the vaginal area and restore the healthy balance of organisms in the vagina. Choose either one and follow the dosage directions on the product label.

■ Use yogurt as a retention douche to get acidophilus culture directly into the vagina. This can be quite soothing to inflamed tissue, and is especially effective for yeast infections. Be sure to buy plain, unflavored nonfat yogurt that contains live cultures. Apply about 1 tablespoon at night.

HERBAL TREATMENT

■ An herbal douche is one of the most helpful treatments for a yeast infection. Try one of the following mixtures (*see* ADMINISTERING A DOUCHE in Part Three).

- Make a standard douche by mixing 40 drops of echinacea, 40 drops of goldenseal, 40 drops of calendula, and 2 tablespoons of aloe vera in a pint of water. Echinacea and goldenseal are antibacterial; calendula helps to soothe and heal inflammation; aloe vera is soothing to the tissues. Any of these herbs may be used separately, but they seem to work best as a combination.

- Add 20 drops of an echinacea and goldenseal combination, 6 drops of tea tree oil, and 1 tablespoon of calendula tincture to 1 pint of water. You can use one or all of these ingredients.

- Add 4 tablespoons of white or apple cider vinegar to 1 cup of water. This can be used as either a standard or a retention douche.

■ An alternative to douching is to prepare a bath with 1½ cups of salt and 1½ cups of apple cider vinegar added to the water. Have your child soak for fifteen to twenty minutes, once or twice a day, for two or three days.

HOMEOPATHY

■ *Cantharis* helps to relieve the burning and sense of urgency (needing to go to the bathroom frequently and quickly) that often accompanies a vaginal infection. Give your child one dose of *Cantharis* 12x or 6c, three times a day, for two to three days.

■ If *Cantharis* is not helpful, or if your daughter suffers from recurrent vaginitis, try *Sulphur*. This remedy will help if the vagina is red, feels hot, and is itchy. It will also help clear up the odor of the vaginal discharge. Give your child one dose of *Sulphur* 30x or 9c, twice a day, for up to five days.

ACUPRESSURE

For the locations of acupressure points, *see* ADMINISTERING AN ACUPRESSURE TREATMENT in Part Three.

■ Bladder 23 and 60 and Kidney 3 all increase circulation to the urinary tract and reproductive organs.

■ Spleen 10 detoxifies the blood.

GENERAL RECOMMENDATIONS

■ Make sure your child wears 100-percent cotton underwear that breathes, and that her underwear is washed in hot water. Heat kills the yeast that cause vaginitis.

■ Have your daughter try a sitz bath. Calendula and goldenseal in a sitz bath will help to soothe burning and itching.

■ Give your child an acidophilus supplement.

■ If your teenager suffers from recurrent vaginitis, she should be tested for diabetes or any other underlying condition. Consult your doctor.

PREVENTION

■ Since the organisms that cause vaginitis are normally present in the vagina, it may not be possible to prevent all infections. However, there are things your child can do to help make the vaginal environment less conducive to the overgrowth of these organisms. Encourage her to wear clothing and underwear that breathes.

White cotton underwear and loose clothing is best. If your daughter must wear pantyhose, make sure the crotch is made of cotton. This is especially important in warm weather.

■ If your child must take antibiotics, give her a *Lactobacillus acidophilus* or *bifidus* supplement to help maintain a healthy balance in the flora of the vagina.

Vaccination Reactions

See IMMUNIZATION-RELATED PROBLEMS.

Vomiting

See NAUSEA AND VOMITING.

Warts

Warts are harmless growths caused by viruses. They occur most often on the hands and feet, but can also appear on the face, neck, and genital area. There are several different kinds of warts. Plantar warts are painful round lumps set into the foot. Plane warts are small, flat, and flesh-colored, and tend to grow in clusters. Genital warts are highly contagious and are usually transmitted through sexual contact.

Warts can occur at any age, but are most common during childhood and adolescence. They have the annoying tendency to recur and can spread from one place to another. Except for genital warts, however, they rarely spread from one person to another.

Common warts (verruca) appear as raised, sharply outlined, hardened, and rough skin. They are brown or gray in color, and may appear in clusters. Warts can be tender or painful.

Childhood warts sometimes spontaneously disappear within two years. But for a child bothered by warts, and perhaps sensitive to teasing by playmates, two years may seem like a very long time.

CONVENTIONAL TREATMENT

■ Acid treatment is commonly prescribed for warts. When applied topically to warts, a solution of salicylic acid (12 percent) or lactic acid (10 to 17 percent) works to soften and loosen the hardened skin. Such solutions are available over the counter as Wart-Off and Occlusal, among others. The usual recommendation is to dab acid on the wart two or three times daily, then cover with an adhesive bandage. Acid treatment is a slow, painless way to remove warts, but acid is drying and irritating to a child's delicate skin. To protect the surrounding skin from contact, it is very important to apply the acid with extreme care.

■ For ease of application, ask your doctor about an acid-impregnated plaster. Sold over the counter as Mediplast, or by prescription as TransPlantar or Trans-Ver-Sal, the plaster is applied to the wart for twenty-four hours at a time, then replaced with a new one every night, for a period of ten to fourteen days (if used consistently).

■ Cryotherapy, also called cryosurgery or "freezing" treatment, must be performed by a physician. This involves exposing the wart to extreme cold to injure and destroy the cells. A probe containing liquid nitrogen is used to cool the tissue to -20°F. The wart usually falls off one or two weeks later. Occasionally several treatments are required, especially for plantar warts. This procedure causes a burning sensation on application, and the area may throb for hours afterward.

■ Bleomycin (Blenoxane), a chemotherapy agent used against cancer, is sometimes used for extremely persistent warts. It is injected directly into the wart, which is painful, but it is highly effective.

■ Warts can be removed surgically by a physician, or by a podiatrist if they are on the foot. This is a relatively painful procedure, however, and may leave a residual scar.

DIETARY GUIDELINES

■ Avoid giving your child foods containing refined sugars and flours. They can foster bacterial and viral growth.

■ Encourage your child to eat green and yellow vegetables. They are high in beta-carotene, which is healing to the skin.

NUTRITIONAL SUPPLEMENTS

For age-appropriate dosages of nutritional supplements, see page 81.

■ Vitamin A can be purchased in liquid form or squeezed out of a capsule. Apply the oil topically, twice daily, for two to three weeks.

■ Beta-carotene, which the body uses to manufacture vitamin A, has antiviral properties. Give your child one dose of beta-carotene, twice a day, for ten days.

■ Vitamin E is a natural antioxidant that is an important maintenance vitamin for a child with chronic warts. Give your child one or two doses per day, for one month, or for one week out of every month, for six months.

HERBAL TREATMENT

■ Banana peel contains a substance that is highly effective for destroying warts. Many dermatologists recommend it. Place a small amount of peel against the wart and hold it in place with silk tape. Change the peel once or twice daily. Repeat for two weeks or until the wart is gone.

■ Podophyllin, an extract of American mandrake root, is very toxic to cells and is primarily used for genital warts. Podophyllin can be applied at home, but should be used only under your doctor's supervision to ensure that surrounding tissues are not injured.

■ Shiitake mushrooms have immune-stimulating and antiviral effects. Give a child over twelve years of age one capsule, twice daily, for one month.

HOMEOPATHY

■ The following homeopathic regimen may help resolve your child's warts.

Days 1–4: Give your child one dose of *Thuja* 30x or 9c, twice daily.
Days 5–9: Discontinue the *Thuja*, and give your child one dose of *Nitricumacidum* 12x or 6c, twice daily.

If the wart has not cleared after nine days, consider one of the symptom-specific remedies that follow.

■ If the wart is dry and itchy, give your child one dose of *Antimonium crudum* 12x or 6c, three times daily, for up to three days.

■ Use *Causticum* for warts that bleed easily, are flat, and are mostly found on your child's fingers. Give your child one dose of *Causticum* 12x or 5c, three times a day, for up to three days.

■ *Mercurius cyanatus* is especially helpful for plantar warts. Give your child one dose of *Mercurius cyanatus* 12x or 5c, twice daily, for up to five days.

■ Apply homeopathic *Thuja* tincture or ointment to your child's warts, once daily, for three weeks.

GENERAL RECOMMENDATIONS

■ Warts, especially the dry, itchy ones, are tempting to pick at. Try to prevent your child from scratching and picking. Explain that it is impossible to "pick off" a wart, and that picking and scratching can only cause infection and may cause the warts to spread.

■ Apply *Thuja* or tea tree oil tincture or ointment to your child's wart two or three times daily. Let an older child make the applications himself. It may satisfy his urge to "do something," and thereby help prevent picking.

■ Use banana peel as outlined above.

■ Follow the homeopathic regime above.

■ Sometimes warts can resolve spontaneously. Try teaching your child visualization techniques, imagining that the warts are melting away. Some studies suggest that this may have an effect. It will also give your child a feeling of connection with his body and a sense of being involved in his health care.

PREVENTION

■ Try giving your child an echinacea and goldenseal combination. Common warts are hard to prevent, but this herbal formula stimulates the immune system. It can help arm your child's defenses against the viral attacks that lead to warts. Give your child one dose, three days a week, for two weeks; discontinue it for two weeks; give it for another two; and so on. (It is important not to give echinacea on a daily basis for more than ten days, or it may lose its effectiveness.)

■ If your child has a tendency to develop warts, give him 5,000 international units of beta-carotene, 50 international units of vitamin E, 250 milligrams of bioflavonoids, and 10 milligrams of zinc each day for two to three months. Although these nutrients cannot resolve warts, they can help warts from recurring.

Note: Excessive amounts of zinc can result in nausea and vomiting. Be careful not to exceed the recommended dosage.

Weight Problems

See OBESITY; UNDERWEIGHT.

Whooping Cough

Whooping cough, medically termed pertussis, is a bacterial infection caused by the microorganism *Bordetella pertussis*. The organism is spread from one person to another through respiratory contact such as coughing, sneezing, or even just talking with an infected person. The incubation period is usually about ten days long, although it can be as short as five or as long as twenty-one days. The total course of the disease is approximately six weeks.

At the beginning of a pertussis infection, a child has the typical symptoms of an upper respiratory infection, including a cough. The cough worsens during the second week of illness. Then, during the next four to six weeks, there are sudden episodes of intense coughing, accompanied by a "whoop" sound, a red or bluish face, large amounts of mucus, vomiting, exhaustion, and possibly anxiety. Then the cough gradually subsides, over a period of two to three weeks, and eventually goes away. Some children have a residual cough for months. Diagnosis is based on symptoms, especially the distinctive cough, and cultures taken from the nose and throat to identify the infecting organism.

Pertussis is a serious disease for infants and babies, less so for older children. In children under two years of age, it is much more likely to cause dangerous respiratory complications, including oxygen deprivation, as well as problems arising from the violent nature of the cough, such as umbilical hernia, convulsions, and hemorrhage. Ear infections and pneumonia are common complications of pertussis.

A child with pertussis is contagious for up to three or four weeks after the beginning of the cough. During this time she must be kept isolated in order to avoid spreading the illness to other children. It is believed that adults may contract the illness from an infected child and experience nothing more than a mild cold with a cough. However, they can still spread the disease to susceptible children.

CONVENTIONAL TREATMENT

■ An infant with pertussis may need to be hospitalized and given respiratory support with a mechanical ventilator. Suctioning of excess mucus from the throat may also be necessary.

EMERGENCY TREATMENT FOR WHOOPING COUGH

✚ A child with pertussis can develop respiratory problems so severe that they can be life threatening. If your child seems to be having serious and/or increasing difficulty breathing, call your doctor immediately or take your child to the emergency room of the nearest hospital.

■ Your child may be given pertussis immune globulin to strengthen her ability to fight the illness. This is most often recommended for children less than two years of age, or for an older child with a particularly serious case of the disease.

■ Antibiotics may be prescribed. Erythromycin is the medication most commonly used for pertussis infection. Even though it kills off the bacteria that cause the disease, the symptoms can last for several weeks after treatment is begun.

■ Your doctor will likely recommend that your child get plenty of bed rest; small, frequent meals; and plenty of fluids.

■ Cough medicines, including expectorants and cough suppressants, have little value in treating pertussis and are not recommended.

DIETARY GUIDELINES

■ Nutrition is very important in treating pertussis. Give your child frequent small but nutrient-dense meals to help maintain her strength during the course of this disease.

■ Encourage your child to take as many fluids as she can. Offer fruit-juice popsicles, spring water, herbal teas, soups, and diluted fruit juices. Immune-boosting astragalus and vegetable soup is an excellent choice (*see* THERAPEUTIC RECIPES in Part Three).

■ Avoid giving your child dairy foods, which tend to increase and thicken mucus.

■ Eliminate fats as much as possible. Fats are difficult to digest under normal circumstances, and are even harder to digest when the body is under stress. Undigested fats inhibit healing by contributing to a toxic internal environment.

NUTRITIONAL SUPPLEMENTS

For age-appropriate dosages of nutritional supplements, see page 81.

■ Vitamin C and bioflavonoids help to stimulate the immune system. Three to four times a day, give your child one dose of vitamin C in mineral ascorbate form, and an equal amount of bioflavonoids, for two or three weeks.

■ Zinc stimulates the immune system and promotes healing. Give your child one dose of zinc, twice a day, for up to two weeks.

Note: Excessive amounts of zinc can result in nausea and vomiting. Be careful not to exceed the recommended dosage.

■ Beta-carotene is the precursor to vitamin A, which helps heal mucous membranes. Give your child one dose, twice daily, for two or three weeks or until the cough subsides.

■ Whooping cough will often adversely affect the bowel. Give your child a *Lactobacillus bifidus* or *acidophilus* supplement twice daily. Follow dosage directions on the product label.

HERBAL TREATMENT

For age-appropriate dosages of herbal remedies, see page 81.

■ Marshmallow root is soothing to the throat and respiratory tract. Make a marshmallow root tea and give your child one dose, three times daily, for up to three days.

■ Slippery elm bark makes a soothing lozenge or tea. Give your child one dose, three times a day, for three to four days.

■ Osha root is healing to the respiratory tract and is a mild cough suppressant. Give your child one dose of osha root tea, two or three times a day, until she is better.

HOMEOPATHY

■ During the early stages of pertussis, give your child one dose of *Aconite* 30c, every two hours, for the first six hours.

■ *Antimonium tartaricum* is for the child with a moist, rattling cough, who is breathless and pale. Give this child one dose of *Antimonium tartaricum* 12x or 6c, three times a day.
   Note: This remedy should not be used in the presence of a fever.

■ *Belladonna* can be given in the early stages if your child heats up and gets a fever. Give one dose of *Belladonna* 30x or 9c, four times a day, for the first twenty-four hours.

■ *Drosera* is for the child with a whooping-type cough that is dry and accompanied by wheezing. Give her one dose of *Drosera* 12x or 6c, three times a day, for up to three days.

■ *Spongia* is good for a child with a crouplike cough who complains that her chest hurts. The cough is worse when the child is excited, and she feels better with hot drinks. Give this child one dose of *Spongia* 12x or 6c, three times a day, for up to three days.

BACH FLOWER REMEDIES

■ Aspen is good to ease a child's anxiety when she is feeling a lot of fear, but neither you nor she can figure out what she is afraid of.

■ Mimulus is helpful for a child who is feeling a lot of fear and can name what the fear is about. (*See* BACH FLOWER REMEDIES in Part One.)

ACUPRESSURE

For the locations of acupressure points on a child's body, *see* ADMINISTERING AN ACUPRESSURE TREATMENT in Part Three.

■ Pericardium 6 helps to relax the chest.

GENERAL RECOMMENDATIONS

■ If your child develops pertussis, keep her isolated from other children, especially infants, until at least four weeks after the onset of the cough, so that she will not infect susceptible children. Parents or other adults who are in contact with susceptible children should also avoid contact with an infected child.

■ Be alert for signs that your child is having difficulty breathing. This is particularly important if your child is under two years of age. If breathing trouble develops, seek emergency medical treatment immediately. Your child may need respiratory support.

■ Make sure your child gets plenty of rest, eats small, frequent meals, and takes as many fluids as possible. Follow the dietary guidelines above.

■ Avoid activities and circumstances that seem to trigger coughing attacks. Protect your child from exposure to secondhand smoke.

■ Give your child slippery elm bark or marshmallow root tea.

■ Select and administer an appropriate homeopathic remedy. If your child is fearful, give her an appropriate Bach Flower Remedy.

■ Give your child vitamin C and bioflavonoids, zinc, and beta-carotene.

PREVENTION

■ A vaccine that protects against the *Bordetella pertussis* bacteria is available. It is usually given in combination with the diphtheria and tetanus vaccines (the DPT vaccine). Physicians normally administer this as a series of injections, given to children at approximately two months, four months, six months, eighteen months, four to six years, and fourteen to sixteen years of age. Thereafter, your doctor may recommend that a booster be given every ten years, or after exposure to the disease. (*See* IMMUNIZATION-RELATED PROBLEMS.)

■ As much as possible, try to keep your child from contact with contagious children, particularly if she is not (or is not yet) immunized against the disease.

Part Three

Therapies and Procedures

Techniques for Using
Conventional and Natural Treatments

Introduction

Part One provided an introduction to conventional and natural approaches to health care, plus important issues in diet, pregnancy and newborn care, and home safety. Part Two provided discussions of specific childhood health problems and available treatments for them. In Part Three, you will find instructions that will help you to implement the various treatments and diagnostic procedures mentioned in Part Two.

Many people, even if they are interested in trying a natural approach to healing, can be put off because it seems so different from the kind of medicine they know—things like poultices, tinctures, and pressure points sound exotic and mysterious. The entries in this section will explain and show how to prepare the various types of herbal treatments, design an elimination diet, and apply acupressure. There are also entries that will show such conventional diagnostic procedures as taking your baby's pulse or temperature.

When you become familiar with the techniques and procedures described here, you will be better able to choose and provide health care for your child that combines the best of conventional and natural approaches.

Administering an Acupressure Treatment

The gentle art of acupressure is something you can do at home for a sick or hurting child. Massaging an acupressure point will help relieve symptoms as well as strengthen your child's body.

Acupressure points are located along lines called meridians that run along the sides of the body. There are twelve of these meridians on each side of the body, each corresponding to and named for a specific organ. Pressure points are identified by numbers that indicate where they fall along a particular meridian. Spleen 6, for example, is the sixth point along the Spleen meridian.

In the entries in Part Two, specific pressure points are recommended for treatment of different disorders. Use the diagrams in Figure 3.1 (pages 424–425) to help you locate specific pressure points on the body. The front view shows points for the Four Gates combination and the Large Intestine, Liver, Spleen, and Stomach meridians. The back view shows points for Neck and Shoulder Release and the Bladder, Gallbladder, and Kidney meridians. The inset of the hand and arm shows points on the Lung and Pericardium meridians.

To give an acupressure treatment, choose a time when your child is relatively calm and relaxed. Make sure he is warm enough. You can apply pressure either directly to his body, or through a shirt or light sheet. Have your child breathe deeply for a few moments to aid relaxation. You may wish to start by giving a back rub, and then move into the acupressure treatment itself.

Expect the acupressure points relevant to your child's condition to be somewhat tender to the touch. Use your judgment. Ask your child what feels good.

When administering acupressure, work the right- and left-side points at the same time whenever possible (if it's not, work one side first and then the other). Using your fingers or thumbs, apply *threshold pressure* to the points. This is firm pressure that is just on the verge of being painful; the point is stimulated but the body doesn't tighten up or retract from the pain. It is a "good hurt" feeling.

Apply from one to three minutes of continuous threshold pressure until the pain is relieved. Or apply pressure for ten seconds, release for ten seconds, apply pressure again for ten seconds, and release again; repeat this sequence ten times.

There are two special acupressure techniques suggested for several of the health problems discussed in Part Two:

• **Four Gates Technique.** Four Gates is a traditional Chinese point combination that has been used by acupuncturists for centuries. Working these points with acupressure will enhance relaxation and help relieve pain, nervousness, anxiety, and sleeplessness. Traditional Chinese doctors believe that working these points "opens the gates" of energy flow in the body. For this technique only, work first on one side of the body and then on the other. Apply pressure simultaneously to Liver 3 and Large Intestine 4.

• **Neck and Shoulder Release.** This is another traditional point combination, used to release the trapezius and other neck and shoulder muscles. Apply threshold pressure to Gallbladder 20 on the right and left sides, until you feel the muscle relax. Then do the same with Gallbladder 21.

Behavior Modification for Weight Control

Willpower alone is rarely an effective tool for losing weight; trying to "just say no" when it comes to controlling one's appetite, especially once a habitual pattern of overeating has been established, is simply not enough. Instead, you should take advantage of the mind's tendency to follow habits by replacing old habits with new, healthy patterns that support a lifestyle more conducive to change. In psychology, this process is called behavior modification.

Following are a number of behavior-modification tricks to try to help your child lose weight. Of course, this technique will probably work best when other family members adopt some or all of these measures as well.

• Permit eating in one room of the house only.

• Require your child to have company when eating; don't let her eat alone.

• Do not let your child do anything else (reading, watching television, etc.) while eating. She should concentrate totally on what is being eaten.

• Permit your child to eat only with utensils.

• Prepare and serve small quantities only.

• Make only good, nutritious foods available.

• Experiment with attractive preparation of the right foods.

• Make sure your child eats slowly and chews thoroughly.

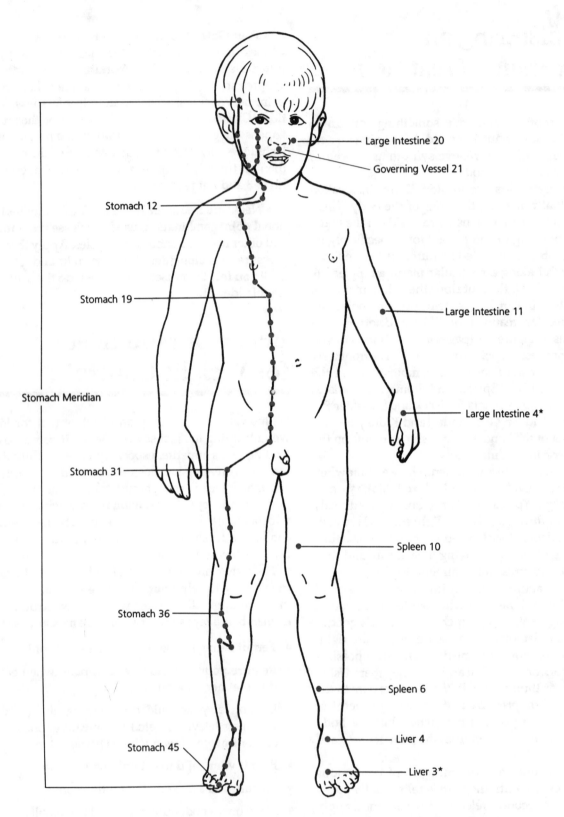

Large Intestine 20

Governing Vessel 21

Stomach 12

Stomach 19

Large Intestine 11

Stomach Meridian

Large Intestine 4*

Stomach 31

Spleen 10

Stomach 36

Spleen 6

Liver 4

Stomach 45

Liver 3*

*half of Four Gates combination.

Figure 3.1 Locations of Common Acupressure Points on a Child's Body
The illustrations above and at right show the locations of the acupressure points recommended in the various entries on common childhood health problems in Part Two. Points on the Governing Vessel, Large Intestine, Liver, Spleen, and Stomach meridians, and the points for the

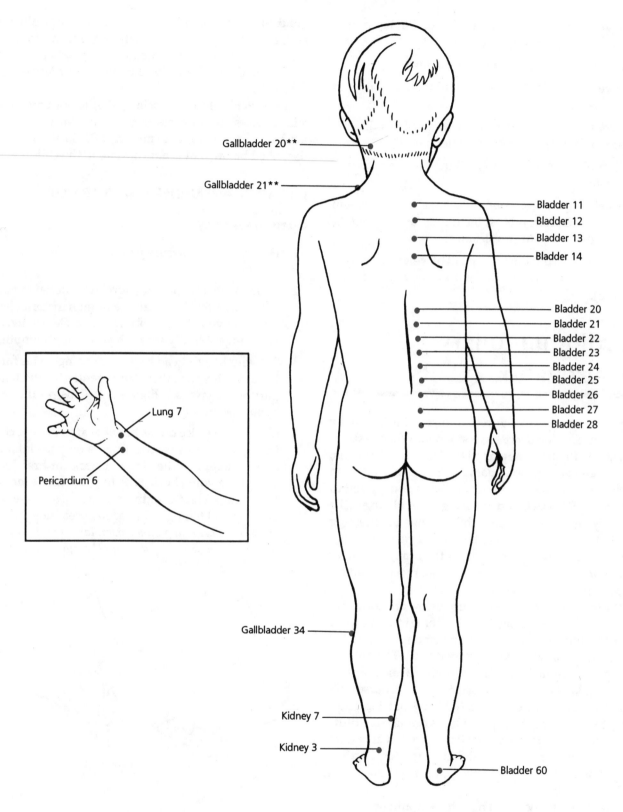

Gallbladder 20**

Gallbladder 21**

Bladder 11
Bladder 12
Bladder 13
Bladder 14

Bladder 20
Bladder 21
Bladder 22
Bladder 23
Bladder 24
Bladder 25
Bladder 26
Bladder 27
Bladder 28

Lung 7

Pericardium 6

Gallbladder 34

Kidney 7

Kidney 3

Bladder 60

*half of Neck and Shoulder Release.

Four Gates technique, are indicated on the front view of the child's body (left). Points on the Bladder, Gallbladder, and Kidney meridians, and the points for Neck and Shoulder Release, are shown on the back view (right).

- Have your child swallow all the food in her mouth before taking another bite.

- Introduce planned delays during meals.

- Have your child save one item from each meal to eat later as a snack.

- Except for the saved item, clear all plates directly into the garbage or compost after meals.

- Keep pictures of desired clothing and/or activities on hand.

- Develop a way for your child to get reinforcement for success from others, including family, friends, other dieters, your physician, etc.

- Plan to reward the achievement of weight-loss goals with a personal gift or a favorite activity (*not* with food!).

Cardiopulmonary Resuscitation (CPR)

These emergency procedures can sustain life if a child's breathing and/or heart have stopped. When respiration stops, the body begins to be deprived of oxygen, which can cause serious damage. Brain cells begin to die within four to six minutes if they are deprived of oxygen. CPR keeps blood and oxygen circulating in the body. By breathing into your child's lungs and pressing on his heart, you can maintain blood flow and oxygen/carbon dioxide exchange to the brain and other organs until he recovers or until emergency medical personnel arrive to take over.

The outlines of CPR procedures below are not meant to teach you everything in a time of crisis, but to be used as a refresher for a course on emergency first aid that includes infant and childhood CPR. The authors strongly recommend that anyone who cares for a child on a regular basis obtain such training. Courses are usually available through the Red Cross or a local hospital. Reading about the procedures cannot substitute for taking a course and practicing on a mannequin under the guidance of a qualified instructor. Further, these practices are constantly being researched and revised. Stay informed.

In addition to the usual mouth-to-mouth breathing, CPR can involve other procedures in special circumstances, such as giving CPR to a patient with a potential spinal-cord injury, mouth-to-nose breathing, mouth-to-nose-and-mouth breathing (as with an infant), and mouth-to-stoma breathing (a stoma is a surgically created opening in the body, such as a tracheostomy or laryngectomy). Only instruction and practice with an instructor in attendance will adequately prepare you to give CPR.

If your child loses consciousness, is not breathing, and/or loses his pulse, assess the situation quickly, call for emergency help, and initiate CPR in the manner described below that is appropriate to the child's age.

FOR AN INFANT UNDER ONE YEAR OLD

Open the Airway

1. Hold your baby securely in the crook of your arm, face up.

2. Look to see if there is any foreign material in your baby's mouth. If you can see foreign material present, use your finger to remove it. *Do not* sweep your finger blindly through your baby's mouth.

3. Tip your baby's head back by pushing on his forehead. With your other hand, gently lift the bony part of the jaw (see Figure 3.2). This positioning opens the airway.

4. Check for a pulse on the brachial artery by placing the tips of your first two fingers on your infant's inner arm above the elbow. Check for breathing by putting your cheek close to your child's mouth to feel for a breath, and watch his chest to see if it is rising and falling as in normal breathing. *If your child is not breathing on his own, take steps to restore breathing (see step 5). If your child has no pulse, initiate full CPR (go to step 9).*

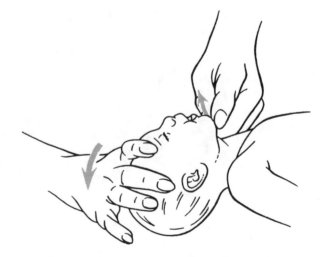

Figure 3.2 Opening the Airway
Gently tip your child's head back and lift the bony part of the jaw.

Restore Breathing

5. With your infant's airway open as described above, cover his nose *and* mouth with your mouth, and give two slow puffs of air, with just enough force to cause your baby's chest to rise and fall as in normal breathing (see Figure 3.3). Be gentle.

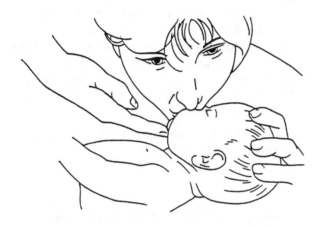

Figure 3.3 Rescue Breathing for an Infant
Cover your baby's mouth *and* nose with your mouth, and give two slow, gentle puffs of air.

6. If your breaths do not cause your child's chest to rise and fall, repeat steps 1 through 3, above, to open the airway again. Give two more puffs of air.

7. If there is still no movement of the chest, the airway is probably blocked. Perform the Heimlich maneuver as follows: Hold your baby securely, resting face down on your forearm. Rest your forearm on your thigh. Using the heel of your other hand, deliver five quick firm blows between the child's shoulder blades. (You will learn precisely how firm these blows need to be by practicing on a mannequin in your first aid class.) Then turn your child over to face you. With your fingers, give five quick firm compressions to the breastbone, just below the nipple line. Repeat these steps, alternating between five back blows and five chest thrusts, until the object is expelled. Do not stop until the foreign material is expelled and your baby begins coughing, breathing, and making normal sounds, *or* another person can take over for you, *or* medical help arrives.

8. *If your child loses his pulse during this procedure, initiate full CPR (see step 9).*

Full CPR

9. Place your baby flat on the floor on his back. Check for a pulse on the brachial artery again. Only if your child's heart has stopped beating and you can't feel a pulse can you safely begin CPR. *Never do chest compressions on a child with a heartbeat.*

10. If your baby is *not* breathing and *does not* have a pulse, give compressions. Locate the spot to give compressions by placing two or three fingers on your infant's chest just below the nipple line (see Figure 3.4). Keep your elbows straight and your shoulders lined up over your infant's body. Maintain this position so that the compressions are done straight up and down on your baby's chest. For each compression, push your baby's breastbone down with your fingers the equivalent of ⅓ to ½ of total chest height (approximately ½–1 inch) straight down. Do not rock your body. Do not move into your child's chest diagonally. Release the pressure between compressions without taking your fingers off his chest.

11. Perform cycles of chest compressions and respirations. For an infant, a complete cycle consists of at least 5 chest compressions followed by 1 breath. Give *at least* 20 breaths per minute (1 breath every 3 seconds) and 100 compressions per minute. Count aloud to help you maintain a steady rhythm: One one-thousand, two one-thousand, three one-thousand, four one-thousand, five one-thousand, and BREATH, and so on.

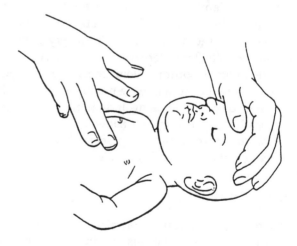

Figure 3.4 Locating the Spot for Compressions on an Infant
Place two or three fingers on your baby's chest just below the nipple line.

12. After giving CPR for one minute, check your infant's brachial pulse again. If you feel a pulse, stop doing chest compressions and check for breathing. If there is no pulse, continue performing CPR. Continue to check for a pulse and breathing every few minutes until emergency medical help arrives. Do not stop CPR until your child starts breathing on his own, *or* someone else can take over for you, *or* emergency help arrives.

13. If your infant begins breathing on his own, discontinue CPR. Once his pulse and breathing have been restored and the immediate crisis is over, check and treat your baby for bleeding, broken bones, or any other injury or problem he might have.

FOR A CHILD OVER ONE YEAR OLD

Open the Airway

1. Place your child on his back on the floor, face up.

2. Look to see if there is any foreign material in your child's mouth. If you can see foreign material in your child's mouth, remove it with your finger, but *do not* sweep your finger blindly through your child's mouth.

3. Tip your child's head back by pushing on his forehead. With your other hand, gently lift the bony part of the jaw (see Figure 3.2, page 426). This positioning opens the airway.

4. Check for a pulse on the carotid artery, located at the side of the neck. Touch your first two fingers to the Adam's apple. Run your fingers across the neck to the depression between the Adam's apple and the large neck muscle. Press very gently so that you don't interfere with blood flow. Check for breathing by putting your cheek close to your child's mouth to feel for a breath, and watch his chest to see if it is rising and falling as in normal breathing. *If your child is not breathing on his own, take steps to restore breathing (see step 5). If there is no pulse, initiate full CPR (go to step 9).*

Restore Breathing

5. Once you have your child's airway open, pinch his nostrils closed, cover his mouth with yours, and give two slow puffs of air with enough force to cause your child's chest to rise and fall as in normal breathing (see Figure 3.5).

6. If your breaths do not cause your child's chest to rise and fall, repeat steps 1 through 3, above, to open the airway again. Give two more puffs of air.

7. If there is still no movement of the chest, the airway is probably blocked. Perform the Heimlich maneuver as follows: Straddle your child, squatting above his knees. Place the heel of your hand against his abdomen, just above the navel and below the rib cage. Place your other hand on top of the first. Use a quick, forceful *upward* push to force air up through the windpipe. If necessary, continue performing these thrusts until your child coughs up all of the foreign material. Do not stop the procedure until the foreign material is expelled and your child begins coughing, breathing, and talking on his own, *or* another person can take over for you, *or* medical help arrives.

8. *If your child loses his pulse during this procedure, initiate full CPR (see step 9).*

Full CPR

9. Place your child flat on the floor on his back. Check for a pulse on the carotid artery again. Only if your child's heart has stopped beating and you can't feel a pulse can you safely begin CPR. *Never do chest compressions on a child with a heartbeat.*

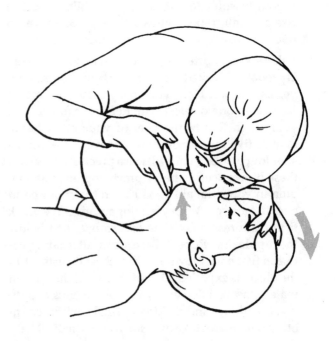

Figure 3.5 Rescue Breathing for a Child
Gently pinch your child's nostrils closed, cover his mouth with yours, and give two slow puffs of air.

10. If your child is *not* breathing and *does not* have a pulse, straddle your child to give compressions. Locate the spot to give compressions by following the rib cage to where the ribs and sternum meet. Put your middle finger on this notch and your index finger right next to your middle finger. Notice the placement of your index finger and place the heel of your hand right next to it (see Figure 3.6). Keep your elbows straight and your shoulders lined up over your child's body. Maintain this position so that the compressions are done straight up and down on his chest. For each compression, push your child's breastbone ⅓ to ½ of total chest height (approximately 1–1½ inches) straight down. Do not rock your body. Do not move into your child's chest diagonally. Release the pressure between compressions without taking your fingers off his chest.

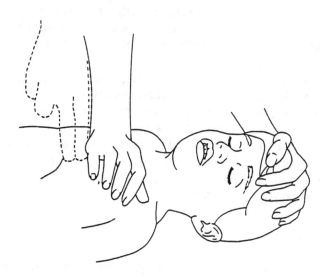

Figure 3.6 Locating the Spot for Compressions on a Child
Place your middle finger where the ribs and sternum meet; place your index finger next to it. Then place the heel of your hand above the spot where your index finger was.

11. Perform cycles of chest compressions and respirations. For a child over one year, give 20 breaths per minute (1 breath every 3 seconds) and 100 compressions per minute. A complete cycle consists of 5 chest compressions followed by 1 breath. Count aloud to help you maintain a steady rhythm: One one-thousand, two one-thousand, three one-thousand, four one-thousand, and BREATH, and so on.

12. After giving CPR for one minute, check your child's carotid pulse again. If you feel a pulse, stop doing chest compressions and check for breathing. If there is no pulse, continue performing CPR. Con-tinue to check for a pulse and breathing every few minutes, until emergency medical help arrives. Do not stop CPR until your child starts breathing on his own, *or* someone else can take over for you, *or* emergency help arrives.

13. If your child begins breathing on his own, discontinue CPR. Once pulse and breathing have been restored and the immediate crisis is over, check and treat your child for bleeding, broken bones, or any other injury or problem he might have.

Administering a Douche

A douche is one of the most helpful treatments for a vaginal infection, because it works right at the site of the problem. Douches can be made from a variety of ingredients, including medicated products such as Betadine or natural products like herbs, yogurt, and white vinegar. Douches should be used only if an infection is present or if recommended by your health care practitioner, however. Excessive douching may actually cause irritation and infection.

When using a commercial product, prepare the solution according to the directions on the product label. When making an herbal douche, you can use either dried herbs or herbal extracts. If you use the dried form, simmer the herb in a pot of water for fifteen minutes, then strain and let the mixture cool to a lukewarm temperature. If you use a tincture, add the recommended dose to a quart of lukewarm water.

Purchase a douche bag or syringe at your local drug store. To administer a standard douche, if using a syringe, squat or sit in an empty bathtub and insert the syringe into the vagina. *Gently* squeeze on the bag to wash the solution over the tissues. If using a bag, sit in an empty bathtub. Hang the bag no more than two feet above the hips. Let the solution fill the tube before inserting the nozzle into the vagina, then allow the solution to flow into and out of the vagina. *Do not* use force or pressure to get the solution into the vagina. The point is to gently cleanse the vaginal tissue.

Some formulas work well as retention douches. These use smaller amounts (no more than about one fluid ounce) of a thicker consistency liquid. As the name implies, a retention douche is retained in the vagina for a period of time. A tampon may be inserted once the solution has been applied to keep it from leaking out. Depending on the formula used, a retention douche may be followed with a standard water douche.

Elimination Diet

An elimination diet can help you determine the particular foods to which your child is most allergic or sensitive. Once you have identified them, you can eliminate from his diet the things that cause trouble.

Begin by eliminating foods you think may be the source of your child's symptoms. If you are not sure exactly where to start, start with the foods that most commonly cause a reaction: wheat, citrus fruits and juices, nuts (including peanut butter), dairy products, corn, soy products, and eggs.

Eliminate the suspect foods from your child's diet for a two-week period. Be aware of the ingredients in manufactured food products. Many of these will probably contain ingredients that are on your list of suspects. Observe your child carefully during this elimination period. How does he feel? Does he seem to be breathing more easily? Are his eyes clear instead of itchy and irritated? Is your child generally happier and less cranky? Does he have more energy?

After the elimination period, test a food, or class of foods, by putting it back on your child's menu. For three days, observe how he reacts (it can take as long as seventy-two hours for a reaction to manifest itself). To make sure you can identify precisely which is the offending food, add only one food or class of foods every three days, and give it to your child in as pure a form as possible. For example, to test wheat, give your child cream of wheat rather than bread, which may contain other allergens.

If eliminating all suspect foods from your child's diet at one time seems too drastic, try eliminating particular classes of foods one at a time. For example, eliminate all wheat products for a two-week period and see how your child reacts. If his symptoms are not relieved, then eliminate all dairy products as well (and continue to keep wheat off the menu) for the next two-week period, and so on. Continue deleting a food or class of foods until your child's symptoms improve, and keep your child off the food throughout the entire trial. Once symptoms have improved, you can assume that your child is sensitive to the food most recently deleted. You can then add the other foods back into your child's diet, one at a time, but be alert for any sensitivity or reaction.

Once you have determined which food or foods are causing your child's reaction, simply keep them off the menu. Read labels carefully to be sure the offending foods are not present as ingredients in the products you buy.

You can also try tracking down food sensitivities by using a diet diary. For three to four weeks, write down everything your child eats and when he eats it, along with how he feels and any reactions he displays. After the four-week period, you should be able to detect patterns in your child's responses to different foods.

For a more detailed approach to uncovering food sensitivities, read *Tracking Down Hidden Food Allergies* by William Crook, M.D. (Professional Books, 1978).

Heimlich Maneuver

The Heimlich maneuver, named for its developer, Dr. H.J. Heimlich, will expel an object that is lodged in the throat and blocking breathing. If a child with something stuck in her throat is talking or coughing forcefully, it means that air is getting through the windpipe and you don't need to interfere. As long as she can breathe, she may be able to expel the material without help. But if your child is unable to speak, making high-pitched sounds or gasping for air, turning blue, or clutching at her throat, intervene quickly. Follow the directions below to perform the Heimlich maneuver in the manner appropriate for your child's age.

Please note that the information in this entry is not meant to serve as a substitute for a hands-on course in first aid, but as a review should you ever be called upon to use your first aid training.

FOR AN INFANT UNDER ONE YEAR OLD

1. Hold your baby securely, resting face down on your forearm. Rest your forearm on your thigh. Using the heel of your other hand, deliver five quick firm blows between the child's shoulder blades (see Figure 3.7). You will learn precisely how firm these blows need to be by practicing on a mannequin in your first aid class.

2. Turn your child over to face you. With your fingers, give five quick firm compressions to the breastbone, just below the nipple line (see Figure 3.7).

3. Repeat steps 1 and 2, alternating between five back blows and five chest thrusts, until the object is expelled.

4. Do not stop the procedure until the foreign material is expelled and your baby begins coughing, breathing, and making normal sounds, *or* another person can take over for you, *or* emergency medical help arrives.

5. Once you have performed the Heimlich maneuver successfully, even if your child seems to be fine, she should be examined by a doctor as soon as possible to make sure there has been no damage to the windpipe or abdomen.

FOR A CHILD OVER ONE YEAR OLD

The Heimlich maneuver, named for its developer, Dr. H.J. Heimlich, will expel an object that is lodged in the throat and blocking breathing.

1. Stand or kneel behind your child, wrapping your arms around her waist. Make a fist with one hand and clasp your other hand over your fist. Using the thumb side of your fist, push into your child's abdomen, just above the navel and below the rib cage. Use a quick, forceful *upward* push to force air up through the windpipe (see Figure 3.8).

2. If necessary, continue performing these thrusts until your child coughs up all of the foreign material.

3. Do not stop the procedure until the foreign material is expelled and your child begins coughing, breathing, and talking on her own, *or* another person can take over for you, *or* emergency medical help arrives.

4. Once you have performed the Heimlich maneuver successfully, even if your child seems to be fine, she should be examined by a doctor as soon as possible to make sure there has been no damage to the windpipe or abdomen.

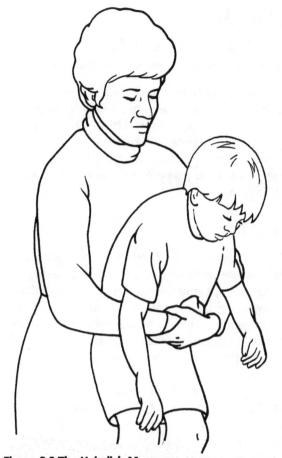

Figure 3.8 The Heimlich Maneuver
Wrap your arms around your child's waist between the navel and rib cage. With your fist, give a forceful upward push.

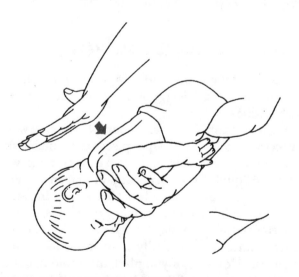
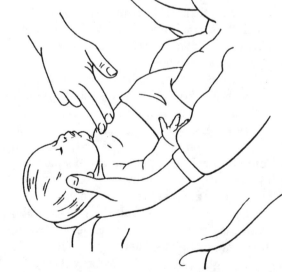

Figure 3.7 First Aid for a Choking Infant
With the heel of your hand, give five quick blows between the shoulder blades (left). Then, using your fingers, give five quick, firm compressions to your baby's breastbone (right).

Preparing Herbal Treatments

The herbal treatments recommended in this book include teas, baths, compresses, poultices, oils, and ointments. Some require that you start from scratch, while others, especially tablets or capsules, are available ready made. The recipes and directions in this section will teach you how to prepare and use a wide variety of herbal treatments.

HERBAL BATHS

An herbal bath is as much of a treat as it is a treatment. There are several ways to prepare an herbal bath.

If you are using a soluble ingredient, such as baking soda or aloe vera gel, simply dissolve it in hot bath water.

If you are using oatmeal, you can either whirl it into a powder in your blender or bag it (see below). Oatmeal seems soft, but it doesn't dissolve completely unless it has first been very finely milled.

If you are using fresh herbs, you can bag them in a square of cheesecloth or a washcloth. A two- or three-thickness square of cheesecloth is ideal. The loose weave permits maximum release of the herbal essence, yet keeps the parts from floating free in the bath water. One method of bagging herbs is to stitch three sides of a cheesecloth square closed and run a drawstring through the top, or tie the bag closed with a sturdy string. An easier and quicker method is to place a suitable quantity of herbs in the middle of a cheesecloth square. Then simply pull the four corners of the square together and secure them with string. (You can do this with a washcloth or small towel, too, but cheesecloth is easier to manage.) For a full bath, use approximately 6 ounces of dried or fresh herbs.

Fill the tub, placing the bagged herbs under a forceful stream of comfortably hot water. As the tub fills, swish the herbs through the bath water. During the bath, gently squeeze an essence-rich stream of water from the herb bag directly on the part of the body you wish to treat. Your child may enjoy soaking and squeezing the bag. If you are treating an itchy skin condition, you may *gently* rub the bag across the affected areas. Unless you can trust your child not to rub itchy places raw, however, you may want to do this gentle scratching yourself. If you are using dried herbs, you will have to guard against rough parts, which may be irritating.

If your child is comforted and soothed by an herbal bath, you may want to be ready with a pre-prepared herbal infusion. Soak 6 tablespoons of dried or fresh herbs overnight in 3 cups of water. Start with very hot water and allow it to cool naturally. The following morning, heat the infusion and strain out the residue. No bag is needed; just pour the strained infusion directly into the bath water.

HERBAL INFUSIONS (TEAS)

Medicinal herbs are most often administered in tea form. The Chinese, who have a 5,000-year history of herbal medicine, teach that the heat of the water and the taste of the herb enhance its effectiveness. Steeping an herb in hot water draws out the therapeutic essence of the plant.

To prepare hot tea from herbs, measure out 2 heaping tablespoons of herb for every cup of tea (unless the label directs otherwise), and place them in a china or glass teapot or cup (plastic and metal containers are not suitable for steeping herbs). For each cup of tea, pour 8 ounces of freshly boiled water over the herbs. Cover the container. As a general rule, teas made with the leaf or flower of the herb should be allowed to steep for five to ten minutes; teas using roots or bark should be simmered for ten minutes and allowed to steep for an additional five minutes. After steeping, strain the tea, cool it to a comfortable temperature, and serve. If you prepare more than one cup of tea at one time, you can keep it at a comfortable sipping temperature in a thermos bottle.

To make an herbal tea from a tincture or extract, put the suggested number of drops of the extract into a hot cup of water. Let the mixture sit for five minutes to allow some of the alcohol to evaporate.

HERBAL JUICES (JUICED FRESH HERBS)

If you are lucky enough to have a reliable source of fresh herbs and a juicer, you may want to prepare a fresh essence.

Wash the fresh herbs well under cold running water. If necessary, scissor them into pieces of a suitable size. Place the wet herb parts in a juice extractor and whiz them into liquid. The fresh juice may be taken internally in the form of a few drops diluted in tea or spring water. For some conditions, the juice may prove valuable when dabbed externally on the affected parts of the body.

Fresh juices are generally used immediately after extraction. However, if you place the liquid in a small glass bottle, cork it tightly, and refrigerate it, it will keep for several days without an appreciable loss of vital properties.

HERBAL OINTMENTS

There are many very fine herbal ointments and salves available. Purchased ointments and salves are often much more attractive and pleasant to use than the homemade variety. But if you wish to emulate yesterday's herbalists, here's how to make your own herbal ointment.

In a double boiler (preferably ceramic or glass), heat 2 ounces of vegetable lanolin or beeswax until it becomes liquid. Once this base is melted, add 80 to 120 drops of each herbal tincture you want in your salve. Mix them together and pour into a glass container. Refrigerate the mixture and allow it to harden. If you prefer, you can use a very strong herbal tea made with your own fresh or dried herbs instead of a store-bought tincture. Keep a record of your recipes for later use.

HERBAL OILS

To prepare a fragrant herbal oil, wash the fresh herbs of your choice and permit them to dry overnight. Place scissored fresh herbs or crumbled dried herbs in a glass bottle or jar. Slowly add light virgin olive oil or almond oil until the oil level is an inch above the herb parts. Cover the container tightly and allow it to stand in a very warm place for two weeks. You may place it near the stove to gather warmth from cooking, or outside in the sun (but remember to bring it in before night cools the air). Strain the oil before using it.

HERBAL POULTICES OR COMPRESSES (PULPED)

Only fresh herbs are suitable for making a pulped poultice. Dried herbs do not pulp well. By pulping the herbs directly onto the poultice cloth, you retain all the juices and improve the effectiveness of the poultice.

Place a quantity of fresh herb parts on a clean white cloth several folds thick (cotton, gauze, linen, and muslin are ideal). Wrap several thicknesses of the cloth over the herbs. Using a rolling pin, thoroughly crush the herbs to a pulp.

Unwrap a layer or two of the cloth, until you uncover a thoroughly wetted area. Apply this to the affected area of the body. To trap the juices and hold the poultice in place, overwrap it well with a woolen cloth or a towel. A pulped compress can remain in place overnight.

HERBAL POULTICES OR COMPRESSES (STEAMED)

A hot herbal poultice can be very comforting to a distressed child. The active ingredients in the herbs will be absorbed through the skin.

Place a steamer, colander, strainer, or sieve over a pot of rapidly boiling water. Layer either chopped fresh or dried herbs in the steamer, reduce the heat to a simmering temperature, and cover the pot. Allow the steam to thoroughly penetrate and wilt the herbs.

After about five minutes, spread the softened and warmed herbs on a clean white, loosely woven cloth, such as cheesecloth, and apply it to the affected area. To hold in the heat, you may overwrap the poultice in a woolen cloth or a towel. The poultice should remain in place for at least twenty minutes, and/or for as long as your child will sit still. If your child feels comforted and soothed by the poultice, you may leave it on overnight.

HERBAL TINCTURES

Tinctures employ alcohol to draw out and preserve the active properties of an herb. Because tinctures concentrate the essence of herbs, they are commonly taken as drops in tea, or diluted in spring water. Tinctures may also be used in a compress or body massage.

To prepare an herbal tincture at home, loosely fill a glass bottle or jar with herbal parts. If you are using fresh herbs, scissor them into manageable pieces. If you are using dried herbs, crumble them into the container. Add pure spirits, such as vodka, to cover the herbs. Seal the container and allow the tincture to stand in a warm place (between 70° and 80°F) for two weeks. While you are waiting for the tincture to mature, shake the container daily. After two weeks, strain out the herbs and squeeze out the residue.

To remove some of the alcohol from a tincture before giving it to your child, add the suitable number of drops of tincture to ¼ cup of very hot water or tea. Most of the alcohol will evaporate away in about five minutes.

HERBAL VAPOR INHALATION TREATMENT

An herbal inhalation treatment is very helpful for respiratory and sinus conditions. It opens up congested sinuses and lung passages, helping your child to discharge mucus, breathe more easily, and heal faster.

Fill your bathroom sink with very hot water and add 2 to 5 drops of herbal oil. To keep the water hot and steaming, allow a small, continuous trickle of hot water to flow into the basin (the overflow outlet in your sink should prevent the water from spilling over). Have your child inhale the steam for at least five minutes. As the treated water becomes diluted, add a few more drops of herbal oil as needed.

If it is not feasible to use the bathroom sink for this purpose, or if you are using dried or whole herbs, use a pot of water heated on the stove to prepare an inhalation treatment. Fill a pot (preferably one that is wide but not too tall) with water. If using whole or dried herbs, add a small handful, heat the water to boiling, and simmer for about five minutes. Then remove the pot from the heat, place it on a hot pad or trivet on a tabletop, and allow it to cool slightly. If using herbal oil, heat the water to just short of boiling, remove it from the heat, place it on a tabletop, and add 4 to 5 drops of the oil. Have your child drape a large towel over his head, forming a tent, and lean over the pot. Have him inhale the steam for at least five minutes. (Be careful that the mixture is not too hot; if it is, it can burn the nasal passages.)

To help clear lung congestion, encourage your child to take several deep, full breaths of air after an inhalation treatment.

Nasal Saline Flush

Nasal saline flushes, or irrigation, are very useful in the treatment of respiratory allergies and sinus infections. They cleanse the sinuses and the tissues that line the nasal passages, as well as soothing the mucous membranes and thinning mucus.

Dissolve ¼ teaspoon of salt and ⅛ teaspoon of baking soda in 4 ounces of water. Spray the mixture inside your child's nose with a bulb syringe, or, for an infant, instill several drops into the nose with an eyedropper. If you are using this technique to clear nasal congestion, you can then suck out the mucus with a bulb syringe. If you are using it to soothe and moisten the mucous membranes, do not suction out mucus afterward.

Applying a Pressure Bandage

If your child is bleeding from a severe external wound, cover it with a clean cloth or gauze and quickly apply firm, steady pressure directly to the site. If there is no clean cloth or gauze immediately available, use your bare hand to apply pressure. Even if your child complains of the pressure you are applying, firm, steady pressure is necessary to stop the bleeding.

If there is no suspicion of a spinal injury or internal bleeding, raise the affected part of the body to above the level of the heart. This will help minimize the amount of blood flowing from the wound. Suspect a spinal cord injury if a child is unresponsive; shows weakness, numbness, or paralysis in the extremities; is found lying flat on her back or seems to have fallen from a high place; or has been in a car accident. Suspect internal bleeding if a child is pale, sweaty, and bleeding from the mouth, nose, or ears; has a very fast or very slow heartbeat; or has a hard, rigid abdomen.

If blood soaks through the cloth pad or gauze, put more cloth or gauze over the old pad and continue applying pressure. It's best not to remove the original blood-soaked pad, as clotting may be disrupted when you try to change the bandage.

If emergency personnel are not available, take your child to the emergency room of the nearest hospital. If you are fortunate enough to have another adult with you, have that person see to the transportation while you hold your child and continue applying pressure to the wound. If you are alone and must transport your child yourself, tie cloth or gauze firmly in place over the wound to maintain the pressure. If you must tie on a bandage, check for a pulse beat below the wound to make sure that the tissues below the wound are receiving an adequate supply of blood.

Taking Your Child's Pulse

Taking your child's pulse is a basic diagnostic procedure that is easily performed. Different techniques are recommended for children under and over one year of age, as outlined below.

FOR AN INFANT UNDER ONE YEAR OLD

To take the pulse of an infant less than one year old, feel for a pulse on the brachial artery, the artery that carries blood to the arm.

Place the tips of your first two fingers on your infant's inner arm above the elbow (see Figure 3.9). Using a precise timer such as the second hand of your watch, count the number of pulses you feel for one minute.

Another useful place to feel for a pulse is the groin, through which the femoral artery passes.

FOR A CHILD OVER ONE YEAR OLD

To take the pulse of a child over one year old, feel for a pulse on the carotid artery, located at the side of the neck.

Touch your first two fingers to your child's Adam's apple, and run your fingers across his neck to the de-

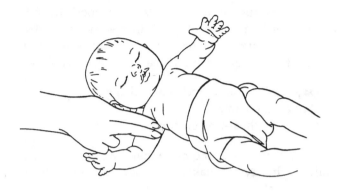

Figure 3.9 Taking an Infant's Pulse on the Brachial Artery

pression between the Adam's apple and the large neck muscle (see Figure 3.10).

Using a precise timer such as the second hand of your watch, count the number of beats you feel for one minute, or count for ten seconds and multiply the result by six.

Another useful place to feel for a pulse is the radial artery, on the thumb side of the wrist.

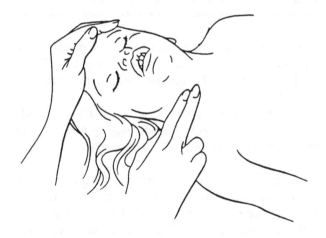

Figure 3.10 Taking a Child's Pulse on the Carotid Artery

Relaxation Techniques

There are a number of different techniques that can be helpful for a child who is restless, ill, under stress (whether physical or mental), or having trouble falling or staying asleep.

RELAXATION AND VISUALIZATION EXERCISES

The goal of these exercises is to cultivate a sense of physical and emotional relaxation. Situations such as

an asthma attack or acute pain can create fear, anxiety, and muscle tension. These reactions in turn make the situation worse. If your child has a chronic illness such as asthma, try practicing the exercises consistently so that when needed, she can readily access the relaxation or visualization.

Have your child sit or lie down in a comfortable position. It is helpful if the environment is quiet. Using a soft voice, speak at a slow, steady pace. The following are examples of things you might say (but whatever scenario you use, your words should make sense and offer comfort to your child).

Try the following words.

Let your eyes close . . . take a deep breath in, and when you blow out, let go of all of your thoughts of the day . . . take another breath in, and when you blow out, let go of all the rest of the thoughts of the day . . . now we will move slowly from your toes to your head, letting go of all the tension . . . starting with your toes, let them feel very heavy and very soft . . . let the floor support your feet . . . let your feet rest . . . let go of all the tension in your toes and feet . . . they are very heavy now . . . now move up to your calves . . . let them feel very heavy and very soft . . . warm and cozy . . . let them rest totally on the floor . . . [continue working your way up through the entire body, finishing with the head].

You can add a visualization to this by suggesting such things as, "Imagine the medicine traveling to your lungs [or your head, or your hurt leg, etc.]," and suggesting that your child imagine that the sensations of pain and/or illness are disappearing and floating away; that her body's defenses are taking care of her by fighting to get rid of an affliction such as eczema or warts; or whatever type of visualization might be appropriate for your child's situation.

THE RELAXATION RESPONSE

An older child can be taught the relaxation response, a natural way to counteract stress. It is also a safe, non-toxic, free, and readily available "tranquilizer" that can be useful for a restless child (or adult!) who is having trouble sleeping. You might want to practice this technique with your child.

1. Have your child sit quietly in a comfortable position.

2. To minimize distraction, have your child close her eyes.

3. Have your child consciously relax all of her muscles, beginning at the feet and progressing upward to the face. To help your child understand how to "let go," have her give a good shake and then relax.

4. Have your child breathe through her nose easily and naturally. On each outgoing breath, have your child say the word *one* silently to herself. Concentrating on the word *one* helps to keep intrusive thoughts away.

5. Once her muscles are relaxed, have your child continue breathing easily and regularly for ten to fifteen minutes. Have her sit quietly for several more minutes when finished, at first with her eyes closed, then with her eyes open.

6. If you are practicing this technique with your child, you may open your eyes to check the elapsed time. Don't set an alarm, which would introduce a jarring note.

If your child doesn't achieve a deep level of relaxation, don't worry. Help her maintain a passive attitude. Relaxation will happen at its own pace. Help your child understand that distracting thoughts will vanish if they are not dwelt upon. Silently repeating the word *one* helps. With practice, the relaxation response will come with little effort. The technique can be practiced during the day, but is the most helpful just before bedtime.

Because digestion can interfere with the relaxation response, the exercise should not be practiced for two hours after eating.

For an excellent discussion of relaxation and visualization techniques you can use with your child, you may wish to consult *Spinning Inward: Using Guided Imagery With Children for Learning, Creativity, and Relaxation* by Maureen Murdock (Shambhala, 1987). Another good resource is *The Relaxation Response* by Dr. H. Benson (William Morrow & Company, 1976).

Rotation Diet

A rotation diet is a diet that can sometimes alleviate problems associated with a food allergy or sensitivity in less time than an elimination diet can. Rather than identifying a particular food allergy or sensitivity, the rotation diet provides a way to plan your child's diet so that he is less at the mercy of food sensitivities. It works on the principle that a child who is allergic to a particular food or class of foods may not show a reaction if those foods are spaced out over a three-day period.

To implement a rotation diet, plan menus so that you do not serve suspect foods or classes of foods to your child more than once during any three-day period. For example, if you suspect that your child may be sensitive to wheat, you might vary the breakfast menu as follows.

Day 1: Wheat toast and poached eggs.
Day 2: Hot oatmeal.
Day 3: A wheat-free muffin.

After three days, the cycle starts again, and your child might have a breakfast of wheat toast or a wheat-based cereal.

By following a three-day rotation diet, you may be able to give your child all classes of foods without triggering the symptoms of food sensitivity. Of course, if your child tends to have a severe reaction, such as hives or wheezing (called *anaphylaxis*), to a particular food, that food must be eliminated from his diet altogether.

Taking Your Child's Temperature

Normal body temperature probably has a much wider range than previously thought. No longer is 98.6°F considered standard. Temperature also varies throughout the day.

In general, any temperature above 101°F is considered elevated. However, it is not usually necessary to treat a temperature under 102°F unless it is making your child uncomfortable.

There are a number of different ways to take a child's temperature: orally, rectally, and under the arm. The way you choose will be determined by your child's age and by her ability to keep still for three minutes or so. In addition to standard thermometers, there are now digital thermometers available that can take a child's temperature in much less time. These are convenient if you have a child who is squirmy and uncomfortable. Ask your nurse or doctor which type or types he or she considers the most reliable. Another option (highly effective but much more expensive) is a device that measures temperature in the ear.

Regardless of which method you choose, *never* leave any child alone with a thermometer. Also, if you notice a crack in the thermometer, throw it out. The mercury it contains is poisonous.

If your child has just eaten or drunk something warm, is dressed very warmly, or has just been exercising, wait thirty minutes before taking her temperature to be sure you get an accurate reading.

ORAL METHOD

If your child is older than five years, take her temperature orally.

Shake down the thermometer so that it registers less than 96°F. Place the silver or red end of the thermometer under your child's tongue or in her cheek. Either you or your child can hold it in place with your fingers. Don't let your child use her teeth to hold it there. Leave the thermometer in place for three minutes, then remove it.

After reading your child's temperature, wash the thermometer with cool water and then rub it with isopropyl rubbing alcohol.

RECTAL METHOD

Because young children are so active, and because babies and younger children cannot hold a thermometer in their mouths, a rectal temperature may be your best (or only) option. To take your child's temperature rectally, use a rectal thermometer, which has a round bulb at the end.

Shake down the thermometer so that it registers less than 96°F. Dip the bulb end of the thermometer in petroleum jelly, and insert it about one inch into your baby's rectum. Hold it in place for three minutes, then remove it. It is a good idea to have a towel or washcloth on hand when taking your child's temperature rectally, in case of "accidents" when removing the thermometer.

When reading your child's temperature, be aware that a rectal temperature is usually about 0.8°F higher than an oral temperature. After reading your child's temperature, wash the thermometer with cool water and then rub it with isopropyl rubbing alcohol.

UNDERARM METHOD

If your child is less than five years old, or unable to hold a thermometer in her mouth, you can try taking her temperature under the arm. This method usually yields a temperature reading approximately 1°F lower than a child's oral temperature. It also does not always give as reliable a reading as the others do, so it is best used only as a general indicator.

Shake down the thermometer so that it registers less than 96°F. Place the silver or red end of the thermometer against your child's armpit. Make sure the armpit is dry before placing the thermometer. Leave the thermometer in place for two minutes.

After reading your child's temperature, wash the thermometer with cool water and then rub it with isopropyl rubbing alcohol.

Therapeutic Recipes

Some of the entries in Part Two recommend certain therapeutic foods that can help your child in different situations. Two of the most useful of these are a soup made with the Chinese herb astragalus and a variety of vegetables, and a digestive remedy made from kuzu powder and umeboshi plum. Both are easy to make.

Astragalus and vegetable soup is excellent for a wide variety of illnesses and conditions. Both astragalus and burdock root help to boost the immune system; barley is very soothing to the digestive tract. Use vegetables that are high in vitamins A and C, such as those suggested in the recipe.

Kuzu cream with salt plum is a stomach-soothing preparation that is both effective and versatile. It works particularly well for nausea associated with overeating or overindulgence in sweets. It is also excellent for acid indigestion, colds, stomach pains, diarrhea, dysentery, and fever. For an upset stomach or diarrhea, you can give your child anywhere from 1 teaspoon to ¼ cup at a time, in small sips. Repeat every one to three hours throughout the day, as needed. Because it has a delicious flavor and a soothing, thick consistency, most children accept the mixture readily.

Astragalus and Vegetable Immune-Boosting Soup

1 astragalus root strip
1 burdock root
10 cups water
½ teaspoon thyme
½ teaspoon sage
6 cups vegetables, cut into bite-sized pieces
(good choices are broccoli, cauliflower, carrots, celery, green peppers, parsley, potatoes, squash, string beans, and zucchini)
1 cup cooked barley

1. In a glass or stainless steel pot, simmer the astragalus and burdock root in the water with the thyme and sage for 20 to 30 minutes. Strain out the herbs and use the resulting tea as a broth for the soup.

2. Add the vegetables and barley to the broth and cook. Allow to simmer slowly for 1 hour.

3. Serve warm. The soup can be strained and served as a broth, or served with all the vegetables. Makes approximately six servings.

Note: Once your child becomes accustomed to herbal tastes, you can combine steps 1 and 2, adding all the ingredients at one time, and pull the astragalus and burdock root out after the soup has simmered and before serving.

Kuzu Cream With Salt Plum

1 cup water
1 salt plum (umeboshi), pitted and minced,
or ½ teaspoon umeboshi paste
1½ tablespoons kuzu powder
¼ cup water
1 teaspoon shoyu (natural soy sauce)
or ¼ teaspoon grated ginger (optional)

1. In a saucepan, combine 1 cup water and the salt plum or umeboshi paste. Bring to a boil.

2. In a small bowl or measuring cup, dissolve 1½ tablespoons kuzu powder in ¼ cup water. (Kuzu powder thickens the mixture. If you find that you prefer a thinner consistency, you may use as little as 1½ teaspoons kuzu powder.)

3. Add the dissolved kuzu powder to the contents of the saucepan, stirring constantly with a fork or wire whisk. Return to a boil.

4. Reduce the heat to low and simmer for 1 minute.

5. Take the mixture off the heat, and allow it to cool sufficiently before serving. Makes about 1½ cups.

6. If desired, you may add shoyu or ginger to the mixture along with the dissolved kuzu powder for flavor. Ginger root also soothes the stomach. If you do not have grated ginger, you may substitute ½ teaspoon powdered ginger root, or 12 drops juice from grated ginger root.

Time-Out

Time-out is a way to deal with behaviors that are unacceptable and need to be addressed and stopped immediately. Temper tantrums, hitting, biting, and other disrespectful and dangerous behaviors can be helped by using time-out. It is most effective for children between eighteen months and ten years old.

Following are the six basic principles of time-out, and the six steps for using the procedure.

PRINCIPLES OF TIME-OUT

1. Establish a place to be used for time-out. Choose a place that is quiet and without stimulation or distraction. Do not use a place that is dark or scary for your child.

2. Explain which behaviors are unacceptable and what the punishment for them is. Explain the house rules, as well as what the consequences are when the rules are broken.

3. Be consistent in your use of time-out. If you say time-out will be for five minutes, be sure it is five minutes, not three or ten. Buy a timer and use it specifically for time-out. Follow through on what you say; use time-out for the behaviors that you say you will use it for.

4. Do not yell, scream, or be judgmental in your use of time-out. When unacceptable behavior occurs, be consistent and matter-of-fact in setting limits.

5. Generally, it is recommended that one minute of time-out be enforced for each year of a child's age, up to a total of five minutes.

6. Do not scold a child who is in time-out. Do not allow other family members to scold or tease a child who is in time-out.

PROCEDURE FOR TIME-OUT

1. When unacceptable behavior happens, name the behavior and ask your child to stop.

2. If the behavior continues, tell your child that if it doesn't stop immediately, time-out will begin.

3. If the behavior continues, with as little effort as possible, take your child to the time-out spot.

4. Set the timer for the agreed amount of time.

5. If your child does not respect the time-out, reset the timer.

6. When the timer goes off, go to your child, let him know that the time-out is over, and ask if he would like to get up. If your child is still angry or disrespectful, reset the timer until you get a positive or neutral response when the timer goes off. Do not call to your child from another room to say that it is okay to get up. It is important to complete the process together. Don't forget that your child is in time-out.

Some parents prefer to give the child responsibility for determining when he is ready to rejoin the group or family activity. In this case, the principles of time-out remain the same, but the child chooses the time frame.

ALTERNATIVE PROCEDURE FOR TIME-OUT

1. When unacceptable behavior happens, name the behavior and ask your child to stop.

2. If the behavior continues, tell your child that if it doesn't stop immediately, time-out will begin.

3. If the behavior continues, with as little effort as possible, take your child to the time-out spot.

4. Explain to your child that when he feels ready to rejoin the family activity in a way that is respectful and that works for everyone, he can come back. His behaviors and choices are up to him.

5. When he rejoins the activity, acknowledge his presence, welcome him back, and be fairly matter-of-fact about it. Don't hold judgments or threats over him; start again with a clean slate.

6. If the unacceptable behavior begins again, repeat the above steps. There may come a point when you have to talk with your child to find out what he needs or why he can't participate in an acceptable way. It is important, however, not to set up a situation in which your child is getting extra attention and support in time-out. This can lead to the child equating acting out or breaking agreements with getting attention.

Appendix

Glossary

acidophilus. *Lactobacillus acidophilus.* A species of bacteria that is normally found in a healthy intestine.

acute illness. An illness that comes on quickly and causes relatively severe symptoms, but is of limited duration.

adenoidectomy. Surgical removal of the adenoids.

adenoids. Clusters of lymphatic tissue situated in the upper throat behind the nose.

adrenal gland. One of two glands located above the kidneys that secrete a number of key hormones, including epinephrine and cortisol.

allergen. An ordinarily harmless substance that provokes an allergic response in a sensitive individual.

allergy. An immunological response to a certain substance or substances that causes an individual to develop sneezing, hives, or some other reaction when she comes into contact with it or ingests it.

amino acid. One of twenty-two known organic acids that contain nitrogen and serve as building blocks for the production of protein in the body; most are synthesized in the liver, but eight of them cannot be. Because they must be taken in through the diet, these are called *essential amino acids.*

analgesic. A substance that alleviates pain.

anemia. A condition in which the blood is incapable of transporting sufficient oxygen to body tissues, caused by an unusually low number of red blood cells, too little hemoglobin in the red blood cells, or low blood volume.

anesthetic. A substance that causes the loss of sensation, especially the ability to feel pain.

antacid. A substance that neutralizes acid in the digestive tract, especially the stomach.

antibiotic. A substance capable of killing or inhibiting the growth of microorganisms, especially bacteria.

antibody. A protein created by the immune system, in response to the presence of a foreign organism or toxin, that is capable of destroying or neutralizing the invader.

anticonvulsant. A substance that prevents or relieves seizures.

antiemetic. A drug designed to ease nausea and stop vomiting.

antigen. A substance that stimulates the production of an antibody.

antihistamine. A medication that blocks the action of histamines, chemicals produced by the immune cells that create allergic symptoms by constricting bronchial passages, dilating small blood vessels, and increasing secretions from mucous membranes.

antioxidant. A substance that blocks oxidation reactions in the body, some of which can lead to cellular dysfunction and destruction. Antioxidant nutrients include beta-carotene, vitamin C, vitamin E, and selenium. Other antioxidants include the amino acid glutathione and the enzymes superoxide dismutase (SOD), peroxidase, and catalase.

antipyretic. A substance that lowers fever.

antispasmodic. A substance that relieves or prevents spasms.

appestat. The area of the brain that controls appetite, probably located in the hypothalamus.

arrhythmia. An irregular heartbeat. Some arrhythmias are benign; others are quite dangerous.

ascorbate. A mineral salt of ascorbic acid (a chemical combination of vitamin C with a mineral). In this form vitamin C is buffered, making it less acidic and therefore less irritating to the intestinal tract.

astringent. A substance that tends to draw together or tighten tissues.

atopic. Used to refer to conditions, especially allergies, that develop as a result of an inherited predisposition.

autoimmune disorder. A condition in which the immune system attacks the body's own tissues and interferes with normal functioning.

bacteremia. A bacterial infection in the blood.

bacteria. Single-celled microorganisms. Some bacteria cause disease; others live in the body and are necessary for normal functioning and help to defend against invasions from harmful microorganisms.

behavior modification. The use of techniques such as conditioning, basic learning, and habit-creation to alter behavior.

beta-carotene. A nutrient related to vitamin A that is used by the body to manufacture vitamin A as needed.

bile. A bitter, yellowish substance manufactured by the liver that is necessary for the digestion and absorption of fats.

biofeedback. A technique that involves monitoring the body's processes, especially involuntary ones such as heartbeat, to make an individual more aware of her physical responses and help her gain mastery over them. It is especially helpful for management of such conditions as migraine and chronic pain.

bioflavonoids. A diverse group of compounds found in most plants—in fruits and vegetables, usually next to the peel; in trees, in the bark. Bioflavonoids can act as antioxidants, immune system regulators, and anti-inflammatory agents.

biopsy. Removal and examination of a sample of living tissue.

blood count. A basic diagnostic test that involves examining a sample of blood to determine the number of red blood cells, white blood cells, and platelets.

botulism. A type of food poisoning caused by the ingestion of botulin, a toxin manufactured by the bacteria *Clostridium botulinum.*

brewer's yeast. A type of yeast that is a source of B-complex vitamins.

bronchi. The two main branches of the trachea (windpipe) that lead to the lungs.

bronchiole. The small, thin-walled air passages that branch off from the bronchi in the lungs.

bronchodilator. A substance that causes the air passages to relax and widen.

candida. Yeastlike fungus that can cause infections, most commonly in the mouth, the digestive tract, and the vagina.

capillaries. Tiny blood vessels that deliver nutrients to the cells and remove wastes from the cells.

carcinogen. An agent that causes the body to develop cancer.

cardiac. Pertaining to the heart.

carditis. An inflammation of the heart tissue.

CAT scan. A diagnostic instrument that uses computers and x-rays to construct a three-dimensional picture of the body's structures and organs (*CAT* stands for computerized *a*xial *t*omography).

cauterization. A procedure in which an electrical current or silver nitrate stick is applied directly to a broken blood vessel to solidify blood and stop bleeding.

cerebral. Pertaining to the brain.

chalazion. A tiny cyst that appears as a small bump on the rim of the eyelid.

chemotherapy. The use of chemicals to treat disease, especially the treatment of cancer by means of toxic chemicals that destroy cancerous cells.

chlorophyll. The green pigment in many plant tissues; taken as a dietary supplement, it is a source of magnesium and trace elements.

cholesterol. A substance that is an important constituent in cell walls and precursor of certain hormones. It also facilitates the transport of fatty acids in the body.

chronic illness. An illness, whether mild or severe, that lasts or recurs consistently for a long period of time, or throughout the life of an individual.

coenzyme. A substance, usually containing a vitamin or mineral, that an enzyme must combine with in order to perform its appointed function in the body.

colic. Spasm in certain organs or structures, such as the intestines, uterus, or bile ducts, that is accompanied by pain.

colic, infantile. A long period of vigorous crying that has no apparent cause and persists despite all efforts at consolation.

complete protein. A source of dietary protein that contains a full complement of amino acids, especially the eight that the body cannot produce on its own.

complex carbohydrate. A carbohydrate that includes fiber, which slows the release of sugar from the carbohydrate into the bloodstream and provides dietary fiber as well. Sources of complex carbohydrate include whole grains, fruits, and vegetables.

complication. A secondary infection, reaction, or other development that occurs during an illness, usually making recovery more difficult and/or longer.

congenital. Present from birth, but not necessarily inherited.

conjunctiva. The transparent mucous membrane that lines the eyeball and the inner surface of the eyelid.

contusion. A bruise or injury in which the skin is not broken.

corticosteroid. A steroid hormone produced by the adrenal gland, or a synthetic version of such a hormone.

coryza. Medical term for the nasal symptoms of the common cold.

cystoscope. An instrument used to examine the ureter and bladder.

cytomegalovirus. A common virus of the herpes family that can cause disease in infants and in people with compromised immune systems.

deciduous teeth. Baby teeth.

decongestant. A drug that reduces nasal congestion and swelling by constricting the blood vessels in the nasal membranes.

demulcent. Soothing, especially to mucous membranes.

dermatitis. Inflammation of the skin.

dermis. The layer of skin that lies underneath the epidermis and contains blood and lymphatic vessels as well as sweat- and oil-producing glands.

desensitization. A treatment sometimes recommended for allergies in which gradually increasing amounts of diluted allergen are injected into the skin with the intent of stimulating the body to develop resistance to it.

developmental disability. A mental or physical problem that impedes a child's normal development.

disinfectant. A substance or agent that kills or neutralizes disease-causing microorganisms.

diuretic. A substance that increases the excretion of urine.

Down's syndrome. Also known as trisomy, a genetic abnormality that causes varying degrees of physical and mental disability.

eardrum. The thin membrane that separates the middle ear from the outer ear.

eating disorder. A disorder characterized by a distorted body image, fear of gaining weight, obsession with food, and/or abnormal habits relating to the handling of food.

echocardiogram. A diagnostic test that uses ultrasound to detect structural and functional abnormalities of the heart.

edema. Swelling that results from an accumulation of fluid.

electrolyte. A form of sodium, magnesium, calcium, potassium, or other mineral that is used by the body to regulate the maintenance of fluid balance in the cells.

emetic. A substance that induces vomiting.

emulsion. A substance that consists of two liquids that do not mix, such as oil and water; the two do not combine, but one is present as small globules in suspension in the other.

encephalitis. An inflammation of the brain.

endocrine system. The system of glands that secrete hormones into the bloodstream to regulate or initiate various bodily processes; these include the pituitary, thyroid, thymus, and adrenal glands, as well as the pancreas, ovaries, and testes.

enteric. Pertaining to the small intestines.

enzyme. A protein that serves as a catalyst, causing or accelerating chemical reactions in the body without being consumed.

epidemic. Used to describe an outbreak of disease that spreads rapidly and extensively, or with unusually high incidence.

epidermis. The outer layer of the skin.

epiglottitis. A rapidly progressing bacterial infection that causes sudden high fever and inflammation of the epiglottis (the structure that covers the windpipe when a person swallows to prevent food from entering the lungs) and can lead to an obstruction of the airway and respiratory failure.

Epstein-Barr virus. A member of the herpes family of viruses and the agent that causes mononucleosis.

erythema. Medical term for reddening of the skin.

erythema toxicum. A benign red, splotchy rash scattered with small white dots that is common in newborns.

eustachian tube. A structure that connects the middle ear to the nasal cavity and the throat, and through which secretions drain away from the ear and into the nose and throat.

expectorant. A substance that thins secretions and makes it easier to expel them from the respiratory tract.

extract. A concentrated essence, as of an herb, made by leaching the active properties out with either alcohol or water.

fat cell. A cell in which fat is stored in the body.

febrile seizure. A seizure induced by fever, usually high fever.

fiber. The indigestible portion of plant foods.

fistula. An opening or passageway between two organs or body parts that should not exist; it may be the result of injury, disease, or a congenital defect.

fontanel. One of an infant's two "soft spots"—gaps between the bones of a baby's skull—that permit molding of the head during birth and allow room for brain growth.

fungus. A low form of plant life, most often a microscopically small organism. Some types of fungus are capable of causing infection. Candidiasis and athlete's foot are two examples of diseases caused by fungal infection.

gastric lavage. Also called stomach pumping, this is a procedure used to remove toxic substances from the stomach by means of a tube that is inserted through the nose and into the stomach.

gastrointestinal tract. A general term for the stomach and intestines, which together make up the digestive system.

genetic. Inherited.

gland. An organ that manufactures and secretes substances, such as hormones, that are not needed for its own functioning but are used in other parts of the body.

globulin. A type of protein found in the blood. Certain globulins contain disease-fighting antibodies.

glucose. A simple sugar that is the principal source of energy for the body's cells.

gluten. A protein found in wheat, rye, barley, and oats.

hematocrit. The percentage of blood volume that is composed of red blood cells.

hematoma. A bulge or swelling that is filled with blood; usually forms as a result of a break in a blood vessel under the skin.

hemoglobin. The iron-containing red pigment in the blood required for the transport of oxygen.

hemorrhage. Profuse or abnormal bleeding.

hepatic. Pertaining to the liver.

hernia. A condition in which part of an internal organ protrudes through an abnormal opening in the wall that is supposed to contain it.

herpes. A group of viruses characterized by their tendency to cause skin eruptions or blisters. They include herpes simplex viruses 1 and 2 (HSV1 and HSV2) as well as the varicella-zoster and Epstein-Barr viruses.

histamine. A chemical produced by the immune system in response to contact with an allergen; histamines cause bronchial tube muscles to constrict, small blood vessels to dilate, and secretions from mucous membranes to increase, all of which result in the sneezing, itching, and discomfort of an allergic reaction.

hormone. A substance produced by one of the endocrine glands to regulate a specific bodily function.

host. An organism in or on which another organism or microorganism lives, and from which the parasite takes its nourishment.

hydrolyzed protein. A common food additive that is a source of hidden gluten in food products, a hazard for people with celiac disease.

hypopituitarism. A condition characterized by insufficient production of pituitary hormones.

hypothalamus. The portion of the brain that regulates body temperature and other metabolic processes, including the hunger response.

hypothyroidism. A condition characterized by insufficient production of thyroid hormone.

idiopathic. Used to refer to a disease whose cause is unknown.

immune deficiency. Failure of the immune system to function normally in response to disease or infection.

immune globulin. A protein manufactured by certain white blood cells and found in body fluids and on mucous membranes. Immune globulins function as antibodies in the body's immune response.

immune system. The complex of organs, cells, tissues, and proteins that work in a coordinated manner to fight off invaders such as viruses and harmful bacteria.

immunity. The condition of being able to resist or overcome infection or disease.

incubation period. The period of time between exposure to a disease and the appearance of symptoms, during which infection is developing.

infection. An invasion of the body by organisms such as viruses, harmful bacteria, or fungi that results in disease.

infestation. An invasion of the body by parasites such as insects, worms, or protozoa.

inflammation. A reaction to illness or injury characterized by swelling and redness.

infusion. A preparation made by steeping herbs in hot water; tea.

inguinal. Concerning or located in the groin.

insulin. A hormone produced by the pancreas that is necessary for the metabolism of carbohydrates, especially sugar.

interaction. A term describing the effects of two different substances in the presence of each other; interactions can occur between one drug and another drug, between drugs and foods, etc.

interferon. A protein produced by the immune system in response to the presence of a virus that can prevent the virus from reproducing or infecting other cells.

international unit (IU). A unit of potency based on an accepted international standard. The potency of vitamin A and E supplements, among others, is usually measured in international units.

intestinal flora. The "friendly" bacteria normally present in the intestines that are necessary for the digestion and absorption of certain nutrients.

intradermal testing. Testing for allergies that is performed by injecting the skin with suspected allergens at timed intervals.

intravenous. A term describing the administration of drugs or fluids by means of a small needle inserted directly in a vein.

intravenous pyelography. A procedure used to diagnose problems of the kidneys and urinary tract. It involves the intravenous injection of a dye followed by x-ray photographs to track its progress through the system.

jaundice. A yellowing of the skin, eyes, etc., that occurs when bile is not processed properly and so accumulates in those tissues.

ketoacidosis. A complication of diabetes, caused by a high blood sugar episode, that can lead to loss of consciousness, coma, or even death if not properly and promptly treated.

laceration. An injury in which tissue is torn.

lactobacilli. "Friendly" bacteria that are capable of fermenting milk sugar; taken as a supplement, they help to establish healthy flora in the intestines, aiding digestion and increasing the body's resistance to certain types of infection.

lanugo. A very fine coating of hair that may be present on the body of a newborn baby.

laxative. A substance that tends to stimulate the bowels to move.

leukemia. A cancer of the blood and lymph system; the most common cancer in children.

limbic system. A group of deep brain structures that, among other things, transmit the perception of pain to the brain and generate an emotional reaction to it.

lipotropic. One of a group of substances, including choline, inositol, and methionine, that prevent the accumulation of abnormal or excessive levels of fat in the liver. They also help to control blood sugar levels and enhance fat and carbohydrate metabolism.

lower respiratory tract. Usually refers to the trachea (the windpipe), the bronchi, the bronchioles, and the lungs.

lymph. The clear fluid in which all of the body's cells are bathed. It provides nourishment to the cells and collects waste products given off by the cells.

lymph gland. One of the glands located in the lymph vessels; lymph glands produce lymphocytes (white blood cells) and remove foreign materials from the lymph stream.

lymphocyte. A type of white blood cell that is a crucial component of the immune system.

lymphoma. A cancer of the lymph system.

magnetic resonance imaging (MRI). A diagnostic technique involving the use of radio waves and magnetic forces to produce detailed images of the body's internal organs and structures.

malignancy. The property of being cancerous and, often, prone to spread.

meconium. A substance that fills the intestines of a fetus in the womb and is excreted as a thick, dark, often greenish stool either during or soon after birth.

menarche. The onset of menstruation.

meninges. The three thin membranes that cover the brain and spinal cord.

metabolic rate. The rate at which the body carries out metabolic functions.

metabolism. The term for the entire complex of physical and chemical processes that are necessary to sustain life; these include the breaking down of certain substances (such as foods, to release energy) and the synthesis of others (such as proteins for growth and repair of tissues).

metabolite. A substance produced as a result of a metabolic process.

microgram (mcg). A measurement of weight equivalent to one one-thousandth of a milligram (or one one-millionth of a gram).

micronutrient. A nutrient required in small amounts, such as a vitamin or mineral.

microorganism. A microscopically small organism, such as a virus, bacterium, fungus, or protozoan.

milligram (mg). A measurement of weight equivalent to one one-thousandth of a gram.

mineral. An inorganic substance, such as calcium, magnesium, or sodium, that is required by the body for proper functioning.

monilia. An infectious fungus also known as candida.

mucous membrane. A membrane that lines one of the hollow organs of the body, such as the nose, mouth, stomach, intestines, bronchial tubes, anus, and vagina.

myringotomy. A surgical procedure in which an incision is made into the tympanic membrane (eardrum). A tiny tube may then be placed in this incision to permit the drainage of fluid.

narcotic. A powerful drug that blocks the perception of pain by binding with receptors in the central nervous system. It is this interaction with body chemistry that makes narcotics addictive.

naturopathy. A system of medicine that uses herbs and other natural methods to stimulate the body to heal itself without the use of drugs.

neurotransmitter. A chemical that transmits nerve impulses between neurons (nerve cells) in the brain and the nerves.

nonsteroidal anti-inflammatory drug. One of a class of drugs often used as painkillers for mild to moderate pain; some are available by prescription only.

organic. A term used to describe foods that are grown without the use of synthetic chemicals, such as pesticides, herbicides, hormones, etc.

otitis media. An infection of the middle ear.

oximeter. A device that is placed on a toe or finger to measure the amount of oxygen being transported by the blood.

parasite. An organism or microorganism that lives in or on, and takes nourishment from, another organism.

parotid gland. One of the two saliva-producing glands located in the back of the mouth, below and in front of the ears.

peak flow meter. An instrument used to measure changes in breathing capacity by determining how much air is exerted with a full exhalation.

peritoneum. The abdominal cavity that holds the abdominal organs.

pharyngitis. A medical term for sore throat.

phenylketonuria. A condition in which the body fails to produce the enzyme required to convert the amino acid phenylalanine into tyrosine, another amino acid, which is part of the process of normal protein metabolism.

pituitary. A gland located at the base of the brain that secretes substances that regulate growth and metabolism, as well as coordinating the actions of other endocrine glands.

postnasal drip. A condition in which nasal mucus flows down through the throat, rather than being discharged through the nostrils, often as a result of allergy or chronic infection.

prognosis. A prediction as to the course and/or outcome of an illness.

projectile vomiting. Vomiting so violent that vomit is ejected in a forceful stream and lands at a distance from the mouth.

propolis. A resinous substance collected by bees; used as a dietary supplement or salve, it has antibacterial properties that aid in fighting infection.

prostaglandins. Hormones that act in extremely low concentrations on local target organs. For example, prostaglandins secreted by the uterine lining cause the smooth muscle of the uterus to contract.

protein. A nitrogen-containing compound that is an essential constituent of all animal and vegetable tissues, necessary for growth and repair.

protocol. A course of medical treatment.

protozoan. One of a group of single-celled microorganisms, such as amoebas.

pruritus. Medical term for itching.

pulmonary. Pertaining to the lungs.

purulent. Containing or causing the production of pus.

radiation therapy. A type of treatment for cancer in which radiation is used to kill cancerous tissues; also called radiotherapy.

rapid eye movement. A term used to describe a phase of the sleep cycle in which the eyes move rapidly and in a jerky motion, and during which dreaming takes place.

RAST. Radioallergosorbent test. A blood test that measures levels of specific antibodies produced by the body's immune system, used to test for allergic reactions.

rebound effect. A situation in which a person who has been treated for a particular symptom or illness, particularly with drug therapy, experiences worse symptoms after the treatment is stopped than he or she had initially.

red blood cells. Blood cells that contain hemoglobin and transport oxygen and carbon dioxide.

reflux. A condition in which a substance flows backward, instead of in the intended direction. For example, urine can flow backwards up through the urethra to the bladder, and sometimes into the kidneys, instead of moving out of the body.

REM. Rapid eye movement.

renal. Pertaining to the kidneys.

saturated fat. A type of fat characterized by its inability to incorporate additional hydrogen atoms. Saturated fats are solid at room temperature, like butter or lard. They are found primarily in foods of animal origin, such as meats and dairy products. A diet high in saturated fats has been implicated in the development of heart disease and certain types of cancer; experts recommend keeping consumption of saturated fats to a minimum.

scratch test. An allergy test that involves placing a small amount of a suspected allergen on a lightly scratched area of skin.

sebaceous glands. Glands in the skin that secrete sebum.

sebum. The oily secretion produced by glands in the skin.

secondary infection. An infection that develops after and is made possible by the presence or effect of a previous infection or inflammation, but is not necessarily directly caused by it.

seizure. A sudden, uncontrollable contraction of a group of muscles that may be accompanied by loss of consciousness, twitching, shaking, clenching of teeth, labored breathing, and/or loss of bladder control.

sensitivity. A tendency to react to the presence of a particular agent or substance.

septic sore throat. A sore throat resulting from bacterial infection; strep throat.

serotonin. A neurotransmitter that, among other things, is responsible for regulating the mechanisms of normal sleep.

simple carbohydrate. A simple sugar, such as glucose or lactose (milk sugar), that is rapidly absorbed into the bloodstream.

sinus. One of four pairs of open spaces within the bones of the skull, located behind the bridge of the nose, back in the upper nose, in the forehead, and under the eyes.

spinal tap. A procedure in which a small amount of spinal fluid is withdrawn for examination by means of a needle inserted into a space between two vertebrae.

spirochete. One of a number of different harmful bacteria characterized by their slender, spiral shape.

stenosis. A narrowing or constriction, especially of a tubelike structure.

steroid. One of a group of fat-soluble organic compounds with a characteristic chemical composition; a number of different hormones, drugs, and other substances—including cholesterol—are classified as steroids.

streptococcus. A genus of bacteria, many members of which cause diseases in humans (including strep throat and scarlet fever) by destroying red blood cells.

symptom-specific. Designed to treat a particular symptom or set of symptoms.

syncope. Temporary loss of consciousness; fainting.

systemic. Pertaining to the entire body.

teratogen. An agent that causes malformation of an embryo or fetus.

tincture. A concentrated essence made by using alcohol to extract and concentrate the active properties of a substance, such as an herb.

tonsillectomy. Surgical removal of the tonsils.

tonsils. Two small masses of lymphatic tissue located at the back of the throat that are believed to help the body defend against respiratory infection.

topical. Applied to the surface of the body.

tourniquet. A tightly tied bandage used as an emergency measure to temporarily stop the flow of blood through a limb. Applying a tourniquet is a drastic measure that should be resorted to only if it is necessary to prevent death from blood loss following a severe injury, such as partial amputation of a limb.

toxin. A substance that is poisonous to the body.

toxoid. An ordinarily poisonous substance that has been treated to remove its dangerous properties, but that remains capable of stimulating the body to develop protective antitoxins.

trace element. A substance, most commonly a mineral, required by the body in minute amounts.

tremor. Involuntary trembling.

tuberculin test. A test used to determine if a person has been exposed to or is infected with tuberculosis.

tumor. An abnormal mass of tissue that serves no function.

ultrasound. The use of ultra-high-frequency sound waves as a diagnostic tool (especially for viewing a developing fetus) or for medical treatment.

upper respiratory tract. Usually refers to the nose and nasal passages, the throat, and the larynx (the voice box).

urticaria. Medical term for hives.

vaccine. A substance administered to induce the body to develop immunity against a disease without developing the disease itself.

vascular. Pertaining to the circulatory system.

venom. A poisonous substance produced by animals, such as certain snakes and insects.

vernix caseosa. A creamy coating that may be present on the body of a newborn baby.

vestibular apparatus. The structure of the inner ear responsible for maintaining the body's sense of balance and equilibrium.

villi. Microscopic hairlike "fingers" lining the walls of the intestinal tract that absorb and transport fluids and nutrients.

virus. One of a large class of minute parasitic organic structures that consist of a protein coat and a core of DNA and/or RNA and are capable of infecting plants and animals by reproducing within their cells. Because it cannot reproduce outside of a host organism's cells, a virus is not technically considered a living organism.

visualization. A technique that involves consciously using the mind to influence the health and functioning of the body.

vitamin. One of approximately fifteen organic micronutrients required by the body that must be obtained through diet.

white blood cells. Blood cells that function in fighting infection and in wound repair. An elevated white blood cell count is often a sign of infection or disease.

yeast. A single-celled organism that can cause infection in various parts of the body, most commonly the mouth (thrush), the vagina (vaginitis), or the gastrointestinal tract (candidiasis).

Common Medical Abbreviations

bid. Two times a day.

BP. Blood pressure.

CAT. Computerized axial tomography.

CBC. Complete blood count.

CMV. Cytomegalovirus.

CNS. Central nervous system.

CPR. Cardiopulmonary resuscitation.

CSF. Cerebrospinal fluid.

CT. Computed tomography.

EBV. Epstein-Barr virus.

EEG. Electroencephalogram.

EKG (or ECG). Electrocardiogram.

ENT. Ear, nose, and throat.

FUO. Fever of unknown origin.

GI. Gastrointestinal.

GU. Genitourinary.

Hb or Hgb. Hemoglobin.

Hct. Hematocrit.

hs. Hour of sleep (i.e., bedtime).

IU. International unit.

IV. Intravenous.

IVP. Intravenous pyelography.

mcg. Microgram.

mg. Milligram.

mL. Milliliter.

mm. Millimeter.

MRI. Magnetic resonance imaging.

NSAID. Nonsteroidal anti-inflammatory drug.

OTC. Over-the-counter.

po. Orally.

ppm. Parts per million.

prn. As needed.

q. Every.

qid. Four times a day.

RBC. Red blood cell.

tid. Three times a day.

URI. Upper respiratory infection.

UTI. Urinary tract infection.

WBC. White blood cell.

Recommended Suppliers

The following list of suppliers is included so that you can find and use the remedies recommended in this book. It is not intended to be an exhaustive list of all possible sources of these products. Rather, the authors recommend them because they have found their products to be of good quality. Also, please be aware that addresses and phone numbers may be subject to change.

HERBAL PRODUCTS

Herbs, Etc.
1340 Rufina Circle
Santa Fe, NM 87501
800-634-3727

Herb-Pharm
P.O. Box 116
William, OR 97544
503-846-6262

McZand Herbal Inc.
P.O. Box 5312
Santa Monica, CA 90409
310-822-0500

Nature's Herbs
P.O. Box 336
Orem, UT 84059
800-HERBALS

Nature's Way Products, Inc.
10 Mountain Springs Parkway
Springville, UT 84663
801-489-1520

Super Salve
606 Lake Mary Road
Flagstaff, AZ 86001
602-774-8910

Wyoming Wildcrafters
Wilson, WY 80304
307-733-6731

HOMEOPATHIC REMEDIES

Boericke and Tafel, Inc.
1011 Arch Street
Philadelphia, PA 19107
215-922-2967

Boiron-Borneman
1208 Amosland Road
Norwood, PA 19074
215-532-2035

Dolisos America, Inc.
3014 Rigel Avenue
Las Vegas, NV 89102
702-871-7153

Hahnemann Pharmacy
828 San Pablo Avenue
Albany, CA 94706
510-527-3003

Homeopathic Educational Services
2124 Kittredge Street
Berkeley, CA 94704
510-649-8930

Luyties Pharmacal Company
4200 Laclede Avenue
St. Louis, MO 63108
800-325-8080

Standard Homeopathic Company
P.O. Box 61604
436 West Eighth Street
Los Angeles, CA 90014
213-321-4284

NUTRITIONAL SUPPLEMENTS

Advanced Medical Nutrition
2247 National Avenue
P.O. Box 5012
Hayward, CA 94540–5012
Products sold only through physicians.

Alacer Corporation
14 Morgan Street
Irvine, CA 92718
714–951–9660

Ethical Nutrients
971 Calle Negocio
San Clemente, CA 92673
714–366–0818

Miracle Exclusives Inc.
3 Elm Street
P.O. Box 349
Locust Valley, NY 11560
516–676–0220

Natren, Inc.
3105 Willow Lane
Westlake Village, CA 91361
805–371–4742

Rainbow Light Nutritional Systems
207 McPherson Street
P.O. Box 3033
Santa Cruz, CA 95060
800–635–1233
408–429–9089

Wakunaga of America Co. Ltd.
23501 Madero
Mission Viejo, CA 92691
714–855–2776

ORGANIC FOODS BY MAIL ORDER

Fresh Meadow Bakery
2610 Lyndale Avenue
Minneapolis, MN 55408
612–870–4740

Gold Mine Natural Food Company
1947 39th Street
San Diego, CA 92102
800–475–3663
619–234–9711

Green Earth Natural Foods
2545 Prairie Avenue
Evanston, IL 60201
800–322–3662

Lundberg Farms
P.O. Box 369
Rockvale, CA 95974
916–882–4551

Mountain Ark Trading Company
120 South East Avenue
Fayetteville, AR 72701
800–643–8909

Organic Foods Express
12050 Parklawn Drive
Rockville, MD 20852
301–816–4944

Walnut Acres
Penns Creek, PA 17862
717–837–0601

OTHER

Biological Rescue Products Inc.
1100 East Hector Street, Suite 130
Conshohocken, PA 19428
215–834–0905
800–882–0505
Manufacturer of Save•A•Tooth solution.

Sawyer Products
P.O. Box 188
Safety Harbor, FL 34695
813–725–1177
Manufacturer of The Extractor venom extraction kit.

Resource Organizations

The following organizations can answer questions, provide referrals, and tell you how to find more information. Some organizations sell literature or offer classes and workshops to help you broaden your understanding of natural medicine. Use them liberally in your investigation of the best ways to care for yourself and your family.

ACUPUNCTURE, ACUPRESSURE, AND MASSAGE

Acupressure Institute
1533 Shattuck Avenue
Berkeley, CA 94709
800–442–2232
In California, call 415–845–1059.

American Association of Acupuncture
  and Oriental Medicine
4101 Lake Boone Trail, Suite 201
Raleigh, NC 27607
919–787–5181

International Association of Infant Massage Instructors
P.O. Box 16103
Portland, OR 97216
503–253–9977

National Commission for Certification
  of Acupuncturists
1424 16th Street, NW, Suite 501
Washington, DC 20036
202–232–1404

ALTERNATIVE MEDICINE (GENERAL)

American Association of Naturopathic Physicians
2366 Eastlake Avenue East
Seattle, WA 98102
206–323–7610

American Holistic Medical Association
4101 Lake Boone Trail, Suite 201
Raleigh, NC 27607
919–787–5181

American Osteopathic Association
142 East Ontario Street
Chicago, IL 60611
312–280–5800

International College of Applied Kinesiology
P.O. Box 905
Lawrence, KS 66044–0905
913–542–1801

John Bastyr College of Naturopathic Medicine
144 NE 54th Street
Seattle, WA 98105
206–523–9585 (administration)
206–632–0354 (clinic)

BACH FLOWER REMEDIES

Ellon Bach USA Inc.
P.O. Box 320
Woodmere, NY 11598
516–593–2206

CHILD SAFETY

The National Child Passenger Safety Association
P.O. Box 841
Ardmore, PA 19003
215–525–4610

National SAFE KIDS Campaign
111 Michigan Avenue, NW
Washington, DC 20010–2970
202–939–4993